CASTLE CONNOLLY
AMERICA'S
TOP DOCTORS®
FOR CANCER

3rd Edition

America's Trusted Source
For Identifying Top Doctors

Text by

John J. Connolly, Ed.D.

&

Jean Morgan, M.D.

A CASTLE CONNOLLY GUIDE

For more information, please contact:

Castle Connolly Medical Ltd., 42 West 24th St, New York, New York 10010
212-367-8400x10
E-mail: info@castleconnolly.com
Web site: http://www.castleconnolly.com.
Library of Congress Catalog Card Number 2007922942
ISBN   1-883769-43-4;   978-1-883769-43-7   (paperback)
ISBN   1-883769-44-2;   978-1-883769-44-4   (hardcover)
Printed in the United States of America

Table of Contents

Table of Contents

Section III: Physician Listings by Medical Specialty

Table of Contents

Table of Contents

Table of Contents

Table of Contents

Table of Contents

Section IV: Appendices

Section V: Indices

About the Publishers

John K. Castle has spent much of the last three decades involved with healthcare institutions and issues. Mr. Castle served as Chairman of the Board of New York Medical College for eleven years, an institution where he served on the Board of Trustees for twenty-two years.

Mr. Castle has been extensively involved in other healthcare and voluntary activities as well. He served for five years as a public commissioner on the Joint Commission on Accredition of Healthcare Organizations (JCAHO), the body which accredits most public and private hospitals throughout the United States. Mr. Castle has also served as a trustee of five different hospitals in the metropolitan New York region, including NewYork-Presbyterian Hospital, where he continues to serve.

Mr. Castle is also the Chairman of the Columbia Presbyterian Science Advisory Council and a Director of the Whitehead Institute for Biomedical Research. He is a Fellow of New York Academy of Medicine and has served as a Trustee of the Academy. He is Chairman of the United Hospital Fund of New York's Capital Campaign. He continues as Director Emeritus of the United Hospital Fund. He is a Life Member of the MIT Corporation, the governing body of the Massachusetts Institute of Technology.

Mr. Castle is the Chairman and Co-Publisher of Castle Connolly Medical Ltd. and affiliated companies which publish *America's Top Doctors*®; *Top Doctors: New York Metro Area* and other books to help people find the best healthcare. Castle Connolly Healthcare Navigation LLC is a company that assists individuals and families obtain the best healthcare from the nation's excellent but confusing healthcare system.

About the Publisher

John J. Connolly, Ed.D. is the President & CEO of Castle Connolly Medical Ltd., and is the nation's foremost authority on identifying top physicians. Dr. Connolly's experience in healthcare is extensive.

For over a decade he served as President of New York Medical College, the nation's second largest private medical college. He is a Fellow of the New York Academy of Medicine, a Fellow of the New York Academy of Sciences, a Director of the New York Business Group on Health, a member of the President's Council of the United States Hospital Fund, and a member of the Board of Advisors of Funding First, a Lasker Foundation initiative. Dr. Connolly has served as a trustee of two hospitals and as Chairman of the Board of one. He is extensively involved in healthcare and community activities and has served on a number of voluntary and corporate boards including the Board of the American Lyme Disease Foundation, of which he is a founder and past chairman, and the Board of Advisors of the Whitehead Institute for Biomedical Research. He is also a Director and Chairman of the Professional Examination Service. He holds a Bachelor of Science degree from Worcester State College, a Master's degree from the University of Connecticut, and a Doctor of Education degree in College and University Administration from Teacher's College, Columbia University.

Dr. Connolly has authored or edited nine books and has been interviewed by more than 100 television and radio stations nationwide including *"Today Show"*, *"Good Morning America,"* *"20/20,"* *"48 Hours,"* *Fox Cable News*, *CNN*, and *"Weekend Today in New York,"* and he and Castle Connolly have been featured in major newspapers and magazines including *The New York Times*, the *Chicago Tribune, the Daily News* and *the Boston Herald, Redbook, Town & Country, Good Housekeeping, Ladies Home Journal, Redbook* and regional magazines including *New York, Chicago, Philadelphia, Memphis, Palm Springs Life, Oakland, Pittsburgh* and *Atlanta* magazines.

Castle Connolly Medical Advisory Board

Castle Connolly Medical Ltd. is pleased to have associated with a distinguished group of medical leaders who offer invaluable advice and wisdom in our efforts to assist consumers in making good healthcare choices. We thank each member of the Medical Advisory Board for their valuable contributions.

Foreword

Vincent T. DeVita, Jr., MD

Director, National Cancer Institute

(1980-1988)

As a physician, I've spent my professional career valuing the ability to find the right information and resources I need - quickly, efficiently and with the confidence that my sources are reliable. Similarly, healthcare consumers need to be able to find reliable information about the very best medical and healthcare services is critical, especially when confronting a diagnosis of cancer. That's why I like Castle Connolly's consumer guide, *America's Top Doctors® for Cancer*.

In creating this guide to more than 2,000 of the nation's leading medical specialists involved in the prevention, diagnosis and treatment of various cancer in both adults and children, Castle Connolly has invested a tremendous amount of time, energy and money in its research, screening and evaluation processes. To illustrate some of the complexity of doing this kind of work, let me share a story with you. In my capacity as Director of the NCI from 1980 to 1988, I was often deluged with phone call requests, frequently from members of Congress or other well-placed individuals, to help them with their own personal problem with cancer or that of a friend or relative - and "pretty damn quick". They were not satisfied with just going to any doctor when their life, or the life of a friend or loved one was at stake - they wanted to know "who was doing what and where" and they wanted suggestions about the top doctors for their particular type of cancer. I often felt guilty that only a privileged few had access to this type of information. (This lack of fundamental information for the average patient is exactly what motivated Castle Connolly to start their "Top Doctors" series in 1991.)

Foreword

The National Cancer Act had been established in 1971 by an Act of the U.S. Congress as part of a national "War on Cancer." Among its mandates for the National Cancer Institute (NCI) was the creation of a cancer information service to get relevant information rapidly to cancer patients. Two unique individuals deserve credit and recognition for the role that they played in creating this information service. This part of the Cancer Act mandate was actually the brainchild of the philanthropist Mary Lasker, who was also one of the main architects of the passage of the Cancer Act itself. She had her finger on the pulse of the American public and was concerned, and correctly so in my view, that researchers and organizations that supported them, like the NIH, had a tendency to ignore the practical applications of their work for the public, despite the fact that their research was paid for by tax dollars. From the time of the passage of the act, Mary Lasker pursued each subsequent National Cancer Institute Director to build this information service. In 1981, Mr. Richard Bloch, of H&R Block, then a member of the National Cancer Advisory Board, and himself a successfully treated lung cancer patient, approached the NCI Director about his dream that a patient could use computerized information services to enter their personal information and get, in return, the most up-to-date management recommendations, and names of doctors using them. He was motivated by his own experience. He had to fight his way through the system, being told by several doctors that he was incurable before he found where to go, and the physicians to provide the treatment that ultimately cured him. It was his goal, to which he dedicated the rest of his life; to see that cancer patients like him got the information they needed.

With the strong advocacy of Mary Lasker and Richard Bloch, in 1984 NCI launched the PDQ system at the National Library of Medicine. It was the first computerized database in the world, aimed at the general public, devoted to a single disease, cancer. PDQ included lists of institutions, treatment protocols, and physicians devoted to managing cancer patients, all geographically matrixed, to allow patients, regardless of their status, to find the most appropriate doctor, treatment, and or clinical trial for them anywhere in the country and in their locale as well. Ironically, this aspect of PDQ - a list of specialists that seemed so logical and necessary - was controversial. From cancer specialists themselves, we heard that since not all cancer specialists (for example Cancer Surgeons) are "certified" by boards that test their qualifications for the cancer part of their work, the PDQ lists did not include " board certification" as a selection criteria. The PDQ physician list was also constructed primarily by using input and lists from specialty organizations. By building our list with assistance from specialty organizations, we were told, we had abrogated peer review and would be including doctors who might be only marginally qualified as specialists. To identify all doctors who were capable of providing modern care for cancer patients, on an individual basis, was not within the capability of the NCI or any government or private institution at the time. And to identify who were among the most qualified to diagnosis and treat specific types of cancers was simply not within our purview. And yet we knew that finding the right doctor at the right time could be a matter of life and death.

Fast-forward to 2005 - PDQ and the Cancer Information Service have played a big part in the decline in national mortality rates from cancer in the U.S. that began in 1990 and has continued since then. PDQ has now become a more complex information system about cancer and NCI cancer programs. But regrettably, the one thing that patients appreciated the most - the list of cancer doctors - is no longer a part of the PDQ system.

Castle Connolly's *America's Top Doctors® for Cancer* represents the much-needed and long-overdue answer for consumers – and physicians - seeking the top cancer specialists. Their physician-led research team has tackled some of the tough issues and developed criteria for selection, built on the foundation of Castle Connolly's well respected national survey process that has enabled them to identify the leading physicians in more than twenty medical specialties associated with the prevention, diagnosis and treatment of cancers. The breadth and depth of the information they offer on each profiled physician will enable readers to be empowered consumers, to make informed decisions about the right doctor for their particular type of cancer. The guide also includes valuable information on some of the nation's most outstanding medical centers and specialty hospitals that are involved in the treatment of cancers.

America's Top Doctors® for Cancer will be an invaluable resource – a user-friendly, trusted source of information from an independent nationally renowned healthcare research and information company. I believe that using Castle Connolly's *America's Top Doctors® for Cancer* as a key source of information will help cancer patients and their loved ones navigate the complexities of the American healthcare system to find – and receive – the highest quality medical care.

Vincent T. DeVita, Jr., MD
Amy and Joseph Perella Professor of Medicine
Yale Cancer Center, Yale School of Medicine
(New Haven, Connecticut) January, 2005
Director, National Cancer Institute (1980-1988)

Section I
Introduction

• 1 •

Cancer in the U.S. Today

If you or someone you love has been diagnosed with cancer, this book is for you. Although almost one in three Americans will be told they have cancer at some point during their lives, it is important to emphasize this no longer automatically carries a grim prognosis. Due to advances in treatment and, more importantly, early detection, people with cancer are living longer as well as healthier and more productive lives. While the overall quality of medical care throughout the United States is generally of very high quality, and in many places is superb, there are still those rare, complex or extremely difficult problems that demand resources beyond the ordinary or that require talents that are exceptional.

There is no denying fear is the most common reaction to the word "cancer," at least initially. Cancer has recently emerged as the leading cause of death of Americans under age 85. Bernadine Healy, M.D., former Director of the National Institutes of Health, wrote in *U.S. News and World Report* (Feb 14, 2005) that cancer is both "sneaky and inexplicably virulent in many of its forms." These characteristics go a long way toward making cancer even more formidable than heart disease, another major killer.

However, Dr. Healy also described how advances in identification and prevention have restrained cancer from "galloping" through our population. We are all familiar with PAP smears which can identify early forms of cervical cancer in women, or the Prostate-Specific Antigen (PSA) test for prostate cancer in men, as well as colonoscopies that permit doctors to remove potentially cancerous polyps from the colon.

Many cancers are potentially curable, provided they are detected in the early stages.

Many cancers are potentially curable, provided they are detected in the early stages. Growing awareness of early warning signs and symptoms, together with advances in screening, have resulted in major improvements in cancer survival.

Prevention is even more important. Jane E. Brody, one of the nation's leading health columnists, wrote in *The New York Times* about life-enhancing changes involving diet and exercise we can make that may enable us to live cancer-free beyond the age of 85.

At the same time that methods of diagnosis and prevention have advanced, so too has our ability to treat cancer. In fact, today, many people are completely cured or are able to cope with their cancer as a chronic disease. There are nearly 10 million cancer survivors in the U.S. alone.

Americans' risk of getting cancer and dying from cancer continues to decline and survival rates for many cancers continue to improve. The Annual Report to the Nation on the Status of Cancer, 1975-2002, which is a collaboration among the American Cancer Society (ACS), the Centers for Disease Control and Prevention (CDC), the National Cancer Institute (NCI), and the North American Association of Central Cancer Registries (NAACCR), provides updated information on cancer rates and trends in the United States, found that overall observed cancer incidence rates increased by 0.3 percent per year from 1987 to 2002, while death rates from all types of cancer combined dropped 1.1 percent per year from 1993 to 2002.

In keeping with the current hopeful climate for cancer patients, the purpose of this book is to help you approach your diagnosis and treatment in the most effective way possible.

Cancer can occur in any cell in the body when the mechanisms that regulate normal cell growth fail. As a result, the cell experiences uncontrolled and excessive growth. These rapidly multiplying cells may go on to invade local tissues or spread (metastasize) to other parts of the body.

The field of cancer research is growing in leaps and bounds. Research is essential, not only to improve current methods of treatment, but also to develop new ways of treating what had previously been considered intractable types of cancer. As medical research and technology advances, more treatments and drugs are being introduced to combat cancer. In fact, every day we can read of new developments which may give renewed hope to many cancer patients.

The huge amount of information now available about all aspects of cancer can be quite daunting. New tests, drugs and technology all may present a bewildering choice for many patients. You need guidance, and also psychological support, as you navigate through this strange new world. That's why it's vital for you to consult and be treated by a physician highly experienced in and knowledgeable about your particular type of cancer.

In certain types of cancer, different specialists may combine their efforts to work together as a team. For example, in successful skull base tumor surgery, the otolaryngologist and neurological surgeon operate together.

Different major medical centers may concentrate on different types of cancer treatments, their physicians working together to provide the "team approach" as needed. In other words, you're not just selecting a single doctor, but an entire hospital for your treatment.

Research is essential, not only to improve on current methods of treatment, but also to develop new ways of treating what had previously been considered intractable types of cancer.

• 2 •

Why Top Doctors
and Top Hospitals?

Finding the best physicians and best hospitals for your care is a major factor in achieving the best possible outcome. The average person may not be familiar with the various medical specialties, or know what constitutes medical education and the specifics of doctor "training," that period of residencies and fellowships that follows medical school. As a result, it is difficult for most Americans to choose physicians or hospitals in a well-informed fashion. Most people still find a doctor by asking a friend for a recommendation, or picking a name from a health plan directory or even a phone book.

In addition to listing excellent physicians identified by the Castle Connolly research team through our surveys, this book will describe the process you can use to find a "top doctor" for any medical problem or need. It will also provide up-to-date information on leading hospitals, and list valuable resources for cancer patients and their families. These resources are found in the appendices.

At times, our healthcare system, while good, may seem less than consumer friendly. The United States (and Canada) has many thousands of exceptionally well-trained and dedicated professionals involved in providing the best healthcare possible. Managed care, despite its shortcomings, has brought some much-needed structure to the healthcare delivery system. Most plans require that you have a primary care physician as well as specify referrals to selected specialists and hospitals. The health plans have the ability to monitor and assess the care delivered to you at all times, regardless of provider or location, because the plan has all your medical records in order to affect appropriate payment.

Unfortunately, the advantages offered by managed care plans have too frequently been directed toward controlling costs rather than enhancing quality. The hospitals and doctors to which patients are referred for more services or complex care are often selected on the basis of cost rather than, more medically relevant criteria. Therefore, even though a health plan directory may list a number of "centers of excellence" and several specialists for a given problem, they may not be the best for your particular needs.

Asking your primary care physician for a referral to a specialist can be a good place to start. However, too many of us don't have a close relationship with that all important "quarterback" of our healthcare, and this type of referral also has its limitations. Is the recommendation being made on the basis of a personal or professional relationship? Is the specialist to whom you are being referred truly the best, or is he or she simply in your primary care physician's group or in the network of your health plan? Even if your primary care physician is making a referral free from outside considerations, how broad is his or her knowledge of this particular specialty? Most primary care physicians have a limited number of referral channels. They are busy caring for their own patients and rarely have the time to devote hours of research to identifying top doctors for referrals. Typically, their referral network is local rather than regional or national

If you are already under the care of an excellent specialist, and he or she refers you to another specialist or sub-specialist for a particular problem, you can be confident of a more "meaningful" referral. When physicians are continually dealing with a specific disease, such as cancer, they are usually more aware of advances in the field, as well as the names of the top practitioners.

As the patient, finding the best physicians and best hospitals for your care is your responsibility. "Get a second opinion" is a common refrain. Everyone has heard stories of patients who were told by one physician (even at a top hospital) that their case was hopeless and yet, when they continued their search, they found another doctor or hospital that provided a different plan of treatment and perhaps even a cure.

Even the best doctors and the best hospitals are not perfect. Cancer treatment, like other medical care, is a combination of art and science. Frequently, opinions on diagnosis and treatment may differ—even among top doctors. That's why it's so important for you to seek second or even third opinions when a diagnosis, even one not involving cancer, is serious or may necessitate major surgery.

Even the best doctors and the best hospitals are not perfect.
Cancer treatment is a combination of
art and science.

One of the best known and inspirational stories of a patient undertaking this kind of search is that of Lance Armstrong, the seven time Tour de France champion cyclist. When Armstrong was first diagnosed with testicular cancer he received a grim prognosis from a number of excellent physicians at some of the nation's leading cancer centers. The recommended courses of treatment would have destroyed his ability to continue competing professionally. Refusing to accept that limitation, he continued his search until he found a physician and institution that offered different treatment options. As most people know, the treatment was successful. Seven of Armstrong's cycling championships (1999-2005) have come since his recovery from cancer.

Of course, there is a difference between seeking additional medical opinions and simply bouncing around from doctor to doctor until you find one that tells you what you want to hear. You need to find a doctor, hospital and treatment plan in which you have confidence, and which you honestly believe, based on extensive research, will work for you. Depending on the circumstances, it may be possible to find another physician or hospital that can offer a superior plan, or it may be that no better treatment options currently exist.

"Hope springs eternal" is not just a trite saying. It is something that should drive every patient and every doctor, simply because there are always unexpected and sometimes unexplainable remissions or cures occurring with cancer, and new breakthroughs in treatment could be just around the corner.

There is a significant amount of evidence that patients who are optimistic and fight, rather than surrender to their disease, have generally better outcomes. A positive attitude and the support of family and friends, as well as physicians and nurses, can be an important factor in your recovery. Knowing as much as possible about your diagnosis and your treatment options is another.

Reaching an initial diagnosis usually involves a number of medical tests including x-rays, MRIs and analysis of tissue samples obtained by a biopsy. It may be necessary to repeat these tests, or perform more specialized ones, in order to gain more thorough information or firmly establish a questionable diagnosis.

In the case of breast cancer, the disease is first likely to be identified either through a mammogram or else the discovery of a lump during a routine self or physician exam. Any breast lumps need to be biopsied for confirmation of cancer. Once that occurs, you will be referred to a surgeon who has special expertise in this field. He or she will recommend one or more possible treatments, including a total mastectomy, a lumpectomy, radiation therapy and chemotherapy.

As the patient, finding the best physicians and best hospitals for your care is your responsibility.

A suspicion of prostate cancer usually occurs following evidence of an enlarged prostate or an elevated PSA test. A urologist will make a definitive diagnosis based on a biopsy and examination of that tissue by a pathologist. Once cancer is found, it can be treated by surgical removal or radioactive seed implants.

Both the breast cancer and prostate cancer patient face the same basic questions: Is the physician treating you the most qualified and, more importantly, is surgery the only or best solution to deal with your disease?

Just like a number of additional options exist for breast cancer, surgery is not the only way to deal with prostate cancer, and may have unwanted side effects. Other alternative treatments include radiation therapy. In addition, since prostate cancer usually develops very slowly, some patients, especially older ones, may choose "watchful waiting." However, because most patients initially see a surgeon at the time of their diagnosis, they may end up having surgery without fully exploring the other alternatives.

Knowledge is not just power; in some instances it can make all the difference in not only your long-term survival, but also the quality of your life. This is why it is essential for you to be an informed consumer and find the best possible healthcare for yourself. This book will help you find the very best doctors and hospitals to treat cancer.

Factors to Consider When Identifying a Top Doctor

1. Medical Education

2. Residency & Fellowships

3. Board Certification

4. Hospital Appointment

5. Academic and Other Professional Titles

6. Insurance Accepted

7. Personality

• 3 •

How Castle Connolly Identified America's Top Doctors® for Cancer

Castle Connolly is best known for its series of consumer guides including *America's Top Doctors®*, and *Top Doctors: New York Metro Area*. These books list "top doctors" in their respective regions. The New York edition profiles primary care physicians as well as other specialists and sub-specialists. *America's Top Doctors®* does not include any primary care physicians, but it lists the nation's top referral specialists. The Castle Connolly Guides are trusted by consumers and physicians alike. In fact, over 50% of the physicians listed in the Guides use them to make referrals.

Doctors do not and cannot pay to be listed in any Castle Connolly Guides. They are selected based on their nomination by peers solicited through mail and phone surveys, and on an extensive review of their credentials by the Castle Connolly physician-led research team.

For *America's Top Doctors® for Cancer* 3rd Edition, Castle Connolly sent nomination forms to all physicians listed in *America's Top Doctors®* and *America's Top Doctors® for Cancer*. In addition, nominations were solicited from the presidents and vice presidents of over 300 of the nation's leading medical centers and specialty hospitals.

The physcians we have identified and listed are clearly among the best as nominated by their peers and screened by our research team.

Thousands of different physicians were nominated by their peers for inclusion in this guide. Of course, most of them received multiple nominations. In addition to the thousands of mail surveys, the Castle Connolly research team made hundreds of phone calls to leading specialists and sought additional nominations as well as using these conversations to reinforce the nominations received through the mail nomination process.

The Castle Connolly physician-led research team reviewed and analyzed the nominations and narrowed the field to those being considered for inclusion in *America's Top Doctors® for Cancer*. They contacted these physicians and asked them to complete an extensive biographical form describing their medical education, residencies, fellowships, hospital appointments and more. Particularly, we were interested in the physicians' area of special expertise; that is, the particular type of cancer (e.g. lung, breast, brain tumors, etc.,) or procedures (e.g. radical prostatectomy laparoscopic surgery) in which the physician had particular experience, interest and expertise.

Finally, the research team checked on the disciplinary histories of the physicians by screening those that may have been disciplined by a medical board or state agency. After this intensive review, the final list was created.

The goal in creating this list was to select physicians viewed by their peers as the best in preventing, diagnosing and treating cancer and its related ramifications. Castle Connolly does not claim these are the only excellent doctors treating cancer in this country. Our nation is fortunate in having a generally excellent cadre of well-trained, dedicated physicians. The physicians we have identified and listed, however, are clearly among the very best as nominated by their peers and screened by our research team. In addition, they practice, for the most part, at major medical centers and leading specialty hospitals where they, and their patients, can receive the support of other highly skilled doctors, nurses and technicians, as well as having access to the sophisticated and expensive equipment, laboratories and other resources that advance the level of cancer treatment and care from good to excellent. Furthermore, many of these physicians are engaged in teaching or research, or both. While the academic nature of their practice can limit the amount of time available to see patients, it keeps them, their colleagues and their institutions on the "cutting edge" of cancer treatment.

One important factor in our selection was geographic coverage. Some patients may be unable to travel long distances to a major medical center or specialty hospital due to financial resources, overall health status or some other reason. For them, a hospital in the immediate region is the only possible alternative. Since this is a guide for consumers and as many physicians use our guide to make referrals, we felt it was important to have broad geographic coverage and attempted to identify the top doctors for cancer in every state.

The reality is that the critical resources, the very best doctors and hospitals, are not dispersed evenly throughout the nation. For good reason they are clustered in large metropolitan areas or at academic medical centers that are part of major universities. It is only in these settings where it is possible to gather the combination of resources necessary to mount and maintain a superior medical program. The laboratories, technicians, intensive care beds, research fellows, scientists, specially trained nursing staff, equipment and, especially, the volume of patients and research subjects so necessary to enable these professional teams to continually develop and hone their skills, typically exist only in metropolitan areas or at university-based medical centers.

Therefore, it may be necessary for many Americans, if they are motivated to seek out the very best doctors and hospitals, to travel many miles, if possible, to obtain their care. It is also this reality that has motivated many outstanding medical centers and specialty hospitals to reach out and establish relationships with community hospitals throughout the nation. While it is not always possible to bring the labs, scientists, equipment and leading physicians to these communities, it is possible to raise the overall level of cancer care through these relationships.

The laboratories, technicians, intensive care beds, research fellows, scientists and specially trained nursing staff, equipment and, especially, the volume of patients and research subjects so necessary to enable these professional teams to continually develop and hone their skills, typically exist only in metropolitan areas or at university-based medical centers.

• 4 •

Judging the Qualifications
of a Physician

The National Cancer Institute has declared its intention to eliminate suffering and death due to cancer by the year 2015. While that is clearly an ambitious goal, and one many may feel is unrealistic, it nonetheless demonstrates the optimism physicians and scientists are beginning to feel about the battle against cancer. As Ellen V. Sigal, Ph.D, founder and chairperson of Friends of Cancer Research in Washington, D.C. and a member of the National Cancer Institute's Board of Scientific Advisors, stated: "The consensus among the science community is that for the first time we understand the genetic underpinnings of this disease."

"How do you identify a top doctor?" is an important question for all Americans, not just those diagnosed with cancer. As we mentioned earlier, too many Americans are incredibly casual in selecting physicians and hospitals. They may pick a name from their health plan directory, or even from a phone book, with the location of the doctor's office being the primary factor in their selection. Others may simply ask a friend or relative and the recommendation they receive may be based on how well the person "likes" the doctor rather than on any particular medical expertise or skill.

The specialists listed in *America's Top Doctors® for Cancer* are clearly among the best in the nation and have been identified through a rigorous research process and thorough screening by the Castle Connolly physician-led research team. Through our extensive surveys and research we have done much of the work in finding a top referral specialist, but they are not the only excellent physicians in the nation.

The goal in creating this guide was to select physicians viewed by their peers as the best in preventing, diagnosing and treating cancer and its consequences.

So, how does one judge the qualifications of a physician who may not be listed in this Guide? If someone was trying to find a specialist on their own, how should they go about it? How can someone tell when a physician has the appropriate training in a specialty and how does one distinguish what is meaningful and what is not from among all those plaques and certificates on a doctor's wall?

The reality is that few of us see only one doctor in our lifetime. Each of us may be cared for by a primary care physician, an ophthalmologist, an orthopaedist, a dermatologist, a surgeon or a number of other specialists. The choices can be many and they can be among the most important choices we make.

The following pages will outline the process for selecting a well-qualified physician. In fact, what is written here reflects much of the logic that underlies the selection of physicians for this book. This section will help not only in finding a top specialist in this guide, but it also should be helpful in choosing among the many specialists, primary care doctors and other physicians, that a person will need to consult throughout his/her life.

Education

The review of a prospective doctor's education and training should begin with medical school. While some may feel that the institution at which a physician earned a bachelor's degree could be an indication of the doctor's quality, most people in the medical field do not believe it plays a major role. A degree from a highly selective undergraduate college or university will help an aspiring doctor gain admission to a medical school, but once there, all students are peers. Furthermore, where a doctor trains (i.e. completes residency) is more important than medical school in judging quality. American medical schools are highly standardized, at least in terms of basic quality standards.

A group known as the Liaison Committee for Medical Education (LCME) accredits all U.S. medical schools that grant medical degrees (MDs) and osteopathic degrees (DOs). Most also are accredited by the appropriate state agency, if one exists, and by regional agencies that accredit colleges and universities of all kinds.

Fortunately, U.S. medical schools have universally high standards for admission, including success on the undergraduate level and on the Medical College Admissions Tests (MCATs). Although frequently criticized for being slow to change and for training too many specialists, the system of medical education in the United States has assured consistent high quality in medical practice. One recent positive change is a strong effort in most medical schools to diversify the composition of the student body. While these schools have been less successful in enrolling racial minorities, the number of women in U.S. medical schools has increased to the point that women now make up about 50 percent of most classes. In certain specialties preferred by women medical graduates (pediatrics, for example), it is possible that in coming years the majority of specialists will be female.

Most doctors practicing in the United States are graduates of U.S. medical schools, but there are two other groups of doctors who make up a significant portion (30+%) of the total physician population. They are (1) foreign nationals who graduated from foreign schools and (2) U.S. nationals who graduated from foreign schools. (Canadian medical schools are not considered foreign.)

Foreign Medical Graduates

Foreign medical schools vary greatly in quality. Even some of the oldest and finest European schools have become virtually "open door," with huge numbers of unscreened students making teaching and learning difficult. Others are excellent and provided the model for our system of medical education.

The fact that someone graduated from a foreign school does not mean that he or she is a poor doctor. Foreign schools, like those in the U.S., produce both good and poor doctors. Foreign medical graduates who wish to practice here must pass the same exam taken by U.S. graduates for licensure. It is true the failure rate for foreign graduates is significantly higher. In the first year of using the new United States Medical Licensing Exam (USMLE), 93 percent of U.S. medical school graduates passed Step II, the clinical exam, as compared with only 39 percent of the foreign graduates. It is clear that the quality of many foreign schools, if not individual doctors, is not the same as U.S. medical schools, at least as measured by our standards. Nonetheless, many communities and patients have been well served by foreign medical graduates practicing in this country—often in areas where it has been difficult to attract graduates of American schools. About 25 percent of practicing physicians in the U.S. today are graduates of foreign medical schools.

In addition, many foreign medical schools and their teaching hospitals are world renowned for their leadership in medical care, research and teaching, and many of the technologies and techniques we utilize in the U.S. today have been developed and perfected in foreign countries.

"How do you identify a top doctor?" is an important question for all Americans, not just those diagnosed with cancer.

Residency

Most doctors practicing today have at least three years of post-graduate training (following the MD or DO) in an approved residency program. This not only is an important step in the process of becoming a competent doctor, but it is also a requirement for board (specialty) certification. Most people assume that a prospective doctor needs to complete a three-year residency program to obtain a medical license. That is not an accurate assumption! New York State, for example, requires only one postgraduate year. However, since all approved residencies last at least three years and some, such as those in neurosurgery, general surgery, orthopaedic surgery and urology, may extend for five or more years, it is important to know the details of a doctor's training. Licensure alone is not enough of a basis on which to choose a physician.

Without undertaking extensive and detailed research on every residency program, the best assessment you can make of a doctor's residency program is to see if it took place in a large medical center whose name you recognize. The more prestigious institutions tend to attract the best medical students, sometimes regardless of the quality of the individual residency program. If in doubt about a doctor's training, ask the doctor if the residency he or she completed was in the specialty of the practice; if not, ask why not.

It is also important to be certain that a doctor completed a residency that has been approved by the appropriate governing board of the specialty, such as the American Board of Surgery, the American Board of Radiology, or the American Osteopathic Board of Pediatrics. These board groups are listed in Appendix A. If you are really concerned about a doctor's training, you should call the hospital that offered the residency and ask if the residency program was approved by the appropriate specialty group. If still in doubt, consult the publication *Directory of Graduate Medical Education Programs*, often called the "green book," found in medical school or hospital libraries, which lists all approved residencies.

If in doubt about a doctor's training, ask the doctor if the residency program he or she completed was in the specialty of the practice; if not, ask why not.

Board Certification

With an MD or DO degree and a license, an individual may practice in any medical specialty with or without additional specialized training. For example, doctors with a license, but no special training, may call themselves a surgeon, oncologist or radiologist. This is why board certification is such an important factor. It assures the physician has had specific training in that specialty and has passed the board exam. The American Board of Medical Specialties (ABMS) recognizes 25 specialties and more than 90 subspecialties. Visit www.abms.org or call 866-275-2267 for more information. Eighteen boards certify in 20 specialties under the aegis of the American Osteopathic Association (AOA). Visit www.osteopathic.org or call 800-621-1773 for more information. Doctors who have qualified for such specialization are called board certified; they have completed an approved residency and passed the board's exam.

(See Appendix A for an approved ABMS and AOA lists). While many doctors who are not board certified call themselves "specialists," board certification is the best standard by which to measure competence and training.

You can be confident that doctors who are board certified have, at a minimum, the proper training in their specialty and have demonstrated their proficiency through supervision and testing. While there are many non-board certified doctors who are highly competent, it is more difficult to assess the level of their training. While board certification alone does not guarantee competence, it is a standard that reflects successful completion of an appropriate training program. If it is impossible to find a doctor in your area who is board certified in a particular subspecialty, for example, Medical Oncology or Radiation Oncology, at least be certain the physician is board certified in a related specialty such as Internal Medicine or Radiology.

Board certified doctors are referred to as Diplomates of the Board. Some of the colleges of medical specialties (e.g., the American College of Radiology, the American College of Surgeons) have multiple levels of recognition. The first is basic membership and the second, more prestigious and difficult to obtain, is status as a Fellow. Fellowship status in the colleges is meaningful and is based on experience, professional achievement and recognition by one's peers, including extensive experience in patient care. It should be viewed as a significant professional qualification.

It is important to know the details of a doctor's training. Licensure alone is not enough of a basis on which to choose a physician.

Board Eligibility

Many doctors who have been more recently trained are waiting to take the boards. They are sometimes described as "board eligible," a common term that the ABMS advocates abandoning because of its ambiguity. Board eligible means that the doctor has completed an approved residency and is qualified to sit for the related board's exam. Another term that is used is "board qualified." Once again, the term has no official standing, but could mean the doctor has completed residency and is awaiting the board exam. It could also mean the doctor took and failed to pass the exam to become board certified.

Each member board of the ABMS has its own policy regarding the use and recognition of the board eligible term. Therefore, the description "board eligible" should not be viewed as a genuine qualification, especially if a doctor has been out of medical school long enough to have taken the certification exam. To the boards, a doctor is either board certified or not. Furthermore, most of the specialty boards permit unlimited attempts to pass the exam and, in some cases, doctors who have failed the exam twice or even ten times, continue to call themselves board eligible. In Osteopathic Medicine, the board eligible status is recognized only for the first six years after completion of a residency.

In addition to the approved lists of specialties and subspecialties of the ABMS and AOA, there are a wide variety of other doctors and groups of doctors who call themselves specialists. At present there are at least 100 such groups called "self-designated medical specialties." They range from doctors who are working to create a recognized body of knowledge and subspecialty training to less formal groups interested in a particular approach to the practice of medicine. These groups may or may not have standards for membership. It may be difficult to determine the true extent of their members' training, and neither the ABMS or the AOA recognizes them. While you should be cautious of doctors who claim they are specialists in these areas, many do have advanced training and the groups at least offer a listing of people interested in a particular approach to medical care. Rely on board certification to assure yourself of basic competence, and use membership in one of these groups to indicate strong interest and possible additional training in a particular aspect of medicine.

You can be confident that doctors who are board certified have, at a minimum, the proper training in their specialty and have demonstrated their proficiency through supervision and testing.

Recertification

A relatively new focus of the specialty boards is the area of recertification. Until recently, board certification lasted for an unlimited time. Now, almost all the boards have put time limits on the certification period. For example, in Internal Medicine and Radiology, the time limit is ten years. These more stringent standards reflect an increasing emphasis on recertification by both the medical boards and state agencies responsible for licensing doctors.

Since the policies of the boards vary widely, it is a good procedure to check a doctor's background to see when certification was awarded. If the date was seven to ten years ago, see if he or she has been recertified. Unfortunately, many boards permit "grandfathering," whereby already certified doctors do not have to be recertified, and recertification requirements apply only to newly certified doctors. Even if recertification is not required, it is good professional practice for doctors to undertake the process. It assures you, the patient, that they are attempting to stay current.

Many states have a continuing medical education requirement for doctors. These states typically require a minimum number of continuing medical education (CME) credits for a doctor to maintain a medical license. Seven states require 150 CME credits over a three-year period. Osteopathic doctors are required to take 120 hours of CME credits within three years to maintain certification.

Fellowships

The purpose of a fellowship is to provide advanced training in the clinical techniques and research of a particular specialty. Fellowships usually, but not always, are designed to lead to board certification in a subspecialty such as medical oncology which is a subspecialty of internal medicine. Many physicians listed in this guide have had fellowship training. In the U.S. there are a variety of fellowship programs available to doctors, which fall into two broad categories: approved and unapproved. Approved fellowships are those that are approved by the appropriate medical specialty board (e.g., the American Board of Radiology) and lead to subspecialty certificates. Fellowship programs that are unapproved are often in the same areas of training as those that are approved, but they do not lead to subspecialty certificates.

Unfortunately, all too often, unapproved fellowships exist only to provide relatively inexpensive labor for the research and/or patient care activities of a clinical department in a medical school or hospital. In such cases, the learning that takes place is secondary and may be a good deal less than in an approved fellowship. On the other hand, any fellowship is better than none at all and some unapproved fellowships have status for a valid reason that should not reflect negatively on the program. For example, the fellowship may have been recently created, with approval being sought. There are also some areas of medicine not yet recognized for sub-specialty certification, such as Transplant Surgery.

Some physicians may have completed more than one fellowship and may be boarded in two or more subspecialties. In addition, some physicians may pursue fellowship training and subspecialty certification but then choose to practice in their primary field of certification. For example, a doctor who is board certified in internal medicine also may have obtained board certification in oncology, but may choose to practice primarily internal medicine. For the most part, the physicians in this guide practice in their sub-specialties.

Professional Reputation

There are practitioners who meet every professional standard on paper, but who are simply not good doctors. In all probability, the medical community has ascertained this and, while the individual may still practice medicine, his or her reputation will reflect that collective assessment. There are also doctors who are outstanding leaders in their fields because of research or professional activities but who are not particularly strong, or perhaps even active, in patient care. It is important to distinguish that kind of professional reputation from a reputation as a competent, caring doctor in delivering patient care or, in the case of this guide, as an outstanding practitioner in a given specialty.

Hospital Appointment

Most doctors are on the medical staff of one or more hospitals and are known as "attendings;" some, however, are not. If a doctor does not have admitting privileges or is not on the attending staff of a hospital, you may wish to consider choosing a different doctor. It can be very difficult to ascertain whether or not the lack of hospital appointment is for a good reason. For example, it is understandable that some doctors who are raising families or heading toward retirement choose not to meet the demands (meetings, committees, etc.) of being an attending. However, if you need care in a hospital, the lack of such an appointment means that another doctor will have to oversee that care. In some specialties, such as dermatology and psychiatry, doctors may conduct their entire practice in the office and a hospital appointment is not as essential, or as good a criterion for assessment, as in other specialties.

If a doctor does not have admitting privileges or is not on the attending staff of a hospital, you may wish to consider choosing a different doctor.

While mistakes are made, most hospitals are quite careful about admissions to their medical staffs. The best hospitals are highly selective, so a degree of screening (or "credentialing") has been done for you. In other words, the best doctors usually practice at the best hospitals. Since caring for a patient in a hospital is often a team effort involving a number of specialists, the reputation of the hospital to which the doctor admits patients carries special weight. Hospital medical staffs review their colleagues' credentials and authorize performance of specific procedures. In addition, they typically review and reappoint their medical staff every two or three years. In effect, this is an additional screening to protect patients. It is especially true of hospitals that have what are known as closed staffs, where it is impossible to obtain admitting privileges unless there is a vacancy that the administration and medical staff deem necessary to fill. If you are having a surgical procedure and are concerned about the doctor's skill or experience, it may be worthwhile to call the Medical Affairs Office at the doctor's hospital to see if he or she is authorized to perform that procedure in that hospital.

The reasons for a hospital's selectivity are easy to understand: no hospital wishes to expose itself to liability and every hospital wants to have the best reputation possible in order to attract patients. Obviously, the quality of the medical staff is immensely important in creating that reputation.

Physicians listed in this guide are primarily on the staffs of major medical centers, university teaching hospitals and leading specialty hospitals. Occasionally, some may be on staff at a community hospital for one or two days a week and spend the majority of their time at the teaching hospital. There are many excellent physicians on the staffs of community hospitals that call themselves "medical centers," but they are typically not physicians who attract complex cases and referrals regionally, nationally and even internationally.

To learn about a hospital, visit its website. It is also useful to review a hospital's accreditation status under the Joint Commission on the Accreditation of Healthcare Organizations at www.JCAHO.com. Also www.hospitalcompare.hhs.gov compares hospital performance in a limited number of cases.

A last and very important reason why a hospital appointment is an essential requirement in your choice of doctor is that some states permit doctors to practice without malpractice insurance. If you are injured as a result of a doctor's poor care, you could be without recourse. However, few hospitals permit doctors to practice in them unless they carry malpractice insurance. This not only protects the hospital, but the patient as well.

The best doctors usually practice at the best hospitals.

Medical School Faculty Appointment

Many doctors have appointments on the faculties of medical schools. There is a range of categories from "straight" appointments, meaning full-time appointment as professor, associate professor, assistant professor or instructor, to clinical ranks that may reflect lesser degrees of involvement in teaching or research. If someone carries what is known as a straight academic rank (e.g. "professor of surgery," without "clinical" in the title), this usually means that the individual is engaged full-time in medical school research, teaching activities and patient care. The title "clinical professor of surgery" usually identifies a part-time or adjunct appointment and less direct involvement in medical school activities such as teaching and research.

Doctors who are full-time academicians are more likely to be in the forefront of new techniques and research, especially when it comes to a disease like cancer. They also have the advantage of the support of other faculty, residents and medical students.

When you are seeking a subspecialist, a doctor's relationship to a medical school becomes more meaningful since medical school faculties tend to be made up of sub-specialists. You are less likely to find large numbers of general or primary care practitioners engaged full-time on a medical school faculty. The newest approaches and techniques in medicine, for the most part, are explored and developed by medical school faculties in their laboratories and clinical practice settings. This is where they practice their sub-specialties, as well as teach and conduct research.

Medical Society Membership

Most medical society memberships sound very prestigious and some are; however, there are many societies that are not selective and virtually any doctor can join. In addition, membership in many of the more prestigious societies is based on research and publication or on leadership in the field and may have little to do with direct patient care. While it is clearly an honor to be invited to join these groups, membership may be less than helpful in discerning whether a doctor can meet your needs.

Physicians listed in this guide are primarily on the staffs of major medical centers, university teaching hospitals and leading specialty hospitals.

Experience

Experience is difficult to assess. Obviously, in most cases, an older doctor has more experience; on the other hand, a younger doctor has been more recently immersed in the challenge of medical school, residency, or even a fellowship, and may be the more up-to-date. If a doctor is board certified, you may assume that assures at least a minimal amount of experience, but since it could be as little as a year, check the date of graduation from medical school or completion of residency to know precisely how long a doctor has been in practice.

There is a good deal of evidence that there is a positive relationship between quantity of experience and quality of care. That is, the more a doctor performs a procedure, the better he or she becomes at it. That is why it is important to ask a doctor about his or her experience with the procedure that you need. Does the doctor see and treat similar cases every day, every week or only rarely? Of course, with some rare diseases, "rarely" is the only possible answer, but it is the relative frequency that is critical. In some states, data is available on volume or numbers of certain procedures performed at hospitals. For volume and outcome information in other states, visit the web site of Healthcare Choices at www.healthcarechoices.org. There is a good deal of controversy, however, on the validity and usefulness of such data. Opponents cite the fact that some of the data is produced from Medicare patient records only and, therefore, is based solely on an elderly population that does not represent the total activity of a hospital or doctor. Proponents of the use of such volume data agree that it is not perfect, but suggest it can be one useful criterion in selecting the best places to receive care for these specific problems. While recognizing the limitations of such data, the healthcare consumer may, nonetheless, find it of interest and use.

The one type of experience you should specifically want to know about is that dealing with any special procedure, particularly a surgical one, that has recently been developed and introduced into practice. For example, in the 1980's many doctors using laparoscopic cholecystectomy, a then new, minimally invasive surgical technique for removing gallbladders, experienced a high percentage of problems because they were not properly trained. This prompted the American Board of Surgery to promulgate new standards for the training of surgeons using this technique. Do not hesitate to ask about your doctor's training in a procedure and how frequently and with what degree of success he or she has performed it. Practice may not lead to perfection, but it does improve skills and enhance the probability of success.

Doctors who are full-time academicians are more likely to be in the forefront of new techniques and research, especially when it comes to a disease like cancer.

In some cases, relatively young doctors have recently completed residency or fellowship training under recognized leaders who have developed new approaches or techniques for dealing with a particular problem. They may have learned the new techniques from their mentors and may be far ahead of the field (and ahead of more senior and distinguished colleagues) in using those approaches. So age and experience must be considered and weighed along with other factors when choosing a physician.

Most doctors will be supportive if you request a second opinion and many will recommend it. In many cases, insurance companies will pay for second opinions, but check ahead of time to make sure your insurance plan does cover them. In an HMO you may have to be more assertive because one way HMOs control costs is by limiting second opinions. Often, the opinion of a second doctor will confirm the opinion of the first, but the reassurance may be worth the time and extra cost. On the other hand, if the second opinion differs from the first, you have two alternatives: seek the opinion of a third doctor, or educate yourself as much as possible by talking to both doctors, reading up on the problem, and trusting your instincts about which diagnosis is correct. Sometimes obtaining a second opinion can be a major challenge. Occasionally, a physician may be offended. Nonetheless, you should not be dissuaded.

The simple logistics of getting a second opinion can be an obstacle. Tara Parker-Pope related in her column "Health Journal" in the *Wall Street Journal* the difficulty gathering her mother's records from five doctors, two radiology offices and the pathology lab. She also cited, in the same piece, a Northwestern University review of 340 breast cancer patients who sought second opinions. They reported that 20 percent of second opinions had no change in pathology or prognosis, but in the remaining 80 percent of patients some change did occur.

Office and Practice Arrangements

Some specialists will only see new patients who are referred to them by another doctor. Therefore, you may need to have your treating physician contact the specialist's office to arrange for your initial visit. Your health plan may also require that your primary care doctor provide a referral.

If English is not your first language, it may be advisable to determine whether someone in the specialist's office speaks your primary language or if a translator can be present during appointments or, perhaps take a bilingual person with you. This will ease communication and assure that all questions, responses and instructions are understood.

Research suggests that there is a positive relationship between quantity of experience and quality of care.

Accessibility of a physician's office may be a concern if you are wheelchair-bound, elderly or cannot climb stairs or negotiate narrow corridors. Convenient parking may also be important to you.

When you are choosing a top specialist, these issues may be of lesser or greater importance, depending on the problem and type of care warranted. If you are traveling a great distance to have a specific procedure performed by a top specialist at a major medical center, continuing long-term monitoring or follow-up care by that physician may not be required or may not be feasible and such things as office practice arrangements are of less importance. On the other hand, if your disease needs to be monitored with follow-up care provided by the same top specialist, then such issues as accessibility of the doctor's office, appointment hours, waiting times and courtesy and professionalism of the staff become more significant.

Often, the opinion of a second doctor will confirm the opinion of the first, but the reassurance may be worth the time and extra cost.

Second Opinions

Second opinions are a valuable medical tool, too infrequently used in many instances and overused in others. Clearly, you do not want to seek another doctor's opinion on every ailment or problem that you face, but a second opinion should be pursued in the following situations:

- Before major surgery

- If a rare disease is diagnosed

- If a diagnosis is uncertain

- If the number of tests or procedures recommended might seem excessive

- If a test result has serious implications (e.g., a positive Pap smear)

- If the treatment suggested is risky or expensive

- If you are uncomfortable with the diagnosis and/or treatment

- If a course of treatment is not successful

- If you question your doctor's competence

- If your insurance company requires it

Personal Chemistry

One element of the doctor-patient relationship that we stress in our guides is chemistry between doctor and patient, a part of which is often referred to as a doctor's "bedside manner." While this factor is of major importance in a long-term relationship such as you would have with your primary care physician, it is of less importance when you see a specialist only once or twice.

It is vital that there is a sense of mutual trust and respect between patient and doctor; this is a judgment that individuals must make for themselves. Among the many talented doctors listed in this guide, there are very likely some to whom you would relate well and others with whom you may not feel as comfortable.

Patients prefer doctors who listen, demonstrate concern, are responsive to patient needs and spend sufficient time with them. The qualities of physicians in this regard, even the excellent ones in this guide, vary widely.

You, the patient, are the only one who can assess these qualities because individuals react differently to various personalities. It is important for you to carefully judge your feelings towards a physician, especially if you are embarking on a long-term relationship. You should feel you can be open, trusting and responsive to your physician and that your relationship will be a positive one. Otherwise, find another doctor, since not doing so could adversely affect your care.

Once you have used this guide to identify the top specialist(s) best suited to treat your condition, there is much you can do to maximize the value of your first visit.

Patients prefer doctors who listen, demonstrate concern, are responsive to patient needs and spend sufficient time with them.

• 5 •

Maximizing Your First Appointment With a Top Doctor

After your research is done and you've secured an appointment for an initial consultation with a top doctor, known for his or her expertise in the diagnosis or treatment of your particular medical condition, what should you do?

Questions Concerning Payment

Other arrangements that may need to be made in advance of your first visit or discussed with the specialist's office staff concern payment. You may wish to ask the following:

- Is the specialist within your plan's network and will you need to make a co-payment? Or, is the specialist out-of-network and will you have to pay for your care out-of-pocket, meet a deductible or submit a form for reimbursement?

- Are credit cards an acceptable mode of payment?

- Does the specialist accept Medicare or Medicaid?

A specialist becoming newly involved in your care needs to learn as much as possible about the state of your health in a very limited time. Since top doctors are extremely busy people with many demands on their time, you should make certain that all relevant records and case summaries are obtained and sent to the specialist well in advance of your appointment.

Lastly, it may be advisable to take a relative or close friend with you for support.

Obtaining Your Records

All healthcare providers, including hospitals, doctors and their staffs, are under legal obligation to maintain the privacy of your medical records. In order to obtain release of those records, you must make a request in writing. If you need to obtain records from a number of providers, you should write one clear and concise letter authorizing release of your records and including your name, address, telephone number, date of birth, and hospital patient I.D. number. You then can make photocopies of this letter, but be sure to sign and date each copy as if it were an original. You also may want to specifically name those test results (e.g., pathology slides) or X-ray films (not just written reports or summaries) that must be included in addition to making a general request for your records. It's also a good idea to indicate the date of your appointment so the office staff can respond in a timely manner.

Although state laws require the timely release of medical records, hospital medical records departments and doctors' offices often take several weeks to pull and review patient charts and get them in the mail either to you or to another doctor. In addition to written authorization, you may be asked to pay the costs involved in copying your records, test results and X-ray films because many doctors' offices will not release the originals. Consider placing a call in advance to determine the procedure for releasing your records, how long you can expect it to take, and the costs involved so that you can save time by including payment with your release authorization letter. Be sure to allow sufficient time in advance of your consultation appointment for your request to be processed. Since you often must wait several weeks for an appointment with a specialist, allow at least that amount of time to obtain your records.

Even after making your written requests, you should follow up each letter with a telephone call to be sure that your records actually are sent. You should not assume that your request for records will be promptly fulfilled by an often overburdened, although well-intentioned, office staff.

> It is vital that there is a sense of mutual trust and respect between patient and doctor; this is a judgment that individuals must make for themselves.

Remember, the more information the specialist has about your condition, the fewer repeat or additional tests or procedures you will need to undergo. This will lower the costs of your consultation and enable the specialist to more easily assess your condition.

The Facts and Only the Facts

Be thorough and organized in documenting your personal and familial medical histories, the medications you take and in relaying information about your condition. Even seemingly minor bits of information may provide subtle clues to the nature of your medical problem and the optimal way in which to treat it. It's also advisable to bring a list with you of names, addresses and telephone numbers of all physicians who have cared for you, especially those you have seen regarding your current medical problem.

Even though thoroughness is essential to presenting a clear picture of your medical condition, bear in mind that the specialist needs to get to your core health concerns as quickly as possible. Therefore, if you have a complex medical history, you may want to ask your current doctors to provide treatment summaries in addition to copies of your medical records. Hospital records should include your admission history and physical exam, dictated consultation and operation notes and discharge summaries for all hospitalizations. You may also be able to get a cumulative lab and X-ray summary for your hospital stays.

Unlike X-rays, which can be copied at reasonable cost, original pathology slides must be transported by mail or hand-carried. Your specialist may wish to have the pathologist with whom he or she works speak directly with the pathologist who initially interpreted your slides as part of the process of evaluating your case.

Being Prepared

To avoid leaving out important details of your condition or past treatment, prepare a concise, chronological summary before your consultation takes place. You may wish to type it and provide a copy to the specialist for inclusion in your chart. Highlight major medical results or significant events in the course of an illness or treatment if these will enlighten the doctor about your condition. Your personal perspective on the state of your health is vital to a full understanding of your medical problem.

You should make certain that all relevant records and case summaries are obtained and sent to the specialist well in advance of your appointment.

It is possible that the specialist will use terminology that you do not understand or may speak quickly assuming certain knowledge on your part about your condition or its treatment. Don't hesitate to ask for clarification as often or repeatedly as you may need to in order to fully comprehend what you are being told. If you are concerned that you may forget what the doctor tells you, ask the doctor's permission to take notes or ask if you might bring along a tape recorder so you can later replay what was said, especially any instructions you are given. You may prefer to bring along a relative or close friend to serve as a "second set of ears," but, again, seek the doctor's permission to do so in advance of your appointment.

Following this process will assure that you and the specialist you are consulting get the most from your appointment. After all, you both have the same goal: restoring you to optimal health and well being.

What To Do If You Can't Get an Appointment

At times it may be difficult, perhaps even impossible, to secure an appointment with the specific specialist you have identified. There are a number of reasons why this may occur. For example, the specialist may not be taking any new patients or may have such a busy schedule that it takes several weeks or months to get an appointment. He or she may only see patients during very limited hours because of teaching, research or other responsibilities or currently may have other limitations related to the acceptance of new patients.

However, bear in mind that the doctors in this guide are the leaders in their fields and therefore they work with and train the very best and brightest in their specialties. So, if you are unable to consult with a particular doctor, consider making an appointment with one of his or her outstanding colleagues. You can do this by asking a member of the doctor's office staff to refer you to an associate who is a member of the practice group or to another excellent physician who is specially trained to address your particular medical issue.

You can be comfortable knowing that you will receive high quality care from another specialist who practices in the same top setting.

Remember, the more information the specialist has about your condition, the fewer repeat or additional tests or procedures you will need to undergo.

Gathering the Facts

Have you done everything you can to prepare yourself and the specialist for the consultation? The following checklist will help you maximize the value of your visit to the specialist and will go a long way toward focusing you on the task at hand—getting the best advice or treatment for your health problem from one of the top doctors in the medical specialty related to your condition.

- Does the specialist have all the information needed to make a diagnosis of or treatment plan for your condition?

- Have your medical records, test results and X-rays been sent ahead of time to allow for their review by the specialist in advance of your first appointment?

- Have you written out your medical history, including that of your siblings, parents and grandparents, emphasizing the particular problem for which you are visiting this specialist?

- Are you prepared with a written list of questions?

- When you ask your questions, have you understood the answers?

• 6 •

Clinical Trials

The following information on special resources has been included to meet the needs of cancer patients and their families. These patients and their physicians may need to search for very new, cutting-edge, perhaps even experimental and not yet approved therapies. In such cases the search may lead to clinical trials, tests of new drugs and new medical devices, or innovative therapeutic approaches. Fortunately, these situations are rare, but when they do occur they are critical.

In addition to the outstanding private and public hospitals recognized in this guide, the U.S. government maintains its own unique, expert source of patient care and clinical research at the National Institutes of Health (NIH). In fact, the NIH operates its own hospital at which the care provided is usually related to clinical studies its researchers are undertaking.

In addition to those at the NIH, clinical trials also are conducted at leading medical centers and other organizations throughout the country. These facilities may be testing a new drug therapy, a new use for an existing medication or a medical device to deal with a problem that is not being resolved through the use of more traditional approaches.

This section will guide you in utilizing these special resources. These is also a listing of selected cancer resources in Appendix C.

If you are unable to consult with a particular doctor, consider making an appointment with one of his or her outstanding colleagues.

The Clinical Trial as a Treatment Option

For some patients the best medical treatment may only be available through clinical trials (also called treatment studies), which are designed to develop improved ways to use current medical treatments or to find new medical treatments by studying their effects on humans. Treatments are studied to determine if they are safe, effective and better treatments than conventional or standard therapies. Only if they meet all three of these criteria are they made available to the general public.

Many people are frightened by the term "clinical trial" because it conveys the notion of being a "guinea pig" in an experiment. Contrary to popular belief, however, new treatments are extensively studied by scientists in the laboratory before they are ever tested by physicians in clinical settings. Among the factors that keep patients from participating in clinical trials are: lack of awareness about clinical trials as a treatment option; fear of side effects or adverse reactions to treatment; refusal of insurance companies to pay for experimental treatments; failure of a physician to inform the patient about clinical trials; difficulty finding suitable clinical trials; unavailability of clinical trials for certain medical problems; distance of the patient from major medical centers conducting clinical trials; disruption of personal and family life; and the decision to stop medical treatment altogether.

Despite these and other obstacles, many people do seek out clinical trials. New medical treatments can offer participants hope for a cure, an extended lifespan, or an improvement in how they feel. Some participants also take comfort in knowing that others may benefit from their contribution to medical knowledge.

Deciding if a clinical trial is the right treatment option for you is no simple matter. Certainly, you will want to talk about it with your doctor(s) and other professionals involved in your care, as well as with family members and friends. But in order to fully benefit from what others have to say — based on either their professional knowledge or personal experience — you need to understand exactly what a clinical trial is and what your role as a volunteer will be.

Understanding Clinical Trials

Clinical trials are conducted for just about every medical condition, including life-threatening diseases such as AIDS or cancer; chronic illnesses such as diabetes and asthma; psychiatric disorders such as depression or anxiety; behavioral problems such as smoking and substance abuse; and even common ailments such as hair loss and acne. Chances are there is at least one trial (and probably more) that may be appropriate for you.

With more than 100 different types of cancer, it is understandable that a large number of clinical trials are cancer-related. Extensive information about clinical trials for cancer can be found on www.cancer.gov, the Web site of the National Cancer Institute (NCI). NCI is part of the National Institutes of Health (NIH). CenterWatch, an online clinical trials listing service, identifies over 14,000 clinical trials that are actively recruiting patients. Veritas Medicine, another useful online organization, allows individuals to perform personalized searches of its clinical trials database. See "Selected Cancer Resources" in Appendix C for more information on clinical trials.

Most clinical trials study new medical treatments, combinations of treatments, or improvements in conventional treatments using drugs, surgery and other medical procedures, medical devices, radiation or other therapies. Newer types of clinical trials, called screening or prevention trials, study how to prevent the incidence or recurrence of disease through the use of medicines, vitamins, minerals or other supplements; and how to screen for disease, especially in its early stages. Another type of trial studies how to improve the quality of life for patients, including both their physical and emotional well-being.

Clinical trials are sponsored both by the federal government (through the National Institutes of Health, the National Cancer Institute and many others) and by private industry through pharmaceutical and biotechnology companies, and through healthcare institutions (hospitals or health maintenance organizations) and community-based physician-investigators. The National Cancer Institute sponsors clinical trials at more than 1,000 sites in the United States. Trials are carried out in major medical research centers such as teaching hospitals as well as in community hospitals, specialized medical clinics and in doctors' offices.

Though clinical trials often involve hospitalized patients, a fair number of trials are conducted on an outpatient basis. Many trials are part of a cooperative network which may include as few as one or two sites or hundreds of locations, although one center generally assumes responsibility for overall coordination of the research. More than 45 research-oriented institutions, recognized for their scientific excellence, have been designated by the NCI as comprehensive or clinical cancer centers. See "Selected Cancer Resources" in Appendix C to find out how to locate these centers.

Clinical research is based on a protocol (established rules or procedures) describing who will be studied, how and when medications, procedures and/or treatments will be administered and how long the study will last. Trials that are conducted simultaneously at different sites use the same protocol to ensure that all patients are treated identically and all data are collected uniformly so that study findings can be compared.

The National Cancer Institute sponsors clinical trials at more than 1,000 sites in the United States.

Clinical trials generally are conducted in three phases, as outlined in the study protocol. The first phase begins testing of the treatment on a small group of human subjects after rigorous and successful animal testing has been concluded. Phases 2 and 3, but usually involves a broader test group and is designed to further evaluate the treatment's safety and more accurately determine appropriate dosage, application methods and side effects. In some trials there may be a fourth phase, conducted after the treatment is in widespread use, to monitor the results of long-term use and the occurrence of any serious side effects.

Some clinical trials test one treatment on one group of subjects, while others compare two or more groups of subjects. In such comparison studies participants are divided into two groups: the control group that receives the standard treatment and the experimental or treatment group which receives the new treatment. For example, the control group may undergo a surgical procedure while the experimental or treatment group undergoes a surgical procedure plus radiation to determine which treatment modality is more effective.

To ensure that patient characteristics do not unduly influence the study findings, patients may be randomly assigned to either the control or the experimental group, meaning that each patient's assignment is based purely on chance. In cases in which a standard treatment does not exist for a particular disease, the experimental group of patients receives the new treatment and the control group receives no treatment at all, or receives a placebo, an inactive medicine or procedure that has no treatment value. It is important to keep in mind that patients are never put into a control group without any treatment if there is a known treatment that could help them. Also, whether a patient is receiving an investigational drug or a placebo, he/she receives the same level and quality of medical care as those receiving the investigational treatment.

One of the most pressing reasons to participate in clinical trials is the opportunity to obtain treatment that might not be available otherwise.

Protecting the Rights of Participants

The safety of those who participate in clinical trials is a serious matter and is the number one priority of medical investigators. All clinical research, regardless of type of sponsorship results of long-term use and the occurrence of any serious side effect is guided by the same ethical and legal codes that govern the medical profession and the practice of medicine. Most clinical research is federally funded or federally regulated (at least in part) with built-in safeguards for patients. According to federal government regulations (and some state laws), every clinical trial in the U.S. must be approved and monitored by an Institutional Review Board (IRB), which is an independent committee of physicians, statisticians, community advocates and others (representing at least five distinct disciplines) to ensure that the protocol is being followed. Government regulations require researchers to fully inform participants about all aspects of a clinical trial before they agree to participate through a process called informed consent. To be sure that you understand your role in a clinical trial, you should jot down any questions beforehand so as not to forget them. You should also consider bringing along a friend or family member for support and additional input, and perhaps even tape recording the conversation (after asking permission to do so) to make sure you do not forget or misunderstand anything. Each participant in a clinical trial must be given a written consent form, which should be available in English and other languages. The consent form explains the issues listed in the box on page 46. Patients also are informed that they may leave the trial, or exclude themselves from any part of it, at any time. Informed consent means exactly what the term implies: you agree to join a clinical trial only after you completely understand exactly what your participation will involve for the duration of the study. By law, each patient must be provided with a copy of the signed consent form, which also must include the name and telephone number of a contact person for questions or additional information. Informed consent is a continuous process, so do not hesitate to ask questions before, during or after the trial.

The investigators must protect the privacy of each participant in a clinical trial by ensuring that all medical records are kept confidential except for inspection by the sponsoring agency, the Food and Drug Administration (FDA) and other agencies involved in regulating the drug or treatment, and all data are collected anonymously by assigning a numeric code or initials to each individual.

During the course of the trial, participants are regularly seen by members of the research team to monitor their health and well-being. Participants also should be responsible for their own health by following the treatment plan (such as taking the proper dosage of medications on time), keeping all scheduled visits and informing members of the healthcare team about any symptoms that occur. If, during the course of the trial, the treatment proves to be ineffective or harmful, the patient is free to leave the study and still obtain conventional care. Conversely, as soon as there is evidence that one treatment modality is better than another, all patients in the trial are given the benefit of the new information.

Questions to Ask Your Doctor and the Trial's Research Team if You are Considering Participating in a Clinical Trial:

- Who is sponsoring the trial?

- How many patients will be involved?

- Will the trial be testing a single treatment or a combination of treatments?

- Will there be one treatment group or more than one treatment group?

- If more than one treatment group, how are patients assigned to each group?

- Has this treatment been studied in previous clinical trials? What were the findings?

- What are the requirements for patient eligibility?

Enrolling in Clinical Trials

Each clinical trial has its own guidelines, called eligibility criteria, for determining who can participate. Treatment studies recruit participants who have a disease or other medical condition, while screening and prevention studies generally recruit healthy volunteers. Inclusion criteria (those that allow you to participate in a study) and exclusion criteria (those that keep you from participating in a study) ensure that the study will answer the research questions posed in the research protocol while maintaining the safety of participants. The disease being studied is a primary factor in selecting suitable patients, but other factors such as the patient's gender, age, treatment history and other diagnosed medical conditions may also be important. Unfortunately, eligibility also may depend upon ability to pay. Many health plans do not cover all of the costs associated with clinical trials because they define these trials as experimental procedures. However, trials sometimes pay volunteers for their time and/or reimburse them for travel, childcare, meals and lodging.

To prevent people who qualify from being excluded from clinical trials for financial reasons, agencies such as the National Cancer Institute (NCI) are working with health plans to find solutions and a growing number of states require insurance companies to pay for all routine patient care costs in cancer trials. To encourage more senior citizens to participate in cancer trials, Medicare plans to revise its payment policy to cover those trials.

When choosing a clinical trial you should determine the factors that are most important to you. For instance, patients generally prefer to participate in trials near their homes so that they can maintain their usual day-to-day activities, be surrounded by family and friends and avoid travel and lodging costs. If travel or temporary relocation becomes necessary, try to find a trial site that is near to some family member or friend or one that is in a locale similar to your own city or town. Many organizations, such as the National Cancer Institute (NCI), will work with patients and their families to identify support networks for them wherever they participate.

Participating in a Clinical Trial

Clinical trials are conducted by a research team led by a principal investigator (usually a physician) and are comprised of physicians, nurses and other health professionals such as social workers, psychologists and nutritionists. As a participant you may be required to commit a fair amount of time to a clinical trial, often within more than one geographic region or state.

Some participants also take comfort in knowing that others may benefit from their contribution to medical knowledge.

Participants in clinical trials should remain under the care of their regular physician(s) since clinical trials tend to provide short-term treatment for a specific medical condition and do not generally provide comprehensive primary care. In fact, some trials require that a patient's regular physician sign a consent form before the patient is enrolled. In addition, your regular physician can collaborate with the research team to make sure there are no adverse reactions between your other medications or treatments and the investigational treatment.

Weighing the Benefits and Risks of a Clinical Trial

If you are considering participation in a clinical trial, you need to consider the medical, emotional and financial ramifications of participation. Of course, the obvious benefit of a clinical trial is the chance that a new treatment may improve your health and prognosis. You will have access to drugs and other medical interventions before they are widely available to the public and you will obtain expert and specialized medical care at leading healthcare facilities. Many patients receive an added psychological benefit by taking an active role in their treatment.

It is important to bear in mind that some medical interventions used in clinical trials may carry potential risks depending upon the type of treatment and the patient's condition. While many side effects or adverse reactions are temporary (such as hair loss and nausea caused by some anti-cancer drugs), other more serious reactions can be permanent and even life-threatening (for example, heart, liver or kidney damage).

Deciding whether or not to participate in a clinical trial is often a matter of determining if the trial's potential benefits outweigh its possible risks. This is a highly personal decision that may be difficult to make in situations involving experimental treatment in which limited medical information may be available.

Getting Information on Clinical Trials

The more information you have about a clinical trial, the easier it will be to make a decision about whether or not it is right for you, and the more confident you will be that you made an appropriate decision. In addition to the "Selected Cancer Resources," Appendix C in this guide, the staff at your local public library, community hospital, or major medical center can assist you in locating the information you need from books, consumer organizations and on the Internet.

It is important to keep in mind that patients are never put into a control group without any treatment if there is a known treatment that could help them.

Questions to Ask the Sponsors About Your Rights as a Participant in a Clinical Trial:

- Who is responsible for approving and monitoring this research? Is there an IRB?

- Who informs me about the trial process? Do I sign a consent form? Will I receive a copy?

- May I leave the trial at any time? Have previous patients dropped out?

- Whom do I contact if I am experiencing any difficulty with this trial?

Learning about the National Institututes of Health (NIH)

The National Institutes of Health (NIH) comprise one the world's leading medical research centers and the Federal government's principal agency for biomedical research. An agency of the United States Department of Health, United States Public Health Service, NIH encompasses 25 separate institutions and centers with its main campus located in Bethesda, Maryland. Research is also conducted at several field units across the country and abroad.

Paitent Care at the NIH

The Warren Grant Magnuson Clinical Center, NIH's principal medical research center and hospital located in Bethesda, Maryland, provides medical care only to patients participating in clinical research programs. Two categories of patients participate in the Clinical Center studies: children and adults who wish to improve their own health, such as those with newly diagnosed medical problems, ongoing medical problems or family history of disease; and healthy volunteers wishing to advance knowledge about the causes, progress and treatment of disease. The patient's case must fit into an ongoing NIH research project for which the patient has the precise kind or stage of illness under investigation. General diagnostic and treatment services common to community hospitals are not available.

The Magnuson Clinical Center is the world's largest biomedical research hospital and ambulatory care facility, housing 1,600 laboratories conducting basic and clinical research. There are 1,200 tenured physicians, dentists and researchers on staff along with 660 nurses and 570 allied healthcare professionals (dieticians, imaging technologists, medical technologists, medical records and clerical staff, pharmacists and therapists).

The Center's hospital is specially designed for medical research and accommodates 540 carefully selected patients who are participating in clinical research programs. Its 350-bed facility has 24 inpatient care units to which 7,000 patients are admitted annually. The Center also has an Ambulatory Care Research Facility (ACRF) that serves 68,000 outpatient visits each year. A new facility, called the Mark O. Hatfield Clinical Research Center, which began accepting patients in early 2005, has 242 beds for inpatient care and 90 day-hospital stations for outpatient care. The Mark O. Hatfield Center carries out the latest biomedical research that results in new forms of disease diagnosis, prevention and treatment, which is then incorporated into improved methods of patient care.

The Consent Form Should Explain the Following:

- Why the research is being done.

- What the researchers hope to accomplish.

- What types of treatment interventions (and other test or procedures) will be performed?

- How long the study will continue.

- What the expected benefits and the possible risks are.

- What other treatments are available.

- What costs will be covered by the study, by the patient or by third-party payers such as Medicare, Medicaid or private insurance.

This is a fine example of Translational Medicine where excellent research discoveries are translated into new and improved methods of clinical treatment. In other words, the laboratory discoveries are brought to the bedside.

The Clinical Center also maintains a Children's Inn for pediatric outpatients and their families. This family-centered residence operates 24 hours a day, 7 days a week, 365 days a year.

In an effort to bring clinical research to the community, NIH supports approximately 80 General Clinical Research Centers (GCRCs) around the country, located within hospitals of major academic medical centers.

It is important to note that, as part of the federal government, the Warren Grant Magnuson Clinical Center provides treatment in clinical trials at no cost to its patients. In some cases, patients receive a stipend to help cover the costs of traveling to Bethesda for treatment and follow-up care. Travel costs for the initial screening visit, however, are not covered.

Areas of Clinical Study at the NIH

At the Magnuson Clinical Center alone, NIH physician-scientists conduct nearly 1,000 studies each year. Among the areas of study are cancer and related diseases.

Not all of these clinical areas are under investigation at any given time, however. The Patient Recruitment and Public Liaison Office (PRPL) at the NIH Clinical Center assists patients, their families and their physicians in obtaining information about participation in NIH clinical trials. Trained nurses are available to answer questions about the research programs and admission procedures.

Cancer Care at the Warren Grant Magnuson Clinical Center

The National Cancer Institute (NCI) is the largest of the biomedical research institutes and centers at NIH. There, clinical studies are designed to evaluate new and promising ways to prevent, detect, diagnose and treat cancer. The Warren Grant Magnuson Clinical Center provides a separate outpatient division for cancer patients and also has several designated inpatient units.

The investigators must protect the privacy of each participant in a clinical trial by ensuring that all medical records are kept confidential.

Questions to Ask the Trial's Sponsor About Eligibility Criteria

- What are the inclusion and exclusion criteria for the clinical trial(s) I am considering?

- How can I improve my chances of being accepted? Pre-existing conditions? Problems?

- If I am not eligible for one trial, what other trials being conducted for my condition?

- Will I be paid for my time or reimbursed for my out-of-pocket expenses?

If you are interested in entering a cancer study at the Magnuson Clinical Center (or at the General Clinical Research Centers), you should first discuss treatment options with a physician. As a general rule, patients interested in participating in clinical studies must be referred by a physician. However, in some instances, self-referral may be permitted.

Patients with medical problems other than cancer or healthy volunteers who wish to participate in a clinical study should contact the particular NIH institute responsible for the clinical area involved.

Cancer Care at the NCI Clinical Centers and Comprehensive Cancer Centers

You may also obtain clinical oncology services (education, screening, diagnosis or treatment) or participate in clinical trials at one of the 21 Cancer Centers or 39 Comprehensive Cancer Centers designated by the NCI for their scientific excellence and extensive resources devoted to cancer and cancer-related problems. Centers are located in 32 states, with the majority of sites in California, New York and Pennsylvania. You can find out about clinical trials at the NCI-designated centers by contacting NCI's Clinical Studies Support Center (CSSC) or by calling each center directly (See Appendix C for contact information). Information about other cancer-related services at these centers also may be obtained from the center itself. For more information, you can visit the National Cancer Institute's website at www.cancer.gov.

Questions to Ask the Research Team or Your Physician About Your Role in a Clinical Trial:

- Who are the members of the health team? Who will be in charge of my care?

- How long will the trial last?

- How does treatment in the trial compare with or differ from the standard treatment?

- Will I be hospitalized? How often? For how long a period of time?

- What will occur during each visit? What treatments or procedures will I be given?

- Will I still be able to see my regular physician(s)?

- Will my doctor and the research team collaborate?

- Can I be put in touch with other patients who have participated in this trial?

To encourage more senior citizens to participate in cancer trials, Medicare plans to revise its payment policy to cover those trials.

If Your Physician Concurs that a Clinical Study Might be Appropriate for you, the NIH Recommends that the Following Steps be Taken:

- Contact NCI's Clinical Studies Support Center (CSSC), which is staffed by trained oncology (cancer) nurses who can identify appropriate clinical studies for you. Summaries of these trials and other pertinent information about the type of treatment being offered and the type of patients eligible for inclusion can be mailed or faxed to you and/or your physician.

- Review the clinical trials summaries and other information with your physician to decide which study or studies you should consider. Your physician also can contact the CSSC to communicate directly with the investigator in charge of the study.

- In cases in which you meet the initial eligibility requirements, it may be necessary for you to schedule a screening visit at the Clinical Center to learn more about the trial and possibly undergo some medical tests.

- If accepted for a clinical trial, make sure that you understand the details about the treatment and any possible risks and benefits.

Section II
Using this Guide to Find a Top Doctor

• 7 •

How to Use This Book

We assume most people who purchase this book have either received a diagnosis of cancer, or know someone who has. Although it would have been possible to arrange the listings by type of cancer, e.g. lung, breast, prostate, etc., that would not have been practical. For any particular type of cancer, a patient may be seeking one or more of a variety of different specialists. For example, any of the cancers mentioned could require, among other specialists, the involvement of pathologists, medical oncologists, surgeons, urologists, radiation oncologists and, possibly, psychiatrists.

Therefore, this guide and its list of physicians is organized first by specialty. Then, because many patients may prefer care as close to home as possible, we organized the lists by region. (See map on page 56)

The Special Expertise Index we include in the book, may also be of great help in locating the specialists a patient needs. We asked physicians making nominations to recommend individuals who were nationally recognized as leaders in the prevention, diagnosis and treatment of particular types of cancer, as well as leaders in various treatment modalities. When physicians selected for inclusion in *America's Top Doctors® for Cancer* completed and submitted their professional biographies, we also asked them to list their areas of special expertise. As a result, the Special Expertise Index lists hundreds of these areas.

The physicians are listed alphabetically within their specialties and then within their regions. A sample biography is presented and explained on the next page.

Smith, John MD [Ped] - **Spec Exp:** Asthma Allergy; **Hospital:** Children's Hosp (page 120);
Name [Specialty] Special Expertise(s) Admitting Hospital & Hospital Information Page

Address: 300 Ridge Road Boston, MA 12345, **Phone:** (617) 555-2343; **Board Cert:** Ped 75;
Office Address Office Phone Board Certification(s)

Med School: Harvard Med Sch 70; **Resid:** Ped, Children's Hosp 73;
Medical School Residency(ies)

Fellow: AM, Children's Hosp 74; **Fac Appt:** Assoc Prof Ped, The Med Sch
Fellowship(s) Faculty Appointment

Step-by-Step Directions for Finding the Specialist you Need

1. Look for a doctor first by specialty. Turn to the Special Cancer Expertise Index on p.573. Review the list which is organized alphabetically, and find the particular disease, organ, procedure or treatment of interest to you. Write down the page numbers of physicians with that expertise and turn to those pages.

2. Look in the area of the country closest to you. Each specialty lists doctors alphabetically within their geographical region. These regions start in New England (northeast) and go around the country in a consistent order to finish the West Coast and Pacific. Each state is grouped into one of these seven geographical regions. See map of the United States and the regions on page 56. If you don't find a doctor in that particular specialty in your first geographic preference, expand your search to other regions.

3. Check further in the Special Expertise Index. If you don't find a doctor to meet your needs, the last chapter contains those specialties which include a small number of doctors. The Special Cancer Expertise Index may include some diseases which are not related to cancer because a physician who treats cancer patients also may treat patients with these diseases.

Locating A Specialist

This guide is organized to make finding the right specialists for you or your loved ones as simple as possible. Physicians' biographies are presented by specialty and are organized by geographic region within each specialty or subspecialty. Thus, you may search for a particular type of specialist or subspecialist in one or more regions or throughout the nation.

A second way to locate the right specialist is to use the **Special Expertise Index** beginning on page 573. This index is organized according to diseases, conditions and procedures or techniques. If you already know a specialist's name, you can find his/her listing by using the **Alphabetical Listing of Doctors** beginning on page 605.

The information reported in each doctor's listing is, for the most part, provided by the doctor or his/her office staff. Castle Connolly attempts to verify the data through other sources but cannot guarantee that in all cases all data has been so verified or accurate. All such information is subject to change from time to time due to changes in physician practices.

Geographic Regions & States

To assist you in using *America's Top Doctors® for Cancer* in the most efficient and effective manner, the Guide is divided into seven geographic regions. This will help you to locate a specialist in your local or neighboring region. For example, if you live in Mississippi in the Southeast region and you are willing and able to travel to Louisiana in the Southwest region to consult with a specialist in medical oncology, you can review just those two regions, under the section headed "Medical Oncology." However, if you prefer to review the information on medical oncologists throughout the country, you can search the entire medical oncology section. Or, you can consult the **Special Expertise Index** in the back of this Guide and choose a medical oncologist who has specific expertise to meet your particular needs.

The geographic regions are as follows:

New England	Great Plains and Mountains
Mid Atlantic	Southwest
Southeast	West Coast and Pacific
Midwest	

The states that are included in each region are listed on the following page and a map of the regions is also provided. Please note that not all regions are represented in all specialties. For example, in "Interventional Radiology" there are no listings in the Southwest region.

Geographic Regions and States

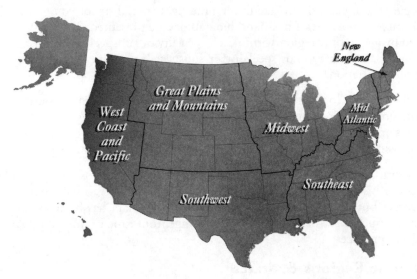

West Coast and Pacific:

Alaska
California
Hawaii
Nevada
Oregon
Washington

Great Plains and Mountains:

Colorado
Idaho
Kansas
Montana
Nebraska
North Dakota
South Dakota
Utah
Wyoming

Southwest:

Arizona
Arkansas
Louisiana
New Mexico
Oklahoma
Texas

Midwest:

Illinois
Indiana
Iowa
Michigan
Minnesota
Missouri
Ohio
Wisconsin

New England:

Connecticut
Maine
Massachusetts
New Hampshire
Rhode Island
Vermont

Mid Atlantic:

Delaware
Maryland
New Jersey
New York
Pennsylvania
Washington, DC
West Virginia

Southeast:

Alabama
Florida
Georgia
Kentucky
Mississippi
North Carolina
South Carolina
Tennessee
Virginia

• 8 •

Medical Specialties

In the pages that follow, each list of doctors in a medical specialty or subspecialty is preceded by a brief description of that specialty (or subspecialty) and the training required for board certification.

Critical Care Medicine has been excluded because in emergency situations there is neither time nor opportunity for choice. A number of other specialities not relevant to most patients (e.g., Forensic Psychiatry) have not been included as well.

The following descriptions of medical specialties and subspecialties were provided by the American Board of Medical Specialties (ABMS), an organization comprised of the 24 medical specialty boards that provide certification in 25 medical specialties. A complete listing of all specialists certified by the ABMS can be found in *The Official ABMS Directory of Board Certified Medical Specialists*, and is published by *Marquis Who's Who*. It is available (either in a multi-volume directory or on CD-ROM) in most public libraries, hospital libraries, university libraries and medical libraries. The ABMS also operates a toll-free phone line at 1-866-275-2267 and a website at www.abms.org to verify the certification status of individual doctors.

The following important policy statement, approved by the ABMS Assembly on March 19, 1987, remains valid.

The Purpose Of Certification

The intent of the certification process, as defined by the member boards of the American Board of Medical Specialties, is to provide assurance to the public that a certified medical specialist has successfully completed an approved educational program and an evaluation, including an examination process designed to assess the knowledge, experience and skills requisite to the provision of high quality patient care in that specialty.

Medical Specialty and Subspecialty Descriptions and Abbreviations

The following medical specialties and subspecialties are indicated in the doctors' listings by their abbreviations. Specialties are indicated in bold, subspecialties in italics, and the four primary care specialties in bold capitals. To review the official American Board of Medical Specialties (ABMS) organization of specialties, refer to Appendix A.

Addiction Psychiatry   *AdP*

Deals with habitual psychological and physiological dependence on a substance or practice which is beyond voluntary control.

Adolescent Medicine   *AM*

Involves the primary care treatment of adolescents and young adults.

Allergy & Immunology   **A&I**

Diagnosis and treatment of allergies, asthma, and skin problems such as hives and contact dermatitis.

Anesthesiology   **Anes**

Provides pain relief in maintenance or restoration of a stable condition during and following an operation. Anesthesiologists also diagnose and treat acute and long standing pain problems.

Cardiac Electrophysiology (Clinical)   *CE*

Involves complicated technical procedures to evaluate heart rhythms and determine appropriate treatment for them.

Cardiovascular Disease   *Cv*

Involves the diagnosis and treatment of disorders of the heart, lungs, and blood vessels.

Child & Adolescent Psychiatry   *ChAP*

Deals with the diagnosis and treatment of mental diseases in children and adolescents.

Child Neurology   *ChiN*

Diagnosis and medical treatment of disorders of the brain, spinal cord, and nervous system in children.

Clinical Genetics   **CG**

Deals with identifying the genetic causes of inherited diseases and ailments and preventing, when possible, their occurrence.

Colon and Rectal Surgery   **CRS**

Surgical treatment of diseases of the intestinal tract, colon and rectum, anal canal, and perianal area.

Critical Care Medicine   *CCM*

Involves diagnosing and taking immediate action to prevent death or further injury of a patient. Examples of critical injuries include shock, heart attack, drug overdose, and massive bleeding.

Dermatology   **D**

Diagnosis and treatment of benign and malignant disorders of the skin, mouth, external genitalia, hair and nails, as well as a number of sexually transmitted diseases.

Diagnostic Radiology   *DR*

Involves the study of all modalities of radiant energy in medical diagnoses and therapeutic procedures utilizing radiologic guidance.

Endocrinology, Diabetes & Metabolism   *EDM*

Involves the study and treatment of patients suffering from hormonal and chemical disorders.

FAMILY MEDICINE   **FP**

Deals with and oversees the total healthcare of individual patients and their family members. Family practitioners are more common in rural areas and may perform procedures more commonly performed by specialists (e.g., minor surgery).

Forensic Psychiatry   *FPsy*

Concerns the evaluation of certain diagnostic groups of patients that include those with sexual disorders, antisocial personality disorders, paranoid disorders, and addictive disorders.

Gastroenterology   *Ge*

The study, diagnosis and treatment of diseases of the digestive organs including the stomach, bowels, liver, and gallbladder.

Geriatric Medicine   *Ger*

Deals with diseases of the elderly and the problems associated with aging.

Geriatric Psychiatry   *GerPsy*

Involves the diagnosis, prevention, and treatment of mental illness in the elderly.

Gynecologic Oncology   *GO*

Deals with cancers of the female genital tract and reproductive systems.

Hand Surgery   *HS*

Involves the treatment of injury to the hand through surgical techniques.

Hematology   *Hem*

Involves the diagnosis and treatment of diseases and disorders of the blood, bone marrow, spleen, and lymph glands.

Infectious Disease   *Inf*

The study and treatment of diseases caused by a bacterium, virus, fungus, or animal parasite.

INTERNAL MEDICINE   **IM**

Diagnosis and nonsurgical treatment of diseases, especially those of adults. Internists may act as primary care specialists, highly trained family doctors, or they may subspecialize in specialties such as cardiology or nephrology.

Maternal & Fetal Medicine   *MF*

Involves the care of women with high-risk pregnancies and their unborn fetuses.

Medical Oncology   *Onc*

Refers to the study and treatment of tumors and other cancers.

Neonatal-Perinatal Medicine   *NP*

Involves the diagnosis and treatments of infants prior to, during, and one month beyond birth.

Nephrology   *Nep*

Concerned with disorders of the kidneys, high blood pressure, fluid and mineral balance, dialysis of body wastes when the kidneys do not function, and consultation with surgeons about kidney transplantation.

Neurological Surgery   **NS**

Involves surgery of the brain, spinal cord, and nervous system.

Neurology   **N**

Diagnosis and medical treatment of disorders of the brain, spinal cord, and nervous system.

Neuroradiology   *NRad*

Involves the utilization of imaging procedures during diagnosis as they relate to the brain, spine and spinal cord, head, neck, and organs of special sense in adults and children.

Nuclear Medicine   **NuM**

Evaluation of the functions of all the organs in the body and treatment of thyroid disease, benign and malignant tumors, and radiation exposure through the use of radioactive substances.

Nuclear Radiology   *NR*

Involves the use of radioactive substances to diagnose and treat certain functions and diseases of the body.

OBSTETRICS & GYNECOLOGY   **ObG**

Deals with the medical aspects of and intervention in pregnancy and labor and the overall health of the female reproductive system.

Occupational Medicine   *OM*

Concentrates on the effect of the work environment on the health of employees.

Ophthalmology   **Oph**

Diagnosis and treatment of diseases of and injuries to the eye.

Orthopaedic Surgery   **OrS**

Involves operations to correct injuries which interfere with the form and function of the extremities, spine, and associated structures.

Otolaryngology   **Oto**

Explores and treats diseases in the interrelated areas of the ears, nose and throat.

Otology/Neurotology   *ON*

Concentrates on the management, prevention, cure and care of patients with diseases of the ear and temporal bone, including disorders of hearing and balance.

Pain Medicine   *PM*

Involves providing a high level of care for patients experiencing problems with acute or chronic pain in both hospital and ambulatory settings.

Pediatric Cardiology   *PCd*

Involves the diagnosis and treatment of heart disease in children.

Pediatric Critical Care Medicine   *PCCM*

Involves the care of children who are victims of life threatening disorders such as severe accidents, shock, and diabetes acidosis.

Pediatric Dermatology   *PD*

Diagnosis and treatment of benign and malignant disorders of the skin, mouth, external genitalia, hair and nails in children.

Pediatric Endocrinology   *PEn*

Involves the study and treatment of children with hormonal and chemical disorders.

Pediatric Gastroenterology   *PGe*

The study, diagnosis, and treatment of diseases of the digestive tract in children.

Pediatric Hematology-Oncology   *PHO*

The study and treatment of cancers of the blood and blood-forming parts of the body in children.

Pediatric Infectious Disease   *PInf*

The study and treatment of diseases caused by a virus, bacterium, fungus, or animal parasite in children.

Pediatric Nephrology   *PNep*

Deals with the diagnosis and treatment of disorders of the kidneys in children.

Pediatric Otolaryngology   *POto*

Involves the diagnosis and treatment of disorders of the ear, nose, and throat which affect children.

Pediatric Pulmonology   *PPul*

Involves the diagnosis and treatment of diseases of the chest, lungs, and chest tissue in children.

Pediatric Radiology   *PR*

Involves diagnostic imaging as it pertains to the newborn, infant, child, and adolescent.

Pediatric Rheumatology   *PRhu*

Involves the treatment of diseases of the joints and connective tissues in children.

Pediatric Surgery   *PS*

Treatment of disease, injury, or deformity in children through surgical techniques.

PEDIATRICS   **Ped**

Diagnosis and treatment of diseases of childhood and monitoring of the growth, development, and well-being of preadolescents.

Physical Medicine & Rehabilitation   **PMR**

The use of physical therapy and physical agents such as water, heat, light electricity, and mechanical manipulations in the diagnosis, treatment, and prevention of disease and body disorders.

Plastic Surgery   **PlS**

Involves reconstructive and cosmetic surgery of the face and other body parts.

Preventive Medicine   **PrM**

A specialty focusing on the prevention of illness and on the health of groups rather than individuals.

Psychiatry   **Psyc**

Examination, treatment, and prevention of mental illness through the use of psychoanalysis and/or drugs.

Public Health & General Preventive Medicine   *PHGPM*

Involves the investigation of the causes of epidemic disease and the prevention of a wide variety of acute and chronic illness.

Pulmonary Disease   *Pul*

Involves the diagnosis and treatment of diseases of the chest, lungs, and airways.

Radiation Oncology   *RadRo*

Involves the use of radiant energy and isotopes in the study and treatment of disease, especially malignant cancer.

Reproductive Endocrinology   *RE*

Deals with the endocrine system (including the pituitary, thyroid, parathyroid, adrenal glands, placenta, ovaries, and testes) and how its failure relates to infertility.

Rheumatology   *Rhu*

Involves the treatment of diseases of the joints, muscles, bones and associated structures.

Sleep Medicine   *Sleep Med*

Involves the investigation and treatment of patients with sleep disorders.

Spinal Cord Injury Medicine   *SpCdInj*

Involves the prevention, diagnosis, treatment and management of traumatic spinal cord injuries.

Sports Medicine   *SM*

Refers to the practice of an orthopaedist or other physician who specializes in injuries to the bone or other soft tissues (muscles, tendons, ligaments) caused by participation in Athletic activity.

Surgery   **S**

Treatment of disease, injury, and deformity by surgical procedures.

Surgery of the Hand   *SHd*

Involves providing appropriate care for all structures in the upper extremity directly affecting the hand and wrist function.

Surgical Critical Care   *SCC*

Involves specialized care in the management of the critically ill patient, particularly the trauma victim and postoperative patient in the emergency department, intensive care unit, trauma unit, burn unit, and other similar settings.

Thoracic Surgery (includes open heart surgery)   **TS**

Involves surgery on the heart, lungs, and chest area.

Urology   **U**

Diagnosis and treatment of diseases of the genitals in men and disorders of the urinary tract and bladder in both men and women.

Vascular & Interventional Radiology   *VIR*

Involves diagnosing and treating diseases by percutaneous methods guided by various radiologic imaging modalities.

Vascular Surgery   *VascS*

Involves the operative treatment of disorders of the blood vessels excluding those to the heart, lungs, or brain.

The Training of a Specialist

Excerpted from *Which Medical Specialist For You?* American Board of Medical Specialties, Evanston, IL, Revised 2000

Everyone knows that a "medical doctor" is a physician who has had years of training to understand the diagnosis, treatment and prevention of disease. The basic training for a physician specialist includes four years of premedical education in a college or university, four years of medical school, and after receiving the M.D. degree, at least three years of specialty training under supervision (called a "residency"). Training in subspecialties can take an additional one to three years.

Some specialists are primary care doctors such as family physicians, general internists and general pediatricians. Other specialists concentrate on certain body systems, specific age groups, or complex scientific techniques developed to diagnose or treat certain types of disorders. Specialties in medicine developed because of the rapidly expanding body of knowledge about health and illness and the constantly evolving new treatment techniques for disease.

A subspecialist is a physician who has completed training in a general medical specialty and then takes additional training in a more specific area of that specialty called a subspecialty. This training increases the depth of knowledge and expertise of the specialist in that particular field. For example, cardiology is a subspecialty of internal medicine and pediatrics, pediatric surgery is a subspecialty of surgery and child and adolescent psychiatry is a subspecialty of psychiatry. The training of a subspecialist within a specialty requires an additional one or more years of full-time education.

The training, or residency, of a specialist begins after the doctor has received the M.D. degree from a medical school. Resident physicians dedicate themselves for three to seven years to full-time experience in hospital and/or ambulatory care settings, caring for patients under the supervision of experienced specialists. Educational conferences and research experience are often part of that training. In years past, the first year of post-medical school training was called an internship, but is now called residency.

Licensure

The legal privilege to practice medicine is governed by state law and is not designed to recognize the knowledge and skills of a trained specialist. A physician is licensed to practice general medicine and surgery by a state board of medical examiners after passing a state or national licensure examination. Each state or territory has its own procedures to license physicians and sets the general standards for all physicians in that state or territory.

Who Credentials a Specialist and/or Subspecialist?

Specialty boards certify physicians as having met certain published standards. There are 24 specialty boards that are recognized by the American Board of Medical Specialties (ABMS) and the American Medical Association (AMA). All of the specialties and subspecialties recognized by the ABMS and the AMA are listed in the brief descriptions that follow. Remember, a subspecialist first must be trained and certified as a specialist.

In order to be certified as a medical specialist by one of these recognized boards a physician must complete certain requirements. See box on the next page.

All of the ABMS Member Boards now, or will soon, issue only time-limited certificates which are valid for six to ten years. In order to retain certification, diplomates must become "recertified," and must periodically go through an additional process involving continuing education in the specialty, review of credentials and further examination. Boards that may not yet require recertification have provided voluntary recertification with similar requirements.

How to Determine If a Physician is a Certified Specialist

Certified specialists are listed in *The Official ABMS Directory of Board Certified Medical Specialists* published by *Marquis Who's Who*. The ABMS Directory can be found in most public libraries, hospital libraries, university libraries and medical libraries, and is also available on CD-ROM. Alternatively, you could ask for that information from your county medical society, the American Board of Medical Specialties, or one of the specialty boards.

The ABMS operates a toll free number (1-866-275-2267) to verify the certification status of individual physicians. Additionally, information about the ABMS organization and links to an electronic directory of certified specialists can be accessed through the ABMS Web site at www.abms.org.

Almost all board certified specialists also are members of their medical specialty societies. These societies are dedicated to furthering standards, practice and professional and public education within individual medical specialties. Some, such as the American College of Surgeons and the American College of Obstetricians and Gynecologists, require board certification for full membership. A physician who has attained full membership is called a "Fellow" of the society and is entitled to use this designation in all formal communications such as certificates, publications, business cards, stationery and signage. Thus, "John Doe, M.D., F.A.C.S. (Fellow of the American College of Surgeons) is a board certified surgeon. Similarly, F.A.A.D. (Fellow of the American Academy of Dermatology) following the M.D. or D.O. in a physician's title would likely indicate board certification in that specialty.

To be Certified as a Medical Specialist by a Recognized Board, a Physician Must Complete Certain Requirements, these Include:

1. Completion of a course of study leading to the M.D. or D.O. (Doctor of Osteopathy) degree from a recognized school of medicine.

2. Completion of three to seven years of full-time training in an accredited residency program designed to train specialists in the field.

3. Many specialty boards require assessments and documentation of individual performance from the residency training director, or from the chief of service in the hospital where the specialist has practiced.

4. All of the ABMS Member Boards require that a person seeking certification have an unrestricted license to practice medicine in order to take the certification examination.

5. Finally, each candidate for certification must pass a written examination given by the specialty board. Fifteen of the 24 specialty boards also require an oral examination conducted by senior specialists in that field. Candidates who have passed the exams and other requirements are then given the status of "Diplomate" and are certified as specialists.

• 9 •

The Partnership for Excellence Program

Among the more than 6,000 acute care and specialty hospitals in the United States, many have extraordinary capabilities for superior patient care. These hospitals, renowned for their use of state-of-the-art equipment and up-to-the-minute technology, also attract outstanding physicians and other healthcare professionals. Many of their physicians are among those in the listings in this guide.

To assist you in your search for top specialists and to supplement the information contained in the physician listings that follow, we invited a select group of these fine institutions to profile their services, special programs and centers of excellence in the *Partnership for Excellence* program. This special section contains pages sponsored by the included hospitals. This paid sponsorship program is totally separate from the physician selection process, which is based upon a completely independent review.

The *Partnership for Excellence* program provides an overview of the programs and services offered by the included hospitals with information related to their accreditation and sponsorship. Most also provide their physician referral numbers, should you wish to ask the hospitals for recommendations of doctors not listed in *America's Top Doctors® for Cancer*.

In addition to the *Partnership for Excellence* program, profiled hospitals were also invited to highlight their special programs or services that focus on a particular disease or medical condition. These can be found in the "Centers of Excellence" sections that are interspersed throughout this book following the medical specialties and/or subspecialties to which they relate. Sponsored pages in the centers of excellence sections reflect the depth of commitment of these hospitals, which provide the staff, resources and financial support necessary to develop these special programs.

By visiting our website **www.castleconnolly.com**, you may also link to the websites of these outstanding hospitals for even more detailed information on their cancer programs.

Participating Hospitals

- **City of Hope Cancer Center**

- **Clarian Health Systems**

- **Cleveland Clinic**

- **Continuum Health Partners**

- **Fox Chase Cancer Center**

- **Hackensack University Medical Center**

- **Maimonides Medical Center**

- **Memorial Sloan-Kettering Cancer Center**

- **Mount Sinai Medical Center**

- **New York Eye & Ear Infirmary**

- **NewYork-Presbyterian Hospital**

- **NYU Medical Center**

- **The University of Texas M.D. Anderson Cancer Center**

- **Thomas Jefferson University Hospital**

- **UCLA Medical Center**

- **University of Pennsylvania Health System**

- **Wake Forest University Baptist Medical Center**

cancer.

At City of Hope Cancer Center, our science is providing answers to cancer. By pioneering minimally invasive treatments, such as robotic-assisted surgery, we're saving patients' lives while preserving their quality of life. As a world leader in cancer research, we are discovering new and promising protocols including the use of adult stem cells, immunotherapy and targeted therapies. And as one of the few U.S. hospitals to offer the unprecedented accuracy of TomoTherapy radiation treatment, we're attaining more positive outcomes for our patients. If you've been diagnosed with any form of cancer, look to the experts. Call City of Hope at 800-826-HOPE or ask your doctor for a referral. Most insurance accepted. At City of Hope, we have answers to cancer.

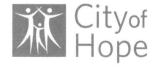

City of
Hope

Science saving lives.
cityofhope.org/topdoctors

Cleveland Clinic

One of the largest and busiest health centers in America. Number one in heart care. National leaders in urology and digestive diseases. Treating all illnesses and disorders of the body. Second opinions a specialty.

General Overview

Founded in 1921, Cleveland Clinic is a 1000-staffed-bed hospital that integrates clinical and hospital care with research and education in a private, non-profit group practice. This group practice model provides an environment that allows our physicians to stay at the cutting edge of medical technology. They pool their expertise and their wisdom for the benefit of the patient and the community.

Vital Statistics

In 2006, more than 1,700 full-time physicians and scientists representing 120 medical specialties and subspecialties provided for 3.3 million outpatient visits, 54,000 hospital admissions and 108,000 surgeries for patients from throughout the United States and more than 80 countries.

One of America's Best

In 2006, Cleveland Clinic was ranked one of the top 3 hospitals in America in the *U.S.News & World Report* annual "America's Best Hospitals" survey. In cardiology and cardiac surgery, we lead the nation. Our Heart Center has been ranked number one in America for twelve years in a row. Cleveland Clinic's Glickman Urological Institute and Digestive Disease Center are ranked second in the nation. Additional specialties rated among America's best include Cancer, Endocrinology, Geriatrics, Gynecology, Nephrology, Neurology and Neurological Surgery, Ophthalmology, Orthopaedics, Otolaryngology, Pediatrics, Psychiatry, Pulmonary, Rehabilitation and Rheumatology.

Global Patient Services

Global Patient Services is a full-service department dedicated to meeting the needs and requirements of both our out-of-state and international patients. The National Center and the International Center, which make up Global Patient Services, provide personalized concierge programs and services to welcome patients and add to their comfort before, during and after their stay.

To schedule an appointment or for more information about Cleveland Clinic, call 800.890.2467 or visit clevelandclinic.org.

Cleveland Clinic | 9500 Euclid Ave. / W14 | Cleveland OH 44195

Mission

"Better care of the sick, investigation of their problems and further education of those who serve."

"Patients first"

"Patients First" is the guiding principle of Cleveland Clinic. It declares the primacy of patient care, patient comfort and patient communication in every activity we undertake. It affirms the importance of research and education for their contributions to clinical medicine and the improvement of patient care. At the same time, "Patients First" demands a relentless focus on measurable quality. By setting standards, collecting data and analyzing the results, Cleveland Clinic puts patients first through improved outcomes and better service, providing a healthier future for all.

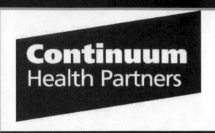

Continuum Health Partners

Phone (800) 420-4004
www.chpnyc.org

Sponsorship: Voluntary Not-for-Profit
Beds: 2,761 certified beds
Accreditation: Joint Commission of Accreditation of Healthcare Organizations (JCAHO). Accreditation
Council for Graduate Medical Education, Medical Society of New York, in conjunction with the
Accreditation Council for Continuing Medical Education

A STRONG PARTNERSHIP WITH A PROUD HERITAGE

Continuum Health Partners, Inc. is a partnership of five venerable health care providers, Beth Israel Medical Center, St. Luke's Hospital, Roosevelt Hospital, Long Island College Hospital, and the New York Eye and Ear Infirmary. Each of the five partner institutions was established more than a century ago by individuals committed to improving health and health care in their communities. Today, the system represents more than 4,000 physicians and dentists and is superbly equipped to respond to the health care needs of the populations we serve. Continuum providers also see patients in group and private practice settings and in ambulatory centers in New York City and Westchester County.

LOCATIONS

Continuum Health Partners has campuses throughout Manhattan and Brooklyn. Beth Israel Medical Center has two divisions: the Milton and Caroll Petrie Division on the East Side, and the Kings Highway Division in Brooklyn. The Phillips Ambulatory Care Center, a state-of-the art outpatient center, is located at Union Square. St. Luke's Hospital is in Morningside Heights and Roosevelt Hospital is in the Columbus Circle and Lincoln Center neighborhoods on the West Side. Long Island College Hospital is located in the Brooklyn Heights/Cobble Hill section of Brooklyn. The New York Eye and Ear Infirmary is located on Second Avenue and 14th Street.

ACADEMIC AFFILIATIONS

Beth Israel Medical Center is the University Hospital and Manhattan Campus for the Albert Einstein College of Medicine. St. Luke's-Roosevelt Hospital Center is the University Hospital for Columbia University College of Physicians and Surgeons. Long Island College Hospital is the primary teaching affiliate of the SUNY-Health Science Center in Brooklyn. The New York Eye and Ear Infirmary is the primary teaching center of the New York Medical College and affiliated teaching hospitals in the areas of ophthalmology and otolaryngology.

Physician Referral For a referral to a doctor in your neighborhood, call (800) 420-4004. Continuum's Referral Service can help you find a primary care physician or specialist affiliated with Beth Israel, St. Luke's, Roosevelt, Long Island College Hospital, or the New York Eye and Ear Infirmary. **Visit our Website at www.chpnyc.org**

FOX CHASE
CANCER CENTER

333 Cottman Avenue
Philadelphia, PA 19111-2497
Phone: 1-888-FOX CHASE • Fax: 215-728-2702
www.fccc.edu

Sponsorship	Independent Nonprofit
Beds	100 licensed beds
Accreditation	The Joint Commission; American Hospital Association; American College of Surgeons Commission on Cancer; College of American Pathology; American College of Radiology

U.S. News & World Report has named Fox Chase Cancer Center the leading cancer center serving eastern Pennsylvania, New Jersey and Delaware and 16th in the entire nation. Fox Chase is also the first hospital in Pennsylvania and the nation's first cancer hospital to earn the Magnet Award for Nursing Excellence from the American Nurses Credentialing Center.

Overview

Fox Chase Cancer Center was founded in 1904 in Philadelphia as the nation's first cancer hospital. In 1974, Fox Chase became one of the first institutions designated as a National Cancer Institute Comprehensive Cancer Center. The mission of Fox Chase is to reduce the burden of human cancer through the highest-quality programs in basic, clinical, population and translational research; programs of prevention, detection and treatment of cancer; and community outreach.

- Fox Chase's 100-bed hospital is one of the few in the country devoted entirely to adult cancer care.
- Annual hospital admissions exceed 4,000 and outpatient visits to physicians total more than 68,700 a year.
- Fox Chase's board-certified specialists are recognized nationally and internationally in medical, radiation and surgical oncology, diagnostic imaging, diagnostic pathology, pain management, oncology nursing and oncology social work.
- The multidisciplinary staff provides a coordinated approach to meet the treatment needs of each patient. Special multidisciplinary centers provide consultations and treatment recommendations for specific types of cancer.
- The nursing staff of specially trained oncology nurses provides one of the best nurse-to-patient ratios in the area.
- Fox Chase investigators have received numerous awards and honors, including Nobel Prizes in medicine and chemistry; a Kyoto Prize, a Lasker Clinical Research Award, memberships in the National Academy of Sciences and General Motors Cancer Research Foundation Prizes.
- Fox Chase is a founding member of the National Comprehensive Cancer Network, an alliance of the nation's leading academic cancer centers, and the hub of Fox Chase Cancer Center Partners, which includes nearly 30 community cancer centers.

**For more about Fox Chase physicians and services,
visit our web site, www.fccc.edu, or call 1-888-FOX CHASE.**

HACKENSACK UNIVERSITY MEDICAL CENTER

30 Prospect Avenue
Hackensack, New Jersey 07601
phone 201-996-3760
fax 201-996-3452

www.humc.com

Sponsorship	A not-for-profit, teaching and research hospital affiliated with the University of Medicine and Dentistry of New Jersey – New Jersey Medical School.
Beds	A 781-bed, Level II Trauma Center, providing tertiary and regional services for the New York/New Jersey metropolitan area.
Accreditation	Joint Commission on the Accreditation of Healthcare Organizations.

BACKGROUND

Founded in 1888 as Bergen County's first hospital, Hackensack University Medical Center (HUMC) has demonstrated more than a century of growth and progress in response to the needs of the communities it serves. The medical center continues to be the largest provider of inpatient and outpatient services in New Jersey and has been ranked as the fourth largest healthcare facility in the nation by number of inpatient admissions. Hackensack University Medical Center is Bergen County's largest employer with a work force of more than 7,200 employees and an annual budget of more than $1 billion.

MEDICAL AND DENTAL STAFF

There are nearly 1,400 members on the medical and dental staff. These physicians and dentists represent a full spectrum of medical and dental specialties and subspecialties.

One of America's 50 Best Hospitals – Hackensack University Medical Center has been recognized as one of America's 50 Best Hospitals by HealthGrades, the nation's leading independent healthcare ratings company. The designation recognizes hospitals that have demonstrated superior clinical quality over a seven-year time period, based upon an analysis of more than 75 million Medicare patient records from 1999-2005. These hospitals have achieved better survival rates and lower complication rates across dozens of medical procedures and diagnoses, from cardiac care to orthopedic surgery, consistently ranking among the top five percent in the nation for overall clinical outcomes. Hackensack University Medical Center is the only healthcare facility in New Jersey, New York, and New England to be named one of America's 50 Best Hospitals.

J.D. Power and Associates Distinguished Hospital Program[SM] **Inpatient, Outpatient, and Emergency Care** – Hackensack University Medical Center was recognized for service excellence by J.D. Power and Associates. The rating was based on five key indicators of patients' satisfaction with their overall hospital experience: dignity and respect; speed and efficiency; comfort; information and communication; and emotional support.

Nursing Excellence – Honored since 1995 as the first hospital in New Jersey to receive the Magnet Award for Nursing Excellence from the American Nurses Credentialing Center. The medical center became the second hospital in the country to receive redesignation of this prestigious award and continues to have this highly honored recognition. HUMC was redesignated again in 2003.

ACCOMPLISHMENTS

The nation's top performer for two years in a row in groundbreaking CMS/Premier pay-for-performance project – Patients treated at hospitals participating in a groundbreaking pay-for-performance project managed by the Premier Inc. healthcare alliance are living longer and receiving recommended treatments more frequently, according to second-year results announced by the Centers for Medicare & Medicaid Services (CMS). For the second year in a row, Hackensack University Medical Center was the top performer in the nation. The medical center's total award across the five clinical areas will be approximately $744,000.

Leapfrog Top Hospitals List – Hackensack University Medical Center is one of 59 U.S. hospitals named to the first Leapfrog Top Hospitals list, based on the most recent results from the Leapfrog Hospital Quality and Safety Survey, a national rating system that offers a broad assessment of a hospital's quality and safety.

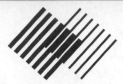

MAIMONIDES MEDICAL CENTER
4802 Tenth Avenue
Brooklyn, New York 11219
Phone: (718) 283-6000
Physician Referral: 1-888 MMC DOCS
http://www.maimonidesmed.org

Sponsorship:	Voluntary, Not-for-Profit
Beds:	705 acute, 70 psychiatric
Accreditation:	Joint Commission on Accreditation of Healthcare Organizations (JCAHO)
	American College of Surgeons
	American Council of Graduate Medical Education (ACGME)

The nation's third largest independent teaching hospital, Maimonides Medical Center is a conductor of clinical trials for new treatments and therapies. Cited for overall clinical excellence by numerous health-care report cards and evaluation services, Maimonides is a celebrated leader in the use of information technology to enhance patient care.

Significant Accomplishments

Maimonides is one of a select few hospitals in the US to meet the criteria for excellence in healthcare established by the Leapfrog Group, a coalition of some of the nation's largest employers.

Excellence in cardiac care is historic: the first successful human heart transplant in the US was performed at Maimonides in 1967, and our current interventional cardiology program provides the best patient outcomes in the state of New York.

Physicians at Maimonides are among the eight percent nationwide who use computers to enter patient orders, thereby reducing the risk of errors, increasing efficiency, and speeding the healing process.

More babies were born at Maimonides in 2006 than at any other facility in the state of New York – due in no small part to its designation as a Regional Perinatal Center with Obstetric and Pediatric services that are unrivaled in this area.

Centers of Excellence

Cancer Center
Provides comprehensive cancer services in a state-of-the-art facility. The Cancer Center at Maimonides utilizes the most advanced imaging technology and radiologic treatments for cancer patients.

Cardiac Institute
Renowned for its Catheterization Lab and pioneering new surgical procedures. The Institute includes an electrophysiology (EP) lab, two ICUs, Chest Pain Observation Unit, Advanced Cardiac Care Unit, and Congestive Heart Failure Program.

Stroke Center
One of only 40 Centers in the nation that provide interventional neuroradiology techniques to remove stroke-causing blood clots from the brain – without surgery – significantly reducing the debilitating effects of stroke.

Infants and Children's Hospital
Accredited by the National Association of Children's Hospitals and Related Institutions (NACHRI), Maimonides Infants and Children's Hospital includes Pediatric ICU, Neonatal ICU, Outpatient Pavilion, and Pediatric ER.

Vascular Institute
The world's top technology and advances in testing, surgery and medical care are offered at The Vascular Institute, which includes a Diagnostic Lab, Wound Center, Vascular Surgery Center and Vein Center.

Stella & Joseph Payson Birthing Center
Delivering the most babies in New York State, the Payson Birthing Center offers patients a home-like setting with doulas and midwives, combined with advanced technology, including a perinatal testing center with 3-D ultrasound.

Geriatrics Program
Serving one of the oldest populations in New York City, the Maimonides Geriatrics Program includes outstanding inpatient and outpatient services, an ACE Unit (Acute Care for Elders) and home-visiting service.

Passionate about medicine. Compassionate about people.

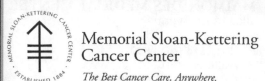

Memorial Sloan-Kettering Cancer Center

The Best Cancer Care. Anywhere.

1275 York Avenue
New York, NY 10021
Phone: (212) 639-2000
Physician Referral: (800) 525-2225
www.mskcc.org

Beds: 432
Sponsorship/Network Affiliation: Private, Non-Profit

THE MSKCC ADVANTAGE: CANCER IS OUR ONLY FOCUS

At Memorial Sloan-Kettering Cancer Center, our sole focus is cancer, and it has been for more than a century. Our doctors have unparalleled expertise in diagnosing and treating all types of cancer, using the latest technology and the most innovative, advanced therapies to increase the chances of a cure. Our designation as a National Cancer Institute (NCI) Comprehensive Cancer Center conveys our position as one of the nation's premier cancer centers.

A MULTIDISCIPLINARY, TEAM APPROACH TO CANCER CARE

Our Disease Management Program features multidisciplinary teams, defined by cancer type (lung, breast, etc.), whose members work together to guide each patient through diagnosis, treatment and recovery. These teams have a depth and breadth of experience that is unsurpassed. Using this approach, treatment plans reflect the combined expertise of many doctors—surgeons, medical oncologists, radiologists, radiation oncologists and pathologists. This approach also ensures that patients who need several different therapies to treat their cancer will receive the best combination for them.

GREATER PRECISION IN DIAGNOSIS

At Memorial Sloan-Kettering, highly sophisticated imaging techniques are used to accurately diagnose and stage cancers. In addition to MRI and CT, we offer the most advanced imaging technologies, such as combination PET/CT imaging, which can more accurately detect cancer and pinpoint its exact location in the body. Our highly specialized pathologists analyze tumor samples to determine a precise diagnosis. They are increasingly able to identify the molecular differences among tumors, providing even greater precision in diagnosis, which means physicians are able to determine the optimal therapy that is available to treat each individual's cancer.

UNPARALLELED SURGICAL EXPERTISE

Recent studies have shown that, for many cancers, patients who have their operations at a hospital that performs large numbers of the procedures are more likely to survive and have fewer complications. Because of their sole focus on cancer, our surgeons are among the most experienced cancer surgeons in the world. Over the years, they have pioneered scores of surgical innovations, including the use of minimally invasive techniques for many cancers. Using several small incisions instead of one large one, this approach results in less post-surgical pain and faster recovery. Our surgeons are also at the forefront of developing surgical procedures to spare organs and preserve function.

LEADERS IN RADIATION THERAPY

Memorial Sloan-Kettering's radiation oncologists pioneered intensity-modulated radiation therapy, a system for delivering radiation that permits unparalleled precision in the shaping and targeting of radiotherapy beams. This allows higher, more effective doses of radiation to be delivered to tumors while minimizing the exposure of surrounding healthy tissues and organs. Our doctors have also developed the use of radiation therapy combined with chemotherapy, which makes tumor cells more sensitive to the effects of radiation, thereby enhancing the success of the treatment.

Physician Referral (800) 525-2225

Access to Tomorrow's Cancer Treatments Today

A ccess to clinical breakthroughs, innovative techniques, leading-edge technologies, the safest and most effective treatment options, and a wide-range of diagnostic, therapeutic, and support services for all types of cancer, including the following specialties:

Head and Neck

Thoracic
(including lung, esophagus)

Gynecologic Oncology

Hematological Malignancies
(including bone marrow transplantation)

Brain Tumors

Radiation Oncology

Prostate/Bladder/Kidney

Medical Oncology

When you're battling cancer, fight smart.

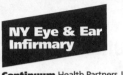

THE NEW YORK EYE AND EAR INFIRMARY

310 East 14th Street
New York, New York 10003
Tel. 212.979.4000   Fax. 212.228.0664
www.nyee.edu

Continuum Health Partners, Inc.

BEDS:	69; Operating Rooms: 17; Surgical Cases: 20,000+ a year
Sponsorship:	Voluntary Not-for-Profit
Accreditation:	Joint Commission on the Accreditation of Healthcare Organizations
	College of American Pathologists

GENERAL OVERVIEW

The New York Eye and Ear Infirmary is one of the world's leading facilities for the diagnosis and treatment of diseases of the eyes, ears, nose, throat and related conditions. Founded in 1820, it is the oldest continuously operating specialty hospital in the nation, as well as one of the busiest.

ACADEMIC AND CLINICAL AFFILIATIONS

A voluntary, not-for-profit institution, the Infirmary is a member of Continuum Health Partners, Inc. and an affiliated teaching hospital of New York Medical College. There are highly regarded residency programs in ophthalmology and otolaryngology, plus some two dozen post-graduate fellowship positions.

THE MEDICAL STAFF

The Medical Staff includes more than 500 board-certified attending physicians and surgeons throughout the metropolitan area. Many are renowned for their breakthrough research introducing widely practiced techniques.

SPECIALTIES

Ophthalmology: Within this area are subspecialties of cataract, glaucoma, retina, cornea and refractive surgery, ocular plastic surgery, pediatric ophthalmology and strabismus, neuro-ophthalmology and ocular tumor. Laser, photography, fluorescein angiography and electrophysiological testing are among the most advanced services available anywhere.

Otolaryngology: The department is in the forefront of treatment modalities using highly sophisticated endoscopic and laser equipment. Subspecialties include rhinology, laryngology, head & neck surgery, otology/neurotology, pediatric otolaryngology, audiology, speech therapy and hearing aid dispensing.

Plastic & Reconstructive Surgery: Microsurgical capabilities and premium patient accommodations provide an optimum environment for facial plasty, liposuction and repair of defects from disease or trauma.

RELATED SERVICES

New York Eye Trauma Center: An advanced program for emergency treatment of eye injuries, it also is the Eye Injury Registry of New York State and leading collector of data which will help develop preventative strategies.

Ambulatory Surgery: A comprehensive Ambulatory Surgery Center is designed to expedite admission testing, pre-op preparation and post-op recovery in an efficient and comfortable setting.

Pediatric Specialty Care: Services of eye and ear, nose and throat specialists are coordinated with other professional and support staff especially sensitive to the youngest patients.

RESEARCH AND EDUCATION

The New York Eye and Ear Infirmary is a national and international leader in research in its specialties, achieving many "firsts" in successful surgical procedures and medical treatments. Laboratories include Cell Culture, Ocular Imaging, and Microsurgical Education. Over a hundred studies and clinical trials are currently being conducted.

Physician Referral: Call 1.800.449.HOPE (4673)

NewYork-Presbyterian
The University Hospital of Columbia and Cornell

Affiliated with Columbia University College of Physicians and Surgeons and Weill Medical College of Cornell University

NewYork-Presbyterian Hospital
Weill Cornell Medical Center
525 East 68th Street
New York, NY 10021

NewYork-Presbyterian Hospital
Columbia University Medical Center
622 West 168th Street
New York, NY 10032

Sponsorship: Voluntary Not-for-Profit
Beds: 2,369
Accreditation: Joint Commission on Accreditation of Healthcare Organizations (JCAHO), Commission on Accreditation of Rehabilitation Facilities (CARF) and College of American Pathologists (CAP)

The *U.S. News & World Report* has ranked NewYork-Presbyterian Hospital higher in more specialties than any other hospital in the New York area. NewYork-Presbyterian Hospital was named to the *Honor Roll of America's Best Hospitals.*

OVERVIEW:

NewYork-Presbyterian Hospital is the largest hospital in New York and one of the most comprehensive healthcare institutions in the world with 5,500 physicians, approximately 96,000 discharges and nearly 1 million outpatient visits annually, and with its affiliated medical schools, more than $330 million in research support.

AMONG ITS RENOWNED CENTERS OF EXCELLENCE ARE:

Morgan Stanley Children's Hospital and the Komansky Center for Children's Health – One of the largest, most comprehensive children's hospitals in the world providing highly sophisticated pediatric medical, surgical and intensive care, including a pediatric cardiovascular center, in a compassionate environment.

NewYork-Presbyterian Cancer Centers – Coordinated, multidisciplinary care and the latest therapeutic options and clinical trials available for all types of cancer.

NewYork-Presbyterian Heart – Expert diagnostic capabilities and medical and surgical innovations for simple to complex heart conditions.

NewYork-Presbyterian Neuroscience Centers – Latest research, diagnosis and treatment capabilities in Alzheimer's disease, Multiple Sclerosis, Parkinson's disease, aneurysms, epilepsy, brain tumors, stokes and other neurological disorders.

NewYork-Presbyterian Psychiatry – World-renowned center of excellence in psychiatric treatment, research and education.

NewYork-Presbyterian Transplant Institute – Adult and pediatric heart, liver, and kidney and adult pancreas and lung transplantation and cutting-edge research.

NewYork-Presbyterian Vascular Care Center – Comprehensive and integrated preventive, diagnostic and treatment program for diverse problems related to arteries and veins throughout the body.

NewYork-Presbyterian Digestive Disease Services – Expert capabilities in the broad range of conditions that affect the organs as well as other components of the digestive system.

William Randolph Hearst Burn Center – Largest and busiest burn center in the nation which also conducts research to improve survival and enhance quality of life for burn victims.

In addition, the Hospital offers extraordinary expertise, comprehensive programs and specialized resources in the fields of AIDS, Complementary Medicine, Gene Therapy, Reproductive Medicine and Infertility, Trauma Center and Women's Health Care.

ACADEMIC AFFILIATIONS:

NewYork-Presbyterian is the only hospital in the world affiliated with two Ivy League medical schools; The Joan and Sanford I Weill Medical College of Cornell University and the Columbia University College of Physicians and Surgeons.

Physician Referral: To find a NewYork-Presbyterian Hospital affiliated physician to meet your needs, call toll free 1-877-NYP-WELL (1-877-697-9355) or visit our website at www.nyp.org

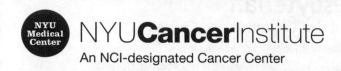

NYU**Cancer**Institute
An NCI-designated Cancer Center

NYU Clinical Cancer Center
160 East 34th Street
New York, New York 10016
www.nyuci.org/atcd

NYU Medical Center
550 First Avenue
(at 31st Street)
New York, New York 10016
www.nyumc.org/atcd

Stephen D. Hassenfeld
Children's Center
for Cancer and Blood
Disorders
160 East 32nd Street
New York, New York 10016
www.nyumc.org/hassenfeld

A Collaborative Approach
The NYU Cancer Institute, an NCI designated center, is a "matrix cancer center" without walls operating within the larger NYU Medical Center. With over 200 members and a research funding base of over $81 million, this structure strengthens our capabilities to forge collaborations across medical and scientific disciplines, which translates to comprehensive care for our patients and discoveries that will influence the future of this disease.

Renowned Expertise
Our highly skilled Magnet™ nursing team not only plays a pivotal role in coordinating direct patient care, but is also a source of invaluable patient education. Team members' compassion and expertise help patients better manage the symptoms of their disease as well as their special needs.

A Patient-Focused Setting
The NYU Clinical Cancer Center, with over 70 faculty members from various disciplines at the New York University School of Medicine, is the principal outpatient facility of the Cancer Institute and serves as home for our patients and their caregivers. The center and its multidisciplinary team of experts provide access to the latest treatment options and clinical trials along with a variety of programs in cancer prevention, screening, diagnostics, genetic counseling, and supportive services. When it comes to kids and cancer, the Stephen D. Hassenfeld Children's Center for Cancer and Blood Disorders offers not just innovation but insight. As a leading member of the NCI-sponsored Children's Oncology Group, our physicians are known for developing new ways to treat childhood cancer. Our affiliation with Bellevue Hospital, the oldest public hospital in the country, affords clinically distinctive opportunities to learn and care for patients with cancer by observing its presentation and behavior in a variety of patient groups.

OUR MISSION

Since 1941, M. D. Anderson Cancer Center has had a single goal – to eliminate cancer. Achieving that goal begins with integrated programs in cancer treatment, clinical trials, education programs and cancer prevention.

More than 60 years of cancer treatment has resulted in unmatched experience in the diagnosis and treatment of all cancer types, as well as expertise in emerging technologies such as proton therapy and robotic surgery. With over 1,600 faculty members, physicians specialize in specific types of cancer while benefiting from collaboration with colleagues in surgery, oncology, pediatrics, and radiation therapy to design individualized treatment plans for every patient.

PATIENT CARE

At M. D. Anderson, we hold ourselves to quality standards higher than the industry requires, and provide a rare breadth of technology, experience, and expertise, all which translate into personalized care and the best outcomes possible.

Our doctors work in teams that include surgeons, medical oncologists, radiation oncologists, and nurses who have expertise in a specific types of cancer. These specialized teams use their experience to create a plan that is individualized for each patient. Therefore, every patient receives the benefit of M. D. Anderson's wide range of cancer expertise combined with personalized care.

CLINICAL RESEARCH

As a federally designated comprehensive cancer center, M. D. Anderson is required to have a strong research program. Many cancer treatments now considered standard had their beginnings at M. D. Anderson, from groundbreaking radiation therapies in the 1950s to designer drugs that target cancer cells today. Patients benefit from M. D. Anderson research through participation in dozens of clinical trials to apply new therapies that may well become tomorrow's standard treatments.

MORE INFORMATION For more information or to make an appointment, call 877-MDA-6789, or visit us online at http://www.mdanderson.org.

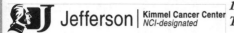

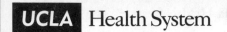

UCLA Medical Center

10883 Le Conte Avenue • Los Angeles, CA 90024
1-800-UCLA-MD1 (1-800-825-2631)
www.uclahealth.org

Beds: 668
Affiliation: UCLA Medical Center, a non-profit hospital, is part of UCLA Health System.
Accreditation: Joint Commission of Healthcare Organizations; American Nurses Credentialing Center-Magnet Recognition Award

UCLA Health System

For more than half a century, UCLA has been recognized as a leader in patient care, medical research and teaching. The legacy that began in 1955 when UCLA Medical Center opened its doors in Westwood has grown to include four hospitals and a network of community offices, known together as UCLA Health System.

UCLA Health System Hospitals

- **UCLA Medical Center**, located in Westwood, offers patients of all ages comprehensive care, from routine to highly specialized medical and surgical treatment.
- **Santa Monica-UCLA Medical Center and Orthopaedic Hospital** became a part of UCLA Health System in 1995 and provides primary and specialty care.
- **Mattel Children's Hospital at UCLA**, located within UCLA Medical Center, offers a wide range of services from well-child care to the treatment of the most difficult and life-threatening illnesses.
- **Stewart and Lynda Resnick Neuropsychiatric Hospital at UCLA** offers programs in geriatric, adult, adolescent and child psychiatry.

Honors and Recognition

- For the 17th consecutive year, UCLA Medical Center ranks number one in the West in *U.S.News & World Report*'s America's Best Hospitals survey.
- *U.S.News* ranks UCLA's Jonsson Cancer Center as best in California for seven consecutive years.

Specialties and Research

- Cancer care through UCLA's Jonsson Comprehensive Cancer Center
- Integrative healthcare through UCLA's East-West Medicine Center
- Advanced care for all neurological disorders, including Alzheimer's disease and neuromuscular problems
- Full range of comprehensive cardiology services from prevention to rehab
- Ophthalmology services through Jules Stein Eye Institute and the Doris Stein Eye Research Center
- World-renowned adult and pediatric organ transplant programs
- Treatment of disorders of the spine and brain through UCLA's neurosurgery services
- The UCLA AIDS Institute for state-of-the-art treatment
- Comprehensive women's health services
- Innovative surgical approaches, including minimally invasive and robotic procedures

Physician Referral   To find the UCLA doctor who best meets your needs, call the
UCLA Physician Referral Service at **1-800-UCLA-MD1** (1-800-825-2631)

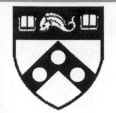

Penn Cancer Services
University of Pennsylvania Health System
Philadelphia, PA
1-800-789-PENN (7366)
pennhealth.com/cancer

University of Pennsylvania Health System Overview

For more than two centuries, Penn physicians and scientists have been committed to the highest standards of patient care, education and research. Our commitment has bee recognized by our peers and by others throughout the greater Philadelphia region and across the nation.

Commitment to Excellence

Our physicians and scientists are united in the health system's mission to expand the frontiers of medicine through new discoveries in the detection, treatment and prevention of human disease. Because we develop and test new treatments through clinical trials, our patients gain access to the very latest advances and future generations will benefit from the work we do today.

Penn continues to lead the way in discovering new treatment methods for diseases once considered incurable, including groundbreaking research in cancer, cardiac, neurosciences, orthopaedics and imaging.

When you choose a University of Pennsylvania Health System physician, you know that all of your health care needs will be met. Our multidisciplinary team of experts is compassionate and passionate about the care they provide.

We Are Medicine

We see daily examples of wonderful achievements in bridging the areas of research and medicine while healing and caring for our patients and families. We take great pride in having America's first hospital, first medical school, first dedicated teaching hospital and many medical breakthroughs and clinical advances that make us a world leader.

Over the past thirty years, Penn physicians and scientists have participated in many important discoveries, including:
The first general vaccine against pneumonia.
The introduction of total intravenous feeding.
The development of magnetic resonance imaging and other imaging technologies.
The discovery of the Philadelphia chromosome, which revolutionized cancer research by making the connection between genetic abnormalities and cancer.

Overview

The University of Pennsylvania Health System is one of the leading health care providers in the country, known for its innovative approaches to cancer diagnosis and treatment as well as the care and compassion of its staff. United in its commitment to clinical excellence and advanced research, the Health System is dedicated to improving the chances for recovery and enhancing the quality of life for its patients.

Locations

Hospital of the University of Pennsylvania
Penn Presbyterian Medical Center
Pennsylvania Hospital
Penn Medicine at Radnor
Penn Medicine at Cherry Hill

To learn more about Penn physicians and services, call 800-789-PENN or visit

847

Section III
Physician Listings by Medical Specialty

Colon & Rectal Surgery

A colon and rectal surgeon is trained to diagnose and treat various diseases of the intestinal tract, colon, rectum, anal canal and perianal area by medical and surgical means. This specialist also deals with other organs and tissues (such as the liver, urinary and female reproductive system) involved with primary intestinal disease.

Colon and rectal surgeons have the expertise to diagnose and often manage anorectal conditions such as hemorrhoids, fissures (painful tears in the anal lining), abscesses and fistulae (infections located around the anus and rectum) in the office setting. They also treat problems of the intestine and colon and perform endoscopic procedures to evaluate and treat problems such as cancer, polyps (pre-cancerous growths) and inflammatory conditions.

Training Required: Six Years (including general surgery)

Colon & Rectal Surgery

New England

Bleday, Ronald MD [CRS] - Spec Exp: Colon & Rectal Cancer; **Hospital:** Brigham & Women's Hosp, Dana-Farber Cancer Inst; **Address:** Brigham & Women's Hosp, Dept Genl Surg, 75 Francis St, ASB II, Boston, MA 02115; **Phone:** 617-732-8460; **Board Cert:** Surgery 1999; Colon & Rectal Surgery 2003; **Med School:** McGill Univ 1982; **Resid:** Surgery, Rhode Island Hosp 1989; Surgical Oncology, Brigham & Womens Hosp 1986; **Fellow:** Endoscopy, Mass Genl Hosp 1990; Colon & Rectal Surgery, Univ Minn 1991; **Fac Appt:** Assoc Prof S, Harvard Med Sch

Coller, John MD [CRS] - Spec Exp: Colon Cancer; Laparoscopic Surgery; Incontinence-Fecal; Sacral Stimulation/Fecal Incontinence; **Hospital:** Lahey Clin; **Address:** Lahey Clinic-Colon & Rectal Surg, 41 Mall Rd, Burlington, MA 01805; **Phone:** 781-744-8581; **Board Cert:** Surgery 1973; Colon & Rectal Surgery 1973; **Med School:** Univ Pennsylvania 1965; **Resid:** Surgery, Hosp Univ Penn 1972; **Fellow:** Colon & Rectal Surgery, Lahey Clinic Fdn 1973; **Fac Appt:** Asst Clin Prof S, Tufts Univ

Harnsberger, Jeffrey R MD [CRS] - Spec Exp: Colon & Rectal Cancer; **Hospital:** Dartmouth - Hitchcock Med Ctr; **Address:** Dartmouth-Hitchcock Manchester, 100 Hitchcock Way, Manchester, NH 03104; **Phone:** 603-695-2840; **Board Cert:** Surgery 2001; Colon & Rectal Surgery 2005; **Med School:** Med Coll OH 1987; **Resid:** Surgery, Dartamouth-Hitchkock Med Ctr 1992; **Fellow:** Colon & Rectal Surgery, St Louis Univ Med Ctr 1993; **Fac Appt:** Asst Prof S, Dartmouth Med Sch

Longo, Walter E MD [CRS] - Spec Exp: Colon & Rectal Cancer; Gastrointestinal Surgery; **Hospital:** Yale - New Haven Hosp; **Address:** Yale Univ School Medicine, Dept Surgery/Gastroenterology, Box 208062, New Haven, CT 06520-8062; **Phone:** 203-785-2616; **Board Cert:** Surgery 2001; Colon & Rectal Surgery 2006; **Med School:** NY Med Coll 1984; **Resid:** Surgery, Yale-New Haven Hosp 1990; **Fellow:** Research, Yale-New Haven Hosp 1988; Colon & Rectal Surgery, Cleveland Clinic 1991; **Fac Appt:** Prof S, Yale Univ

Nagle, Deborah A MD [CRS] - Hospital: Beth Israel Deaconess Med Ctr - Boston; **Address:** Beth Israel Deaconess Med Ctr, 330 Brookline Ave Stoneman Bldg - rm 932, Boston, MA 02215; **Phone:** 617-667-4170; **Board Cert:** Colon & Rectal Surgery 2006; Surgery 2004; **Med School:** Thomas Jefferson Univ 1988; **Resid:** Surgery, Thos Jefferson U Hosp 1993; Colon & Rectal Surgery, Thos Jefferson U Hosp 1994

Roberts, Patricia L MD [CRS] - Spec Exp: Colon & Rectal Cancer; **Hospital:** Lahey Clin; **Address:** 41 Mall Rd, Burlington, MA 01805; **Phone:** 781-744-8243; **Board Cert:** Surgery 1996; Colon & Rectal Surgery 2003; **Med School:** Boston Univ 1981; **Resid:** Surgery, Boston City Hosp 1986; **Fellow:** Colon & Rectal Surgery, Lahey Clinic 1988; **Fac Appt:** Assoc Prof S, Tufts Univ

Schoetz, David MD [CRS] - Spec Exp: Colon & Rectal Cancer; Incontinence-Fecal; **Hospital:** Lahey Clin; **Address:** Lahey Clinic Med Ctr, Dept Colon & Rectal Surg, 41 Mall Rd, Burlington, MA 01805-0001; **Phone:** 781-744-8889; **Board Cert:** Surgery 2001; Colon & Rectal Surgery 1983; **Med School:** Med Coll Wisc 1974; **Resid:** Surgery, Boston Univ Med Ctr 1981; **Fellow:** Colon & Rectal Surgery, Lahey Clin Med Ctr 1982; **Fac Appt:** Prof S, Tufts Univ

Shellito, Paul C MD [CRS] - Spec Exp: Colon & Rectal Cancer; Anorectal Disorders; **Hospital:** Mass Genl Hosp; **Address:** 15 Parkman St, Ste 460, Boston, MA 02114-3117; **Phone:** 617-724-0365; **Board Cert:** Surgery 1992; Colon & Rectal Surgery 1994; **Med School:** Harvard Med Sch 1977; **Resid:** Surgery, Mass Genl Hosp 1983; Surgery, Auckland Univ Med Sch 1981; **Fellow:** Colon & Rectal Surgery, Univ Minn 1985; **Fac Appt:** Asst Prof S, Harvard Med Sch

Mid Atlantic

Eisenstat, Theodore E MD [CRS] - Spec Exp: Colon & Rectal Cancer; **Hospital:** Robert Wood Johnson Univ Hosp - New Brunswick, JFK Med Ctr - Edison; **Address:** 3900 Park Ave, Ste 101, Edison, NJ 08820-3032; **Phone:** 732-494-6640; **Board Cert:** Surgery 1974; Colon & Rectal Surgery 1994; **Med School:** NY Med Coll 1968; **Resid:** Surgery, Thomas Jefferson Univ Hosp 1971; Surgery, Pennsylvania Hosp 1973; **Fellow:** Colon & Rectal Surgery, Muhlenberg Med Ctr 1978; **Fac Appt:** Clin Prof S, UMDNJ-RW Johnson Med Sch

Fry, Robert D MD [CRS] - Spec Exp: Colon & Rectal Cancer; **Hospital:** Pennsylvania Hosp (page 84), Hosp Univ Penn - UPHS (page 84); **Address:** Pennsylvania Hospital, Div Colon & Rectal Surgery, 700 Spruce St, Ste 305, Philadelphia, PA 19106; **Phone:** 215-829-5333; **Board Cert:** Surgery 1996; Colon & Rectal Surgery 1998; **Med School:** Washington Univ, St Louis 1972; **Resid:** Surgery, Barnes Jewish Hosp 1977; **Fellow:** Colon & Rectal Surgery, Cleveland Clinic 1978; **Fac Appt:** Prof S, Univ Pennsylvania

Gorfine, Stephen MD [CRS] - Spec Exp: Rectal Cancer; Anal Cancer; **Hospital:** Mount Sinai Med Ctr (page 77), Lenox Hill Hosp; **Address:** 25 E 69th St, New York, NY 10021-4925; **Phone:** 212-517-8600; **Board Cert:** Internal Medicine 1981; Surgery 1996; Colon & Rectal Surgery 1988; **Med School:** Univ Mass Sch Med 1978; **Resid:** Internal Medicine, Mount Sinai Hosp 1981; Surgery, Mount Sinai Hosp 1985; **Fellow:** Colon & Rectal Surgery, Ferguson Hosp 1987; **Fac Appt:** Clin Prof S, Mount Sinai Sch Med

Guillem, Jose MD [CRS] - Spec Exp: Colon & Rectal Cancer; Rectal Cancer/Sphincter Preservation; Minimally Invasive Surgery; Colon & Rectal Cancer-Familial Polyposis; **Hospital:** Meml Sloan Kettering Cancer Ctr (page 76); **Address:** Meml Sloan Kettering Cancer Ctr, 1275 York Ave, rm C1077, New York, NY 10021; **Phone:** 212-639-8278; **Board Cert:** Colon & Rectal Surgery 2004; Surgery 2004; **Med School:** Yale Univ 1983; **Resid:** Surgery, Columbia-Presby Med Ctr 1990; **Fellow:** Colon & Rectal Surgery, Lahey Clinic 1991; **Fac Appt:** Prof CRS, Cornell Univ-Weill Med Coll

Medich, David MD [CRS] - Spec Exp: Colon & Rectal Cancer; **Hospital:** Allegheny General Hosp; **Address:** Allegheny General Hosp, South Tower, 320 E North Ave Fl 5, Pittsburgh, PA 15212; **Phone:** 412-359-3901; **Board Cert:** Surgery 2004; Colon & Rectal Surgery 2006; **Med School:** Ohio State Univ 1987; **Resid:** Surgery, Univ Pittsburgh Med Ctr 1990; **Fellow:** Research, Univ Pittsburgh 1993; Colon & Rectal Surgery, Cleveland Clin Fdn 1994; **Fac Appt:** Assoc Prof CRS, Drexel Univ Coll Med

Milsom, Jeffrey W MD [CRS] - Spec Exp: Laparoscopic Surgery; Colon & Rectal Cancer; **Hospital:** NY-Presby Hosp (page 79); **Address:** NY Cornell Med Ctr, Div Colorectal Surgery, 1315 York Ave Fl 2, New York, NY 10021-4870; **Phone:** 212-746-6030; **Board Cert:** Colon & Rectal Surgery 1986; **Med School:** Univ Pittsburgh 1979; **Resid:** Surgery, Roosevelt Hosp 1981; Surgery, Univ Virginia Med Ctr 1984; **Fellow:** Colon & Rectal Surgery, Ferguson Hosp 1985; **Fac Appt:** Prof S, Columbia P&S

Colon & Rectal Surgery

Read, Thomas E MD [CRS] - **Spec Exp:** Colon & Rectal Cancer; Laparoscopic Surgery; **Hospital:** Western Penn Hosp; **Address:** 4815 Liberty Ave, Ste GR-59, Mellon Pavilion, Pittsburgh, PA 15224; **Phone:** 412-578-1425; **Board Cert:** Surgery 2005; Colon & Rectal Surgery 2006; **Med School:** UCSF 1988; **Resid:** Surgery, UCSF Med Ctr 1995; **Fellow:** Colon & Rectal Surgery, Lahey Clinic 1996; **Fac Appt:** Assoc Prof S, Temple Univ

Rombeau, John L MD [CRS] - **Spec Exp:** Colon & Rectal Cancer; **Hospital:** Temple Univ Hosp; **Address:** Department of Surgery, 3401 N Broad St, Parkinson Pavilion Fl 4, Philadelphia, PA 19104; **Phone:** 215-707-3133; **Board Cert:** Colon & Rectal Surgery 1977; **Med School:** Loma Linda Univ 1967; **Resid:** Surgery, Good Samaritan Hosp 1971; Surgery, LAC-USC Med Ctr 1975; **Fellow:** Colon & Rectal Surgery, Cleveland Clinic 1976; **Fac Appt:** Prof S, Temple Univ

Smith, Lee MD [CRS] - **Spec Exp:** Colon & Rectal Cancer; Anorectal Disorders; **Hospital:** Washington Hosp Ctr, Georgetown Univ Hosp; **Address:** 106 Irving St NW, Ste 2100, Washington, DC 20010-2975; **Phone:** 202-877-8484; **Board Cert:** Surgery 1971; Colon & Rectal Surgery 1973; **Med School:** UCSF 1962; **Resid:** Surgery, Naval Hosp 1970; Colon & Rectal Surgery, Univ Minn 1973; **Fac Appt:** Prof S, Georgetown Univ

Steinhagen, Randolph MD [CRS] - **Spec Exp:** Colostomy Avoidance; Colon & Rectal Cancer; **Hospital:** Mount Sinai Med Ctr (page 77); **Address:** Div Colon & Rectal Surgery, 5 E 98th St Fl 14, Box 1259, New York, NY 10029-6501; **Phone:** 212-241-3547; **Board Cert:** Surgery 2002; Colon & Rectal Surgery 1985; **Med School:** Wayne State Univ 1977; **Resid:** Surgery, Mount Sinai Hosp 1982; **Fellow:** Colon & Rectal Surgery, Cleveland Clinic 1983; **Fac Appt:** Assoc Prof S, Mount Sinai Sch Med

Whelan, Richard L MD [CRS] - **Spec Exp:** Laparoscopic Surgery; Colon & Rectal Cancer; **Hospital:** NY-Presby Hosp (page 79); **Address:** 161 Ft Washington Ave, rm 820, New York, NY 10032; **Phone:** 212-342-1155; **Board Cert:** Surgery 1997; Colon & Rectal Surgery 1989; **Med School:** Columbia P&S 1982; **Resid:** Surgery, Columbia Presby Hosp 1987; **Fellow:** Colon & Rectal Surgery, Univ Minn Med Ctr 1988; **Fac Appt:** Assoc Clin Prof S, Columbia P&S

Wong, W Douglas MD [CRS] - **Spec Exp:** Rectal Cancer/Sphincter Preservation; Colon & Rectal Cancer; Anal Disorders & Reconstruction; **Hospital:** Meml Sloan Kettering Cancer Ctr (page 76); **Address:** Meml Sloan Kettering Cancer Ctr, 1275 York Ave, rm C-1067, New York, NY 10021-6094; **Phone:** 212-639-5117; **Board Cert:** Surgery 1997; Colon & Rectal Surgery 2004; **Med School:** Canada 1972; **Resid:** Surgery, Univ Manitoba Hosp 1977; **Fellow:** Colon & Rectal Surgery, Univ Minn Med Ctr 1984; **Fac Appt:** Prof S, Cornell Univ-Weill Med Coll

Southeast

Foley, Eugene F MD [CRS] - **Spec Exp:** Colon & Rectal Cancer; **Hospital:** Univ Virginia Med Ctr; **Address:** Univ Va Hlth Sys, Dept Surg, PO Box 800709, Charlottesville, VA 22908-0709; **Phone:** 434-924-9304; **Board Cert:** Surgery 1993; Colon & Rectal Surgery 1994; **Med School:** Harvard Med Sch 1985; **Resid:** Surgery, New England Deaconess Hosp 1991; **Fellow:** Colon & Rectal Surgery, Lahey Clinic 1993; **Fac Appt:** Assoc Prof S, Univ VA Sch Med

Galandiuk, Susan MD [CRS] - **Spec Exp:** Colon & Rectal Cancer; **Hospital:** Univ of Louisville Hosp, Norton Hosp; **Address:** 601 S Floyd St, Ste 700, Louisville, KY 40202; **Phone:** 502-583-8303; **Board Cert:** Surgery 1998; Colon & Rectal Surgery 1999; **Med School:** Germany 1982; **Resid:** Surgery, Cleveland Clinic Fdtn 1988; **Fellow:** Research, Univ Louisville Hosp 1989; Colon & Rectal Surgery, Mayo Clinic 1990; **Fac Appt:** Prof CRS, Univ Louisville Sch Med

Golub, Richard MD [CRS] - Spec Exp: Colon & Rectal Cancer; Laparoscopic Surgery; **Hospital:** Sarasota Meml Hosp, Doctors Hosp - Sarasota; **Address:** Sarasota Memorial Hospital, 3333 Cattlemen Rd, Ste 206, Sarasota, FL 34232; **Phone:** 941-341-0042; **Board Cert:** Surgery 2000; Colon & Rectal Surgery 2003; **Med School:** Albert Einstein Coll Med 1984; **Resid:** Surgery, Univ Hosp Stony Brook 1990; **Fellow:** Colon & Rectal Surgery, Grant Medical Center 1991

Ludwig, Kirk A MD [CRS] - Spec Exp: Colon & Rectal Cancer & Surgery; Rectal Cancer/Sphincter Preservation; Incontinence-Fecal; Colon & Rectal Cancer-Familial Polyposis; **Hospital:** Duke Univ Med Ctr; **Address:** Duke University Medical Ctr-Dept Surgery, Box 3262, Durham, NC 27710; **Phone:** 919-681-3977; **Board Cert:** Colon & Rectal Surgery 1998; Surgery 2005; **Med School:** Univ Cincinnati 1988; **Resid:** Surgery, Med Coll Wisc 1994; **Fellow:** Colon & Rectal Surgery, Cleveland Clinic 1996; **Fac Appt:** Asst Prof S, Duke Univ

Nogueras, Juan J MD [CRS] - Spec Exp: Colon & Rectal Cancer; Incontinence-Fecal; **Hospital:** Cleveland Clin - Weston (page 71); **Address:** Cleveland Clinic, Dept Colorectal Surgery, 2950 Cleveland Clinic Blvd, Weston, FL 33331; **Phone:** 954-659-5251; **Board Cert:** Surgery 1997; Colon & Rectal Surgery 2003; **Med School:** Jefferson Med Coll 1982; **Resid:** Surgery, Columbia Presby Med Ctr 1987; **Fellow:** Colon & Rectal Surgery, Univ Minn Med Ctr 1991

Vernava III, Anthony M MD [CRS] - Spec Exp: Colon & Rectal Cancer; Incontinence-Fecal; **Hospital:** Physicians Regl Med Ctr; **Address:** Medical Surgical Specialists, 6101 Pine Ridge Rd, Naples, FL 34119; **Phone:** 239-348-4000; **Board Cert:** Surgery 1997; Colon & Rectal Surgery 1989; **Med School:** St Louis Univ 1982; **Resid:** Surgery, St Louis Univ Med Ctr 1988; Colon & Rectal Surgery, Univ Minnesota Med Ctr 1989; **Fellow:** Colon & Rectal Surgery, St Marks Hosp 1990

Wexner, Steven MD [CRS] - Spec Exp: Colon & Rectal Cancer; Laparoscopic Surgery; **Hospital:** Cleveland Clin - Weston (page 71); **Address:** 2950 Cleveland Clinic Blvd, Weston, FL 33331-3609; **Phone:** 954-659-5278; **Board Cert:** Surgery 2005; Colon & Rectal Surgery 2006; **Med School:** Cornell Univ-Weill Med Coll 1982; **Resid:** Surgery, Roosevelt Hosp 1987; **Fellow:** Colon & Rectal Surgery, Univ Minn 1988; **Fac Appt:** Prof S, Cleveland Cl Coll Med/Case West Res

Midwest

Abcarian, Herand MD [CRS] - Spec Exp: Rectal Cancer/Sphincter Preservation; Incontinence-Fecal; **Hospital:** Univ of IL Med Ctr at Chicago, Gottlieb Meml Hosp; **Address:** 675 W North Ave, Ste 406, Melrose Park, IL 60160; **Phone:** 708-450-5075; **Board Cert:** Surgery 1972; Colon & Rectal Surgery 1972; **Med School:** Iran 1965; **Resid:** Surgery, Cook County Hosp 1971; Colon & Rectal Surgery, Cook County Hosp 1972; **Fac Appt:** Prof S, Univ IL Coll Med

Delaney, Conor P MD/PhD [CRS] - Spec Exp: Laparoscopic Surgery; Colon & Rectal Cancer; **Hospital:** Univ Hosps Case Med Ctr; **Address:** Univ Hosp of Cleveland, 11100 Euclid Ave, MS 5047, Cleveland, OH 44106-5047; **Phone:** 216-844-8087; **Board Cert:** Surgery 1998; Colon & Rectal Surgery 1998; **Med School:** Ireland 1989; **Resid:** Surgery, Univ Hosp 1993, Surgery, Univ Hosp 1999; **Fellow:** Research, Univ of Pittsburgh 1995; Colon & Rectal Surgery, Cleveland Clinic 2000; **Fac Appt:** Prof S, Cleveland Cl Coll Med/Case West Res

Colon & Rectal Surgery

Fleshman, James MD [CRS] - **Spec Exp:** Colon & Rectal Cancer; Laparoscopic Surgery; **Hospital:** Barnes-Jewish Hosp, Barnes-Jewish West County Hosp; **Address:** Wash Univ Sch Med, Div Col Rectal Surgery, 660 S Euclid Ave, Box 8109, St Louis, MO 63110; **Phone:** 314-454-7177; **Board Cert:** Colon & Rectal Surgery 1988; Surgery 1996; **Med School:** Washington Univ, St Louis 1980; **Resid:** Surgery, Jewish Hospital 1986; **Fellow:** Colon & Rectal Surgery, Univ Toronto 1987; **Fac Appt:** Prof S, Washington Univ, St Louis

Kodner, Ira J MD [CRS] - **Spec Exp:** Colon & Rectal Cancer; Laparoscopic Surgery; **Hospital:** Barnes-Jewish Hosp; **Address:** Wash Univ Sch Med, Div Col Rectal Surgery, 660 S Euclid Ave, Box 8109, St. Louis, MO 63110; **Phone:** 314-454-7177; **Board Cert:** Surgery 1975; Colon & Rectal Surgery 1975; **Med School:** Washington Univ, St Louis 1967; **Resid:** Surgery, Barnes-Jewish Hosp 1974; **Fellow:** Colon & Rectal Surgery, Cleveland Clinic 1975; **Fac Appt:** Prof S, Washington Univ, St Louis

Lavery, Ian C MD [CRS] - **Spec Exp:** Colon & Rectal Cancer; **Hospital:** Cleveland Clin Fdn (page 71); **Address:** Cleveland Clinic, Desk A30, 9500 Euclid Ave, Cleveland, OH 44195; **Phone:** 216-444-6930; **Board Cert:** Colon & Rectal Surgery 1998; **Med School:** Australia 1967; **Resid:** Surgery, Princess Alexandra Hosp 1974; Colon & Rectal Surgery, Cleveland Clinic 1977; **Fac Appt:** Prof S, Case West Res Univ

MacKeigan, John MD [CRS] - **Spec Exp:** Rectal Cancer; **Hospital:** Spectrum Hlth Blodgett Campus, Spectrum Hlth Butterworth Campus; **Address:** The Ferguson Clinic, 4100 Lake SE, Ste 205, Grand Rapids, MI 49546-8292; **Phone:** 616-356-4100; **Board Cert:** Colon & Rectal Surgery 1974; **Med School:** Dalhousie Univ 1969; **Resid:** Surgery, Dalhousie Univ 1973; Colon & Rectal Surgery, Ferguson Hosp 1974; **Fac Appt:** Assoc Prof S, Mich State Univ

Madoff, Robert D MD [CRS] - **Spec Exp:** Colon & Rectal Cancer; **Hospital:** Univ Minn Med Ctr, Fairview - Univ Campus; **Address:** 420 Delaware St SE, MMC 450, Minneapolis, MN 55455; **Phone:** 612-624-9708; **Board Cert:** Surgery 1995; Colon & Rectal Surgery 2002; **Med School:** Columbia P&S 1979; **Resid:** Surgery, Univ Minn Hosps 1987; **Fellow:** Colon & Rectal Surgery, Univ Minn Hosps 1988; **Fac Appt:** Prof S, Univ Minn

Nelson, Heidi MD [CRS] - **Spec Exp:** Colon & Rectal Cancer; Gastrointestinal Cancer; **Hospital:** Mayo Med Ctr & Clin - Rochester, Rochester Meth Hosp; **Address:** Mayo Clinic, Div Colon & Rectal Surg, 200 First St SW, Rochester, MN 55905; **Phone:** 507-284-3329; **Board Cert:** Surgery 1995; Colon & Rectal Surgery 1989; **Med School:** Univ Wash 1981; **Resid:** Surgery, Oregon Hlth Sci Univ Hosp 1987; Colon & Rectal Surgery, Oregon Hlth Sci Univ Hosp 1985; **Fellow:** Colon & Rectal Surgery, Mayo Clinic 1988; **Fac Appt:** Prof S, Mayo Med Sch

Pemberton, John MD [CRS] - **Spec Exp:** Colon & Rectal Cancer; **Hospital:** St Mary's Hosp - Rochester, Rochester Meth Hosp; **Address:** Mayo Clinic, Div Colon & Rectal Surg, 200 First St SW, Gonda 9-S, Rochester, MN 55905; **Phone:** 507-284-2359; **Board Cert:** Surgery 2001; Colon & Rectal Surgery 1985; **Med School:** Tulane Univ 1976; **Resid:** Surgery, Mayo Clinic 1983; **Fellow:** Colon & Rectal Surgery, Mayo Clinic 1984; **Fac Appt:** Prof S, Mayo Med Sch

Rothenberger, David A MD [CRS] - **Spec Exp:** Colon & Rectal Cancer; **Hospital:** Univ Minn Med Ctr, Fairview - Univ Campus; **Address:** Dept Surg, 420 Delaware St SE, MMC 195, Minneapolis, MN 55455; **Phone:** 612-626-6666; **Board Cert:** Colon & Rectal Surgery 2005; **Med School:** Tufts Univ 1973; **Resid:** Surgery, St Paul-Ramsey Med Ctr 1978; **Fellow:** Colon & Rectal Surgery, Univ Minnesota Hosps 1979; **Fac Appt:** Prof S, Univ Minn

Saclarides, Theodore J MD [CRS] - **Spec Exp:** Rectal Cancer/Sphincter Preservation; Incontinence-Fecal; **Hospital:** Rush Univ Med Ctr, Rush N Shore Med Ctr; **Address:** University Surgeons, 1725 W Harrison St, Ste 810, Chicago, IL 60612-3832; **Phone:** 312-942-6543; **Board Cert:** Surgery 1996; Colon & Rectal Surgery 1989; **Med School:** Univ Miami Sch Med 1982; **Resid:** Surgery, Rush Presby-St Luke's Hosp 1987; **Fellow:** Colon & Rectal Surgery, Mayo Clinic 1988; **Fac Appt:** Prof S, Rush Med Coll

Senagore, Anthony MD [CRS] - **Spec Exp:** Laparoscopic Surgery; Colon & Rectal Cancer; Anorectal Disorders; **Hospital:** Spectrum Hlth Blodgett Campus; **Address:** Spectrum Health, 100 Michigan St NE, MC 005, Grand Rapids, MI 49503; **Phone:** 616-391-2467; **Board Cert:** Surgery 1995; Colon & Rectal Surgery 2001; **Med School:** Mich State Univ 1981; **Resid:** Surgery, Butterworth Hosp 1987; Colon & Rectal Surgery, Ferguson Hosp 1989; **Fac Appt:** Prof S, Med Univ Ohio at Toledo

Stryker, Steven J MD [CRS] - **Spec Exp:** Colon & Rectal Cancer; Laparoscopic Surgery; **Hospital:** Northwestern Meml Hosp; **Address:** 676 N Saint Clair St, Ste 1525A, Chicago, IL 60611-2862; **Phone:** 312-943-5427; **Board Cert:** Surgery 2004; Colon & Rectal Surgery 1986; **Med School:** Northwestern Univ 1978; **Resid:** Surgery, Northwestern Meml Hosp 1983; **Fellow:** Colon & Rectal Surgery, Mayo Clinic 1985; **Fac Appt:** Clin Prof S, Northwestern Univ

Wolff, Bruce G MD [CRS] - **Spec Exp:** Colon & Rectal Cancer; **Hospital:** Mayo Med Ctr & Clin - Rochester; **Address:** Mayo Clinic, Div Colon & Rectal Surg, 200 First St SW, Rochester, MN 55905; **Phone:** 507-284-0800; **Board Cert:** Surgery 2000; Colon & Rectal Surgery 2001; **Med School:** Duke Univ 1973; **Resid:** Surgery, NY Hosp-Cornell Med Ctr 1981; **Fellow:** Colon & Rectal Surgery, Mayo Clinic 1982; **Fac Appt:** Prof S, Mayo Med Sch

Great Plains and Mountains

Thorson, Alan MD [CRS] - **Spec Exp:** Colon & Rectal Cancer; Laparoscopic Surgery; Incontinence-Fecal; **Hospital:** Nebraska Meth Hosp, Archbishop Bergen Mercy Med Ctr; **Address:** 9850 Nicholas St, Ste 100, Omaha, NE 68114-2191; **Phone:** 402-343-1122; **Board Cert:** Surgery 1994; Colon & Rectal Surgery 1999; **Med School:** Univ Nebr Coll Med 1979; **Resid:** Surgery, Univ Nebraska 1984; Colon & Rectal Surgery, Univ Minn 1985; **Fac Appt:** Assoc Clin Prof S, Creighton Univ

Colon & Rectal Surgery

Southwest

Adkins, Terrance P MD [CRS] - **Spec Exp:** Colon & Rectal Cancer; **Hospital:** Tucson Med Ctr; **Address:** Southwestern Surgery Assoc, 1951 N Wilmot Rd Bldg 2, Tucson, AZ 85712; **Phone:** 520-795-5845; **Board Cert:** Surgery 2001; Colon & Rectal Surgery 2004; **Med School:** Univ Tex SW, Dallas 1985; **Resid:** Surgery, Univ Utah Med Ctr 1991; **Fellow:** Colon & Rectal Surgery, Univ Texas Med Ctr 1992; **Fac Appt:** Asst Clin Prof S, Univ Ariz Coll Med

Bailey, Harold Randolph MD [CRS] - **Spec Exp:** Rectal Cancer/Sphincter Preservation; Incontinence-Fecal; **Hospital:** Methodist Hosp - Houston, St Luke's Episcopal Hosp - Houston; **Address:** Colon & Rectal Clinic, Smith Twr, 6550 Fannin St, Ste 2307, Houston, TX 77030-2717; **Phone:** 713-790-9250; **Board Cert:** Surgery 1974; Colon & Rectal Surgery 2004; **Med School:** Univ Tex SW, Dallas 1968; **Resid:** Surgery, Hermann Hosp-Univ Tex Med Sch 1973; **Fellow:** Colon & Rectal Surgery, Ferguson-Droste Hosp 1974; **Fac Appt:** Clin Prof S, Univ Tex, Houston

Beck, David E MD [CRS] - **Spec Exp:** Colon & Rectal Cancer; Minimally Invasive Surgery; **Hospital:** Ochsner Fdn Hosp, Summit Hosp-Baton Rouge; **Address:** Ochsner Clinic Fdn, Colorectal Surgery, 1514 Jefferson Hwy, 4th Fl, rm 04 East, New Orleans, LA 70121; **Phone:** 504-842-4060; **Board Cert:** Colon & Rectal Surgery 1987; **Med School:** Univ Miami Sch Med 1979; **Resid:** Surgery, Wilford Hall USAF Med Ctr 1984; **Fellow:** Colon & Rectal Surgery, Cleveland Clinic Fdn 1986; **Fac Appt:** Assoc Clin Prof S, Louisiana State Univ

Efron, Jonathan E MD [CRS] - **Spec Exp:** Colon & Rectal Cancer; Incontinence-Fecal; Anorectal Disorders; **Hospital:** Mayo Clin Hosp - Scottsdale; **Address:** Mayo Clinic, Concourse B, 13400 E Shea Blvd, Scottsdale, AZ 85259; **Phone:** 480-342-2697; **Board Cert:** Surgery 1999; Colon & Rectal Surgery 2000; **Med School:** Univ MD Sch Med 1993; **Resid:** Surgery, LIJ Medical Ctr 1999; **Fellow:** Colon & Rectal Surgery, Cleveland Clinic 2000; Research, Cleveland Clinic 2001; **Fac Appt:** Assoc Prof S, Mayo Med Sch

Heppell, Jacques P MD [CRS] - **Spec Exp:** Colon & Rectal Cancer; Anorectal Disorders; **Hospital:** Mayo - Phoenix; **Address:** Mayo Clinic, ATTN: GENS/CB/Distribution 13, 5777 E Mayo Blvd, Phoenix, AZ 85259-5404; **Phone:** 480-342-2697; **Board Cert:** Surgery 2004; Colon & Rectal Surgery 1995; **Med School:** Univ Montreal 1974; **Resid:** Surgery, Univ Montreal Med Ctr 1979; **Fellow:** Colon & Rectal Surgery, Mayo Clinic 1983; **Fac Appt:** Prof S, Mayo Med Sch

Huber Jr, Philip J MD [CRS] - **Spec Exp:** Colon & Rectal Cancer; **Hospital:** Med City Dallas Hosp, Presby Hosp of Dallas; **Address:** 7777 Forest Lane, Ste C-760, Dallas, TX 75230; **Phone:** 972-566-8039; **Board Cert:** Surgery 1997; Colon & Rectal Surgery 1993; **Med School:** Columbia P&S 1972; **Resid:** Surgery, Parkland Hosp 1977; Colon & Rectal Surgery, Presby Hosp 1978

West Coast and Pacific

Beart Jr, Robert W MD [CRS] - **Spec Exp:** Colon & Rectal Cancer; **Hospital:** USC Norris Comp Cancer Ctr, USC Univ Hosp - R K Eamer Med Plz; **Address:** USC Comprehensive Cancer Center, Topping Tower Suite 7418, 1441 Eastlake Ave, Los Angeles, CA 90033; **Phone:** 323-865-3690; **Board Cert:** Surgery 1993; Colon & Rectal Surgery 1995; **Med School:** Harvard Med Sch 1971; **Resid:** Surgery, Univ Colo Med Ctr 1976; Colon & Rectal Surgery, Mayo Clinic 1978; **Fellow:** Transplant Surgery, Univ Colo Med Ctr 1975; **Fac Appt:** Prof S, USC Sch Med

Stamos, Michael J MD [CRS] - **Spec Exp:** Rectal Cancer/Sphincter Preservation; Laparoscopic Surgery; Colon & Rectal Cancer; Anorectal Disorders; **Hospital:** UC Irvine Med Ctr; **Address:** UC Irvine Med Ctr, Div Colon & Rectal Surg, 333 City Blvd W, Ste 850, Orange, CA 92868; **Phone:** 714-456-8511; **Board Cert:** Surgery 2000; Colon & Rectal Surgery 2003; **Med School:** Case West Res Univ 1985; **Resid:** Surgery, Jackson Meml Hosp 1990; Colon & Rectal Surgery, Ochsner Clinic 1991; **Fac Appt:** Prof S, UC Irvine

Volpe, Peter A MD [CRS] - **Spec Exp:** Colon Cancer; Colonoscopy; Anorectal Disorders; **Hospital:** CA Pacific Med Ctr - Pacific Campus, St Mary's Med Ctr - San Fran; **Address:** 3838 California St, Ste 616, San Francisco, CA 94118; **Phone:** 415-668-0411; **Board Cert:** Surgery 1970; Colon & Rectal Surgery 1971; **Med School:** Ohio State Univ 1961; **Resid:** Surgery, UCSF Hosps 1969; Colon & Rectal Surgery, ABCRS Preceptorship 1971; **Fac Appt:** Clin Prof S, UCSF

Welton, Mark L MD [CRS] - **Spec Exp:** Colon & Rectal Cancer; Anal Cancer; **Hospital:** Stanford Univ Med Ctr; **Address:** Stanford Univ - Colon & Rectal Surgery, 300 Pasteur Drive, rm H 3680, Stanford, CA 94305-5655; **Phone:** 650-723-5461; **Board Cert:** Surgery 2000; Colon & Rectal Surgery 2005; **Med School:** UCLA 1984; **Resid:** Surgery, UCLA Med Ctr 1992; **Fellow:** Colon & Rectal Surgery, Barnes Jewish Hosp 1993; **Fac Appt:** Assoc Prof S, Stanford Univ

Cleveland Clinic

National Leader in Colorectal Surgery

Cleveland Clinic's Digestive Disease Center is one of the largest in the country and one of the first to fully integrate its departments of Colorectal Surgery and Gastroenterology & Hepatology. Combining these disciplines in one location facilitates unprecedented patient care, multidisciplinary education, and collaborative research.

Cleveland Clinic colorectal surgeons have performed more than 1,800 laparoscopic intestinal resections and currently average eight to ten cases each week, which demonstrates their expertise in performing minimally invasive intestinal surgery. Although colon surgery is one of the more difficult procedures to perform laparoscopically, the latest research suggests that laparoscopic surgery – even for colorectal cancer – offers an equally good outcome as open surgery when performed by experienced surgeons.

Additionally, the Digestive Disease Center is a recognized leader in many areas, including pelvic pouch procedures. Cleveland Clinic colorectal surgeons have performed more than 3,500 pelvic pouch procedures and are the established leaders in pouch salvage. Furthermore, a comprehensive Pelvic Floor Center has three surgeons dedicated to the subspecialty of rectal function and fecal incontinence. Over the years, the staff of the Digestive Disease Center has pioneered many new technologies and procedures for treating digestive disorders, including:

- Continent ileostomy/stapled pouch to valve
- Stapled pelvic pouch procedures
- Surgery for ostomy complications
- Advancement flap/sleeves for perianal fistulas and Crohn's disease
- Coloplasty for enhanced function after rectal resection
- Strictureplasty for Crohn's disease
- Salvage surgery for apparently "failed" ileal pelvic (J) pouches
- Surgery for fecal incontinence

For patients with advanced disease, a multi-disciplinary team collaborates with the staff of Cleveland Clinic Taussig Cancer Center to provide state-of-the-art clinical trials, novel therapeutics, and innovative diagnostic techniques. Genetic counseling and participation in national studies of familial cancer are part of our routinely available services. The largest registry in the United States for inherited forms of colorectal cancer is part of the Digestive Disease Center.

Cleveland Clinic's Digestive Disease Center is ranked #2 in the nation by *U.S.News & World Report's* 2006 "America's Best Hospitals" Survey.

To schedule an appointment or for more information about the Cleveland Clinic Digestive Disease Center, call 800.890.2467 or visit www.clevelandclinic.org/colorectaltopdocs.

Digestive Disease Center | 9500 Euclid Ave. / W14 | Cleveland, OH 44195

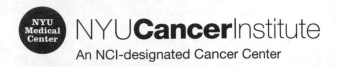

NYU**Cancer**Institute
An NCI-designated Cancer Center

A Collaborative Approach
The NYU Cancer Institute, an NCI designated center, is a "matrix cancer center" without walls operating within the larger NYU Medical Center. With over 200 members and a research funding base of over $81 million, this structure strengthens our capabilities to forge collaborations across medical and scientific disciplines, which translates to comprehensive care for our patients and discoveries that will influence the future of this disease.

Renowned Expertise
Our highly skilled Magnet™ nursing team not only plays a pivotal role in coordinating direct patient care, but is also a source of invaluable patient education. Team members' compassion and expertise help patients better manage the symptoms of their disease as well as their special needs.

A Patient-Focused Setting
The NYU Clinical Cancer Center, with over 70 faculty members from various disciplines at the New York University School of Medicine, is the principal outpatient facility of the Cancer Institute and serves as home for our patients and their caregivers. The center and its multidisciplinary team of experts provide access to the latest treatment options and clinical trials along with a variety of programs in cancer prevention, screening, diagnostics, genetic counseling, and supportive services. When it comes to kids and cancer, the Stephen D. Hassenfeld Children's Center for Cancer and Blood Disorders offers not just innovation but insight. As a leading member of the NCI-sponsored Children's Oncology Group, our physicians are known for developing new ways to treat childhood cancer. Our affiliation with Bellevue Hospital, the oldest public hospital in the country, affords clinically distinctive opportunities to learn and care for patients with cancer by observing its presentation and behavior in a variety of patient groups.

Dermatology

A dermatologist is trained to diagnose and treat pediatric and adult patients with benign and malignant disorders of the skin, mouth, external genitalia, hair and nails, as well as a number of sexually transmitted diseases. The dermatologist has had additional training and experience in the diagnosis and treatment of skin cancers, melanomas, moles and other tumors of the skin, the management of contact dermatitis and other allergic and non-allergic skin disorders, and in the recognition of the skin manifestations of systemic (including internal malignancy) and infectious diseases.

Dermatologists may have special training in dermatopathology and in the surgical techniques used in dermatology. They also have expertise in the management of cosmetic disorders of the skin such as hair loss and scars, and the skin changes associated with aging.

Training Required: Four years

Dermatology

New England

Braverman, Irwin MD [D] - **Spec Exp:** Cutaneous Lymphoma; **Hospital:** Yale - New Haven Hosp; **Address:** Yale Dermatology, 2 Church St S, Ste 305, New Haven, CT 06519; **Phone:** 203-789-1249; **Board Cert:** Dermatology 1963; Dermatopathology 1982; **Med School:** Yale Univ 1955; **Resid:** Internal Medicine, Yale-New Haven Hosp 1956; Internal Medicine, Yale-New Haven Hosp 1959; **Fellow:** Dermatology, Yale-New Haven Hosp 1962; **Fac Appt:** Prof D, Yale Univ

Del Giudice, Stephen M MD [D] - **Spec Exp:** Skin Cancer; **Hospital:** Concord Hospital; **Address:** Dartmouth Hitchcock Concord - Dermatology, 253 Pleasant St, Concord, NH 03301; **Phone:** 603-226-6119; **Board Cert:** Dermatology 1987; **Med School:** Tufts Univ 1981; **Resid:** Dermatology, Yale-New Haven Hosp 1987

Edelson, Richard L MD [D] - **Spec Exp:** Cutaneous Lymphoma; **Hospital:** Yale - New Haven Hosp; **Address:** 2 Church St S, Ste 305, New Haven, CT 06519; **Phone:** 203-789-1249; **Board Cert:** Dermatology 1977; **Med School:** Yale Univ 1970; **Resid:** Dermatology, Mass Genl Hosp 1972; Dermatology, Natl Inst Hlth 1975; **Fac Appt:** Prof D, Yale Univ

Fewkes, Jessica L MD [D] - **Spec Exp:** Mohs' Surgery; Skin Cancer-Head & Neck; Melanoma-Head & Neck; **Hospital:** Mass Eye & Ear Infirmary; **Address:** Mass Eye & Ear Infirmary, 243 Charles St Fl 9, Boston, MA 02114; **Phone:** 617-573-3789; **Board Cert:** Dermatology 1982; **Med School:** UCSF 1978; **Resid:** Dermatology, Mass General Hosp 1982; **Fellow:** Mohs Surgery, Duke Univ Med Ctr 1983; **Fac Appt:** Asst Prof D, Harvard Med Sch

Gilchrest, Barbara MD [D] - **Spec Exp:** Melanoma; Skin Cancer; **Hospital:** Boston Med Ctr; **Address:** 609 Albany St Bldg J - Ste 507, Boston, MA 02118-2394; **Phone:** 617-638-5538; **Board Cert:** Internal Medicine 1975; Dermatology 1978; **Med School:** Harvard Med Sch 1971; **Resid:** Internal Medicine, Boston City Hosp 1973; Dermatology, Harvard Med Sch 1976; **Fellow:** Photo Biology, Harvard Med Sch 1975; **Fac Appt:** Prof D, Boston Univ

Kupper, Thomas S MD [D] - **Spec Exp:** Melanoma; Cutaneous Lymphoma; Skin Cancer; **Hospital:** Brigham & Women's Hosp, Dana-Farber Cancer Inst; **Address:** Brigham & Women's Hosp, Dept Dermatology, 77 Avenue Louis Pasteur, Ste 671, Boston, MA 02115; **Phone:** 617-525-5550; **Board Cert:** Dermatology 1989; **Med School:** Wright State Univ 1981; **Resid:** Surgery, Yale-New Haven Hosp 1984; Dermatology, Yale-New Haven Hosp 1989; **Fac Appt:** Prof D, Harvard Med Sch

Leffell, David J MD [D] - **Spec Exp:** Mohs' Surgery; Melanoma; Skin Cancer; Skin Laser Surgery; **Hospital:** Yale - New Haven Hosp, Hosp of St Raphael; **Address:** New Haven Hosp-Dept Dermatology, 40 Temple St, Ste 5A, PO Box 208059, New Haven, CT 06520; **Phone:** 203-785-3466; **Board Cert:** Internal Medicine 1984; Dermatology 1987; **Med School:** McGill Univ 1981; **Resid:** Internal Medicine, New York Hosp 1984; Dermatology, Yale-New Haven Hosp 1986; **Fellow:** Dermatology, Yale-New Haven Hosp 1987; Dermatologic Surgery, Univ Michigan Med Ctr 1988; **Fac Appt:** Prof D, Yale Univ

Maloney, Mary MD [D] - **Spec Exp:** Mohs' Surgery; Skin Laser Surgery; **Hospital:** UMass Memorial Med Ctr; **Address:** Univ Mass Med Ctr, Dept Derm, 281 Lincoln St Fl 4, Worcester, MA 01605; **Phone:** 508-334-5962; **Board Cert:** Dermatology 1982; **Med School:** Univ VT Coll Med 1977; **Resid:** Internal Medicine, Hartford Hospital 1979; Dermatology, Dartmouth-Hitchcock Med Ctr 1982; **Fellow:** Dermatologic Surgery, UCSF Med Ctr 1983; **Fac Appt:** Prof D, Univ Mass Sch Med

McDonald, Charles J MD [D] - **Spec Exp:** Cutaneous Lymphoma; Autoimmune Disease; **Hospital:** Rhode Island Hosp; **Address:** Rhode Island Hosp, Dept Dermatology, 593 Eddy St, APC-10, Providence, RI 02903-4923; **Phone:** 401-444-7959; **Board Cert:** Dermatology 1966; **Med School:** Howard Univ 1960; **Resid:** Internal Medicine, Hosp St Raphael 1963; Dermatology, Yale New Haven Hosp 1965; **Fellow:** Clinical Oncology, Yale New Haven Hosp 1966; **Fac Appt:** Prof D, Brown Univ

Mihm Jr, Martin C MD [D] - **Spec Exp:** Melanoma; Dermatopathology; **Hospital:** Mass Genl Hosp; **Address:** Mass General Hosp, 55 Fruit St, Warren Bldg 827, Boston, MA 02114-2926; **Phone:** 617-724-1350; **Board Cert:** Dermatology 1969; Dermatopathology 1974; Anatomic Pathology 1974; **Med School:** Univ Pittsburgh 1961; **Resid:** Internal Medicine, Mt Sinai Hosp 1964; Dermatology, Mass Genl Hosp 1967; **Fellow:** Anatomic Pathology, Mass Genl Hosp 1972; **Fac Appt:** Clin Prof Path, Harvard Med Sch

Sober, Arthur MD [D] - **Spec Exp:** Melanoma; Skin Cancer; **Hospital:** Mass Genl Hosp; **Address:** Mass General Hospital, 50 Staniford St, Ste 200, Boston, MA 02114; **Phone:** 617-726-2914; **Board Cert:** Dermatology 1975; Internal Medicine 1974; **Med School:** Geo Wash Univ 1968; **Resid:** Internal Medicine, Beth Israel Hosp 1970; Dermatology, Mass General Hosp 1974; **Fellow:** Immunology, Peter Bent Brigham Hosp 1976; **Fac Appt:** Prof D, Harvard Med Sch

Mid Atlantic

Ackerman, A Bernard MD [D] - **Spec Exp:** Dermatopathology; Melanoma Consultation; **Hospital:** SUNY Downstate Med Ctr; **Address:** 145 E 32nd St Fl 10, New York, NY 10016; **Phone:** 212-889-6225; **Board Cert:** Dermatology 1970; Dermatopathology 1974; **Med School:** Columbia P&S 1962; **Resid:** Dermatology, Columbia Presby Hosp 1964; Dermatology, Univ Penn Hosp 1967; **Fellow:** Dermatopathology, Mass Genl Hosp 1969

Braun III, Martin MD [D] - **Spec Exp:** Mohs' Surgery; Skin Cancer; **Hospital:** G Washington Univ Hosp; **Address:** 2112 F St NW, Ste 701, Washington, DC 20037; **Phone:** 202-293-7618; **Board Cert:** Dermatology 1977; Dermatopathology 1982; **Med School:** Univ MD Sch Med 1970; **Resid:** Dermatology, Univ Mich Med Ctr 1976; **Fellow:** Mohs Surgery, Precept w/ Dr Frederic Mohs 1975; **Fac Appt:** Clin Prof D, Geo Wash Univ

Brodland, David MD [D] - **Spec Exp:** Mohs' Surgery; Skin Cancer; Reconstructive Surgery-Skin; **Hospital:** UPMC Shadyside, Jefferson Hosp - Pittsburgh; **Address:** South Hills Med Bldg, 575 Coal Valley Rd, Ste 360, Clairton, PA 15025; **Phone:** 412-466-9400; **Board Cert:** Dermatology 1989; **Med School:** Southern IL Univ 1985; **Resid:** Dermatology, Mayo Grad Sch Med 1989; **Fellow:** Mohs Surgery, John A Zitelli MD 1990; **Fac Appt:** Asst Clin Prof D, Univ Pittsburgh

Dermatology

Bystryn, Jean Claude MD [D] - **Spec Exp:** Melanoma; Skin Cancer; **Hospital:** NYU Med Ctr (page 80); **Address:** 530 1st Ave, Ste 7F, New York, NY 10016; **Phone:** 212-889-3846; **Board Cert:** Dermatology 1970; Clinical & Laboratory Dematologic Immunology 1985; **Med School:** NYU Sch Med 1962; **Resid:** Internal Medicine, Montefiore Hosp 1964; Dermatology, NYU Med Ctr 1969; **Fellow:** Immunology, New York Univ 1972; **Fac Appt:** Prof D, NYU Sch Med

Dzubow, Leonard MD [D] - **Spec Exp:** Mohs' Surgery; **Hospital:** Bryn Mawr Hosp, Riddle Meml Hosp; **Address:** 101 Chesley Drive, Media, PA 19063; **Phone:** 484-621-0082; **Board Cert:** Internal Medicine 1978; Dermatology 1980; **Med School:** Univ Pennsylvania 1975; **Resid:** Internal Medicine, Hosp Univ Penn 1978; Dermatology, NYU-Skin Cancer Unit 1980; **Fellow:** Mohs Surgery, NYU-Skin Cancer Unit; **Fac Appt:** Clin Prof D, Univ Pennsylvania

Geronemus, Roy MD [D] - **Spec Exp:** Skin Laser Surgery; Mohs' Surgery; Skin Cancer; **Hospital:** NYU Med Ctr (page 80), New York Eye & Ear Infirm (page 78); **Address:** 317 E 34 St, Ste 11N, New York, NY 10016-4974; **Phone:** 212-686-7306; **Board Cert:** Dermatology 1983; **Med School:** Univ Miami Sch Med 1979; **Resid:** Dermatology, NYU-Skin Cancer Unit 1983; **Fellow:** Mohs Surgery, NYU-Skin Cancer Unit 1984; **Fac Appt:** Clin Prof D, NYU Sch Med

Granstein, Richard D MD [D] - **Spec Exp:** Autoimmune Disease; Skin Cancer; **Hospital:** NY-Presby Hosp (page 79); **Address:** 520 E 70th St Fl 3 - Ste 326, New York, NY 10021; **Phone:** 212-746-2007; **Board Cert:** Dermatology 1983; Clinical & Laboratory Dematologic Immunology 1985; **Med School:** UCLA 1978; **Resid:** Dermatology, Mass Genl Hosp 1981; **Fellow:** Research, Natl Cancer Inst 1982; Dermatology, Mass Genl Hosp 1983; **Fac Appt:** Prof D, Cornell Univ-Weill Med Coll

Halpern, Allan C MD [D] - **Spec Exp:** Skin Cancer; Melanoma; Melanoma Early Detection/Prevention; **Hospital:** Meml Sloan Kettering Cancer Ctr (page 76); **Address:** 160 E 53rd St, New York, NY 10022; **Phone:** 212-610-0766; **Board Cert:** Internal Medicine 1984; Dermatology 1988; **Med School:** Albert Einstein Coll Med 1981; **Resid:** Dermatology, Hosp Univ Penn 1988; **Fellow:** Epidemiology, Hosp Univ Penn 1989; **Fac Appt:** Assoc Prof Med, Cornell Univ-Weill Med Coll

Kriegel, David MD [D] - **Spec Exp:** Mohs' Surgery; Skin Laser Surgery; **Hospital:** Mount Sinai Med Ctr (page 77); **Address:** 250 W 57th St, Ste 825, New York, NY 10107; **Phone:** 212-489-6669; **Board Cert:** Dermatology 2003; **Med School:** Boston Univ 1987; **Resid:** Dermatology, New England Med Ctr 1991; **Fellow:** Mohs Surgery, Stony Brook Univ Hosp 1993; **Fac Appt:** Assoc Prof D, Mount Sinai Sch Med

Lebwohl, Mark MD [D] - **Spec Exp:** Skin Cancer; Cutaneous Lymphoma; **Hospital:** Mount Sinai Med Ctr (page 77); **Address:** 5 E 98th St Fl 5, New York, NY 10029-6501; **Phone:** 212-241-9728; **Board Cert:** Internal Medicine 1981; Dermatology 1983; **Med School:** Harvard Med Sch 1978; **Resid:** Internal Medicine, Mount Sinai Hosp 1981; **Fellow:** Dermatology, Mount Sinai Hosp 1983; **Fac Appt:** Prof D, Mount Sinai Sch Med

Lessin, Stuart R MD [D] - **Spec Exp:** Melanoma; Skin Cancer; Cutaneous Lymphoma; Melanoma Risk Assessment; **Hospital:** Fox Chase Cancer Ctr (page 73); **Address:** Fox Chase Cancer Ctr, Dept Dermatology, 333 Cottman Ave, Philadelphia, PA 19111; **Phone:** 215-728-2191; **Board Cert:** Dermatology 1986; **Med School:** Temple Univ 1982; **Resid:** Dermatology, Hosp Univ Penn 1986; **Fac Appt:** Prof D, Temple Univ

Miller, Stanley MD [D] - Spec Exp: Skin Cancer; Mohs' Surgery; **Hospital:** Johns Hopkins Hosp - Baltimore; **Address:** Charles Towson Bldg, Ste 201, 1104 Kenilworth Drive, Ste 201, Towson, MD 21204; **Phone:** 443-279-0340; **Board Cert:** Dermatology 1989; **Med School:** Univ VT Coll Med 1984; **Resid:** Dermatology, UCSD Med Ctr 1989; **Fellow:** Dermatologic Surgery, Hosp Univ Penn 1991; **Fac Appt:** Prof D, Johns Hopkins Univ

Nigra, Thomas P MD [D] - Spec Exp: Skin Cancer; **Hospital:** Washington Hosp Ctr; **Address:** Washington Hosp Ctr, Derm Assocs, 110 Irving St NW, 2B44, Washington, DC 20010; **Phone:** 202-877-6227; **Board Cert:** Dermatology 1973; **Med School:** Univ Pennsylvania 1967; **Resid:** Dermatology, Mass Genl Hosp 1973; **Fac Appt:** Clin Prof D, Geo Wash Univ

Ramsay, David L MD [D] - Spec Exp: Cutaneous Lymphoma; Skin Cancer; **Hospital:** NYU Med Ctr (page 80); **Address:** 530 1st Ave, Ste 7G, New York, NY 10016-6402; **Phone:** 212-683-6283; **Board Cert:** Dermatology 1974; **Med School:** Indiana Univ 1969; **Resid:** Dermatology, New York Univ Med Ctr 1973; **Fellow:** Dermatology, Univ Ill Hosp 1973; **Fac Appt:** Clin Prof D, NYU Sch Med

Rigel, Darrell S MD [D] - Spec Exp: Melanoma; Skin Cancer; **Hospital:** NYU Med Ctr (page 80), Mount Sinai Med Ctr (page 77); **Address:** 35 E 35th Street, Ste 208, New York, NY 10016-3823; **Phone:** 212-684-5964; **Board Cert:** Dermatology 1983; **Med School:** Geo Wash Univ 1978; **Resid:** Dermatology, NYU Med Ctr 1982; **Fellow:** Dermatologic Surgery, NYU Med Ctr 1983; **Fac Appt:** Clin Prof D, NYU Sch Med

Robins, Perry MD [D] - Spec Exp: Mohs' Surgery; Skin Cancer; Melanoma; **Hospital:** NYU Med Ctr (page 80), Bellevue Hosp Ctr; **Address:** 530 First Ave, Ste 7H, New York, NY 10016; **Phone:** 212-263-7222; **Med School:** Germany 1961; **Resid:** Dermatology, VA Med Ctr 1964; **Fellow:** Dermatology, NYU Med Ctr 1967; **Fac Appt:** Prof D, NYU Sch Med

Rook, Alain H MD [D] - Spec Exp: Cutaneous Lymphoma; **Hospital:** Hosp Univ Penn - UPHS (page 84); **Address:** Hosp Univ Penn, Dept Dermatology, 3400 Spruce St Rhoades Bldg, Philadelphia, PA 19104; **Phone:** 215-662-6751; **Board Cert:** Internal Medicine 1979; Nephrology 1980; Dermatology 2001; **Med School:** Univ Mich Med Sch 1975; **Resid:** Internal Medicine, McGill Univ Med Ctr 1977; Dermatology, Hosp Univ Penn 1989; **Fellow:** Nephrology, McGill Univ Med Ctr 1979; Immunology, NIH 1986; **Fac Appt:** Prof D, Univ Pennsylvania

Safai, Bijan MD [D] - Spec Exp: Skin Cancer; **Hospital:** Metropolitan Hosp Ctr - NY, Westchester Med Ctr; **Address:** 625 Park Ave, New York, NY 10021-6545; **Phone:** 212-988-8918; **Board Cert:** Dermatology 1974; **Med School:** Iran 1965; **Resid:** Internal Medicine, VA Med Ctr 1970; Dermatology, NYU Med Ctr 1973; **Fellow:** Immunology, Mem Sloan-Kettering Cancer Ctr 1974; **Fac Appt:** Prof D, NY Med Coll

Vonderheid, Eric C MD [D] - Spec Exp: Cutaneous Lymphoma; Skin Cancer; **Hospital:** Johns Hopkins Hosp - Baltimore; **Address:** Johns Hopkins Dept Dermatology, 550 N Broadway, Ste 1002, Baltimore, MD 21205; **Phone:** 410-955-5933; **Board Cert:** Dermatology 1976; **Med School:** Temple Univ 1968; **Resid:** Internal Medicine, St Louis Univ Med Ctr 1972; Dermatology, Temple Univ Med Ctr 1975; **Fac Appt:** Prof D, Johns Hopkins Univ

Dermatology

Zitelli, John MD [D] - **Spec Exp:** Mohs' Surgery; Skin Cancer; Melanoma; **Hospital:** UPMC Shadyside, Jefferson Hosp - Pittsburgh; **Address:** Shadyside Med Ctr, 5200 Centre Ave, Ste 303, Pittsburgh, PA 15232-1312; **Phone:** 412-681-9400; **Board Cert:** Dermatology 1980; **Med School:** Univ Pittsburgh 1976; **Resid:** Dermatology, Univ Hlth Ctr Hosp 1979; **Fellow:** Mohs Surgery, Univ Wisconsin 1980; **Fac Appt:** Assoc Clin Prof D, Univ Pittsburgh

Southeast

Amonette, Rex A MD [D] - **Spec Exp:** Skin Cancer; Mohs' Surgery; **Hospital:** Methodist Univ Hosp - Memphis, Baptist Memorial Hospital - Memphis; **Address:** Memphis Dermatology Clinic, 1455 Union Ave, Memphis, TN 38104-6727; **Phone:** 901-726-6655; **Board Cert:** Dermatology 1974; **Med School:** Univ Ark 1966; **Resid:** Dermatology, Univ Tenn Med Ctr 1971; **Fellow:** Mohs Surgery, NYU Med Ctr 1972; **Fac Appt:** Clin Prof D, Univ Tenn Coll Med, Memphis

Cook, Jonathan L MD [D] - **Spec Exp:** Skin Cancer; Mohs' Surgery; Reconstructive Surgery-Skin; **Hospital:** Duke Univ Med Ctr; **Address:** Duke Univ Med Ctr, 1300 Morreene Rd, Box 3915, Durham, NC 27710; **Phone:** 919-684-6805; **Board Cert:** Dermatology 2005; **Med School:** Med Univ SC 1992; **Resid:** Dermatology, Emory Univ Hosp 1996; **Fellow:** Dermatology, Hosp Univ Penn 1997; **Fac Appt:** Assoc Prof D, Duke Univ

Eichler, Craig MD [D] - **Spec Exp:** Skin Cancer; **Hospital:** Physicians Regl Med Ctr; **Address:** 6101 Pine Ridge Rd, Naples, FL 34119-3900; **Phone:** 239-348-4335; **Board Cert:** Dermatology 2003; **Med School:** Univ Fla Coll Med 1989; **Resid:** Dermatology, Univ Texas Med Branch 1993

Elmets, Craig A MD [D] - **Spec Exp:** Phototherapy in Skin Disease; Skin Cancer; **Hospital:** Univ of Ala Hosp at Birmingham, VA Med Ctr; **Address:** Univ of Alabama-Birmingham-Derm Dept, 1530 Third Ave S, EFH 414, Birmingham, AL 35294; **Phone:** 205-996-7546; **Board Cert:** Dermatology 1980; Internal Medicine 1978; Clinical & Laboratory Immunology 1989; **Med School:** Univ Iowa Coll Med 1975; **Resid:** Internal Medicine, Kansas Med Ctr 1978; Dermatology, Univ Iowa Hosps 1980; **Fellow:** Immunological Dermatology, Univ Texas Hlth Sci Ctr 1982; **Fac Appt:** Prof D, Univ Ala

Fenske, Neil A MD [D] - **Spec Exp:** Skin Cancer; Melanoma; **Hospital:** H Lee Moffitt Cancer Ctr & Research Inst, Tampa Genl Hosp; **Address:** 12901 Bruce B Downs Blvd, MDC-79, Tampa, FL 33612-4742; **Phone:** 813-974-2920; **Board Cert:** Dermatology 1977; Dermatopathology 1984; **Med School:** St Louis Univ 1973; **Resid:** Dermatology, Wisconsin Hlth Sci Ctr 1977; **Fac Appt:** Prof Med, Univ S Fla Coll Med

Flowers, Franklin P MD [D] - **Spec Exp:** Mohs' Surgery; Dermatopathology; **Hospital:** Shands Hlthcre at Univ of FL; **Address:** Shands Healthcare, PO Box 100383, Gainesville, FL 32610; **Phone:** 352-265-8001; **Board Cert:** Dermatology 1976; Dermatopathology 1981; **Med School:** Univ Fla Coll Med 1971; **Resid:** Dermatology, Ohio State Univ 1975; **Fellow:** Mohs Surgery, Univ Alabama 1993; **Fac Appt:** Prof Med, Univ Fla Coll Med

Garrett, Algin MD [D] - **Spec Exp:** Skin Cancer; Mohs' Surgery; **Hospital:** Med Coll of VA Hosp; **Address:** Stonypoint Medical Park, 9000 Stonypoint Pkwy Fl 2, Richmond, VA 23235; **Phone:** 804-560-8919; **Board Cert:** Dermatology 1983; **Med School:** Penn State Univ-Hershey Med Ctr 1978; **Resid:** Internal Medicine, VA Med Ctr 1980; Dermatology, Med Col VA 1983; **Fellow:** Mohs Surgery, Cleveland Clinic Found 1988; **Fac Appt:** Prof D, Va Commonwealth Univ

Green, Howard MD [D] - **Spec Exp:** Mohs' Surgery; Skin Cancer; **Hospital:** St Mary's Med Ctr - W Palm Bch, JFK Med Ctr - Atlantis; **Address:** 120 Butler St, Ste A, West Palm Beach, FL 33407-6106; **Phone:** 561-659-1510; **Board Cert:** Internal Medicine 1988; Dermatology 2004; **Med School:** Boston Univ 1985; **Resid:** Internal Medicine, Jefferson Univ Hosp 1988; Dermatology, Harvard Med Sch 1992; **Fellow:** Mohs Surgery, Boston Univ Med Ctr 1993

Grichnik, James M MD/PhD [D] - **Spec Exp:** Melanoma; Skin Cancer; **Hospital:** Duke Univ Med Ctr; **Address:** Duke Univ Med Ctr-Dept Surgery, Box 3135, Durham, NC 27710; **Phone:** 919-684-3270; **Board Cert:** Dermatology 2003; **Med School:** Harvard Med Sch 1990; **Resid:** Dermatology, Duke Univ Med Ctr 1994; **Fac Appt:** Assoc Prof D, Duke Univ

Johr, Robert MD [D] - **Spec Exp:** Pigmented Lesions; Melanoma; **Hospital:** Univ of Miami Hosp & Clins/Sylvester Comp Canc Ctr, Boca Raton Comm Hosp; **Address:** 1050 NW 15th St, Ste 201A, Boca Raton, FL 33486-1341; **Phone:** 561-368-4545; **Board Cert:** Dermatology 1981; **Med School:** Mexico 1975; **Resid:** Dermatology, Roswell Park Cancer Ctr 1977; Dermatology, Metro Med Ctr/Case Western Reserve 1979; **Fac Appt:** Clin Prof D, Univ Miami Sch Med

Leshin, Barry MD [D] - **Spec Exp:** Skin Cancer; Mohs' Surgery; **Address:** 125 Sunnynoll Ct, Ste 100, Winston-Salem, NC 27106; **Phone:** 336-724-2434; **Board Cert:** Dermatology 1985; **Med School:** Univ Tex, Houston 1981; **Resid:** Dermatology, Univ Iowa Hosp 1985; **Fellow:** Dermatologic Surgery, Univ Iowa Hosp 1986; **Fac Appt:** Clin Prof PlS, Wake Forest Univ

Olsen, Elise A MD [D] - **Spec Exp:** Cutaneous Lymphoma; **Hospital:** Duke Univ Med Ctr; **Address:** Duke Univ Med Ctr, Box 3294, Durham, NC 27710; **Phone:** 919-684-3432; **Board Cert:** Dermatology 1983; **Med School:** Baylor Coll Med 1978; **Resid:** Internal Medicine, Univ NC Meml Hosp 1980; Dermatology, Duke Univ Med Ctr 1983; **Fac Appt:** Prof D, Duke Univ

Sobel, Stuart MD [D] - **Spec Exp:** Skin Cancer; **Hospital:** Meml Regl Hosp - Hollywood, Joe Di Maggio Chldns Hosp; **Address:** 4340 Sheridan St, Ste 101, Hollywood, FL 33021-3511; **Phone:** 954-983-5533; **Board Cert:** Dermatology 1977; **Med School:** Tufts Univ 1972; **Resid:** Dermatology, Mt Sinai Hosp 1976

Sokoloff, Daniel MD [D] - **Spec Exp:** Skin Cancer; **Hospital:** St Mary's Med Ctr - W Palm Bch, Good Sam Med Ctr - W Palm Beach; **Address:** Palm Beach Dermatology, 1000 45th St, Ste 1, West Palm Beach, FL 33407-2416; **Phone:** 561-863-1000; **Board Cert:** Dermatology 1982; **Med School:** Geo Wash Univ 1977; **Resid:** Dermatology, Baylor Coll Med 1982

Thiers, Bruce H MD [D] - **Spec Exp:** Cutaneous Lymphoma; Skin Cancer; **Hospital:** MUSC Med Ctr; **Address:** MUSC Dept Dermatology, 135 Rutledge Ave Fl 11, Box 250578, Charleston, SC 29425; **Phone:** 843-792-5858; **Board Cert:** Dermatology 1978; **Med School:** SUNY Buffalo 1974, **Resid:** Dermatology, SUNY Buffalo Med Ctr 1978; **Fac Appt:** Prof D, Med Univ SC

Dermatology

Midwest

Alam, Murad MD [D] - **Spec Exp:** Mohs' Surgery; Skin Cancer; Melanoma; **Hospital:** Northwestern Meml Hosp; **Address:** 676 N St. Clair, Galter Pavilion, Ste 1600, Chicago, IL 60611; **Phone:** 312-695-8106; **Board Cert:** Dermatology 2001; **Med School:** Yale Univ 1996; **Resid:** Dermatology, Columbia Univ Coll of P&S 2000; **Fellow:** Dermatology, Harvard Univ/Skin Care Phys 2001; Dermatology 2003; **Fac Appt:** Asst Prof D, Northwestern Univ-Feinberg Sch Med

Bailin, Philip L MD [D] - **Spec Exp:** Mohs' Surgery; Skin Laser Surgery; Skin Cancer; **Hospital:** Cleveland Clin Fdn (page 71); **Address:** Cleveland Clinic Fdn, 9500 Euclid Ave, Desk A61, Cleveland, OH 44195-5032; **Phone:** 216-444-2115; **Board Cert:** Dermatology 1975; **Med School:** Northwestern Univ 1968; **Resid:** Dermatology, Cleveland Clin Fdn 1974; **Fellow:** Dermatopathology, Armed Forces Inst Pathology 1975; Mohs Surgery, Univ Wisc Hosp & Clin

Cornelius, Lynn A MD [D] - **Spec Exp:** Melanoma; **Hospital:** Barnes-Jewish Hosp, St Louis Chldns Hosp; **Address:** 660 S Euclid, Box 8123, St Louis, MO 63110; **Phone:** 314-362-8187; **Board Cert:** Dermatology 1989; **Med School:** Univ MO-Columbia Sch Med 1984; **Resid:** Dermatology, Barnes Jewish Hosp-Wash Univ 1989; **Fellow:** Immunological Dermatology, Emory Univ Med Ctr 1992; **Fac Appt:** Assoc Prof D, Washington Univ, St Louis

Hanke, C William MD [D] - **Spec Exp:** Mohs' Surgery; Skin Laser Surgery; Photodynamic Therapy; **Hospital:** St Vincent Carmel Hosp, Clarian Hlth Ptrs (page 70); **Address:** Laser & Skin Surgery Ctr of Indiana, 13450 N Meridian St, Ste 355, Carmel, IN 46032-1486; **Phone:** 317-582-8484; **Board Cert:** Dermatology 1978; Dermatopathology 1982; **Med School:** Univ Iowa Coll Med 1971; **Resid:** Dermatology, Cleveland Clinic 1978; Dermatopathology, Indiana Univ 1982; **Fellow:** Cutaneous Oncology, Cleveland Clinic 1979; **Fac Appt:** Clin Prof D, Indiana Univ

Hruza, George J MD [D] - **Spec Exp:** Skin Laser Surgery; Mohs' Surgery; **Hospital:** St Luke's Hosp - Chesterfield, MO, St Louis Univ Hosp; **Address:** Laser & Derm Surg Ctr, 14377 Woodlake Drive, Ste 111, St. Louis, MO 63017-5735; **Phone:** 314-878-3839; **Board Cert:** Dermatology 1986; **Med School:** NYU Sch Med 1982; **Resid:** Dermatology, NYU Med Ctr-Skin Cancer Unit 1986; **Fellow:** Laser Surgery, Mass Genl Hosp-Harvard 1987; Surgery, Univ Wisc 1988; **Fac Appt:** Assoc Clin Prof D, St Louis Univ

Johnson, Timothy M MD [D] - **Spec Exp:** Melanoma; Mohs' Surgery; **Hospital:** Univ Michigan Hlth Sys; **Address:** Univ Michigan Hlth System, Dept Dermatology, 1910 Taubman Ctr, Ann Arbor, MI 48109-0314; **Phone:** 734-936-4190; **Board Cert:** Dermatology 1988; **Med School:** Univ Tex, Houston 1984; **Resid:** Dermatology, Univ Texas Med Ctr 1988; **Fellow:** Cutaneous Oncology, Univ Mich Med Ctr 1989; Mohs Surgery, Univ Oregon Hlth Sci Ctr 1990; **Fac Appt:** Prof D, Univ Mich Med Sch

Lim, Henry W MD [D] - **Spec Exp:** Cutaneous Lymphoma; Skin Cancer; **Hospital:** Henry Ford Hosp; **Address:** Henry Ford Hosp, Dept Derm, 3031 W Grand Blvd, Ste 800, Detroit, MI 48202-3141; **Phone:** 313-916-4060; **Board Cert:** Dermatology 2005; Clinical & Laboratory Dematologic Immunology 1985; **Med School:** SUNY Downstate 1975; **Resid:** Dermatology, NYU Med Ctr 1979; **Fellow:** Immunological Dermatology, NYU Med Ctr 1980; **Fac Appt:** Prof Path, Wayne State Univ

Lowe, Lori MD [D] - **Spec Exp:** Dermatopathology; Skin Cancer; **Hospital:** Univ Michigan Hlth Sys; **Address:** Univ Michigan Dept Pathology, 1301 Catherine Rd, M3261-Med Sci I, Ann Arbor, MI 48109-0602; **Phone:** 734-764-4460; **Board Cert:** Dermatology 1990; Dermatopathology 1991; **Med School:** Univ Tex, Houston 1985; **Resid:** Dermatology, Univ Tex Hlth Sci Ctr 1990; **Fellow:** Dermatopathology, Univ Colo Hlth Sci Ctr 1991; **Fac Appt:** Prof D, Univ Mich Med Sch

Neuburg, Marcelle MD [D] - **Spec Exp:** Mohs' Surgery; Skin Cancer; **Hospital:** Froedtert Meml Lutheran Hosp; **Address:** Dept Dermatology, 9200 W Wisconsin Ave, Milwaukee, WI 53226; **Phone:** 414-805-5300; **Board Cert:** Internal Medicine 1985; Dermatology 1988; **Med School:** Oregon Hlth Sci Univ 1982; **Resid:** Internal Medicine, Georgetown Univ Hosp 1985; Dermatology, Boston Univ Sch Med Ctr 1988; **Fellow:** Mohs Surgery, Tufts New England Med Ctr 1990; **Fac Appt:** Assoc Prof D, Med Coll Wisc

Otley, Clark C MD [D] - **Spec Exp:** Mohs' Surgery; Skin Cancer; Skin Cancer in Transplant Patients; **Hospital:** Mayo Med Ctr & Clin - Rochester; **Address:** Mayo Clinic, 200 1st St SW, Rochester, MN 55905; **Phone:** 507-284-3579; **Board Cert:** Dermatology 2004; **Med School:** Duke Univ 1991; **Resid:** Dermatology, Mass Genl Hosp 1995; **Fellow:** Dermatologic Surgery, Mayo Clinic 1996; **Fac Appt:** Assoc Prof D, Mayo Med Sch

Wood, Gary S MD [D] - **Spec Exp:** Cutaneous Lymphoma; Melanoma; Skin Cancer; **Hospital:** Univ WI Hosp & Clins, VA Hospital, Madison; **Address:** Univ Wisconsin Health, Dept Dermatology, 1 S Park St Fl 7, Madison, WI 53715-1375; **Phone:** 608-287-2620; **Board Cert:** Anatomic Pathology 1983; Dermatology 1986; Dermatopathology 1987; **Med School:** Univ IL Coll Med 1979; **Resid:** Anatomic Pathology, Stanford Univ Med Ctr 1983; Dermatology, Stanford Univ Med Ctr 1985; **Fellow:** Immunopathology, Stanford Univ Med Ctr 1981; **Fac Appt:** Prof D, Univ Wisc

Great Plains and Mountains

Bowen, Glen M MD [D] - **Spec Exp:** Melanoma; Cutaneous Lymphoma; Clinical Trials; Mohs' Surgery; **Hospital:** Univ Utah Hosps and Clins, Cottonwood Hosp & Med Ctr; **Address:** Huntsman Cancer Inst, 500 N Medical Drive, 4B454-SOM, Salt Lake City, UT 84132; **Phone:** 801-585-0197; **Board Cert:** Dermatology 1995; **Med School:** Univ Utah 1990; **Resid:** Dermatology, Univ Michigan Med Ctr 1993; **Fellow:** Immunological Dermatology, Univ Michigan Med Ctr 1995; Mohs Surgery, Univ Utah 2001; **Fac Appt:** Asst Prof D, Univ Utah

Southwest

Butler, David F MD [D] - **Spec Exp:** Skin Cancer; **Hospital:** Scott & White Mem Hosp; **Address:** Scott White Meml Hosp, Dept Dermatology, 409 W Adams St, Temple, TX 76501; **Phone:** 254-742-3724; **Board Cert:** Dermatology 1985; **Med School:** Univ Tex Med Br, Galveston 1980; **Resid:** Dermatology, Walter Reed Army Med Ctr 1985; **Fac Appt:** Assoc Prof D, Texas Tech Univ

Carney, John M MD [D] - **Spec Exp:** Mohs' Surgery; Skin Cancer; **Hospital:** UAMS Med Ctr; **Address:** Southwest Med Arts Bldg, 11321 Interstate 30, Ste 201, Little Rock, AR 72209; **Phone:** 501-455-4700; **Board Cert:** Dermatology 1984; **Med School:** Northwestern Univ 1979; **Resid:** Dermatology, Univ Hosps 1984; **Fellow:** Physiology, Harvard Med Sch 1985; Dermatologic Surgery, Univ Tenn Med Ctr 1986; **Fac Appt:** Clin Prof D, Univ Ark

Dermatology

Duvic, Madeleine MD [D] - **Spec Exp:** Cutaneous Lymphoma; Skin Cancer; **Hospital:** UT MD Anderson Cancer Ctr (page 81); **Address:** MD Anderson Cancer Ctr, Dept Dermatology, 1515 Holcombe Blvd, Unit 434, Houston, TX 77030; **Phone:** 713-745-1113; **Board Cert:** Dermatology 1981; Internal Medicine 1982; **Med School:** Duke Univ 1977; **Resid:** Dermatology, Duke Univ Med Ctr 1980; Internal Medicine, Duke Univ Med Ctr 1982; **Fellow:** Geriatric Medicine, Duke Univ Med Ctr 1984; **Fac Appt:** Prof D, Univ Tex, Houston

Horn, Thomas D MD [D] - **Spec Exp:** Skin Cancer; Graft vs Host Disease; **Hospital:** UAMS Med Ctr; **Address:** UAMS, Dept Derm, 4301 W Markham Street, Slot 576, Little Rock, AR 72205; **Phone:** 501-686-5110; **Board Cert:** Dermatology 2001; Dermatopathology 1988; **Med School:** Univ VA Sch Med 1982; **Resid:** Dermatology, Univ Maryland Med Ctr 1987; **Fellow:** Dermatopathology, Johns Hopkins Hosp 1989; **Fac Appt:** Prof D, Univ Ark

Orengo, Ida F MD [D] - **Spec Exp:** Melanoma; Mohs' Surgery; **Hospital:** St Luke's Episcopal Hosp - Houston, DeBakey VA Med Ctr-Houston; **Address:** Baylor College of Medicine, 6620 Main St, Ste 1425, Houston, TX 77030; **Phone:** 713-798-6925; **Board Cert:** Dermatology 2001; **Med School:** Harvard Med Sch 1988; **Resid:** Dermatology, Baylor Coll Med 1991; **Fac Appt:** Assoc Prof D, Baylor Coll Med

Taylor, R Stan MD [D] - **Spec Exp:** Mohs' Surgery; Melanoma; Skin Cancer; **Hospital:** UT Southwestern Med Ctr - Dallas, Parkland Meml Hosp - Dallas; **Address:** Univ Tex SW Med Sch, Dept Derm, 5323 Harry Hines Blvd, MC 9192, Dallas, TX 75390-9192; **Phone:** 214-645-8950; **Board Cert:** Dermatology 1989; **Med School:** Univ Tex Med Br, Galveston 1985; **Resid:** Dermatology, Univ Mich Med Ctr 1989; **Fellow:** Immunological Dermatology, Univ Mich 1990; Mohs Surgery, Oregon Hlth Sci Univ 1991; **Fac Appt:** Prof D, Univ Tex SW, Dallas

Wheeland, Ronald MD [D] - **Spec Exp:** Skin Laser Surgery; Mohs' Surgery; **Hospital:** Univ Med Ctr - Tucson; **Address:** Univ Arizona, Sect Dermatology, 535 N Wilmot, Ste 101, Tucson, AZ 85711; **Phone:** 520-694-8888; **Board Cert:** Dermatology 1977; Dermatopathology 1978; **Med School:** Univ Ariz Coll Med 1973; **Resid:** Dermatology, Univ Ok Hlth Sci Ctr 1977; **Fellow:** Dermatopathology, Univ Ok Hlth Sci Ctr 1978; Dermatologic Surgery, Cleveland Clin Fnd 1984; **Fac Appt:** Prof D, Univ Ariz Coll Med

West Coast and Pacific

Bennett, Richard G MD [D] - **Spec Exp:** Mohs' Surgery; Skin Cancer; **Hospital:** UCLA Med Ctr (page 83), USC Univ Hosp - R K Eamer Med Plz; **Address:** 1301 20th St, Ste 570, Santa Monica, CA 90404-2080; **Phone:** 310-315-0171; **Board Cert:** Dermatology 1975; **Med School:** Case West Res Univ 1970; **Resid:** Dermatology, Hosp Univ Penn 1974; **Fellow:** Chemosurgery, NYU Med Ctr 1977; **Fac Appt:** Clin Prof D, UCLA

Berg, Daniel MD [D] - **Spec Exp:** Skin Laser Surgery; Skin Cancer; **Hospital:** Univ Wash Med Ctr; **Address:** 4225 Roosevelt Way NE, Seattle, WA 98105; **Phone:** 206-598-6647; **Board Cert:** Dermatology 1999; **Med School:** Univ Toronto 1985; **Resid:** Internal Medicine, Sunnybrook Med Ctr 1988; Dermatology, Duke Univ Med Ctr 1991; **Fellow:** Dermatologic Surgery, Univ Toronto 1993; Dermatologic Surgery, Univ British Columbia 1994; **Fac Appt:** Prof D, Univ Wash

Conant, Marcus A MD [D] - **Spec Exp:** AIDS/HIV-Kaposi's Sarcoma; **Hospital:** UCSF Med Ctr, CA Pacific Med Ctr; **Address:** 470 Castro St, Ste 202, San Francisco, CA 94114; **Phone:** 415-575-7500; **Board Cert:** Dermatology 1969; **Med School:** Duke Univ 1961; **Resid:** Dermatology, UCSF Med Ctr 1967; **Fac Appt:** Clin Prof D, UCSF

Glogau, Richard G MD [D] - **Spec Exp:** Skin Laser Surgery; Mohs' Surgery; **Hospital:** UCSF Med Ctr; **Address:** 350 Parnassus Ave, Ste 400, San Francisco, CA 94117; **Phone:** 415-564-1261; **Board Cert:** Dermatology 1978; Dermatopathology 1982; **Med School:** Harvard Med Sch 1973; **Resid:** Dermatology, UCSF Med Ctr 1977; **Fellow:** Chemosurgery, UCSF Med Ctr 1978; **Fac Appt:** Clin Prof D, UCSF

Greenway, Hubert T MD [D] - **Spec Exp:** Skin Cancer; Mohs' Surgery; Melanoma; **Hospital:** Scripps Green Hosp; **Address:** Scripps Clinic, Dept Mohs' Surgery, 10666 N Torrey Pines Rd, MS 112A, La Jolla, CA 92037; **Phone:** 858-554-8646; **Board Cert:** Dermatology 1982; **Med School:** Med Coll GA 1974; **Resid:** Dermatology, Naval Hosp 1982; **Fellow:** Chemosurgery, Univ Wisconsin Med Ctr 1983

Kim, Youn-Hee MD [D] - **Spec Exp:** Cutaneous Lymphoma; Skin Cancer; **Hospital:** Stanford Univ Med Ctr; **Address:** 900 Blake Wilbur Drive, rm W0010, MC 5334, Stanford Univ Med Ctr, Dept Dermatology, Stanford, CA 94305-5334; **Phone:** 650-723-6316; **Board Cert:** Dermatology 1989; **Med School:** Stanford Univ 1985; **Resid:** Dermatology, Metropolitan Hospital 1989

Swanson, Neil MD [D] - **Spec Exp:** Skin Cancer; **Hospital:** OR Hlth & Sci Univ, VA Medical Center - Portland; **Address:** Oregon HSU, Center for Health & Healing, 3303 SW Bond Ave, CH16D, Portland, OR 97239; **Phone:** 503-418-3376; **Board Cert:** Dermatology 1980; **Med School:** Univ Rochester 1976; **Resid:** Dermatology, Univ Michigan Med Ctr 1979; **Fellow:** Dermatology, UCSF Med Ctr 1980; **Fac Appt:** Prof D, Oregon Hlth Sci Univ

Swetter, Susan M MD [D] - **Spec Exp:** Melanoma; Melanoma Early Detection/Prevention; Skin Cancer; **Hospital:** VA Hlth Care Sys - Palo Alto, Stanford Univ Med Ctr; **Address:** Stanford U Medical Ctr, Dept Dermatology, 900 Blake Wilbur Dr, W0069, Stanford, CA 94305; **Phone:** 650-852-3494; **Board Cert:** Dermatology 2001; **Med School:** Univ Pennsylvania 1990; **Resid:** Dermatology, Stanford U Med Ctr 1994; **Fac Appt:** Assoc Prof D, Stanford Univ

Tabak, Brian MD [D] - **Spec Exp:** Skin Cancer; **Hospital:** Long Beach Meml Med Ctr; **Address:** 3918 Long Beach Blvd, Ste 200, Long Beach, CA 90807; **Phone:** 562-989-5512; **Board Cert:** Dermatology 1981; **Med School:** McGill Univ 1977; **Resid:** Dermatology, USC Med Ctr 1981; **Fac Appt:** Asst Clin Prof Med, USC Sch Med

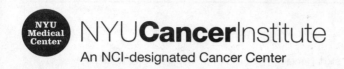

NYU**Cancer**Institute
An NCI-designated Cancer Center

NYU Clinical Cancer Center
160 East 34th Street
New York, New York 10016
www.nyuci.org/atcd

NYU Medical Center
550 First Avenue
(at 31st Street)
New York, New York 10016
www.nyumc.org/atcd

Stephen D. Hassenfeld
Children's Center
for Cancer and Blood
Disorders
160 East 32nd Street
New York, New York 10016
www.nyumc.org/hassenfeld

A Collaborative Approach
The NYU Cancer Institute, an NCI designated center, is a "matrix cancer center" without walls operating within the larger NYU Medical Center. With over 200 members and a research funding base of over $81 million, this structure strengthens our capabilities to forge collaborations across medical and scientific disciplines, which translates to comprehensive care for our patients and discoveries that will influence the future of this disease.

Renowned Expertise
Our highly skilled Magnet™ nursing team not only plays a pivotal role in coordinating direct patient care, but is also a source of invaluable patient education. Team members' compassion and expertise help patients better manage the symptoms of their disease as well as their special needs.

A Patient-Focused Setting
The NYU Clinical Cancer Center, with over 70 faculty members from various disciplines at the New York University School of Medicine, is the principal outpatient facility of the Cancer Institute and serves as home for our patients and their caregivers. The center and its multidisciplinary team of experts provide access to the latest treatment options and clinical trials along with a variety of programs in cancer prevention, screening, diagnostics, genetic counseling, and supportive services. When it comes to kids and cancer, the Stephen D. Hassenfeld Children's Center for Cancer and Blood Disorders offers not just innovation but insight. As a leading member of the NCI-sponsored Children's Oncology Group, our physicians are known for developing new ways to treat childhood cancer. Our affiliation with Bellevue Hospital, the oldest public hospital in the country, affords clinically distinctive opportunities to learn and care for patients with cancer by observing its presentation and behavior in a variety of patient groups.

Endocrinology

a subspecialty of Internal Medicine

An internist who concentrates on disorders of the internal
(endocrine) glands such as the thyroid and adrenal glands. This
specialist also deals with disorders such as diabetes, metabolic and
nutritional disorders, pituitary diseases, menstrual and
sexual problems.

Training Required: Three years in internal medicine *plus* additional
training and examination for certification in endocrinology,
diabetes, and metabolism.

Endocrinology, Diabetes & Metabolism

New England

Levine, Robert A MD [EDM] - **Spec Exp:** Thyroid Cancer; Thyroid Disorders; **Hospital:** St Joseph Hosp; **Address:** Thyroid Center of New Hampshire, 5 Coliseum Ave, Nashua, NH 03060; **Phone:** 603-881-7141; **Board Cert:** Internal Medicine 1984; Endocrinology, Diabetes & Metabolism 1987; **Med School:** Univ Conn 1981; **Resid:** Internal Medicine, Mt Auburn Hosp 1984; **Fellow:** Endocrinology, Yale Univ 1987

Mid Atlantic

Ball, Douglas W MD [EDM] - **Spec Exp:** Thyroid Cancer; **Hospital:** Johns Hopkins Hosp - Baltimore; **Address:** Sidney Kimmel Cancer Ctr, 1830 E Monument St, Ste 333, Baltimore, MD 21287; **Phone:** 410-955-8964; **Board Cert:** Internal Medicine 1987; **Med School:** Geo Wash Univ 1984; **Resid:** Internal Medicine, Univ Pittsburgh 1987; **Fellow:** Endocrinology, Diabetes & Metabolism, Johns Hopkins Hosp 1991; **Fac Appt:** Assoc Prof Med, Johns Hopkins Univ

Ladenson, Paul W MD [EDM] - **Spec Exp:** Thyroid Disorders; Thyroid Cancer; **Hospital:** Johns Hopkins Hosp - Baltimore; **Address:** Johns Hopkins-Div Endocrinology & Metabolism, 1830 E Monument St, rm 333, Baltimore, MD 21287; **Phone:** 410-955-3663; **Board Cert:** Internal Medicine 1978; Endocrinology, Diabetes & Metabolism 1981; **Med School:** Harvard Med Sch 1975; **Resid:** Internal Medicine, Mass Genl Hosp 1978; **Fellow:** Endocrinology, Diabetes & Metabolism, Mass Genl Hosp 1980; **Fac Appt:** Prof Med, Johns Hopkins Univ

Snyder, Peter J MD [EDM] - **Spec Exp:** Pituitary Tumors; **Hospital:** Hosp Univ Penn - UPHS (page 84); **Address:** Univ Pennsylvania Med Group, 3400 Spruce St, Philadelphia, PA 19104; **Phone:** 215-898-0208; **Board Cert:** Internal Medicine 1972; Endocrinology, Diabetes & Metabolism 1972; **Med School:** Harvard Med Sch 1965; **Resid:** Internal Medicine, Beth Israel Hosp 1967; Internal Medicine, Beth Israel Hosp 1970; **Fellow:** Endocrinology, Diabetes & Metabolism, Hosp Univ Penn 1971; **Fac Appt:** Prof Med, Univ Pennsylvania

Tuttle, Robert Michael MD [EDM] - **Spec Exp:** Thyroid Cancer; Nuclear Medicine; **Hospital:** Meml Sloan Kettering Cancer Ctr (page 76); **Address:** Memorial Sloane Kettering Cancer Ctr, 1275 York St, Box 419, New York, NY 10021; **Phone:** 212-639-6042; **Board Cert:** Endocrinology, Diabetes & Metabolism 2004; **Med School:** Univ Louisville Sch Med 1987; **Resid:** Internal Medicine, DD Eisenhower Army Med Ctr 1990; **Fellow:** Endocrinology, Diabetes & Metabolism, Madigan Army Med Ctr 1993; **Fac Appt:** Assoc Prof Med, Cornell Univ-Weill Med Coll

Wartofsky, Leonard MD [EDM] - **Spec Exp:** Thyroid Cancer; Thyroid Disorders; **Hospital:** Washington Hosp Ctr; **Address:** 110 Irving St NW, Ste 2A62, Washington, DC 20010-2975; **Phone:** 202-877-3109; **Board Cert:** Internal Medicine 1971; Endocrinology, Diabetes & Metabolism 1972; **Med School:** Geo Wash Univ 1964; **Resid:** Internal Medicine, Barnes Hosp 1966; Internal Medicine, Bronx Muni Hosp Ctr 1967; **Fellow:** Endocrinology, Diabetes & Metabolism, Boston City Hosp 1969; **Fac Appt:** Prof Med, Georgetown Univ

Southeast

Ain, Kenneth B MD [EDM] - **Spec Exp:** Thyroid Cancer; Thyroid Disorders; **Hospital:** Univ of Kentucky Chandler Hosp, VA Med Ctr - Lexington; **Address:** Markey Cancer Center, 800 Rose St, rm CC455, Lexington, KY 40536; **Phone:** 859-323-3778; **Board Cert:** Internal Medicine 1984; Endocrinology, Diabetes & Metabolism 1987; **Med School:** Brown Univ 1981; **Resid:** Internal Medicine, Hahnemann Univ 1984; **Fellow:** Endocrinology, Univ Chicago 1986; Thyroid Oncology, NIDDK, Natl Inst Hlth 1990; **Fac Appt:** Prof Med, Univ KY Coll Med

Earp III, H Shelton MD [EDM] - **Spec Exp:** Cancer-Hormonal Influences; **Hospital:** Univ NC Hosps; **Address:** UNC Lineberger Comprehensive Cancer Center, 102 Mason Farm Rd, CB 7295, Chapel Hill, NC 27599-7295; **Phone:** 919-966-3036; **Board Cert:** Internal Medicine 1976; Endocrinology, Diabetes & Metabolism 1977; **Med School:** Univ NC Sch Med 1970; **Resid:** Internal Medicine, NC Memorial Hosp 1975; **Fellow:** Endocrinology, Diabetes & Metabolism, Univ North Carolina Hosp 1977; **Fac Appt:** Prof Med, Univ NC Sch Med

Koch, Christian A MD [EDM] - **Spec Exp:** Endocrine Cancers; Thyroid Cancer; **Hospital:** Univ Hosps & Clins - Jackson; **Address:** 2500 N State St, Jackson, MS 39216; **Phone:** 601-984-5525; **Board Cert:** Internal Medicine 1999; Endocrinology, Diabetes & Metabolism 2000; **Med School:** Germany 1991; **Resid:** Internal Medicine, Ohio State Univ Hosp 1997; **Fellow:** Endocrinology, Natl Inst Hlth 2001; **Fac Appt:** Prof Med, Univ Miss

Vance, Mary Lee MD [EDM] - **Spec Exp:** Adrenal Tumors & Disorders; **Hospital:** Univ Virginia Med Ctr; **Address:** Univ Virginia Hlth Sys, PO Box 800601, Charlottesville, VA 22908-0601; **Phone:** 434-924-2284; **Board Cert:** Internal Medicine 1980; **Med School:** Louisiana State Univ 1977; **Resid:** Internal Medicine, Baylor Univ Med Ctr 1980; **Fellow:** Endocrinology, Univ Virginia Med Ctr 1983; **Fac Appt:** Prof Med, Univ VA Sch Med

Midwest

Clutter, William E MD [EDM] - **Spec Exp:** Endocrine Cancers; **Hospital:** Barnes-Jewish Hosp; **Address:** Barnes Jewish Hosp, Dept Internal Medicine, 4921 Parkview Pl Fl 5 - Ste B, St Louis, MO 63110; **Phone:** 314-362-3500; **Board Cert:** Internal Medicine 1978; Endocrinology, Diabetes & Metabolism 1981; **Med School:** Ohio State Univ 1975; **Resid:** Internal Medicine, Barnes Jewish Hosp 1978; **Fellow:** Endocrinology, Diabetes & Metabolism, Barnes Jewish Hosp 1980; **Fac Appt:** Prof Med, Washington Univ, St Louis

Kloos, Richard MD [EDM] - **Spec Exp:** Thyroid Cancer; **Hospital:** Ohio St Univ Med Ctr; **Address:** 446 McCampbell Hall, 1581 Dodd Drive, Columbus, OH 43210; **Phone:** 614-292-3800; **Board Cert:** Nuclear Medicine 2005; Internal Medicine 2002; Endocrinology, Diabetes & Metabolism 2005; **Med School:** Case West Res Univ 1989; **Resid:** Internal Medicine, MetroHealth MC 1992; **Fellow:** Endocrinology, Diabetes & Metabolism, Univ Michigan 1995; Nuclear Medicine, Univ Michigan 1996; **Fac Appt:** Assoc Prof Med, Ohio State Univ

Kopp, Peter A MD [EDM] - **Spec Exp:** Thyroid Cancer; **Hospital:** Northwestern Meml Hosp; **Address:** Northwestern Meml Hospital, 675 N St Clair St, Ste 14-100, Chicago, IL 60611; **Phone:** 312-695-7970; **Board Cert:** Internal Medicine 2003; Endocrinology, Diabetes & Metabolism 2004; **Med School:** Switzerland 1985; **Resid:** Internal Medicine, Regl Hosp 1992; Endocrinology, Diabetes & Metabolism, Univ Berne 1990; **Fellow:** Endocrinology, Diabetes & Metabolism, Northwestern Univ Hosp 1997; **Fac Appt:** Assoc Prof Med, Northwestern Univ-Feinberg Sch Med

Endocrinology

Great Plains and Mountains

Ridgway, E Chester MD [EDM] - **Spec Exp:** Thyroid Cancer; **Hospital:** Univ Colorado Hosp, VA Med Ctr; **Address:** UCHSC at Fitzsimons, Endocrinology, 1635 N Ursula St, Box 6510, MS F732, Aurora, CO 80045; **Phone:** 720-848-2650; **Board Cert:** Internal Medicine 1972; Endocrinology 1973; **Med School:** Univ Colorado 1968; **Resid:** Internal Medicine, Mass Genl Hosp 1970; **Fellow:** Endocrinology, Mass Genl Hosp 1972; **Fac Appt:** Prof Med, Univ Colorado

Southwest

Gagel, Robert F MD [EDM] - **Spec Exp:** Thyroid Cancer; **Hospital:** UT MD Anderson Cancer Ctr (page 81); **Address:** MD Anderson Cancer Ctr, 1515 Holcombe Blvd, Unit 433, Houston, TX 77030; **Phone:** 713-792-6517; **Board Cert:** Internal Medicine 1975; Endocrinology 1977; **Med School:** Ohio State Univ 1971; **Resid:** Internal Medicine, New England Med Ctr 1973; **Fellow:** Endocrinology, New England Med Ctr 1975; Research, Harvard Med Sch 1981; **Fac Appt:** Prof Med, Univ Tex, Houston

Robbins, Richard MD [EDM] - **Spec Exp:** Thyroid Cancer; Pituitary Tumors; **Hospital:** Methodist Hosp - Houston; **Address:** The Methodist Hosp, 6550 Fannin St, Ste 10001, Houston, TX 77030; **Phone:** 713-441-6640; **Board Cert:** Internal Medicine 1978; Endocrinology, Diabetes & Metabolism 1983; **Med School:** Creighton Univ 1975; **Resid:** Internal Medicine, New York Hosp-Cornell Med Ctr 1978; **Fellow:** Endocrinology, New England Med Ctr 1981; **Fac Appt:** Prof Med, Cornell Univ-Weill Med Coll

Rubenfeld, Sheldon MD [EDM] - **Spec Exp:** Thyroid Cancer; **Hospital:** St Luke's Episcopal Hosp - Houston, Methodist Hosp - Houston; **Address:** 7515 S Main St, Ste 690, Houston, TX 77030; **Phone:** 713-795-5750; **Board Cert:** Internal Medicine 1976; Endocrinology, Diabetes & Metabolism 1979; **Med School:** Georgetown Univ 1971; **Resid:** Internal Medicine, Baylor Affil Hosps 1976; **Fellow:** Endocrinology, Baylor Affil Hosps 1978; **Fac Appt:** Clin Prof Med, Baylor Coll Med

Sherman, Steven I MD [EDM] - **Spec Exp:** Thyroid Cancer; Endocrine Cancers; **Hospital:** UT MD Anderson Cancer Ctr (page 81); **Address:** MD Anderson Cancer Ctr, 1515 Holcombe Blvd, Unit 435, Houston, TX 77030; **Phone:** 713-792-2840; **Board Cert:** Internal Medicine 1988; **Med School:** Johns Hopkins Univ 1985; **Resid:** Internal Medicine, Johns Hopkins Hosp 1988; **Fellow:** Endocrinology, Diabetes & Metabolism, Johns Hopkins Hosp 1991

Waguespack, Steven G MD [EDM] - **Spec Exp:** Thyroid Cancer; Pituitary Tumors; Adrenal Tumors & Disorders; **Hospital:** UT MD Anderson Cancer Ctr (page 81); **Address:** MD Anderson Cancer Ctr, Dept Endocrine Neoplasia, 1400 Holcombe Blvd, Unit 435, Houston, TX 77030; **Phone:** 713-563-4400; **Board Cert:** Internal Medicine 1998; Pediatrics 1999; Endocrinology, Diabetes & Metabolism 2002; Pediatric Endocrinology 2003; **Med School:** Univ Tex, Houston 1994; **Resid:** Internal Medicine & Pediatrics, Indiana Univ Hosp 1998; **Fellow:** Endocrinology, Indiana Univ 2002; **Fac Appt:** Asst Prof Med, Univ Tex, Houston

West Coast and Pacific

Chait, Alan MD [EDM] - **Spec Exp:** Nutrition & Cancer/Disease Prevention; **Hospital:** Univ Wash Med Ctr; **Address:** Univ Washington Med Ctr, 1959 NE Pacific St, Box 356166, Seattle, WA 98195; **Phone:** 206-598-4615; **Med School:** South Africa 1967; **Resid:** Internal Medicine, Hammersmith Hosp 1971; **Fellow:** Endocrinology, Diabetes & Metabolism, Hammersmith Hosp 1973; Endocrinology, Diabetes & Metabolism, Univ Washington 1977; **Fac Appt:** Prof Med, Univ Wash

Darwin, Christine H MD [EDM] - **Spec Exp:** Pituitary Tumors; **Hospital:** UCLA Med Ctr (page 83); **Address:** 200 UCLA Medical Plaza, Ste 365 C1, Box 951693, Los Angeles, CA 90095-7065; **Phone:** 310-794-5584; **Board Cert:** Geriatric Medicine 1994; Endocrinology, Diabetes & Metabolism 1997; **Med School:** India 1980; **Resid:** Internal Medicine, UC Irvine Med Ctr 1987; **Fellow:** Endocrinology, VA Hosp 1988; Endocrinology, USC Med Ctr 1993; **Fac Appt:** Assoc Prof Med, UCLA

Fitzgerald, Paul Anthony MD [EDM] - **Spec Exp:** Thyroid Cancer; Pituitary Tumors; Adrenal Tumors & Disorders; **Hospital:** UCSF Med Ctr; **Address:** 350 Parnassus Ave, Ste 710, San Francisco, CA 94117; **Phone:** 415-665-1136; **Board Cert:** Internal Medicine 1975; Endocrinology, Diabetes & Metabolism 1981; **Med School:** Jefferson Med Coll 1972; **Resid:** Internal Medicine, Presby Med Ctr-Univ Colo 1975; **Fellow:** Endocrinology, Diabetes & Metabolism, UCSF Med Ctr 1978; **Fac Appt:** Clin Prof Med, UCSF

Heber, David MD [EDM] - **Spec Exp:** Nutrition & Cancer Prevention; Nutrition & Disease Prevention/Control; **Hospital:** UCLA Med Ctr (page 83); **Address:** 900 Veteran Ave, Rm 12-217, UCLA Center for Human Nutrition, Los Angeles, CA 90095-1742; **Phone:** 310-206-1987; **Board Cert:** Internal Medicine 1976; Endocrinology, Diabetes & Metabolism 1977; **Med School:** Harvard Med Sch 1973; **Resid:** Internal Medicine, LA Co Harbor Genl Hosp 1975; **Fellow:** Endocrinology, Diabetes & Metabolism, LA Co Harbor Genl Hosp 1978; **Fac Appt:** Prof Med, UCLA

Hoffman, Andrew R MD [EDM] - **Spec Exp:** Pituitary Tumors; **Hospital:** Stanford Univ Med Ctr, VA Hlth Care Sys - Palo Alto; **Address:** 300 Pastur Drive Boswell Bldg - rm A-175, Stanford, CA 94305; **Phone:** 650-723-6961; **Board Cert:** Internal Medicine 1979; Endocrinology 1981; **Med School:** Stanford Univ 1976; **Resid:** Internal Medicine, Mass Genl Hosp 1978; **Fellow:** Pharmacology, Mass Genl Hosp 1980; Endocrinology, Diabetes & Metabolism, Mass Genl Hosp 1982; **Fac Appt:** Prof Med, Stanford Univ

Kandeel, Fouad MD/PhD [EDM] - **Spec Exp:** Thyroid Cancer; Endocrine Cancers; **Hospital:** City of Hope Natl Med Ctr & Beckman Rsch (page 69); **Address:** City of Hope Cancer Ctr, 1500 E Duarte Rd, Duarte, CA 91010; **Phone:** 626-256-4673 x62251; **Med School:** Egypt 1969; **Fac Appt:** Assoc Clin Prof Med, UCLA

Melmed, Shlomo MD [EDM] - **Spec Exp:** Pituitary Tumors; **Hospital:** Cedars-Sinai Med Ctr; **Address:** Cedars Sinai Med Ctr, 8700 Beverly Blvd, Ste 2015, Los Angeles, CA 90048; **Phone:** 310-423-4691; **Board Cert:** Internal Medicine 1979; Endocrinology, Diabetes & Metabolism 1983; **Med School:** South Africa 1970; **Resid:** Internal Medicine, Sheba Med Ctr 1976; **Fellow:** Endocrinology, Diabetes & Metabolism, Wadsworth VA Hosp 1980; **Fac Appt:** Prof Med, UCLA

Gastroenterology

a subspecialty of Internal Medicine

An internist who specializes in diagnosis and treatment of diseases of the digestive organs including the stomach, bowels, liver, and gallbladder. This specialist treats conditions such as abdominal pain, ulcers, diarrhea, cancer and jaundice and performs complex diagnostic and therapeutic procedures using endoscopes to see internal organs.

Training Required: Three years in internal medicine plus additional training and examination for certification in gastroenterology.

Gastroenterology

New England

Levine, Joel B MD [Ge] - **Spec Exp:** Colon & Rectal Cancer Detection; Colonoscopy; **Hospital:** Univ of Conn Hlth Ctr, John Dempsey Hosp; **Address:** Univ Connecticut, Colon Cancer Prevention Program, 263 Farmington Ave, Farmington, CT 06030-2813; **Phone:** 860-679-4567; **Board Cert:** Internal Medicine 1973; Gastroenterology 1977; **Med School:** SUNY Downstate 1969; **Resid:** Internal Medicine, Univ Chicago Hosps 1971; Internal Medicine, Mass Genl Hosp 1974; **Fellow:** Gastroenterology, Mass Genl Hosp 1977; **Fac Appt:** Prof Med, Univ Conn

Mason, Joel B MD [Ge] - **Spec Exp:** Nutrition & Cancer Prevention; **Hospital:** Tufts-New England Med Ctr; **Address:** Tufts-New England Med Ctr, Dept Gastro, 750 Washington St, Boston, MA 02111; **Phone:** 617-636-1621; **Board Cert:** Internal Medicine 1984; Gastroenterology 1987; **Med School:** Univ Chicago-Pritzker Sch Med 1981; **Resid:** Internal Medicine, Univ Iowa Hosps 1984; **Fellow:** Gastroenterology, Univ Chicago Hosps 1986; Nutrition, Univ Chicago Hosps 1986; **Fac Appt:** Assoc Prof Med, Tufts Univ

Mid Atlantic

Gerdes, Hans MD [Ge] - **Spec Exp:** Endoscopy; Endoscopic Ultrasound; Barrett's Esophagus; Gastrointestinal Cancer; **Hospital:** Meml Sloan Kettering Cancer Ctr (page 76); **Address:** 1275 York Ave, rm Howard 504, New York, NY 10021-6007; **Phone:** 212-639-7108; **Board Cert:** Internal Medicine 1987; Gastroenterology 1989; **Med School:** Cornell Univ-Weill Med Coll 1983; **Resid:** Internal Medicine, New York Hosp 1986; **Fellow:** Gastroenterology, Meml Sloan Kettering Cancer Ctr 1989

Goggins, Michael MD [Ge] - **Spec Exp:** Pancreatic Cancer-Early Detection; **Hospital:** Johns Hopkins Hosp - Baltimore; **Address:** Johns Hopkins Univ Sch Med, Dept Med-GE, 1550 Orleans St CRB-2 Bldg - rm 341, Baltimore, MD 21231; **Phone:** 410-955-3511; **Med School:** Ireland 1988; **Resid:** Internal Medicine, St Jame's Hosp 1990; **Fellow:** Gastroenterology, St Jame's Hosp 1992; **Fac Appt:** Assoc Prof Med, Johns Hopkins Univ

Greenwald, Bruce D MD [Ge] - **Spec Exp:** Endoscopic Ultrasound; Barrett's Esophagus; Esophageal Cancer/Dysplasia; Gastroesophageal Reflux Disease (GERD); **Hospital:** Univ of MD Med Sys; **Address:** Univ of Maryland Hosp, Gastroenterology, 22 S Greene St Fl 3 - rm N3W62, Baltimore, MD 21201-1595; **Phone:** 410-328-8731; **Board Cert:** Internal Medicine 2000; Gastroenterology 2000; **Med School:** Univ MD Sch Med 1987; **Resid:** Internal Medicine, Univ of Virginia Hosp 1990; **Fellow:** Gastroenterology, Univ of Maryland Hosp 1992; **Fac Appt:** Assoc Prof Med, Univ MD Sch Med

Haluszka, Oleh MD [Ge] - **Spec Exp:** Pancreatic/Biliary Endoscopy (ERCP); Gastrointestinal Cancer; Endoscopic Ultrasound; Endoscopy; **Hospital:** Fox Chase Cancer Ctr (page 73); **Address:** Fox Chase Cancer Ctr, 333 Cottman Ave, Ste C307, Philadelphia, PA 19111; **Phone:** 215-214-1424; **Board Cert:** Internal Medicine 1987; Gastroenterology 2001; **Med School:** Uniformed Srvs Univ, Bethesda 1982; **Resid:** Internal Medicine, US Naval Hosp 1987; **Fellow:** Gastroenterology, US Naval Hosp 1990; Endoscopy, Med Coll Wisconsin 1993; **Fac Appt:** Assoc Clin Prof Med, Temple Univ

Itzkowitz, Steven H MD [Ge] - **Spec Exp:** Colon & Rectal Cancer; Colon & Rectal Cancer Detection; **Hospital:** Mount Sinai Med Ctr (page 77); **Address:** 5 E 98th St, Box 1625, New York, NY 10029; **Phone:** 212-241-4299; **Board Cert:** Internal Medicine 1982; Gastroenterology 1985; **Med School:** Mount Sinai Sch Med 1979; **Resid:** Internal Medicine, Bellevue Hosp/ NYU Med Ctr 1982; **Fellow:** Gastroenterology, UCSF Med Ctr 1984; **Fac Appt:** Prof Med, Mount Sinai Sch Med

Kurtz, Robert C MD [Ge] - **Spec Exp:** Gastrointestinal Cancer; Pancreatic Cancer; Endoscopy; Nutrition & Cancer Prevention/Control; **Hospital:** Meml Sloan Kettering Cancer Ctr (page 76); **Address:** Meml Sloan Kettering Cancer Ctr, 1275 York Ave, rm H510, New York, NY 10021-6007; **Phone:** 212-639-7620; **Board Cert:** Internal Medicine 1971; Gastroenterology 1977; **Med School:** Jefferson Med Coll 1968; **Resid:** Internal Medicine, NY Hosp/Meml Sloan Kettering Cancer Ctr 1971; **Fellow:** Gastroenterology, Meml Sloan Kettering Cancer Ctr 1973; **Fac Appt:** Prof Med, Cornell Univ-Weill Med Coll

Lightdale, Charles MD [Ge] - **Spec Exp:** Barrett's Esophagus; Gastrointestinal Cancer; Endoscopic Ultrasound; **Hospital:** NY-Presby Hosp (page 79); **Address:** Columbia-Presby Med Ctr, Irving Pavilion, 161 Fort Washington Ave, rm 812, New York, NY 10032-3713; **Phone:** 212-305-3423; **Board Cert:** Internal Medicine 1972; Gastroenterology 1973; **Med School:** Columbia P&S 1966; **Resid:** Internal Medicine, Yale-New Haven Hosp 1968; Internal Medicine, New York Hosp 1969; **Fellow:** Gastroenterology, New York Hosp-Cornell 1973; **Fac Appt:** Prof Med, Columbia P&S

Lipshutz, William H MD [Ge] - **Spec Exp:** Colon Cancer; Esophageal Disorders; **Hospital:** Pennsylvania Hosp (page 84); **Address:** 230 W Washington Sq, Farm Journal Bldg, Fl 4, Philadelphia, PA 19106; **Phone:** 215-829-3561; **Board Cert:** Internal Medicine 1972; Gastroenterology 1973; **Med School:** Univ Pennsylvania 1967; **Resid:** Internal Medicine, Pennsylvania Hosp 1972; **Fellow:** Gastroenterology, Hosp Univ Penn 1971; **Fac Appt:** Clin Prof Med, Univ Pennsylvania

Pochapin, Mark B MD [Ge] - **Spec Exp:** Pancreatic Cancer; Endoscopic Ultrasound; Colon & Rectal Cancer Detection; Colon Cancer; **Hospital:** NY-Presby Hosp (page 79); **Address:** The Jay Monahan Ctr for GI Hlth, 1315 York Ave, New York, NY 10022; **Phone:** 212-746-4014; **Board Cert:** Gastroenterology 2004; **Med School:** Cornell Univ-Weill Med Coll 1988; **Resid:** Internal Medicine, NY Hosp-Cornell Med Ctr 1991; **Fellow:** Gastroenterology, Montefiore Med Ctr 1993; **Fac Appt:** Assoc Clin Prof Med, Cornell Univ-Weill Med Coll

Shike, Moshe MD [Ge] - **Spec Exp:** Gastrointestinal Cancer; Nutrition & Cancer Prevention; Endoscopy; **Hospital:** Meml Sloan Kettering Cancer Ctr (page 76), NY-Presby Hosp (page 79); **Address:** 1275 York Ave, rm S-536, New York, NY 10021; **Phone:** 212-639-7230; **Board Cert:** Internal Medicine 1977; Gastroenterology 1981; **Med School:** Israel 1975; **Resid:** Internal Medicine, Mt Auburn Hosp 1977; **Fellow:** Gastroenterology, Toronto Genl Hosp 1981; **Fac Appt:** Prof Med, Cornell Univ-Weill Med Coll

Waye, Jerome MD [Ge] - **Spec Exp:** Endoscopy; Colon Cancer; Colonoscopy; **Hospital:** Mount Sinai Med Ctr (page 77), Lenox Hill Hosp; **Address:** 650 Park Ave, New York, NY 10021-6115; **Phone:** 212-439-7779; **Board Cert:** Internal Medicine 1965; Gastroenterology 1970; **Med School:** Boston Univ 1958; **Resid:** Internal Medicine, Mount Sinai Hosp 1961; **Fellow:** Gastroenterology, Mount Sinai Hosp 1962; **Fac Appt:** Clin Prof Med, Mount Sinai Sch Med

Gastroenterology

Winawer, Sidney J MD [Ge] - **Spec Exp:** Colonoscopy; Colon Cancer; Cancer Prevention; **Hospital:** Meml Sloan Kettering Cancer Ctr (page 76); **Address:** 1275 York Ave, Box 90, New York, NY 10021-6094; **Phone:** 212-639-7678; **Board Cert:** Internal Medicine 1965; Gastroenterology 1973; **Med School:** SUNY Downstate 1956; **Resid:** Internal Medicine, VA Hosp 1961; Internal Medicine, Maimonides Hosp 1962; **Fellow:** Gastroenterology, Boston City Hosp 1964; **Fac Appt:** Prof Med, Cornell Univ-Weill Med Coll

Southeast

Barkin, Jamie S MD [Ge] - **Spec Exp:** Gastrointestinal Cancer; Endoscopy; **Hospital:** Mount Sinai Med Ctr - Miami, Univ of Miami Hosp & Clins/Sylvester Comp Canc Ctr; **Address:** Mount Sinai Medical Center, Gumenick Bldg, 4300 Alton Rd, Ste 2522, Miami Beach, FL 33140-2800; **Phone:** 305-674-2240; **Board Cert:** Internal Medicine 1973; Gastroenterology 1975; **Med School:** Univ Miami Sch Med 1970; **Resid:** Internal Medicine, Univ Miami Hosp 1973; **Fellow:** Gastroenterology, Univ Miami Hosp 1975; **Fac Appt:** Prof Med, Univ Miami Sch Med

Boyce Jr, H Worth MD [Ge] - **Spec Exp:** Esophageal Disorders; Barrett's Esophagus; Esophageal Cancer; **Hospital:** H Lee Moffitt Cancer Ctr & Research Inst, Tampa Genl Hosp; **Address:** Ctr for Swallowing Disorders, 12901 Bruce B Downs Blvd, MDC 72, Tampa, FL 33612-4742; **Phone:** 813-974-3374; **Board Cert:** Internal Medicine 1977; Gastroenterology 1965; **Med School:** Wake Forest Univ 1955; **Resid:** Internal Medicine, Brooke Army Hosp 1959; Gastroenterology, Brooke Army Hosp 1960; **Fac Appt:** Prof Med, Univ S Fla Coll Med

Eloubeidi, Mohamad A MD [Ge] - **Spec Exp:** Gastrointestinal Cancer; Colon & Rectal Cancer; Pancreatic Cancer; Lung Cancer; **Hospital:** Univ of Ala Hosp at Birmingham; **Address:** 1530 3rd Ave S, Ste LHRB-408, Birmingham, AL 35294-0007; **Phone:** 205-934-7955; **Board Cert:** Gastroenterology 2000; **Med School:** Lebanon 1993; **Resid:** Internal Medicine, Duke Univ Med Ctr 1996; **Fellow:** Gastroenterology, Duke Univ Med Ctr 1999; Advanced Endoscopy, Med Univ South Carolina 2000; **Fac Appt:** Assoc Prof Med, Univ Ala

Hoffman, Brenda J MD [Ge] - **Spec Exp:** Endoscopic Ultrasound; Gastrointestinal Cancer; Colon & Rectal Cancer-Familial Polyposis; **Hospital:** MUSC Med Ctr; **Address:** Digestive Disease Center, 210 CSB, 96 Jonathan Lucas St, Box 250327, Charleston, SC 29425; **Phone:** 843-792-6999; **Board Cert:** Internal Medicine 1986; Gastroenterology 1989; **Med School:** Univ KY Coll Med 1983; **Resid:** Internal Medicine, MUSC Med Ctr 1987; **Fellow:** Gastroenterology, MUSC Med Ctr 1989; **Fac Appt:** Prof Med, Univ SC Sch Med

Liddle, Rodger Alan MD [Ge] - **Spec Exp:** Gastrointestinal Cancer; **Hospital:** Duke Univ Med Ctr, VA Med Ctr - Durham; **Address:** Duke University Medical Ctr, Div Gastroenterology, Box 3913, Durham, NC 27710; **Phone:** 919-681-6380; **Board Cert:** Internal Medicine 1981; Gastroenterology 1983; **Med School:** Vanderbilt Univ 1978; **Resid:** Internal Medicine, UCSF Med Ctr 1981; **Fellow:** Gastroenterology, UCSF Med Ctr 1984; **Fac Appt:** Prof Med, Duke Univ

Raiford, David S MD [Ge] - **Spec Exp:** Liver Tumors; **Hospital:** Vanderbilt Univ Med Ctr; **Address:** Vanderbilt Hepatology, 1660 The Vanderbilt Clinic, Nashville, TN 37232-5280; **Phone:** 615-322-0128; **Board Cert:** Internal Medicine 1989; Gastroenterology 2001; **Med School:** Johns Hopkins Univ 1985; **Resid:** Internal Medicine, Johns Hopkins Hosp 1988; **Fellow:** Hepatology, Johns Hopkins Hosp 1991; **Fac Appt:** Prof Med, Vanderbilt Univ

Midwest

Brown, Kimberly A MD [Ge] - **Spec Exp:** Transplant Medicine-Liver; Liver Cancer; **Hospital:** Henry Ford Hosp; **Address:** Henry Ford Hosp, Dept Gastroenterology, 2799 W Grand Blvd Bldg K Fl 7, Detroit, MI 48202-2608; **Phone:** 313-916-8632; **Board Cert:** Internal Medicine 1988; Gastroenterology 2002; **Med School:** Wayne State Univ 1985; **Resid:** Internal Medicine, Univ Michigan Med Ctr 1989; **Fellow:** Gastroenterology, Univ Michigan Med Ctr 1992

Crippin, Jeffrey S MD [Ge] - **Spec Exp:** Transplant Medicine-Liver; Gastrointestinal Cancer; **Hospital:** Barnes-Jewish Hosp; **Address:** Barnes Jewish Hosp, Div Gastroenterology, 660 S Euclid Ave Campus Box 8124, St Louis, MO 63110; **Phone:** 314-454-8160; **Board Cert:** Internal Medicine 1987; Gastroenterology 2001; **Med School:** Univ Kans 1984; **Resid:** Internal Medicine, Kansas Univ Med Ctr 1988; **Fellow:** Gastroenterology, Mayo Clinic 1991; **Fac Appt:** Assoc Prof Med, Washington Univ, St Louis

Di Bisceglie, Adrian Michael MD [Ge] - **Spec Exp:** Liver Cancer; **Hospital:** St Louis Univ Hosp; **Address:** St Louis Univ Hosp, Dept. Gastroenterology, 3635 Vista Ave, PO Box 15250, St. Louis, MO 63110-0250; **Phone:** 314-577-8764; **Board Cert:** Internal Medicine 2002; Gastroenterology 2002; **Med School:** South Africa 1977; **Resid:** Internal Medicine, Baragwanath Hosp 1984; **Fellow:** Hepatology, Natl Inst Hlth 1988; **Fac Appt:** Prof Med, St Louis Univ

Goldberg, Michael MD [Ge] - **Spec Exp:** Colon Cancer; Pancreatic/Biliary Endoscopy (ERCP); Pancreatic Cancer; **Hospital:** Evanston Hosp, Glenbrook Hosp; **Address:** 2650 Ridge Ave, Ste G-208, Evanston, IL 60201; **Phone:** 847-657-1900; **Board Cert:** Internal Medicine 1978; Gastroenterology 1981; **Med School:** Univ IL Coll Med 1975; **Resid:** Internal Medicine, Univ Illinois Hosp 1978; **Fellow:** Gastroenterology, Tufts-New England Med Ctr 1980; **Fac Appt:** Assoc Clin Prof Med, Northwestern Univ

Waxman, Irving MD [Ge] - **Spec Exp:** Gastrointestinal Cancer; Pancreatic Cancer; Endoscopy; **Hospital:** Univ of Chicago Hosps; **Address:** University of Chicago Hospitals, 5758 S Maryland Ave, MC 9028, Chicago, IL 60637; **Phone:** 773-702-1459; **Board Cert:** Internal Medicine 1988; Gastroenterology 2003; **Med School:** Mexico 1986; **Resid:** Internal Medicine, New England Deaconess Hosp 1988; **Fellow:** Gastroenterology, Georgetown Univ Med Ctr 1991; Endoscopy, Academic Med Ctr-Univ Amsterdam 1991; **Fac Appt:** Prof Med, Univ Chicago-Pritzker Sch Med

Great Plains and Mountains

Burt, Randall W MD [Ge] - **Spec Exp:** Colon Cancer; Colon & Rectal Cancer-Familial Polyposis; **Hospital:** Univ Utah Hosps and Clins; **Address:** Huntsman Cancer Institute, 2000 Circle of Hope, Salt Lake City, UT 84112; **Phone:** 801-585-3281; **Board Cert:** Internal Medicine 1977; Gastroenterology 1979; **Med School:** Univ Utah 1974; **Resid:** Internal Medicine, Barnes Hosp 1977; **Fellow:** Gastroenterology, Univ Utah Med Ctr 1979; **Fac Appt:** Prof Med, Univ Utah

Gastroenterology

Southwest

Boland, C Richard MD [Ge] - **Spec Exp:** Colon & Rectal Cancer Detection; Cancer Genetics; **Hospital:** Baylor Univ Medical Ctr; **Address:** GI Cancer Research Lab H-250, 3500 Gaston Ave, Dallas, TX 75246; **Phone:** 214-820-2692; **Board Cert:** Internal Medicine 1978; Gastroenterology 1981; **Med School:** Yale Univ 1973; **Resid:** Internal Medicine, USPHS Hosp 1978; **Fellow:** Gastroenterology, UCSF 1981; **Fac Appt:** Clin Prof Med, Univ Tex SW, Dallas

Bresalier, Robert MD [Ge] - **Spec Exp:** Gastrointestinal Cancer; **Hospital:** UT MD Anderson Cancer Ctr (page 81); **Address:** MD Anderson Canc Ctr, GI Med & Nutrition, 1515 Holcombe Blvd - Unit 436, Houston, TX 77030-4009; **Phone:** 713-745-4340; **Board Cert:** Internal Medicine 1981; Gastroenterology 1983; **Med School:** Univ Chicago-Pritzker Sch Med 1978; **Resid:** Internal Medicine, Barnes Hosp-Washington Univ 1981; **Fellow:** Gastroenterology, UCSF Med Ctr 1983; **Fac Appt:** Prof Med, Univ Tex, Houston

Fleischer, David MD [Ge] - **Spec Exp:** Barrett's Esophagus; Esophageal Cancer; **Hospital:** Mayo Clin Hosp - Scottsdale; **Address:** Mayo Clinic - Scottsdale, 13400 E Shea Blvd, Div Gastroenterology 2A, Scottsdale, AZ 85259; **Phone:** 480-301-8484; **Board Cert:** Internal Medicine 1975; Gastroenterology 1977; **Med School:** Vanderbilt Univ 1970; **Resid:** Internal Medicine, Metro General Hosp 1975; **Fellow:** Gastroenterology, LA Co Harbor-UCLA Med Ctr 1977; **Fac Appt:** Prof Med, Mayo Med Sch

Levin, Bernard MD [Ge] - **Spec Exp:** Gastrointestinal Cancer; Colon & Rectal Cancer; Cancer Prevention; **Hospital:** UT MD Anderson Cancer Ctr (page 81); **Address:** Univ Tex MD Anderson Cancer Ctr, 1515 Holcombe Blvd Unit #1370, Houston, TX 77030-4095; **Phone:** 713-792-3900; **Board Cert:** Internal Medicine 1972; Gastroenterology 1972; **Med School:** South Africa 1964; **Resid:** Internal Medicine, Rush Presby-St Lukes Hosp 1968; **Fellow:** Pathology, Univ Chicago 1970; Gastroenterology, Univ Chicago 1972

West Coast and Pacific

Gish, Robert MD [Ge] - **Spec Exp:** Liver Cancer; Transplant Medicine-Liver; Clinical Trials; **Hospital:** CA Pacific Med Ctr - Pacific Campus; **Address:** 2340 Clay St Fl 2, San Francisco, CA 94115; **Phone:** 415-600-1020; **Board Cert:** Internal Medicine 1984; Gastroenterology 1987; **Med School:** Univ Kans 1980; **Resid:** Internal Medicine, UCSD Med Ctr 1983; **Fellow:** Gastroenterology, UCLA Med Ctr 1988; **Fac Appt:** Assoc Clin Prof Med, UCSF

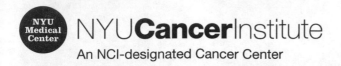

NYU**Cancer**Institute
An NCI-designated Cancer Center

Hematology & Medical Oncology
a subspecialty of Internal Medicine

Hematology: An internist with additional training who specializes in diseases of the blood, spleen and lymph glands. This specialist treats conditions such as anemia, clotting disorders, sickle cell disease, hemophilia, leukemia and lymphoma.

Medical Oncology: An internist who specializes in the diagnosis and treatment of all types of cancer and other benign and malignant tumors. This specialist decides on and administers chemotherapy for malignancy, as well as consulting with surgeons and radiotherapists on other treatments for cancer.

Training Required: Three years in internal medicine *plus* additional training and examination for certification in hematology or medical oncology.

Hematology

New England

Benz Jr, Edward MD [Hem] - **Spec Exp:** Bone Marrow Transplant; **Hospital:** Brigham & Women's Hosp, Children's Hospital - Boston; **Address:** 44 Binney St, rm D-1628, Boston, MA 02115; **Phone:** 617-632-2159; **Board Cert:** Internal Medicine 1979; Hematology 1982; **Med School:** Harvard Med Sch 1973; **Resid:** Internal Medicine, Peter Bent Brigham Hosp 1975; Hematology, Yale New Haven Hosp 1980; **Fellow:** Hematology, Natl Inst of Hlth 1978; **Fac Appt:** Prof Med, Harvard Med Sch

Berliner, Nancy MD [Hem] - **Spec Exp:** Leukemia; Multiple Myeloma; Hodgkin's Disease; **Hospital:** Yale - New Haven Hosp; **Address:** Sect of Hematology, Dpt of Internal Med, 333 Cedar St, Box 208021, New Haven, CT 06520-8021; **Phone:** 203-785-4144; **Board Cert:** Internal Medicine 1982; Hematology 1984; **Med School:** Yale Univ 1979; **Resid:** Internal Medicine, Brigham Womens Hosp 1982; **Fellow:** Hematology, Brigham Womens Hosp 1985; **Fac Appt:** Prof Med, Yale Univ

Dezube, Bruce J MD [Hem] - **Spec Exp:** AIDS Related Cancers; Clinical Trials; **Hospital:** Beth Israel Deaconess Med Ctr - Boston; **Address:** BIDMC-Division of Hematology/Oncology, 330 Brookline Ave, Shapiro 9, Boston, MA 02215; **Phone:** 617-667-7082; **Board Cert:** Internal Medicine 1986; Medical Oncology 1989; Hematology 1988; **Med School:** Tufts Univ 1983; **Resid:** Internal Medicine, New England Med Ctr 1986; **Fellow:** Hematology & Oncology, Beth Israel Deaconess Hosp 1989; **Fac Appt:** Assoc Prof Med, Harvard Med Sch

Groopman, Jerome E MD [Hem] - **Spec Exp:** AIDS Related Cancers; **Hospital:** Beth Israel Deaconess Med Ctr - Boston; **Address:** Beth Israel Deaconess Medical Ctr, 330 Brookline Ave, Boston, MA 02215; **Phone:** 617-667-0070; **Board Cert:** Internal Medicine 1979; Medical Oncology 1981; Hematology 1984; **Med School:** Columbia P&S 1976; **Resid:** Internal Medicine, Mass Genl Hosp 1978; **Fellow:** Hematology & Oncology, UCLA Med Ctr 1979; Research, Dana Farber Cancer Ctr 1980; **Fac Appt:** Prof Med, Harvard Med Sch

Meehan, Kenneth MD [Hem] - **Spec Exp:** Bone Marrow Transplant; **Hospital:** Dartmouth - Hitchcock Med Ctr; **Address:** Norris Cotton Cancer Ctr-Dartmouth-Hitchcock MC, 1 Medical Center Drive, Lebanon, NH 03756; **Phone:** 603-650-4628; **Board Cert:** Internal Medicine 1989; Hematology 2003; Medical Oncology 1991; **Med School:** Georgetown Univ 1986; **Resid:** Internal Medicine, Georgetown Univ 1989; **Fellow:** Hematology & Oncology, Dartmouth-Hitchcock Med Ctr 1992; **Fac Appt:** Assoc Prof Med, Dartmouth Med Sch

Miller, Kenneth B MD [Hem] - **Spec Exp:** Bone Marrow Transplant; Leukemia; **Hospital:** Beth Israel Deaconess Med Ctr - Boston; **Address:** 330 Brookline Ave, Kirstein Bldg, rm 121, Boston, MA 02215; **Phone:** 617-667-9920 x2; **Board Cert:** Internal Medicine 1976; Hematology 1980; **Med School:** NY Med Coll 1972; **Resid:** Internal Medicine, NYU Med Ctr/VA Hosp 1976; Internal Medicine, NYU Med Ctr 1976; **Fellow:** Hematology, New England Med Ctr 1979; **Fac Appt:** Assoc Prof Med, Harvard Med Sch

Spitzer, Thomas R MD [Hem] - **Spec Exp:** Bone Marrow Transplant; Leukemia; **Hospital:** Mass Genl Hosp; **Address:** Mass Genl Hosp-Bone Marrow Tranplant Program, 55 Fruit St, Ste 118, Boston, MA 02114; **Phone:** 617-724-1124; **Board Cert:** Internal Medicine 1977; Medical Oncology 1983; Hematology 1984; **Med School:** Univ Rochester 1974; **Resid:** Internal Medicine, NYew York Hosp-Cornell Med Ctr 1977; **Fellow:** Hematology & Oncology, Case West Res Univ 1983; **Fac Appt:** Prof Med, Harvard Med Sch

Stone, Richard M MD [Hem] - **Spec Exp:** Leukemia; **Hospital:** Dana-Farber Cancer Inst, Brigham & Women's Hosp; **Address:** Dana Farber Cancer Inst, Adult Leukemia Prog, 44 Binney St, Ste M1B17, Boston, MA 02115-6084; **Phone:** 617-632-2214; **Board Cert:** Internal Medicine 1984; Medical Oncology 1987; Hematology 1988; **Med School:** Harvard Med Sch 1981; **Resid:** Internal Medicine, Brigham & Womens Hosp 1984; **Fellow:** Medical Oncology, Dana Farber Cancer Inst 1987; **Fac Appt:** Assoc Prof Med, Harvard Med Sch

Mid Atlantic

Baer, Maria MD [Hem] - **Spec Exp:** Leukemia; **Hospital:** Roswell Park Cancer Inst; **Address:** Roswell Park Cancer Inst, Elm & Carlton Sts, Buffalo, NY 14263; **Phone:** 716-845-8546; **Board Cert:** Internal Medicine 1983; Hematology 1984; **Med School:** Johns Hopkins Univ 1979; **Resid:** Internal Medicine, Vanderbilt Univ Hosp 1982; **Fellow:** Hematology, Vanderbilt Univ Hosp 1984; **Fac Appt:** Prof Med, SUNY Buffalo

Cheson, Bruce D MD [Hem] - **Spec Exp:** Leukemia; Hematologic Malignancies; **Hospital:** Georgetown Univ Hosp; **Address:** GUMC - Lombardi Cancer Ctr, 3800 Reservoir Rd NW, Podium A, Washington, DC 20007; **Phone:** 202-444-2223; **Board Cert:** Internal Medicine 1974; Hematology 1976; **Med School:** Tufts Univ 1971; **Resid:** Internal Medicine, Univ Virginia Hosp 1974; **Fellow:** Hematology, New England Med Ctr Hosp 1976

Emerson, Stephen G MD/PhD [Hem] - **Spec Exp:** Leukemia; Lymphoma; **Hospital:** Hosp Univ Penn - UPHS (page 84); **Address:** Hospital U Penn, 510 Maloney Bldg, 3400 Spruce St, Philadelphia, PA 19104; **Phone:** 215-573-3002; **Board Cert:** Internal Medicine 1983; Hematology 1986; Medical Oncology 1987; **Med School:** Yale Univ 1980; **Resid:** Internal Medicine, Mass Genl Hosp 1982; **Fellow:** Hematology & Oncology, Brigham & Women's Hosp 1986; **Fac Appt:** Prof Med, Univ Pennsylvania

Fruchtman, Steven M MD [Hem] - **Spec Exp:** Myeloproliferative Disorders; Stem Cell Transplant; **Hospital:** Mount Sinai Med Ctr (page 77); **Address:** 1111 Park Ave, New York, NY 10029; **Phone:** 212-427-7700; **Board Cert:** Internal Medicine 1980; Hematology 1984; **Med School:** NY Med Coll 1977; **Resid:** Internal Medicine, Univ Hosp 1981; **Fellow:** Hematology, Mount Sinai Med Ctr 1984; Hematology, Meml Sloan Kettering Cancer Ctr 1985; **Fac Appt:** Assoc Prof Med, NY Med Coll

Gewirtz, Alan M MD [Hem] - **Spec Exp:** Leukemia; Gene Therapy; **Hospital:** Hosp Univ Penn - UPHS (page 84); **Address:** Univ Penn - Div Hem/Onc, 421 Curie Blvd, 716BRB, Philadelphia, PA 19104; **Phone:** 215-662-3914; **Board Cert:** Internal Medicine 1979; Hematology 1982; Medical Oncology 1981; **Med School:** SUNY Buffalo 1976; **Resid:** Internal Medicine, Mt Sinai Hosp 1979; **Fellow:** Oncology, Yale New Haven Hosp 1981; **Fac Appt:** Prof Med, Univ Pennsylvania

Goldberg, Jack MD [Hem] - **Spec Exp:** Bleeding Disorders; Leukemia & Lymphoma; Solid Tumors; **Hospital:** Penn Presby Med Ctr - UPHS (page 84), Virtua West Jersey Hosp - Voorhees (page 73); **Address:** 409 Route 70 E, Cherry Hill, NJ 08034; **Phone:** 856-429-1519; **Board Cert:** Internal Medicine 1976; Hematology 1980; Medical Oncology 1989; **Med School:** SUNY Upstate Med Univ 1973; **Resid:** Internal Medicine, Boston Univ Hosp 1975; **Fellow:** Hematology & Oncology, SUNY Syracuse Med Ctr 1977; **Fac Appt:** Clin Prof Med, Univ Pennsylvania

Kempin, Sanford Jay MD [Hem] - **Spec Exp:** Bleeding/Coagulation Disorders; Leukemia; Lymphoma; **Hospital:** St Vincent Cath Med Ctrs - Manhattan; **Address:** St Vincents Cancer Ctr, 325 W 15th St, New York, NY 10011; **Phone:** 212-604-6010; **Board Cert:** Internal Medicine 1976; Medical Oncology 1977; Hematology 1978; **Med School:** Belgium 1971; **Resid:** Internal Medicine, Lemuel Shattuck Hosp 1972; **Fellow:** Hematology, St Jude Chldns Hosp 1975; Medical Oncology, Meml Sloan Kettering Cancer Ctr 1976

Kessler, Craig M MD [Hem] - **Spec Exp:** Bleeding/Coagulation Disorders; Hematologic Malignancies; **Hospital:** Georgetown Univ Hosp; **Address:** GUMC, Lombardi Cancer Ctr, 3800 Reservoir Rd NW, Washington, DC 20007; **Phone:** 202-444-7094; **Board Cert:** Internal Medicine 1976; Hematology 1980; **Med School:** Tulane Univ 1973; **Resid:** Internal Medicine, Ochsner Fdn Hosp 1976; **Fellow:** Hematology, Johns Hopkins Hosp 1978; **Fac Appt:** Prof Med, Georgetown Univ

Kopel, Samuel MD [Hem] - **Spec Exp:** Hematologic Malignancies; Solid Tumors; **Hospital:** Maimonides Med Ctr (page 75); **Address:** MMC Hematology/Oncology, 6300 8th Ave, Brooklyn, NY 11220; **Phone:** 718-765-2600; **Board Cert:** Internal Medicine 1975; Hematology 1978; Medical Oncology 1979; **Med School:** Italy 1972; **Resid:** Internal Medicine, Jewish Hosp 1975; **Fellow:** Hematology & Oncology, Mt Sinai Med Ctr 1978; **Fac Appt:** Asst Prof Med, SUNY Downstate

Mears, John G MD [Hem] - **Spec Exp:** Lymphoma; Leukemia; Multiple Myeloma; Breast Cancer; **Hospital:** NY-Presby Hosp (page 79); **Address:** 161 Ft Washington Ave, Ste 923, New York, NY 10032; **Phone:** 212-305-3506; **Board Cert:** Internal Medicine 1976; Hematology 1978; **Med School:** Columbia P&S 1973; **Resid:** Internal Medicine, Boston Univ Med Ctr 1975; **Fellow:** Hematology & Oncology, Columbia-Presby Med Ctr 1978; **Fac Appt:** Clin Prof Med, Columbia P&S

Millenson, Michael M MD [Hem] - **Spec Exp:** Leukemia & Lymphoma; Thromboembolic Disorders; **Hospital:** Fox Chase Cancer Ctr (page 73); **Address:** Fox Chase Cancer Center, 7701 Burholme Ave, Ste C307, Philadelphia, PA 19111; **Phone:** 215-728-6900; **Board Cert:** Medical Oncology 2000; Hematology 2000; **Med School:** Temple Univ 1984; **Resid:** Internal Medicine, Temple Univ Hosp 1987; **Fellow:** Hematology & Oncology, Beth Israel Hosp 1991

Nimer, Stephen D MD [Hem] - **Spec Exp:** Bone Marrow Transplant; Myelodysplastic Syndromes; Leukemia; Stem Cell Transplant; **Hospital:** Meml Sloan Kettering Cancer Ctr (page 76); **Address:** Memorial Sloan Kettering Cancer Ctr, 1275 York Ave, Box 575, New York, NY 10021; **Phone:** 212-639-7871; **Board Cert:** Internal Medicine 1982; Hematology 1986; Medical Oncology 1985; **Med School:** Univ Chicago-Pritzker Sch Med 1979; **Resid:** Internal Medicine, UCLA Med Ctr 1982; **Fellow:** Hematology & Oncology, UCLA Med Ctr 1986; **Fac Appt:** Prof Med, Cornell Univ-Weill Med Coll

Porter, David L MD [Hem] - **Spec Exp:** Leukemia; Bone Marrow Transplant; **Hospital:** Hosp Univ Penn - UPHS (page 84); **Address:** Hosp Univ Penn, Div Hem/Oncology, 3400 Spruce St, 16 Penn Twr, Philadelphia, PA 19104; **Phone:** 215-662-2862; **Board Cert:** Internal Medicine 1990; Medical Oncology 1993; Hematology 1994; **Med School:** Brown Univ 1987; **Resid:** Internal Medicine, Univ Hosp 1990; **Fellow:** Hematology & Oncology, Brigham & Womens Hosp 1992; **Fac Appt:** Assoc Prof Med, Univ Pennsylvania

Rai, Kanti MD [Hem] - **Spec Exp:** Leukemia; Lymphoma; Multiple Myeloma; **Hospital:** Long Island Jewish Med Ctr; **Address:** 270-05 76th Ave, New Hyde Park, NY 11040-1433; **Phone:** 718 470 7135; **Board Cert:** Pediatrics 1961; **Med School:** India 1955; **Resid:** Pediatrics, Lincoln Hosp 1958; Pediatrics, North Shore Univ Hosp 1959; **Fellow:** Hematology, LI Jewish Med Ctr 1960; **Fac Appt:** Prof Med, Albert Einstein Coll Med

Raphael, Bruce MD [Hem] - **Spec Exp:** Lymphoma; Leukemia; Multiple Myeloma; **Hospital:** NYU Med Ctr (page 80), NY Downtown Hosp; **Address:** 160 E 34th Street Ave Fl 7, NYU Clinical Cancer Ctr, New York, NY 10016-6402; **Phone:** 212-731-5185; **Board Cert:** Internal Medicine 1978; Hematology 1980; Medical Oncology 1981; **Med School:** McGill Univ 1975; **Resid:** Internal Medicine, Jewish Genl Hosp 1977; **Fellow:** Medical Oncology, Meml Sloan Kettering Cancer Ctr 1978; Hematology, NYU Med Ctr 1980; **Fac Appt:** Assoc Prof Med, NYU Sch Med

Roodman, G David MD [Hem] - **Spec Exp:** Multiple Myeloma; **Hospital:** UPMC Shadyside, VA Pittsburgh Hlth Care Sys; **Address:** VA Pittsburgh Healthcare System, 151-U, rm 2E113, University Drive C, Pittsburgh, PA 15240; **Phone:** 412-688-6571; **Board Cert:** Internal Medicine 1978; Hematology 1980; **Med School:** Univ KY Coll Med 1973; **Resid:** Internal Medicine, Univ Minnesota Hosp 1978; **Fellow:** Hematology, Univ Minnesota Hosp 1980; **Fac Appt:** Prof Med, Univ Pittsburgh

Savage, David G MD [Hem] - **Spec Exp:** Stem Cell Transplant; Multiple Myeloma; Lymphoma; **Hospital:** NY-Presby Hosp (page 79); **Address:** 177 Fort Washington Ave, Millstein Bldg Fl 6 - rm 435, New York, NY 10032; **Phone:** 212-305-9783; **Board Cert:** Internal Medicine 1977; Hematology 1982; Medical Oncology 1985; **Med School:** Columbia P&S 1971; **Resid:** Internal Medicine, Harlem Hosp/Columbia Presby Med Ctr 1975; **Fellow:** Hematology & Oncology, Harlem Hosp/Columbia Presby Med Ctr 1977; **Fac Appt:** Assoc Prof Med, Columbia P&S

Schuster, Michael W MD [Hem] - **Spec Exp:** Bone Marrow Transplant; **Hospital:** NY-Presby Hosp (page 79); **Address:** NY Weill Cornell Medical Ctr, 525 E 68th St, Starr 341, New York, NY 10021; **Phone:** 212-746-2119; **Board Cert:** Internal Medicine 1984; Hematology 1986; **Med School:** Dartmouth Med Sch 1980; **Resid:** Internal Medicine, New England Deaconess Hosp 1983; **Fellow:** Hematology & Oncology, Beth Israel Med Ctr 1987; **Fac Appt:** Assoc Prof Med, Cornell Univ-Weill Med Coll

Spivak, Jerry L MD [Hem] - **Spec Exp:** Myeloproliferative Disorders; Leukemia; **Hospital:** Johns Hopkins Hosp - Baltimore; **Address:** 720 Rutland Ave Bldg Ross - Ste 1025, Baltimore, MD 21205; **Phone:** 410-614-0167; **Board Cert:** Internal Medicine 1971; Hematology 1974; **Med School:** Cornell Univ-Weill Med Coll 1964; **Resid:** Internal Medicine, Johns Hopkins Hosp 1966; Internal Medicine, Johns Hopkins Hosp 1972; **Fellow:** Hematology, Natl Cancer Inst 1968; Hematology, Johns Hopkins Hosp 1971; **Fac Appt:** Prof Med, Johns Hopkins Univ

Wisch, Nathaniel MD [Hem] - **Spec Exp:** Lymphoma; Breast Cancer; Leukemia; **Hospital:** Lenox Hill Hosp, Mount Sinai Med Ctr (page 77); **Address:** 12 E 86th St, New York, NY 10028-0506; **Phone:** 212-861-6660; **Board Cert:** Internal Medicine 1965; Hematology 1972; Medical Oncology 1977; **Med School:** Northwestern Univ 1958; **Resid:** Internal Medicine, VA Hosp 1960; Internal Medicine, Montefiore Hosp 1961; **Fellow:** Hematology, Mount Sinai Hosp 1962; **Fac Appt:** Clin Prof Med, Mount Sinai Sch Med

Zalusky, Ralph MD [Hem] - **Spec Exp:** Leukemia; Lymphoma; **Hospital:** Beth Israel Med Ctr - Petrie Division (page 72); **Address:** Beth Israel Med Ctr, First Ave at 16th St, New York, NY 10003; **Phone:** 212-420-4185; **Board Cert:** Internal Medicine 1964; Hematology 1972; **Med School:** Boston Univ 1957; **Resid:** Internal Medicine, Duke Univ Med Ctr 1962; **Fellow:** Hematology, Boston Med Ctr 1961; **Fac Appt:** Prof Med, Albert Einstein Coll Med

Hematology

Southeast

Abramson, Neil MD [Hem] - **Spec Exp:** Breast Cancer; Hematologic Malignancies; **Hospital:** Baptist Medical Center - Jacksonville; **Address:** 1235 San Marco Blvd, Ste 3, Jacksonville, FL 32207; **Phone:** 904-202-7051; **Board Cert:** Internal Medicine 1970; Hematology 1972; Medical Oncology 1975; **Med School:** Albert Einstein Coll Med 1963; **Resid:** Internal Medicine, Presbyterian Univ Hosp 1965; **Fellow:** Hematology, Thorndike Meml Lab-Harvard 1969; **Fac Appt:** Clin Prof Med, Univ Fla Coll Med

Bigelow, Carolyn L MD [Hem] - **Spec Exp:** Bone Marrow Transplant; **Hospital:** Univ Hosps & Clins - Jackson; **Address:** Univ Mississippi Med Ctr-Div Hematology, 2500 N State St, Jackson, MS 39216; **Phone:** 601-984-5615; **Board Cert:** Internal Medicine 1982; Hematology 1988; **Med School:** Univ Miss 1979; **Resid:** Internal Medicine, Univ Mississippi Med Ctr 1982; **Fellow:** Hematology & Oncology, Univ Washington Med Ctr 1987; **Fac Appt:** Prof Med, Univ Miss

Buadi, Francis K MD [Hem] - **Spec Exp:** Lymphoma; Stem Cell Transplant; **Hospital:** Univ of Tennesee Mem Hosp; **Address:** UT Cancer Inst, 1331 Union Ave, Ste 800, Memphis, TN 38104; **Phone:** 901-725-1785; **Board Cert:** Internal Medicine 1999; Hematology 2002; Medical Oncology 2003; **Med School:** Ghana 1991; **Resid:** Internal Medicine, St Agnes Hosp 1997; **Fellow:** Hematology & Oncology, Univ Maryland Hosp 1999; Bone Marrow Transplant, Mayo Clinic 2001

Djulbegovic, Benjamin MD [Hem] - **Spec Exp:** Multiple Myeloma; Lymphoma; Myeloproliferative Disorders; **Hospital:** H Lee Moffitt Cancer Ctr & Research Inst; **Address:** H Lee Moffitt Cancer Ctr, 12902 Magnolia Drive, MRC Bldg - Ste 2067H, Tampa, FL 33612; **Phone:** 813-745-4605; **Board Cert:** Internal Medicine 2002; Hematology 2004; **Med School:** Bosnia 1976; **Resid:** Internal Medicine, Univ Med Ctr 1983; Internal Medicine, Univ Louisville Med Ctr 1988; **Fellow:** Univ Manchester 1985; Hematology & Oncology, Univ Louisville 1990; **Fac Appt:** Prof Med, Univ S Fla Coll Med

Emanuel, Peter D MD [Hem] - **Spec Exp:** Lymphoma; Leukemia; Hodgkin's Disease; Multiple Myeloma; **Hospital:** Univ of Ala Hosp at Birmingham; **Address:** 1802 6th Ave S, 2555 N Pavilion, Birmingham, AL 35294-3300; **Phone:** 205-934-5077; **Board Cert:** Internal Medicine 1988; **Med School:** Univ Wisc 1985; **Resid:** Internal Medicine, Univ Alabama Hosp 1988; **Fellow:** Hematology & Oncology, Univ Alabama 1991; **Fac Appt:** Prof Med, Univ Ala

Files, Joe C MD [Hem] - **Spec Exp:** Bone Marrow Transplant; Stem Cell Transplant; Leukemia; **Hospital:** Univ Hosps & Clins - Jackson; **Address:** Univ Miss Med Ctr-Div Hematology, 2500 N State St, Jackson, MS 39216; **Phone:** 601-984-5615; **Board Cert:** Internal Medicine 1976; Hematology 1980; **Med School:** Univ Miss 1972; **Resid:** Internal Medicine, Univ Miss Med Ctr 1976; **Fellow:** Hematology, Univ Wash Sch Med 1979; **Fac Appt:** Prof Med, Univ Miss

Greer, John P MD [Hem] - **Spec Exp:** Leukemia & Lymphoma; Myelodysplastic Syndromes; Stem Cell Transplant; **Hospital:** Vanderbilt Univ Med Ctr; **Address:** 2665 The Vanderbilt Clinic, 1301 22nd Ave S, Nashville, TN 37232-5505; **Phone:** 615-936-1803; **Board Cert:** Pediatrics 1985; Internal Medicine 1979; Hematology 1984; Medical Oncology 1985; **Med School:** Vanderbilt Univ 1976; **Resid:** Internal Medicine, Tulane Univ Med Ctr 1979; Pediatrics, Med Coll Virginia 1981; **Fellow:** Hematology & Oncology, Vanderbilt Univ Med Ctr 1984; **Fac Appt:** Prof Med, Vanderbilt Univ

Lilenbaum, Rogerio MD [Hem] - **Spec Exp:** Lung Cancer; **Hospital:** Mount Sinai Med Ctr - Miami; **Address:** Mount Sinai Cancer Ctr, 4306 Alton Rd, Ste 3, Miami, FL 33140-2840; **Phone:** 305-535-3310; **Board Cert:** Internal Medicine 1995; Hematology 1998; Medical Oncology 1997; **Med School:** Brazil 1986; **Resid:** Internal Medicine, Univ Hosp-Rio de Janeiro 1989; **Fellow:** Hematology & Oncology, Washington Univ Sch Med 1992; Oncology, UCSD 1994; **Fac Appt:** Assoc Clin Prof Med, Univ Miami Sch Med

Lin, Weei-Chin MD/PhD [Hem] - **Spec Exp:** Hematologic Malignancies; **Hospital:** Univ of Ala Hosp at Birmingham; **Address:** Univ of Alabama, 1530 3rd Ave S, Ste 520A, Birmingham, AL 35294; **Phone:** 205-934-3980; **Board Cert:** Internal Medicine 1996; Hematology 1999; Medical Oncology 1999; **Med School:** Taiwan 1986; **Resid:** Internal Medicine, Duke Univ Med Ctr 1996; **Fellow:** Hematology & Oncology, Duke Univ Med Ctr 1999

List, Alan F MD [Hem] - **Spec Exp:** Myelodysplastic Syndromes; Leukemia; **Hospital:** H Lee Moffitt Cancer Ctr & Research Inst; **Address:** 12902 Magnolia Drive, SRB 4, Tampa, FL 33612-9497; **Phone:** 813-745-6086; **Board Cert:** Internal Medicine 1983; Medical Oncology 1985; Hematology 1986; **Med School:** Univ Pennsylvania 1980; **Resid:** Internal Medicine, Good Samaritan Hosp 1983; Oncology, Vanderbilt Univ Med Ctr 1985; **Fellow:** Hematology, Vanderbilt Univ Med Ctr 1986

Powell, Bayard L MD [Hem] - **Spec Exp:** Leukemia; Myelodysplastic Syndromes; **Hospital:** Wake Forest Univ Baptist Med Ctr (page 85); **Address:** Wake Forest Univ Baptist Med Ctr, Med Ctr Blvd-Cancer Center, Winston-Salem, NC 27157; **Phone:** 336-716-7970; **Board Cert:** Internal Medicine 1983; Medical Oncology 1985; **Med School:** Univ NC Sch Med 1980; **Resid:** Internal Medicine, NC Baptist Hospital 1983; **Fellow:** Hematology & Oncology, Wake Forest Univ Sch Med 1986; **Fac Appt:** Prof Med, Wake Forest Univ

Rosenblatt, Joseph D MD [Hem] - **Spec Exp:** Lymphoma; Leukemia; Multiple Myeloma; **Hospital:** Univ of Miami Hosp & Clins/Sylvester Comp Canc Ctr, Jackson Meml Hosp; **Address:** Sylvester Comprehensive Cancer Ctr, 1475 NW 12th Ave, D8-4, Ste 3300, Miami, FL 33136; **Phone:** 305-243-4909; **Board Cert:** Internal Medicine 1983; Hematology 1990; Medical Oncology 1985; **Med School:** UCLA 1980; **Resid:** Internal Medicine, UCLA Medical Ctr 1983; **Fellow:** Hematology & Oncology, UCLA Medical Ctr 1986; **Fac Appt:** Prof Med, Univ Miami Sch Med

Schwartzberg, Lee S MD [Hem] - **Spec Exp:** Breast Cancer; Lung Cancer; Stem Cell Transplant; **Hospital:** Baptist Hosp Nashville; **Address:** The West Clinic, 100 N Humphreys Blvd, Memphis, TN 38120; **Phone:** 901-683-0055; **Board Cert:** Internal Medicine 1983; Hematology 1986; Medical Oncology 1985; **Med School:** NY Med Coll 1980; **Resid:** Internal Medicine, North Shore Univ Hosp 1983; Internal Medicine, Meml Sloan Kettering Cancer Ctr 1985; **Fellow:** Hematology & Oncology, Meml Sloan Kettering Cancer Ctr 1984; Hematology & Oncology, Meml Sloan Kettering Cancer Ctr 1987; **Fac Appt:** Assoc Prof Med, Univ Tenn Coll Med, Memphis

Solberg, Lawrence MD/PhD [Hem] - **Spec Exp:** Bone Marrow Transplant; Myeloproliferative Disorders; **Hospital:** Mayo - Jacksonville, St Luke's Hosp - Jacksonville; **Address:** Mayo Clinic-Dept Hem-Onc, 4500 San Pablo Rd Fl 8, Jacksonville, FL 32224; **Phone:** 904-953-7292; **Board Cert:** Internal Medicine 1978; Hematology 1980; **Med School:** St Louis Univ 1975; **Resid:** Internal Medicine, Mayo Clinic 1978; **Fellow:** Hematology, Mayo Clinic 1980; **Fac Appt:** Prof Med, Mayo Med Sch

Hematology

Zuckerman, Kenneth S MD [Hem] - **Spec Exp:** Myeloproliferative Disorders; Myelodysplastic Syndromes; Leukemia; Lymphoma; **Hospital:** H Lee Moffitt Cancer Ctr & Research Inst, Tampa Genl Hosp; **Address:** H Lee Moffitt Cancer Ctr, 12902 Magnolia Drive, MS SRB 4, Tampa, FL 33612-9416; **Phone:** 813-745-8090; **Board Cert:** Internal Medicine 1975; Hematology 1978; **Med School:** Ohio State Univ 1972; **Resid:** Internal Medicine, Ohio State Univ Hosps 1975; **Fellow:** Hematology, Brigham Hosp/Harvard Univ 1978; **Fac Appt:** Prof Med, Univ S Fla Coll Med

Midwest

Baron, Joseph M MD [Hem] - **Spec Exp:** Lymphoma; Myeloproliferative Disorders; **Hospital:** Univ of Chicago Hosps; **Address:** 5841 S Maryland Ave, MC 2115, Chicago, IL 60637-1463; **Phone:** 773-702-6149; **Board Cert:** Internal Medicine 1969; Hematology 1972; Medical Oncology 1975; **Med School:** Univ Chicago-Pritzker Sch Med 1962; **Resid:** Internal Medicine, Univ Chicago Hosps 1964; **Fellow:** Hematology, Univ Chicago Hosps 1968; **Fac Appt:** Assoc Prof Med, Univ Chicago-Pritzker Sch Med

Bockenstedt, Paula MD [Hem] - **Spec Exp:** Bleeding/Coagulation Disorders; Leukemia; **Hospital:** Univ Michigan Hlth Sys; **Address:** Div Hematology, 1500 E Med Ctr Dr, MIB, rm C-344, Ann Arbor, MI 48109-8048; **Phone:** 734-647-8921; **Board Cert:** Internal Medicine 1981; Hematology 1984; **Med School:** Harvard Med Sch 1978; **Resid:** Internal Medicine, Brigham-Womens Hosp 1981; **Fellow:** Hematology, Brigham-Womens Hosp 1984; **Fac Appt:** Assoc Clin Prof Med, Univ Mich Med Sch

Erba, Harry P MD/PhD [Hem] - **Spec Exp:** Leukemia; Myelodysplastic Syndromes; Lymphoma; **Hospital:** Univ Michigan Hlth Sys; **Address:** Univ Michigan Medical Ctr, 1500 Medical Center Dr, rm C348 MIB, Ann Arbor, MI 48109-0848; **Phone:** 734-647-8901; **Board Cert:** Internal Medicine 2004; Hematology 2004; Medical Oncology 2005; **Med School:** Stanford Univ 1988; **Resid:** Internal Medicine, Brigham & Womens Hosp 1990; **Fellow:** Hematology & Oncology, Brigham & Womens Hosp 1993; **Fac Appt:** Prof Med, Univ Mich Med Sch

Flynn, Patrick MD [Hem] - **Spec Exp:** Hematologic Malignancies; Colon & Rectal Cancer; Clinical Trials; **Hospital:** Abbott - Northwestern Hosp, Fairview Southdale Hosp; **Address:** 800 E 28th St, Piper Bldg, Ste 405, Minneapolis, MN 55407; **Phone:** 612-863-8585; **Board Cert:** Internal Medicine 1978; Medical Oncology 1981; Hematology 1982; **Med School:** Univ Minn 1975; **Resid:** Internal Medicine, Hennepin Co Med Ctr 1978; **Fellow:** Hematology & Oncology, Univ Minnesota Hosp 1981

Gaynor, Ellen MD [Hem] - **Spec Exp:** Lymphoma; Genitourinary Cancer; Breast Cancer; **Hospital:** Loyola Univ Med Ctr; **Address:** Loyola Univ Med Ctr, Dept Hematology, 2160 S First Ave Bldg 112 - rm 108, Maywood, IL 60153; **Phone:** 708-327-3214; **Board Cert:** Internal Medicine 1982; Hematology 1986; Medical Oncology 1985; **Med School:** Univ Wisc 1978; **Resid:** Internal Medicine, Loyola Univ Med Ctr 1982; **Fellow:** Medical Oncology, Loyola Univ Med Ctr 1981; Hematology & Oncology, Univ Chicago Hosp 1984; **Fac Appt:** Prof Med, Loyola Univ-Stritch Sch Med

Gertz, Morris MD [Hem] - **Spec Exp:** Multiple Myeloma; Waldenstrom's Macroglobulinemia; Plasma Cell Disorders; **Hospital:** Mayo Med Ctr & Clin - Rochester, Rochester Meth Hosp; **Address:** 200 SW 1st St Fl W10, Rochester, MN 55905; **Phone:** 507-284-2511; **Board Cert:** Internal Medicine 1979; Hematology 1982; Medical Oncology 1983; **Med School:** Loyola Univ-Stritch Sch Med 1975; **Resid:** Internal Medicine, St Lukes Hosp 1979; **Fellow:** Hematology & Oncology, Mayo Clin 1982; **Fac Appt:** Prof Med, Mayo Med Sch

Godwin, John MD [Hem] - **Spec Exp:** Leukemia in Elderly; **Hospital:** St John's Hosp - Springfield; **Address:** Southern IL University Med Ctr, Carol Jo Vecchie Center, PO Box 19678, Springfield, IL 62794; **Phone:** 217-545-5817; **Board Cert:** Internal Medicine 1981; Hematology 1986; **Med School:** Univ Ala 1978; **Resid:** Internal Medicine, Baylor Coll Med 1981; Internal Medicine, Baylor Coll Med 1982; **Fellow:** Hematology, Baylor Coll Med 1983; Hematology, North Carolina Meml Hosp 1985; **Fac Appt:** Prof Med, Southern IL Univ

Gordon, Leo I MD [Hem] - **Spec Exp:** Lymphoma, Non-Hodgkin's; Hodgkin's Disease; Bone Marrow Transplant; **Hospital:** Northwestern Meml Hosp; **Address:** 675 N St Clair St, Ste 850, Chicago, IL 60611-3124; **Phone:** 312-695-0990; **Board Cert:** Internal Medicine 1976; Hematology 1978; Medical Oncology 1979; **Med School:** Univ Cincinnati 1973; **Resid:** Internal Medicine, Univ Chicago Hosps 1976; **Fellow:** Hematology, Univ Minnesota Hosps 1978; Hematology & Oncology, Univ Chicago Hosps 1979; **Fac Appt:** Prof Med, Northwestern Univ

Gregory, Stephanie A MD [Hem] - **Spec Exp:** Lymphoma; Leukemia; Plasma Cell Disorders; Multiple Myeloma; **Hospital:** Rush Univ Med Ctr; **Address:** 1725 W Harrison St, Ste 834, Rush Professional Office Building, Chicago, IL 60612-3861; **Phone:** 312-563-2320; **Board Cert:** Internal Medicine 1972; Hematology 1972; **Med School:** Med Coll PA Hahnemann 1965; **Resid:** Internal Medicine, Rush/Presby-St Luke's Med Ctr 1969; **Fellow:** Hematology, Rush/Presby-St Luke's Med Ctr 1972; **Fac Appt:** Prof Med, Rush Med Coll

Greipp, Philip R MD [Hem] - **Spec Exp:** Multiple Myeloma; **Hospital:** Mayo Med Ctr & Clin - Rochester; **Address:** Mayo Clinic, Div Hematology, 200 First St SW Bldg Mayo Fl W-10, Rochester, MN 55905-0001; **Phone:** 507-284-3159; **Board Cert:** Internal Medicine 1974; Hematology 1994; **Med School:** Georgetown Univ 1968; **Resid:** Internal Medicine, Mayo Clinic 1973; **Fellow:** Hematology, Mayo Clinic 1975; **Fac Appt:** Prof Med, Mayo Med Sch

Grever, Michael R MD [Hem] - **Spec Exp:** Hematologic Malignancies; Leukemia; Drug Development; Clinical Trials; **Hospital:** Ohio St Univ Med Ctr; **Address:** 215 Means Hall, 1654 Upham Drive, Columbus, OH 43210; **Phone:** 614-293-8724; **Board Cert:** Internal Medicine 1975; Hematology 1988; Medical Oncology 1979; **Med School:** Univ Pittsburgh 1971; **Resid:** Internal Medicine, Presby-Univ Hosp 1974; **Fellow:** Hematology & Oncology, Ohio State Univ 1978; **Fac Appt:** Prof Med, Ohio State Univ

Habermann, Thomas M MD [Hem] - **Spec Exp:** Lymphoma; Hodgkin's Disease; Leukemia; **Hospital:** Mayo Med Ctr & Clin - Rochester; **Address:** Mayo Clinic, 200 1st St SW, Rochester, MN 55905; **Phone:** 507-284-0923; **Board Cert:** Internal Medicine 1982; Hematology 1984; **Med School:** Creighton Univ 1979; **Resid:** Internal Medicine, Mayo Clinic 1982; **Fellow:** Hematology, Mayo Clinic 1985; **Fac Appt:** Prof Med, Mayo Med Sch

Kraut, Eric H MD [Hem] - **Spec Exp:** Hematologic Malignancies, Leukemia; Drug Development; Clinical Trials; **Hospital:** Ohio St Univ Med Ctr; **Address:** B405 Starling Loving Hall, 320 W 10th Ave, Columbus, OH 43210; **Phone:** 614-293-8726; **Board Cert:** Internal Medicine 1975; Hematology 1978; Medical Oncology 1977; **Med School:** Temple Univ 1972; **Resid:** Internal Medicine, Univ Pittsburgh 1975; **Fellow:** Hematology & Oncology, Ohio State Univ Hosp 1977; **Fac Appt:** Prof Med, Ohio State Univ

Kuzel, Timothy M MD [Hem] - **Spec Exp:** Kidney Cancer; Testicular Cancer; Bladder Cancer; Lymphoma; **Hospital:** Northwestern Meml Hosp; **Address:** Northwestern Meml Hosp, 676 N St Clair, Ste 100, Chicago, IL 60611; **Phone:** 312-695-8697; **Board Cert:** Internal Medicine 1987; Hematology 2000; Medical Oncology 1989; **Med School:** Univ Mich Med Sch 1984; **Resid:** Internal Medicine, McGraw MC-Northwestern Univ 1987; **Fellow:** Hematology & Oncology, McGraw MC-Northwestern Univ 1990; **Fac Appt:** Prof Med, Northwestern Univ

Larson, Richard A MD [Hem] - **Spec Exp:** Leukemia & Lymphoma; Bone Marrow Transplant; Myelodysplastic Syndromes; **Hospital:** Univ of Chicago Hosps; **Address:** Univ Chicago Hospitals, 5841 S Maryland Ave, MC 2115, Chicago, IL 60637; **Phone:** 773-702-6149; **Board Cert:** Internal Medicine 1980; Hematology 1982; Medical Oncology 1983; **Med School:** Stanford Univ 1977; **Resid:** Internal Medicine, Univ Chicago Hosps 1980; **Fellow:** Hematology & Oncology, Univ Chicago Hosps 1983; **Fac Appt:** Prof Med, Univ Chicago-Pritzker Sch Med

Laughlin, Mary J MD [Hem] - **Spec Exp:** Bone Marrow Transplant; **Hospital:** Univ Hosps Case Med Ctr; **Address:** 2103 Cornell Rd, WRB 2-129, Cleveland, OH 44106; **Phone:** 216-844-5182; **Board Cert:** Internal Medicine 2003; Hematology 1994; **Med School:** SUNY Buffalo 1988; **Resid:** Internal Medicine, Duke Univ Med Ctr 1991; **Fellow:** Hematology & Oncology, Duke Univ Med Ctr 1992; Bone Marrow Transplant, Rosewell Park Cancer Inst 1994; **Fac Appt:** Assoc Prof Med, Case West Res Univ

Lazarus, Hillard M MD [Hem] - **Spec Exp:** Bone Marrow Transplant; Stem Cell Transplant; Leukemia; **Hospital:** Univ Hosps Case Med Ctr; **Address:** Univ Hosp Med Ctr, 11100 Euclid Ave, Cleveland, OH 44106-5065; **Phone:** 216-844-3629; **Board Cert:** Internal Medicine 1977; Medical Oncology 1979; Hematology 1980; **Med School:** Univ Rochester 1974; **Resid:** Internal Medicine, Univ Hosps 1977; **Fellow:** Hematology & Oncology, Univ Hosps 1979; **Fac Appt:** Prof Med, Case West Res Univ

Litzow, Mark Robert MD [Hem] - **Spec Exp:** Bone Marrow Transplant; Leukemia; **Hospital:** Mayo Med Ctr & Clin - Rochester; **Address:** Mayo Clinic, Div Hematology, 200 First St SW, Rochester, MN 55905; **Phone:** 507-284-0923; **Board Cert:** Internal Medicine 1983; Hematology 1988; Medical Oncology 1989; **Med School:** Univ Chicago-Pritzker Sch Med 1980; **Resid:** Internal Medicine, Mayo Clinic 1984; **Fellow:** Medical Oncology, Mayo Clinic 1990; **Fac Appt:** Asst Prof Med, Mayo Med Sch

Maciejewski, Jaroslow P MD/PhD [Hem] - **Spec Exp:** Anemia-Aplastic; Hematologic Malignancies; Stem Cell Transplant; **Hospital:** Cleveland Clin Fdn (page 71); **Address:** Cleveland Clinic, 9500 Euclid Ave, Desk R40, Cleveland, OH 44195; **Phone:** 216-445-5962; **Board Cert:** Internal Medicine 1999; Hematology 2001; **Med School:** Germany 1987; **Resid:** Internal Medicine, Univ Nevada Med Ctr 1997; **Fellow:** Hematology, Natl Inst Hlth 2000

McGlave, Philip B MD [Hem] - **Spec Exp:** Leukemia; Bone Marrow Transplant; **Hospital:** Univ Minn Med Ctr, Fairview - Univ Campus; **Address:** Univ Minn, Dept Med - Div Hem/Onc, 420 Delaware St SE, MMC 480, Minneapolis, MN 55455; **Phone:** 612-626-2446; **Board Cert:** Internal Medicine 1977; Hematology 1980; **Med School:** Univ IL Coll Med 1974; **Resid:** Internal Medicine, Univ Minn 1977; **Fellow:** Hematology & Oncology, Univ Minn 1980; **Fac Appt:** Prof Med, Univ Minn

Nand, Sucha MD [Hem] - **Spec Exp:** Myelodysplastic Syndromes; Myeloproliferative Disorders; Leukemia; **Hospital:** Loyola Univ Med Ctr; **Address:** Cardinal Bernardin Cancer Ctr, 2160 S First Ave Bldg 112 - rm 342, Maywood, IL 60153-3304; **Phone:** 708-327-3217; **Board Cert:** Internal Medicine 1979; Medical Oncology 1981; Hematology 1982; **Med School:** India 1971; **Resid:** Physical Medicine & Rehabilitation, Northwestern Meml Hosp 1976; Internal Medicine, North Chicago VA Hosp 1978; **Fellow:** Medical Oncology, Northwestern Meml Hosp 1981; **Fac Appt:** Prof Med, Loyola Univ-Stritch Sch Med

Porcu, Pierluigi MD [Hem] - **Spec Exp:** Lymphoma; Lymphoma, Non-Hodgkin's; Immunotherapy; **Hospital:** Ohio St Univ Med Ctr; **Address:** 320 W 10th Ave, B320 Starling Loving Hall, Columbus, OH 43210; **Phone:** 614-293-9273; **Board Cert:** Internal Medicine 1996; Hematology 1999; Medical Oncology 1999; **Med School:** Italy 1987; **Resid:** Internal Medicine, Indiana Univ Hosp 1996; **Fellow:** Hematology & Oncology, Indiana Univ Hosp 1999; **Fac Appt:** Asst Prof Med, Ohio State Univ

Singhal, Seema MD [Hem] - **Spec Exp:** Multiple Myeloma; **Hospital:** Northwestern Meml Hosp; **Address:** 675 N St Claire St, Ste 21-100, Chicago, IL 60611; **Phone:** 312-695-0990; **Board Cert:** Internal Medicine 2005; **Med School:** India 1988; **Resid:** Internal Medicine, King Edward Meml Hosp 1991; Hematology, King Edward Meml Hosp 1991; **Fellow:** Bone Marrow Transplant, Hadassah Univ Hosp 1992; **Fac Appt:** Prof Med, Northwestern Univ

Stiff, Patrick J MD [Hem] - **Spec Exp:** Bone Marrow Transplant; Lymphoma, Non-Hodgkin's; Leukemia; **Hospital:** Loyola Univ Med Ctr; **Address:** Cardinal Bernadin Cancer Ctr, 2160 S First Ave Bldg 112 - rm 342, Maywood, IL 60153; **Phone:** 708-327-3216; **Board Cert:** Internal Medicine 1978; Medical Oncology 1981; Hematology 1982; **Med School:** Loyola Univ-Stritch Sch Med 1975; **Resid:** Internal Medicine, Cleveland Clinic 1978; **Fellow:** Hematology & Oncology, Meml Sloan Kettering Cancer Ctr 1981; **Fac Appt:** Prof Med, Loyola Univ-Stritch Sch Med

Tallman, Martin S MD [Hem] - **Spec Exp:** Bone Marrow Transplant; Leukemia; Lymphoma; **Hospital:** Northwestern Meml Hosp; **Address:** 675 N St Clair St, Ste 21-100, Chicago, IL 60611; **Phone:** 312-695-0990; **Board Cert:** Internal Medicine 1983; Medical Oncology 1987; Hematology 1988; **Med School:** Ros Franklin Univ/Chicago Med Sch 1980; **Resid:** Internal Medicine, Evanston Hosp 1983; **Fellow:** Medical Oncology, Fred Hutchinson Cancer Ctr 1987; **Fac Appt:** Prof Med, Northwestern Univ

van Besien, Koen W MD [Hem] - **Spec Exp:** Lymphoma; Stem Cell Transplant; **Hospital:** Univ of Chicago Hosps; **Address:** Univ Chicago Stem Cell Transplant Program, 5841 S Maryland Ave, MC 2115, Chicago, IL 60637; **Phone:** 773-702-4400; **Board Cert:** Internal Medicine 2005; Medical Oncology 2005; Hematology 1996; **Med School:** Belgium 1984; **Resid:** Internal Medicine, Univ Leuven Med Ctr 1987; **Fellow:** Hematology & Oncology, Indiana Univ Med Ctr 1990; **Fac Appt:** Prof Med, Univ Chicago-Pritzker Sch Med

Winter, Jane N MD [Hem] - **Spec Exp:** Lymphoma, Non-Hodgkin's; Hodgkin's Disease; Bone Marrow Transplant; **Hospital:** Northwestern Meml Hosp; **Address:** Northwestern Univ - Div Hem/Oncology, 675 N St Clair St, Ste 21-100, Chicago, IL 60611; **Phone:** 312-695-0990; **Board Cert:** Internal Medicine 1980; Hematology 1982; Medical Oncology 1983; **Med School:** Univ Pennsylvania 1977; **Resid:** Internal Medicine, Univ Chicago Hosps 1980; **Fellow:** Hematology & Oncology, Columbia Presby Hosp 1981; Hematology & Oncology, Northwestern Univ 1983; **Fac Appt:** Prof Med, Northwestern Univ

Hematology

Great Plains and Mountains

Vose, Julie M MD [Hem] - Spec Exp: Lymphoma; **Hospital:** Nebraska Med Ctr; **Address:** Univ Nebraska Med Assoc, Emile @ 42nd St, Omaha, NE 68198; **Phone:** 402-559-5600; **Board Cert:** Internal Medicine 1987; Hematology 2000; Medical Oncology 2000; **Med School:** Univ Nebr Coll Med 1987; **Resid:** Internal Medicine, Univ Nebraska Med Ctr 1987; **Fellow:** Hematology & Oncology, Univ Nebraska Med Ctr 1990; **Fac Appt:** Prof Med, Univ Nebr Coll Med

Walters, Theodore MD [Hem] - Spec Exp: Myeloproliferative Disorders; Lymphoma; **Hospital:** St. Luke's Reg Med Ctr - Boise, St Alphonsus Regl Med Ctr; **Address:** 520 S Eagle Rd, Lower Level, Meridian, ID 83642; **Phone:** 208-706-5651; **Board Cert:** Internal Medicine 1972; Hematology 1976; **Med School:** Oregon Hlth Sci Univ 1963; **Resid:** Internal Medicine, Univ Oregon Med Ctr 1970; **Fellow:** Hematology, Univ Oregon Med Ctr 1972; **Fac Appt:** Asst Clin Prof Med, Univ Wash

Southwest

Barlogie, Bart MD/PhD [Hem] - Spec Exp: Bone Marrow Transplant; Plasma Cell Disorders; Multiple Myeloma; **Hospital:** UAMS Med Ctr; **Address:** UAMS-Myeloma Inst Rsch & Therapy, 4301 West Markham St, Slot 816, Little Rock, AR 72205; **Phone:** 501-603-1583; **Med School:** Germany 1969; **Resid:** Internal Medicine, Univ Muenster Med Sch; **Fellow:** Medical Oncology, MD Anderson Cancer Ctr-Tumor Inst 1976; **Fac Appt:** Prof Med, Univ Ark

Boldt, David H MD [Hem] - Spec Exp: Leukemia; Lymphoma; Multiple Myeloma; **Hospital:** Univ Hlth Sys - Univ Hosp; **Address:** UT Hlth Sci Ctr, Div Hematology, 7703 Floyd Curl Drive, MC 7880, San Antonio, TX 78229; **Phone:** 210-567-4848; **Board Cert:** Internal Medicine 1973; Hematology 1974; Medical Oncology 1975; **Med School:** Tufts Univ 1969; **Resid:** Internal Medicine, Barnes Hosp-Wash Univ 1971; **Fellow:** Hematology & Oncology, Barnes Hosp 1973; **Fac Appt:** Prof Med, Univ Tex, San Antonio

Brenner, Malcolm K MD/PhD [Hem] - Spec Exp: Gene Therapy; Bone Marrow Transplant; **Hospital:** Methodist Hosp - Houston, Texas Chldns Hosp - Houston; **Address:** 6621 Fannin St, rm 3-3320, Houston, TX 77030; **Phone:** 832-824-4671; **Med School:** England 1975; **Resid:** Internal Medicine, Cambridge Univ 1979; **Fellow:** Immunology, Clinical Research Ctr 1984; Hematology & Oncology, Royal Free Hospital 1986; **Fac Appt:** Prof Med, Baylor Coll Med

Champlin, Richard E MD [Hem] - Spec Exp: Bone Marrow Transplant; Stem Cell Transplant; Leukemia & Lymphoma; **Hospital:** UT MD Anderson Cancer Ctr (page 81); **Address:** MD Anderson Cancer Ctr, Div Hematology, 1515 Holcombe Blvd, Box 0423, Houston, TX 77030; **Phone:** 713-792-3618; **Board Cert:** Internal Medicine 1978; Hematology 1980; Medical Oncology 1981; **Med School:** Univ Chicago-Pritzker Sch Med 1975; **Resid:** Internal Medicine, LA Co Harbor/UCLA Med Ctr 1978; **Fellow:** Hematology & Oncology, LA Co Harbor/UCLA Med Ctr 1980; **Fac Appt:** Prof Med, Univ Tex, Houston

Cobos, Everardo MD [Hem] - Spec Exp: Bone Marrow Transplant; **Hospital:** Univ Med Ctr - Lubbock; **Address:** Texas Tech Univ Med Sch, Dept Med, 3601 4th St, MS 9410, Lubbock, TX 79430; **Phone:** 806-743-3155; **Board Cert:** Internal Medicine 1985; Medical Oncology 1987; Hematology 1988; **Med School:** Univ Tex, San Antonio 1981; **Resid:** Internal Medicine, Letterman Army Med Ctr 1985; **Fellow:** Hematology & Oncology, Letterman Army Med Ctr 1988; **Fac Appt:** Prof Med, Texas Tech Univ

Cooper, Barry MD [Hem] - **Spec Exp:** Leukemia; Lymphoma; **Hospital:** Baylor Univ Medical Ctr; **Address:** 3535 Worth St, Ste 200, Dallas, TX 75246-2096; **Phone:** 214-370-1002; **Board Cert:** Internal Medicine 1974; Medical Oncology 1977; Hematology 1978; **Med School:** Johns Hopkins Univ 1971; **Resid:** Internal Medicine, Johns Hopkins Hosp 1973; **Fellow:** Metabolism, Natl Inst of Health 1975; Hematology, Peter Bent Brigham Hosp 1977; **Fac Appt:** Clin Prof Med, Univ Tex SW, Dallas

Fields, Karen MD [Hem] - **Spec Exp:** Bone Marrow & Stem Cell Transplant; Breast Cancer; **Hospital:** Univ Hlth Sys - Univ Hosp, Christus Santa Rosa Children's Hosp; **Address:** Cancer Therapy & Rsch Ctr, 7979 Wurzbach, Urschel Twr, Ste 600, San Antonio, TX 78229-3264; **Phone:** 210-450-1405; **Board Cert:** Internal Medicine 1984; Medical Oncology 1989; Hematology 1990; **Med School:** Ohio State Univ 1981; **Resid:** Internal Medicine, The Jewish Hospital 1984; Medical Oncology, University of Cincinnati 1988; **Fellow:** Hematology & Oncology, University Hospital 1989

Fonseca, Rafael MD [Hem] - **Spec Exp:** Multiple Myeloma; **Hospital:** Mayo Clin Hosp - Scottsdale; **Address:** 13400 E Shea Blvd, MCCRB 3-001, Scottsdale, AZ 85259; **Phone:** 480-301-6118; **Board Cert:** Internal Medicine 1994; Hematology 1998; Medical Oncology 1997; **Med School:** Mexico 1991; **Resid:** Internal Medicine, Jackson Meml Hosp 1994; **Fellow:** Hematology & Oncology, Mayo Clinic 1998; **Fac Appt:** Assoc Prof Med, Mayo Med Sch

Kantarjian, Hagop M MD [Hem] - **Spec Exp:** Leukemia; **Hospital:** UT MD Anderson Cancer Ctr (page 81); **Address:** 1400 Holcombe Blvd, Unit 428, Houston, TX 77030; **Phone:** 713-792-7026; **Board Cert:** Internal Medicine 1983; Medical Oncology 1985; **Med School:** Lebanon 1979; **Resid:** Internal Medicine, Univ Tex MD Anderson Cancer Ctr 1983; **Fellow:** Hematology & Oncology, Univ Tex MD Anderson Cancer Ctr 1983; **Fac Appt:** Prof Med, Univ Tex, Houston

Keating, Michael MD [Hem] - **Spec Exp:** Leukemia; **Hospital:** UT MD Anderson Cancer Ctr (page 81); **Address:** MD Anderson Cancer Ctr, 1515 Holcombe Blvd, Box 428, Houston, TX 77030; **Phone:** 713-745-2376; **Med School:** Australia 1966; **Resid:** Internal Medicine, St Vincents Hosp 1973; **Fellow:** Hematology, MD Anderson Cancer Ctr 1975; **Fac Appt:** Prof Med, Univ Tex, Houston

Lyons, Roger M MD [Hem] - **Spec Exp:** Leukemia & Lymphoma; Multiple Myeloma; **Hospital:** SW TX Meth Hosp, Methodist Spec & Transpl Hosp; **Address:** 4411 Medical Drive, Ste 100, San Antonio, TX 78229-3325; **Phone:** 210-595-5300; **Board Cert:** Internal Medicine 1981; Hematology 1982; **Med School:** Canada 1967; **Resid:** Internal Medicine, Winnipeg Genl Hosp 1969; Internal Medicine, Barnes-Wohl Hosps 1972; **Fellow:** Hematology, Washington Univ Hosps 1975; **Fac Appt:** Clin Prof Med, Univ Tex, San Antonio

Maddox, Anne Marie MD [Hem] - **Spec Exp:** Hematologic Malignancies; Lung Cancer; Head & Neck Cancer; Clinical Trials; **Hospital:** UAMS Med Ctr; **Address:** Univ Arkansas Med Ctr, 4301 W Markham St, Slot 74-5, Little Rock, AR 72205; **Phone:** 501-686-8530; **Board Cert:** Internal Medicine 1979; Medical Oncology 1985, Hematology 2004; **Med School:** Dalhousie Univ 1975; **Resid:** Internal Medicine, Univ Toronto 1978; **Fellow:** Medical Oncology, MD Anderson Cancer Ctr 1982; **Fac Appt:** Prof, Univ Ark

Strauss, James F MD [Hem] - **Spec Exp:** Bleeding/Coagulation Disorders; Leukemia; Lymphoma; **Hospital:** Presby Hosp of Dallas; **Address:** Texas Oncology, Professional Bldg 2, 8220 Walnut Hill Ln, Ste 700, Dallas, TX 75231; **Phone:** 214-739-4175; **Board Cert:** Internal Medicine 1976; Hematology 1978; Medical Oncology 1981; **Med School:** NYU Sch Med 1972; **Resid:** Internal Medicine, Baylor Univ Medical Ctr 1976; **Fellow:** Hematology, Univ Texas SW Medical Ctr 1977

Hematology

Yeager, Andrew M MD [Hem] - **Spec Exp:** Bone Marrow & Stem Cell Transplant; Leukemia; **Hospital:** Univ Med Ctr - Tucson; **Address:** Arizona Cancer Ctr, 1515 N Campbell Ave, Ste 2956, Tuscon, AZ 85724-0001; **Phone:** 520-626-0662; **Board Cert:** Pediatrics 1979; Pediatric Hematology-Oncology 1980; **Med School:** Johns Hopkins Univ 1975; **Resid:** Pediatrics, Johns Hopkins Hosp 1978; **Fellow:** Pediatric Hematology-Oncology, Johns Hopkins Hosp 1980; **Fac Appt:** Prof Med, Univ Ariz Coll Med

West Coast and Pacific

Coutre, Steven E MD [Hem] - **Spec Exp:** Leukemia; Multiple Myeloma; **Hospital:** Stanford Univ Med Ctr; **Address:** Stanford Univ Med Ctr, Hematology Clinic, 875 Blake Wilbur Drive, MC 5820, Stanford, CA 94305; **Phone:** 650-723-9729; **Med School:** Stanford Univ 1986; **Resid:** Internal Medicine, Yale-New Haven Hosp 1989; **Fellow:** Hematology, Stanford Univ Med Ctr 1992; **Fac Appt:** Assoc Prof Med, Stanford Univ

Damon, Lloyd E MD [Hem] - **Spec Exp:** Multiple Myeloma; Hematologic Malignancies; Stem Cell Transplant; **Hospital:** UCSF Med Ctr; **Address:** UCSF Comprehensive Cancer Ctr, 400 Parnassus Ave, Ste A502, San Francisco, CA 94143; **Phone:** 415-353-2421; **Board Cert:** Internal Medicine 1985; Hematology 1988; Medical Oncology 1987; **Med School:** Univ Mich Med Sch 1982; **Resid:** Internal Medicine, UCSF Med Ctr 1985; **Fellow:** Hematology & Oncology, UCSF Med Ctr 1988; **Fac Appt:** Clin Prof Med, UCSF

Feinstein, Donald I MD [Hem] - **Spec Exp:** Hematologic Malignancies; **Hospital:** USC Norris Comp Cancer Ctr, USC Univ Hosp - R K Eamer Med Plz; **Address:** USC Keck Sch Med, Topping Tower, 1441 Eastlake Ave, Ste 3436, Los Angeles, CA 90033-9172; **Phone:** 323-865-3964; **Board Cert:** Internal Medicine 1965; Hematology 1974; **Med School:** Stanford Univ 1958; **Resid:** Internal Medicine, LAC-USC Med Ctr 1962; **Fellow:** Hematology, NYU Med Ctr 1966; **Fac Appt:** Prof Med, USC Sch Med

Forman, Stephen J MD [Hem] - **Spec Exp:** Lymphoma; Leukemia; Bone Marrow Transplant; **Hospital:** City of Hope Natl Med Ctr & Beckman Rsch (page 69); **Address:** City Hope National Medical Ctr, 1500 E Duarte Rd, rm 3002, Duarte, CA 91010-3012; **Phone:** 626-256-4673 x62403; **Board Cert:** Internal Medicine 1977; **Med School:** USC Sch Med 1974; **Resid:** Internal Medicine, LAC-Harbor-UCLA Med Ctr 1976; **Fellow:** Hematology, LAC-USC Med Ctr 1978; Hematology, City of Hope Med Ctr 1979; **Fac Appt:** Clin Prof Med, USC Sch Med

Heinrich, Michael C MD [Hem] - **Spec Exp:** Hematologic Malignancies; Sarcoma; Gastrointestinal Stromal Tumors; **Hospital:** VA Medical Center - Portland, OR Hlth & Sci Univ; **Address:** 3710 SW Veteran's Hospital Rd, Bldg 103 - rm E211, MC RND19, Portland, OR 97239; **Phone:** 503-220-8262; **Board Cert:** Internal Medicine 1987; Hematology 2000; Medical Oncology 2001; **Med School:** Johns Hopkins Univ 1984; **Resid:** Internal Medicine, Oreg Hlth Scis Univ 1987; **Fellow:** Hematology & Oncology, Oreg Hlth Scis Univ 1991; **Fac Appt:** Prof Med, Oregon Hlth Sci Univ

Levine, Alexandra M MD [Hem] - **Spec Exp:** Leukemia & Lymphoma; AIDS Related Cancers; **Hospital:** City of Hope Natl Med Ctr & Beckman Rsch (page 69); **Address:** 1500 E Duarte Rd, Needleman 213, Duarte, CA 91010; **Phone:** 626-256-4673; **Med School:** USC Sch Med 1971; **Resid:** Internal Medicine, LAC-USC Med Ctr 1974; **Fellow:** Hematology & Oncology, Grady Meml Hosp-Emory Univ 1975; Hematology, LAC-USC Med Ctr 1978; **Fac Appt:** Prof Med, USC Sch Med

Lill, Michael MD [Hem] - **Spec Exp:** Lymphoma; Leukemia; Stem Cell Transplant; Bone Marrow Transplant; **Hospital:** Cedars-Sinai Med Ctr; **Address:** Cedars-Sinai Med Ctr- Outpt Cancer Ctr, 8700 Beverly Blvd, Ste AC 1070, Los Angeles, CA 90048; **Phone:** 310-423-1160; **Med School:** Australia 1982; **Resid:** Internal Medicine, Sir Charles Gairdner Hospital 1985; **Fellow:** Hematology, Royal Perth Hospital 1988; **Fac Appt:** Assoc Prof Med, UCLA

Linenberger, Michael MD [Hem] - **Spec Exp:** Bone Marrow Transplant; Leukemia & Lymphoma; Multiple Myeloma; **Hospital:** Univ Wash Med Ctr; **Address:** 825 Eastlake Ave E, MS G6-800, Seattle, WA 98109; **Phone:** 206-288-1260; **Board Cert:** Internal Medicine 1985; Hematology 1988; **Med School:** Univ Kans 1982; **Resid:** Internal Medicine, Rhode Island Hosp 1985; **Fellow:** Hematology, Univ Wash Med Ctr 1989; **Fac Appt:** Assoc Prof Med, Univ Wash

Linker, Charles A MD [Hem] - **Spec Exp:** Leukemia; Bone Marrow Transplant; Multiple Myeloma; **Hospital:** UCSF Med Ctr, St Francis Memorial Hosp; **Address:** 400 Parnassus Ave, Ste A502, San Francisco, CA 94143; **Phone:** 415-353-2421; **Board Cert:** Internal Medicine 1978; Hematology 1980; Medical Oncology 1981; **Med School:** Stanford Univ 1974; **Resid:** Internal Medicine, Stanford Univ Hosp 1978; **Fellow:** Hematology & Oncology, UCSF Med Ctr 1981; **Fac Appt:** Clin Prof Med, UCSF

Maziarz, Richard MD [Hem] - **Spec Exp:** Leukemia; Immunotherapy; Bone Marrow Transplant; Lymphoma; **Hospital:** OR Hlth & Sci Univ; **Address:** OHSU Ctr Hematologic Malignancies, 3181 SW Sam Jackson Park Rd, UHN 73C, Portland, OR 97239; **Phone:** 503-494-5058; **Board Cert:** Internal Medicine 1982; Hematology 1988; Medical Oncology 1989; **Med School:** Harvard Med Sch 1979; **Resid:** Internal Medicine, Univ Hosp 1982; **Fellow:** Hematology & Oncology, Brigham & Womens Hosp 1988; **Fac Appt:** Prof Med, Oregon Hlth Sci Univ

Negrin, Robert S MD [Hem] - **Spec Exp:** Bone Marrow Transplant; **Hospital:** Stanford Univ Med Ctr; **Address:** BMT Program, 300 Pasteur Drive, rm H3249, MC 5623, Stanford, CA 94305; **Phone:** 650-723-0822; **Board Cert:** Internal Medicine 1987; Hematology 1992; **Med School:** Harvard Med Sch 1984; **Resid:** Internal Medicine, Stanford Univ Hosp 1987; **Fellow:** Hematology, Stanford Univ Hosp 1990; **Fac Appt:** Prof Med, Stanford Univ

O'Donnell, Margaret R MD [Hem] - **Spec Exp:** Leukemia; Clinical Trials; **Hospital:** City of Hope Natl Med Ctr & Beckman Rsch (page 69); **Address:** City of Hope National Med Ctr, 1500 E Duarte Rd, MOB-rm 3001, Duarte, CA 91010; **Phone:** 626-359-8111 x62405; **Board Cert:** Internal Medicine 1980; Hematology 1980; Medical Oncology 1979; **Med School:** Med Coll PA 1974; **Resid:** Internal Medicine, Montreal Genl Hosp 1976; Hematology, Royal Victoria Hosp 1977; **Fellow:** Hematology & Oncology, Fred Hutchinson Cancer Ctr 1979

Saven, Alan MD [Hem] - **Spec Exp:** Leukemia; Lymphoma; **Hospital:** Scripps Green Hosp; **Address:** Scripps Green Hosp, 10666 N Torrey Pines Rd, MS 217, La Jolla, CA 92037; **Phone:** 858-554-9489; **Board Cert:** Internal Medicine 1987; Medical Oncology 1989; Hematology 1990; **Med School:** South Africa 1982; **Resid:** Internal Medicine, Albert Einstein Med Ctr 1986; **Fellow:** Hematology & Oncology, Scripps Clinic 1987

Schiller, Gary J MD [Hem] - **Spec Exp:** Leukemia; **Hospital:** UCLA Med Ctr (page 83); **Address:** UCLA Med Ctr, 10833 Le Conte Ave, rm 42-121 CHS, Los Angeles, CA 90095; **Phone:** 310-825-5513; **Board Cert:** Internal Medicine 1987; Hematology 2000; Medical Oncology 1989; **Med School:** USC Sch Med 1984; **Resid:** Internal Medicine, UCLA Med Ctr 1987; **Fellow:** Hematology & Oncology, UCLA Med Ctr 1990; **Fac Appt:** Prof Med, UCLA

Snyder, David S MD [Hem] - **Spec Exp:** Leukemia; Bone Marrow Transplant; **Hospital:** City of Hope Natl Med Ctr & Beckman Rsch (page 69); **Address:** 1500 E Duarte Rd, Duarte, CA 91010-3012; **Phone:** 626-256-4673; **Board Cert:** Internal Medicine 1980; Hematology 1984; **Med School:** Harvard Med Sch 1977; **Resid:** Internal Medicine, Beth Israel Hosp 1980; **Fellow:** Immunology, Harvard Med Sch 1982; Hematology & Oncology, New England Med Ctr 1984

Medical Oncology

New England

Anderson, Kenneth C MD [Onc] - **Spec Exp:** Multiple Myeloma; **Hospital:** Dana-Farber Cancer Inst, Brigham & Women's Hosp; **Address:** Dana Farber Cancer Inst, 44 Binney St Mayer Bldg - rm 557, Boston, MA 02115; **Phone:** 617-632-2144; **Board Cert:** Internal Medicine 1980; **Med School:** Johns Hopkins Univ 1977; **Resid:** Internal Medicine, Johns Hopkins Hosp 1980; **Fellow:** Hematology & Oncology, Dana Farber Cancer Inst 1983; **Fac Appt:** Prof Med, Harvard Med Sch

Antin, Joseph Harry MD [Onc] - **Spec Exp:** Bone Marrow Transplant; Stem Cell Transplant; Leukemia; **Hospital:** Brigham & Women's Hosp, Dana-Farber Cancer Inst; **Address:** 44 Binney St, rm D1B12, Boston, MA 02115-6013; **Phone:** 617-632-3667; **Board Cert:** Internal Medicine 1981; Medical Oncology 1983; Hematology 1984; **Med School:** Cornell Univ-Weill Med Coll 1978; **Resid:** Internal Medicine, Peter Bent Brigham Hosp 1981; **Fellow:** Hematology & Oncology, Brigham & Womens Hosp/Dana Farber 1984; **Fac Appt:** Prof Med, Harvard Med Sch

Atkins, Michael B MD [Onc] - **Spec Exp:** Melanoma; Kidney Cancer; Immunotherapy; **Hospital:** Beth Israel Deaconess Med Ctr - Boston; **Address:** Beth Israel Deaconess Med Ctr, Cancer Clinical Trials, 330 Brookline Ave, E-157, Boston, MA 02215; **Phone:** 617-667-1930; **Board Cert:** Internal Medicine 1983; Medical Oncology 1987; **Med School:** Tufts Univ 1980; **Resid:** Internal Medicine, New England Med Ctr 1983; **Fellow:** Hematology & Oncology, New England Med Ctr 1987; **Fac Appt:** Prof Med, Harvard Med Sch

Burstein, Harold J MD [Onc] - **Spec Exp:** Breast Cancer; **Hospital:** Dana-Farber Cancer Inst, Brigham & Women's Hosp; **Address:** Dana Farber Cancer Inst, 44 Binney St, Boston, MA 02115; **Phone:** 617-632-4587; **Board Cert:** Internal Medicine 1997; Medical Oncology 2000; **Med School:** Harvard Med Sch 1994; **Resid:** Internal Medicine, Mass Genl Hosp 1996; **Fellow:** Medical Oncology, Dana Farber Cancer Inst 1999; **Fac Appt:** Asst Prof Med, Harvard Med Sch

Canellos, George P MD [Onc] - **Spec Exp:** Lymphoma; Leukemia; Breast Cancer; **Hospital:** Dana-Farber Cancer Inst, Brigham & Women's Hosp; **Address:** 44 Binney St, Boston, MA 02115; **Phone:** 617-632-3470; **Board Cert:** Internal Medicine 1967; Hematology 1972; Medical Oncology 1973; **Med School:** Columbia P&S 1960; **Resid:** Internal Medicine, Mass Genl Hosp 1963; Internal Medicine, Mass Genl Hosp 1966; **Fellow:** Medical Oncology, Natl Cancer Inst 1965; Hematology, Hammersmith Hosp 1967; **Fac Appt:** Prof Med, Harvard Med Sch

Chabner, Bruce A MD [Onc] - Spec Exp: Colon & Rectal Cancer; Breast Cancer; **Hospital:** Mass Genl Hosp; **Address:** Mass General Hospital, 55 Fruit St, Lawrence House 214, Boston, MA 02114; **Phone:** 617-724-3200; **Board Cert:** Internal Medicine 1971; Medical Oncology 1973; **Med School:** Harvard Med Sch 1965; **Resid:** Internal Medicine, Peter Bent Brigham Hosp 1967; Internal Medicine, Yale-New Haven Hosp 1970; **Fellow:** Medical Oncology, Natl Inst Hlth 1969; **Fac Appt:** Prof Med, Harvard Med Sch

Chu, Edward MD [Onc] - Spec Exp: Colon & Rectal Cancer; Gastrointestinal Cancer; Clinical Trials; **Hospital:** Yale - New Haven Hosp, VA Conn Hlthcre Sys; **Address:** Yale Cancer Ctr, 333 Cedar St, PO Box 208032, rm WWW221, New Haven, CT 06520-8032; **Phone:** 203-785-6879; **Board Cert:** Internal Medicine 1986; Medical Oncology 1989; **Med School:** Brown Univ 1983; **Resid:** Internal Medicine, Roger Williams Hosp 1987; **Fellow:** Hematology & Oncology, Natl Cancer Inst 1990; Internal Medicine, Natl Cancer Inst 1992; **Fac Appt:** Prof Med, Yale Univ

Come, Steven E MD [Onc] - Spec Exp: Breast Cancer; Hodgkin's Disease; **Hospital:** Beth Israel Deaconess Med Ctr - Boston, Dana-Farber Cancer Inst; **Address:** Beth Israel Deaconess Hosp, 330 Brookline Ave, Boston, MA 02215-5400; **Phone:** 617-667-4599; **Board Cert:** Internal Medicine 1975; Medical Oncology 1979; **Med School:** Harvard Med Sch 1972; **Resid:** Internal Medicine, Beth Israel Hosp 1977; **Fellow:** Medical Oncology, Natl Cancer Inst 1976; **Fac Appt:** Assoc Prof Med, Harvard Med Sch

Demetri, George D MD [Onc] - Spec Exp: Sarcoma; **Hospital:** Dana-Farber Cancer Inst; **Address:** Dana Farber Cancer Inst, 44 Binney St, Shields-Warren 530, Boston, MA 02115; **Phone:** 617-632-3985; **Board Cert:** Internal Medicine 1986; Medical Oncology 1989; **Med School:** Stanford Univ 1983; **Resid:** Internal Medicine, Univ Wash Med Ctr 1986; **Fellow:** Medical Oncology, Dana Farber Cancer Inst 1989; **Fac Appt:** Assoc Prof Med, Harvard Med Sch

DeVita Jr, Vincent T MD [Onc] - Spec Exp: Lymphoma Consultation; Hodgkin's Disease Consultation; **Hospital:** Yale - New Haven Hosp; **Address:** Yale Cancer Ctr, 333 Cedar St, rm WWW-211B, New Haven, CT 06520-8028; **Phone:** 203-737-1010; **Board Cert:** Internal Medicine 1974; Hematology 1972; Medical Oncology 1973; **Med School:** Geo Wash Univ 1961; **Resid:** Internal Medicine, Geo Wash Hosp 1963; Internal Medicine, Yale-New Haven Hosp 1966; **Fellow:** Medical Oncology, Natl Cancer Inst 1965; **Fac Appt:** Prof Med, Yale Univ

Earle, Craig C MD [Onc] - Spec Exp: Gastrointestinal Cancer; **Hospital:** Dana-Farber Cancer Inst; **Address:** Dana Farber Cancer Institute, 44 Binney St, Boston, MA 02115; **Phone:** 617-632-5564; **Board Cert:** Internal Medicine 2004; Medical Oncology 2000; **Med School:** Univ Ottawa 1990; **Resid:** Internal Medicine, Univ Ottawa 1994; **Fellow:** Medical Oncology, Univ Ottawa 1996; **Fac Appt:** Assoc Prof Med, Harvard Med Sch

Erban III, John K MD [Onc] - Spec Exp: Breast Cancer; Hematologic Malignancies; Stem Cell Transplant; **Hospital:** Tufts-New England Med Ctr; **Address:** Tufts-New England Med Ctr, 750 Washington St, Box 245, Boston, MA 02111; **Phone:** 617-636-5147; **Board Cert:** Internal Medicine 1984; Medical Oncology 1989; Hematology 1999; **Med School:** Tufts Univ 1981; **Resid:** Internal Medicine, Hosp Univ Penn 1984; **Fellow:** Hematology & Oncology, New England Med Ctr 1990; **Fac Appt:** Assoc Prof Med, Tufts Univ

Medical Oncology

Fuchs, Charles S MD [Onc] - **Spec Exp:** Gastrointestinal Cancer; **Hospital:** Dana-Farber Cancer Inst, Brigham & Women's Hosp; **Address:** 44 Binney St, Dana 1220, Boston, MA 02115; **Phone:** 617-632-5840; **Board Cert:** Internal Medicine 1989; Medical Oncology 2002; Hematology 1996; **Med School:** Harvard Med Sch 1986; **Resid:** Internal Medicine, Brigham & Womens Hosp 1989; **Fellow:** Hematology & Oncology, Dana Farber Cancer Inst 1992; **Fac Appt:** Assoc Prof Med, Harvard Med Sch

Garber, Judy E MD [Onc] - **Spec Exp:** Breast Cancer; **Hospital:** Dana-Farber Cancer Inst; **Address:** Dana Farber Cancer Inst, 44 Binney St, Smith 209, Boston, MA 02115; **Phone:** 617-632-5770; **Board Cert:** Internal Medicine 1984; Medical Oncology 1987; Hematology 1988; **Med School:** Yale Univ 1981; **Resid:** Internal Medicine, Brigham & Womens Hosp 1984; **Fellow:** Medical Oncology, Dana Farber Cancer Inst 1988; Epidemiology, Dana Farber Cancer Inst 1990; **Fac Appt:** Assoc Prof Med, Harvard Med Sch

Garnick, Marc B MD [Onc] - **Spec Exp:** Prostate Cancer; Urologic Cancer; **Hospital:** Beth Israel Deaconess Med Ctr - Boston; **Address:** Beth Israel Deaconess Medical Ctr, SCC9, 330 Brookline Ave, Boston, MA 02215; **Phone:** 617-667-9187; **Board Cert:** Internal Medicine 1976; Medical Oncology 1979; **Med School:** Univ Pennsylvania 1972; **Resid:** Internal Medicine, Univ Penn Hosp 1974; **Fellow:** Research, Natl Inst Hlth 1976; Medical Oncology, Dana-Farber Cancer Inst 1978; **Fac Appt:** Clin Prof Med, Harvard Med Sch

Grunberg, Steven Marc MD [Onc] - **Spec Exp:** Lung Cancer; Head & Neck Cancer; **Hospital:** FAHC - UHC Campus; **Address:** FAHC-UHC Campus, St Joseph-3, 1 S Prospect St, Burlington, VT 05401; **Phone:** 802-847-8400; **Board Cert:** Internal Medicine 1978; Medical Oncology 1983; **Med School:** Cornell Univ-Weill Med Coll 1975; **Resid:** Internal Medicine, Mofitt Hosp-U Calif 1978; **Fellow:** Medical Oncology, Sidney Farber Cancer Ctr 1981; **Fac Appt:** Prof Med, Univ VT Coll Med

Haluska, Frank G MD/PhD [Onc] - **Spec Exp:** Melanoma; **Hospital:** Tufts-New England Med Ctr; **Address:** Tufts-New England Med Ctr, 750 Washington St, Box 245, Boston, MA 02111; **Phone:** 617-636-5147; **Board Cert:** Internal Medicine 2002; Medical Oncology 1995; **Med School:** Univ Pennsylvania 1989; **Resid:** Internal Medicine, Mass Genl Hosp 1991; **Fellow:** Medical Oncology, Dana-Farber Cancer Inst 1994; **Fac Appt:** Prof Med, Tufts Univ

Hammond, Denis B MD [Onc] - **Spec Exp:** Breast Cancer; Prostate Cancer; **Hospital:** Elliot Hosp, Catholic Med Ctr; **Address:** NH Oncology-Hematology, 200 Technology Drive, Hooksett, NH 03106; **Phone:** 603-622-6484; **Board Cert:** Internal Medicine 1977; Hematology 1978; **Med School:** Tufts Univ 1973; **Resid:** Internal Medicine, SUNY Buffalo Affil Hosps 1976; **Fellow:** Hematology, Mass Genl Hosp 1977; Medical Oncology, Dartmouth Med Sch 1978

Johnson, Bruce E MD [Onc] - **Spec Exp:** Lung Cancer; Thoracic Cancers; Merkel Cell Carcinoma; **Hospital:** Dana-Farber Cancer Inst, Brigham & Women's Hosp; **Address:** Lowe Ctr Thoracic Oncology, 44 Binney St, Ste D-1234, Boston, MA 02115; **Phone:** 617-632-4790; **Board Cert:** Internal Medicine 1982; Medical Oncology 1985; **Med School:** Univ Minn 1979; **Resid:** Internal Medicine, Univ Chicago Hosps 1982; **Fellow:** Medical Oncology, Natl Cancer Inst 1985; **Fac Appt:** Assoc Prof Med, Harvard Med Sch

Kaelin, William G MD [Onc] - **Spec Exp:** Drug Discovery & Development; **Hospital:** Dana-Farber Cancer Inst; **Address:** Dana Farber Cancer Inst, 44 Binney St, rm MA-457, Boston, MA 02115; **Phone:** 617-632-4747; **Board Cert:** Internal Medicine 1987; Medical Oncology 1989; **Med School:** Duke Univ 1982; **Resid:** Internal Medicine, Johns Hopkins Hosp 1986; **Fellow:** Medical Oncology, Dana Farber Cancer Inst 1989; **Fac Appt:** Prof Med, Harvard Med Sch

Kantoff, Philip W MD [Onc] - **Spec Exp:** Genitourinary Cancer; Prostate Cancer; **Hospital:** Dana-Farber Cancer Inst, Brigham & Women's Hosp; **Address:** 44 Binney St, Ste D-1230, Boston, MA 02115; **Phone:** 617-632-3466; **Board Cert:** Internal Medicine 1982; Medical Oncology 1989; **Med School:** Brown Univ 1979; **Resid:** Internal Medicine, NYU/Bellevue Hosp 1983; **Fellow:** Gene Therapy Research, NIH 1986; **Fac Appt:** Prof Med, Harvard Med Sch

Kaufman, Peter A MD [Onc] - **Spec Exp:** Breast Cancer; Clinical Trials; **Hospital:** Dartmouth - Hitchcock Med Ctr; **Address:** Dartmouth-Hitchcock Med Ctr, Dept Hem/Onc, One Medical Center Drive, Lebanon, NH 03756; **Phone:** 603-653-6181; **Board Cert:** Internal Medicine 1986; Medical Oncology 1989; **Med School:** NYU Sch Med 1983; **Resid:** Internal Medicine, Duke Univ Med Ctr 1986; **Fellow:** Hematology & Oncology, Duke Univ Med Ctr 1989; **Fac Appt:** Assoc Prof Med, Dartmouth Med Sch

Lacy, Jill MD [Onc] - **Spec Exp:** Colon & Rectal Cancer; Brain Tumors; Gastrointestinal Cancer; **Hospital:** Yale - New Haven Hosp; **Address:** Yale Univ Sch Med - Div Medical Oncology, 333 Cedar St, PO Box 208032, New Haven, CT 06520-8032; **Phone:** 203-785-4191; **Board Cert:** Internal Medicine 1982; Medical Oncology 2005; **Med School:** Yale Univ 1978; **Resid:** Internal Medicine, Yale-New Haven Hosp 1981; **Fellow:** Medical Oncology, Yale-New Haven Hosp 1985; **Fac Appt:** Assoc Prof Med, Yale Univ

Lynch, Thomas MD [Onc] - **Spec Exp:** Lung Cancer; Thoracic Cancers; **Hospital:** Mass Genl Hosp; **Address:** Mass Genl Hosp, Dept Hem/Onc, 55 Fruit St, Yawkey Bldg - Ste 7B, Boston, MA 02114-2617; **Phone:** 617-724-1136; **Board Cert:** Internal Medicine 1989; Medical Oncology 2003; **Med School:** Yale Univ 1986; **Resid:** Internal Medicine, Mass Genl Hosp 1989; **Fellow:** Medical Oncology, Dana-Farber Cancer Inst 1991; **Fac Appt:** Asst Prof Med, Harvard Med Sch

Matulonis, Ursula A MD [Onc] - **Spec Exp:** Gynecologic Cancer; Ovarian Cancer; Breast Cancer; Drug Development; **Hospital:** Dana-Farber Cancer Inst; **Address:** Dana Farber Cancer Institute, 44 Binney St, Ste Dana 1210, Boston, MA 02115; **Phone:** 617-632-2334; **Board Cert:** Internal Medicine 2000; Medical Oncology 2000; **Med School:** Albany Med Coll 1987; **Resid:** Internal Medicine, Univ Pittsburgh Hosp 1990; **Fellow:** Medical Oncology, Dana Farber Cancer Inst 1993; **Fac Appt:** Asst Prof Med, Harvard Med Sch

Mayer, Robert J MD [Onc] - **Spec Exp:** Colon & Rectal Cancer; Gastrointestinal Cancer; **Hospital:** Dana-Farber Cancer Inst, Brigham & Women's Hosp; **Address:** Dana Farber Cancer Inst, 44 Binney St, rm D1608, Boston, MA 02115-6084; **Phone:** 617-632-34/4; **Board Cert:** Internal Medicine 1973; Medical Oncology 1975; Hematology 1976; **Med School:** Harvard Med Sch 1969; **Resid:** Internal Medicine, Mt Sinai Hosp 1971; Hematology & Oncology, Natl Cancer Inst 1974; **Fellow:** Dana Farber Cancer Inst 1976; **Fac Appt:** Prof Med, Harvard Med Sch

Muss, Hyman B MD [Onc] - **Spec Exp:** Breast Cancer; **Hospital:** FAHC - Med Ctr Campus; **Address:** Fletcher Allen Health Care-UHC Campus, 1 S Prospect St, Joseph 3, Burlington, VT 05401-1429; **Phone:** 802-847-3827; **Board Cert:** Internal Medicine 1973; Hematology 1974; Medical Oncology 1975; **Med School:** SUNY Downstate 1968; **Resid:** Internal Medicine, Peter Bent Brigham Hosp 1970; **Fellow:** Hematology & Oncology, Peter Bent Brigham Hosp 1974; **Fac Appt:** Prof Med, Univ VT Coll Med

Nadler, Lee M MD [Onc] - **Spec Exp:** Lymphoma; **Hospital:** Dana-Farber Cancer Inst, Brigham & Women's Hosp; **Address:** Dana Farber Cancer Inst, 44 Binney St, SM 339, Boston, MA 02115; **Phone:** 617-632-3331; **Board Cert:** Internal Medicine 1976; **Med School:** Harvard Med Sch 1973; **Resid:** Internal Medicine, Columbia-Presby Hosp 1975; **Fellow:** Medical Oncology, Natl Cancer Inst 1977; Medical Oncology, Dana-Farber Cancer Inst 1978; **Fac Appt:** Prof Med, Harvard Med Sch

Posner, Marshall R MD [Onc] - **Spec Exp:** Head & Neck Cancer; Skin Cancer-Head & Neck; **Hospital:** Dana-Farber Cancer Inst, Beth Israel Deaconess Med Ctr - Boston; **Address:** Dana-Farber Cancer Inst-H&N Cancer Ctr, 44 Binney St, rm G430, Brookline, MA 02115; **Phone:** 617-632-3090; **Board Cert:** Internal Medicine 1978; Medical Oncology 1981; **Med School:** Tufts Univ 1975; **Resid:** Internal Medicine, Boston City Hosp 1978; **Fellow:** Oncology, Dana-Farber Cancer Inst 1981; **Fac Appt:** Assoc Prof Med, Harvard Med Sch

Schnipper, Lowell E MD [Onc] - **Spec Exp:** Breast Cancer; **Hospital:** Beth Israel Deaconess Med Ctr - Boston; **Address:** Beth Israel Deaconess Med Ctr, 330 Brookline Ave, Boston, MA 02215; **Phone:** 617-667-1198; **Board Cert:** Internal Medicine 1973; Medical Oncology 1983; **Med School:** SUNY Downstate 1968; **Resid:** Internal Medicine, Yale-New Haven Hosp 1970; Medical Oncology, Natl Cancer Inst 1973; **Fellow:** Hematology & Oncology, Barnes Jewish Hosp 1974; **Fac Appt:** Prof Med, Harvard Med Sch

Seiden, Michael MD/PhD [Onc] - **Spec Exp:** Ovarian Cancer; Gynecologic Cancer; **Hospital:** Mass Genl Hosp; **Address:** Mass General Hospital, 55 Fruit St, LRH 108, Boston, MA 02114; **Phone:** 617-724-3123; **Board Cert:** Internal Medicine 1989; Medical Oncology 2004; **Med School:** Washington Univ, St Louis 1986; **Resid:** Internal Medicine, Mass Genl Hosp 1990; **Fellow:** Medical Oncology, Dana Farber Cancer Ctr 1992; **Fac Appt:** Assoc Prof Med, Harvard Med Sch

Shulman, Lawrence N MD [Onc] - **Spec Exp:** Breast Cancer; Lymphoma; **Hospital:** Dana-Farber Cancer Inst; **Address:** Dana-Farber Cancer Inst, 44 Binney St, rm Dana-1608, Boston, MA 02115; **Phone:** 617-632-2277; **Board Cert:** Internal Medicine 1978; Medical Oncology 1981; Hematology 1982; **Med School:** Harvard Med Sch 1975; **Resid:** Internal Medicine, Beth Israel Hosp 1977; **Fellow:** Hematology & Oncology, Beth Israel Hosp 1980; **Fac Appt:** Assoc Prof Med, Harvard Med Sch

Taplin, Mary-Ellen MD [Onc] - **Spec Exp:** Prostate Cancer; Genitourinary Cancer; **Hospital:** Dana-Farber Cancer Inst, Brigham & Women's Hosp; **Address:** Dana Farber Cancer Inst, 44 Binney St, rm D1230, Boston, MA 02115; **Phone:** 617-632-3237; **Board Cert:** Internal Medicine 1989; Hematology 1996; Medical Oncology 2003; **Med School:** Univ Mass Sch Med 1986; **Resid:** Internal Medicine, U Mass Med Ctr 1990; **Fellow:** Hematology & Oncology, Beth Israel Deaconess Hosp 1993; **Fac Appt:** Assoc Prof Med

Treon, Steven P MD/PhD [Onc] - **Spec Exp:** Waldenstrom's Macroglobulinemia; Multiple Myeloma; **Hospital:** Dana-Farber Cancer Inst; **Address:** Dana-Farber Cancer Inst, 44 Binney St, Mayer 548B, Boston, MA 02115; **Phone:** 617-632-2681; **Board Cert:** Internal Medicine 1995; Medical Oncology 1997; **Med School:** Boston Univ 1993; **Resid:** Internal Medicine, Boston Univ Med Ctr 1995; **Fellow:** Hematology & Oncology, Mass Genl Hosp 1996; Research, Dana Farber Cancer Inst 1997; **Fac Appt:** Asst Prof Med, Harvard Med Sch

Weisberg, Tracey MD [Onc] - **Spec Exp:** Breast Cancer; **Hospital:** Maine Med Ctr; **Address:** 100 Campus Drive, Unit 108, Scarborough, ME 04074; **Phone:** 207-885-7600; **Board Cert:** Internal Medicine 1987; Medical Oncology 1989; **Med School:** SUNY Stony Brook 1983; **Resid:** Internal Medicine, Mount Sinai Hosp 1985; Internal Medicine, Hartford Hosp 1986; **Fellow:** Medical Oncology, Yale Univ Hosp 1988

Winer, Eric P MD [Onc] - **Spec Exp:** Breast Cancer; **Hospital:** Dana-Farber Cancer Inst, Brigham & Women's Hosp; **Address:** Dana Farber Cancer Inst, 44 Binney St, Mayer 2, Boston, MA 02115; **Phone:** 617-632-2175; **Board Cert:** Internal Medicine 1987; Medical Oncology 1989; **Med School:** Yale Univ 1983; **Resid:** Internal Medicine, Yale-New Haven Hosp 1987; **Fellow:** Hematology & Oncology, Duke Univ 1989; **Fac Appt:** Assoc Prof Med, Harvard Med Sch

Mid Atlantic

Abeloff, Martin MD [Onc] - **Spec Exp:** Breast Cancer; **Hospital:** Johns Hopkins Hosp - Baltimore; **Address:** 401 N Broadway, Ste 1100, Baltimore, MD 21231; **Phone:** 410-955-8822; **Board Cert:** Internal Medicine 1973; Medical Oncology 1973; **Med School:** Johns Hopkins Univ 1966; **Resid:** Internal Medicine, Beth Israel Hosp 1970; **Fellow:** Hematology, New England Med Ctr 1971; **Fac Appt:** Prof Med, Johns Hopkins Univ

Agarwala, Sanjiv MD [Onc] - **Spec Exp:** Melanoma; Melanoma Clinical Trials; Head & Neck Cancer; **Hospital:** St Luke's Hosp - Bethlehem; **Address:** St Luke's Cancer Ctr, 801 Ostrum St, Bethlehem, PA 18015; **Phone:** 610-954-2145; **Board Cert:** Internal Medicine 1994; Hematology 1996; Medical Oncology 1995; **Med School:** India 1985; **Resid:** Internal Medicine, Univ Pittsburgh Med Ctr 1993; **Fellow:** Hematology & Oncology, Univ Pittsburgh Med Ctr 1994; **Fac Appt:** Asst Prof Med, Univ Pittsburgh

Ahlgren, James D MD [Onc] - **Spec Exp:** Gastrointestinal Cancer; **Hospital:** G Washington Univ Hosp; **Address:** Geo Wash Univ Med Ctr, Div Hem/Oncology, 2150 Pennsylvania Ave NW, Ste 3-428, Washington, DC 20037-3201; **Phone:** 202-741-2478; **Board Cert:** Internal Medicine 1980; Medical Oncology 1989; **Med School:** Georgetown Univ 1977; **Resid:** Internal Medicine, Georgetown Univ Hosp 1979; **Fellow:** Medical Oncology, Georgetown Univ Hosp 1981; **Fac Appt:** Prof Med, Geo Wash Univ

Aisner, Joseph MD [Onc] - **Spec Exp:** Lung Cancer; Solid Tumors; **Hospital:** Robert Wood Johnson Univ Hosp - New Brunswick; **Address:** Cancer Inst of New Jersey, 195 Little Albany St, rm 2012, New Brunswick, NJ 08903-2681; **Phone:** 732-235-6777; **Board Cert:** Internal Medicine 1973; Medical Oncology 1975; **Med School:** Wayne State Univ 1970; **Resid:** Internal Medicine, Georgetown Univ Hosp 1972; **Fellow:** Medical Oncology, Natl Cancer Inst 1975

Algazy, Kenneth M MD [Onc] - **Spec Exp:** Lung Cancer; Mesothelioma; Hematologic Malignancies; **Hospital:** Hosp Univ Penn - UPHS (page 84), VA Med Ctr; **Address:** Hosp Univ Pennsylvania, 3400 Spruce St, 12 Penn Tower, Philadelphia, PA 19104; **Phone:** 215-614-1858; **Board Cert:** Internal Medicine 1972; Hematology 1974; Medical Oncology 1979; **Med School:** Temple Univ 1969; **Resid:** Internal Medicine, Univ Rochester-Strong Meml Hosp 1972; **Fellow:** Hematology & Oncology, Johns Hopkins Med Ctr 1974; **Fac Appt:** Clin Prof Med, Univ Pennsylvania

Ambinder, Richard F MD/PhD [Onc] - **Spec Exp:** Lymphoma; Hodgkin's Disease; AIDS Related Cancers; **Hospital:** Johns Hopkins Hosp - Baltimore; **Address:** Cancer Research Bldg, 1650 Orleans St, rm CRB 389, Baltimore, MD 21231; **Phone:** 410-955-8964; **Board Cert:** Internal Medicine 1982; Medical Oncology 1985; **Med School:** Johns Hopkins Univ 1979; **Resid:** Internal Medicine, Johns Hopkins Hosp 1981; **Fellow:** Internal Medicine, Johns Hopkins Hosp 1982; Medical Oncology, Johns Hopkins Hosp 1985; **Fac Appt:** Prof Med, Johns Hopkins Univ

Medical Oncology

Bashevkin, Michael MD [Onc] - Spec Exp: Solid Tumors; Hematologic Malignancies; **Hospital:** Maimonides Med Ctr (page 75); **Address:** 1660 E 14st St, Ste 501, Brooklyn, NY 11229; **Phone:** 718-382-8500 x501; **Board Cert:** Internal Medicine 1976; Hematology 1978; Medical Oncology 1979; **Med School:** SUNY Downstate 1973; **Resid:** Internal Medicine, VA Med Ctr 1976; Hematology & Oncology, Maimonides Med Ctr 1979

Belani, Chandra MD [Onc] - Spec Exp: Lung Cancer; Drug Discovery; **Hospital:** UPMC Shadyside, UPMC Presby, Pittsburgh; **Address:** UPMC Cancer Pavilion, 5150 Centre Ave Fl 5, Pittsburgh, PA 15232; **Phone:** 412-648-6619; **Board Cert:** Internal Medicine 1986; Medical Oncology 1987; **Med School:** India 1978; **Resid:** Internal Medicine, SMS Med Hosp 1981; Internal Medicine, Good Samaritan/Univ MD Hosp 1984; **Fellow:** Hematology & Oncology, Univ Maryland Hosp 1987; **Fac Appt:** Prof Med, Univ Pittsburgh

Bosl, George MD [Onc] - Spec Exp: Testicular Cancer; Head & Neck Cancer; **Hospital:** Meml Sloan Kettering Cancer Ctr (page 76); **Address:** 1275 York Ave, rm C1289, New York, NY 10021; **Phone:** 212-639-8473; **Board Cert:** Internal Medicine 1976; Medical Oncology 1979; **Med School:** Creighton Univ 1973; **Resid:** Internal Medicine, New York Hosp 1975; Internal Medicine, Memorial Sloan-Kettering Cancer Ctr 1977; **Fellow:** Medical Oncology, Univ Minn Hosps 1979; **Fac Appt:** Prof Med, Cornell Univ-Weill Med Coll

Brufsky, Adam MD/PhD [Onc] - Spec Exp: Breast Cancer; **Hospital:** Magee-Womens Hosp - UPMC, UPMC Presby, Pittsburgh; **Address:** Univ Pitt Cancer Inst/Magee-Women's Hosp, 300 Halket St, Ste 4628, Pittsburgh, PA 15213; **Phone:** 412-641-4530; **Board Cert:** Internal Medicine 2004; Medical Oncology 2005; **Med School:** Univ Conn 1990; **Resid:** Internal Medicine, Brigham & Womens Hosp 1992; **Fellow:** Medical Oncology, Dana Farber Cancer Inst 1995; Medical Microbiology, Brigham & Womens Hosp 1995; **Fac Appt:** Asst Prof Med, Univ Pittsburgh

Carducci, Michael A MD [Onc] - Spec Exp: Urologic Cancer; Drug Discovery & Development; Vaccine Therapy; Clinical Trials; **Hospital:** Johns Hopkins Hosp - Baltimore; **Address:** Sidney Kimmel Cancer Ctr, 1650 Orleans St IM59 BB Bldg, Baltimore, MD 21231; **Phone:** 410-614-3977; **Board Cert:** Internal Medicine 2001; Medical Oncology 2005; **Med School:** Washington Univ, St Louis 1988; **Resid:** Internal Medicine, Univ Colorado Hlth Sci Ctr 1992; **Fellow:** Medical Oncology, Johns Hopkins Hosp 1995; **Fac Appt:** Assoc Prof Med, Johns Hopkins Univ

Chanan-Khan, Asher A A MD [Onc] - Spec Exp: Multiple Myeloma; Leukemia; **Hospital:** Roswell Park Cancer Inst; **Address:** Roswell Park Cancer Inst, Elm & Carlton Sts, Buffalo, NY 14263; **Phone:** 716-845-3221; **Board Cert:** Internal Medicine 1997; Medical Oncology 2001; **Med School:** Pakistan 1993; **Resid:** Internal Medicine, Harlem Hosp Ctr 1997; **Fellow:** Hematology & Oncology, NYU Med Ctr 1999; **Fac Appt:** Asst Prof Med, SUNY Buffalo

Chapman, Paul MD [Onc] - Spec Exp: Melanoma; Immunotherapy; **Hospital:** Meml Sloan Kettering Cancer Ctr (page 76); **Address:** 1275 York Ave, New York, NY 10021; **Phone:** 646-888-2378; **Board Cert:** Internal Medicine 1984; Medical Oncology 1987; **Med School:** Cornell Univ-Weill Med Coll 1981; **Resid:** Internal Medicine, Univ Chicago Hosps 1984; **Fellow:** Medical Oncology, Meml Sloan-Kettering Cancer Ctr 1987; **Fac Appt:** Prof Med, Cornell Univ-Weill Med Coll

Cohen, Philip MD [Onc] - **Spec Exp:** Breast Cancer; **Hospital:** Georgetown Univ Hosp; **Address:** Georgetown Univ Hosp, Lombardi Cancer Ctr, 3800 Reservoir Rd NW, Washington, DC 20007; **Phone:** 202-444-2198; **Board Cert:** Internal Medicine 1973; Medical Oncology 1975; Hematology 1976; **Med School:** Harvard Med Sch 1970; **Resid:** Internal Medicine, Mass Genl Hosp 1972; **Fellow:** Medical Oncology, Natl Cancer Inst 1974; **Fac Appt:** Assoc Prof Med, Geo Wash Univ

Cohen, Roger MD [Onc] - **Spec Exp:** Drug Discovery & Development; Clinical Trials; **Hospital:** Fox Chase Cancer Ctr (page 73); **Address:** Fox Chase Cancer Ctr, 333 Cottman Ave, Ste C307, Philadelphia, PA 19111; **Phone:** 215-214-1676; **Board Cert:** Internal Medicine 1984; Medical Oncology 1993; Hematology 1986; **Med School:** Harvard Med Sch 1980; **Resid:** Internal Medicine, Mt Sinai Hosp 1982; **Fellow:** Research, Sloan Kettering Cancer Inst 1985; Hematology, Mt Sinai Hosp 1986

Cohen, Seymour M MD [Onc] - **Spec Exp:** Melanoma; Breast Cancer; Lung Cancer; Merkel Cell Carcinoma; **Hospital:** Mount Sinai Med Ctr (page 77); **Address:** 1045 5th Ave, New York, NY 10028-0138; **Phone:** 212-249-9141; **Board Cert:** Internal Medicine 1971; Medical Oncology 1973; **Med School:** Univ Pittsburgh 1962; **Resid:** Internal Medicine, Montefiore Med Ctr 1964; Internal Medicine, Mount Sinai Med Ctr 1965; **Fellow:** Hematology, Mount Sinai Med Ctr 1966; Hematology & Oncology, LI Jewish Hosp 1969; **Fac Appt:** Assoc Clin Prof Med, Mount Sinai Sch Med

Coleman, Morton MD [Onc] - **Spec Exp:** Lymphoma; Hodgkin's Disease; Multiple Myeloma; Waldenstrom's Macroglobulinemia; **Hospital:** NY-Presby Hosp (page 79); **Address:** 407 E 70th St, FL 3, New York, NY 10021-5302; **Phone:** 212-517-5900; **Board Cert:** Internal Medicine 1971; Hematology 1972; Medical Oncology 1973; **Med School:** Med Coll VA 1963; **Resid:** Internal Medicine, Grady Meml Hosp-Emory 1965; Internal Medicine, New York Hosp-Cornell 1968; **Fellow:** Hematology & Oncology, New York Hosp-Cornell 1970; **Fac Appt:** Clin Prof Med, Cornell Univ-Weill Med Coll

Comis, Robert L MD [Onc] - **Spec Exp:** Lung Cancer; **Hospital:** Hahnemann Univ Hosp; **Address:** 1818 Market St, Ste 1100, Philadelphia, PA 19103; **Phone:** 215-789-3609; **Board Cert:** Internal Medicine 1975; Medical Oncology 1977; **Med School:** SUNY Upstate Med Univ 1971; **Resid:** Internal Medicine, SUNY Upstate Med Ctr 1975; **Fac Appt:** Prof Med, Drexel Univ Coll Med

Cullen, Kevin MD [Onc] - **Spec Exp:** Head & Neck Cancer; **Hospital:** Univ of MD Med Sys; **Address:** Univ Md Greenbaum Cancer Ctr, 22 S Greene St, rm N9E22, Baltimore, MD 21201; **Phone:** 410-328-5506; **Board Cert:** Internal Medicine 1986; Medical Oncology 1989; **Med School:** Harvard Med Sch 1983; **Resid:** Internal Medicine, Beth Israel Hosp 1986; Internal Medicine, Hammersmith Hosp; **Fellow:** Medical Oncology, Natl Cancer Inst 1988

Czuczman, Myron MD [Onc] - **Spec Exp:** Lymphoma; Multiple Myeloma; Leukemia; **Hospital:** Roswell Park Cancer Inst; **Address:** Roswell Park Cancer Inst, Elm & Carlton Sts, Buffalo, NY 14263; **Phone:** 716-845-7695; **Board Cert:** Internal Medicine 1988; Medical Oncology 1991; **Med School:** Penn State Univ-Hershey Med Ctr 1985; **Resid:** Internal Medicine, North Shore Univ Hosp 1988; **Fellow:** Hematology & Oncology, Meml Sloan-Kettering Cancer Ctr 1992; **Fac Appt:** Assoc Prof Med, SUNY Buffalo

Medical Oncology

Daly, Mary B MD/PhD [Onc] - **Spec Exp:** Breast Cancer; Breast Cancer Risk Assessment; Cancer Prevention; Ovarian Cancer Risk Assessment; **Hospital:** Fox Chase Cancer Ctr (page 73); **Address:** Fox Chase Cancer Ctr, 333 Cottman Ave, P1054, Philadelphia, PA 19111; **Phone:** 215-728-2791; **Board Cert:** Internal Medicine 1981; Medical Oncology 1983; **Med School:** Univ NC Sch Med 1978; **Resid:** Internal Medicine, Univ Texas Hlth Sci Ctr 1981; **Fellow:** Medical Oncology, Univ Texas Hlth Sci Ctr 1983; **Fac Appt:** Clin Prof Med, Temple Univ

Davidson, Nancy E MD [Onc] - **Spec Exp:** Breast Cancer; **Hospital:** Johns Hopkins Hosp - Baltimore; **Address:** Johns Hopkins Oncology Center, 1650 Orleans St, Baltimore, MD 21231-1000; **Phone:** 410-955-8964; **Board Cert:** Internal Medicine 1982; Medical Oncology 1985; **Med School:** Harvard Med Sch 1979; **Resid:** Internal Medicine, Johns Hopkins Hosp 1982; **Fellow:** Medical Oncology, Natl Cancer Inst 1986; **Fac Appt:** Prof Med, Johns Hopkins Univ

Dawson, Nancy MD [Onc] - **Spec Exp:** Prostate Cancer; Kidney Cancer; Bladder Cancer; **Hospital:** Univ of MD Med Sys; **Address:** Univ Maryland - Greenbaum Cancer Ctr, 22 S Greene St, Baltimore, MD 21201; **Phone:** 410-328-2565; **Board Cert:** Internal Medicine 1982; Medical Oncology 1985; Hematology 1984; **Med School:** Georgetown Univ 1979; **Resid:** Internal Medicine, Walter Reed AMC 1982; **Fellow:** Hematology & Oncology, Walter Reed AMC 1985; **Fac Appt:** Prof Med, Univ MD Sch Med

Dickler, Maura MD [Onc] - **Spec Exp:** Breast Cancer; **Hospital:** Meml Sloan Kettering Cancer Ctr (page 76); **Address:** Meml Sloan Kettering Cancer Ctr, 1275 York Ave, New York, NY 10021; **Phone:** 212-639-5456; **Board Cert:** Internal Medicine 1994; Medical Oncology 1998; **Med School:** Univ Chicago-Pritzker Sch Med 1991; **Resid:** Internal Medicine, Univ Chicago Hosps 1994; **Fellow:** Medical Oncology, Meml Sloan Kettering Cancer Ctr 1998; **Fac Appt:** Asst Prof Med, Cornell Univ-Weill Med Coll

Donehower, Ross Carl MD [Onc] - **Spec Exp:** Pancreatic Cancer; Colon Cancer; Prostate Cancer; **Hospital:** Johns Hopkins Hosp - Baltimore; **Address:** Hopkins Kimmel Cancer Ctr, 1650 Orleans St, CRB-187, Baltimore, MD 21231-1000; **Phone:** 410-955-8838; **Board Cert:** Internal Medicine 1977; Medical Oncology 1979; **Med School:** Univ Minn 1974; **Resid:** Internal Medicine, Johns Hopkins Hosp 1976; **Fellow:** Medical Oncology, Natl Inst Hlth 1980; **Fac Appt:** Prof Med, Johns Hopkins Univ

Doroshow, James H MD [Onc] - **Spec Exp:** Drug Discovery & Development; Colon Cancer; Breast Cancer; **Hospital:** Natl Inst of Hlth - Clin Ctr; **Address:** National Cancer Institute, Div Cancer Treatment & Diagnosis, 31 Center, Bldg 31-rm 3A44, Bethesda, MD 20892; **Phone:** 301-496-4291; **Board Cert:** Internal Medicine 1976; Medical Oncology 1977; **Med School:** Harvard Med Sch 1973; **Resid:** Internal Medicine, Mass Genl Hosp 1975; **Fellow:** Medical Oncology, Natl Cancer Inst 1978

Dutcher, Janice P MD [Onc] - **Spec Exp:** Kidney Cancer; Melanoma; Breast Cancer; **Hospital:** Our Lady of Mercy Med Ctr; **Address:** Our Lady of Mercy Cancer Ctr, 600 E 233rd St, Bronx, NY 10466-2697; **Phone:** 718-304-7219; **Board Cert:** Internal Medicine 1978; Medical Oncology 1983; **Med School:** UC Davis 1975; **Resid:** Internal Medicine, Rush Presbyterian Med Ctr 1978; **Fellow:** Medical Oncology, National Cancer Inst 1981; **Fac Appt:** Prof Med, NY Med Coll

Eisenberger, Mario MD [Onc] - **Spec Exp:** Prostate Cancer; **Hospital:** Johns Hopkins Hosp - Baltimore; **Address:** 1650 Orleans St, rm 1M51, Baltimore, MD 21231; **Phone:** 410-614-3511; **Board Cert:** Internal Medicine 1976; Medical Oncology 1979; **Med School:** Brazil 1972; **Resid:** Internal Medicine, Michael Reese Hosp 1975; **Fellow:** Hematology, Michael Reese Hosp 1976; Medical Oncology, Jackson Meml Hosp/Univ Miami 1979; **Fac Appt:** Prof Med, Johns Hopkins Univ

Ettinger, David S MD [Onc] - **Spec Exp:** Lung Cancer; Sarcoma; Clinical Trials; **Hospital:** Johns Hopkins Hosp - Baltimore; **Address:** Bunting Blaustein Cancer Rsrch Bldg, 1650 Orleans St, rm G88, Baltimore, MD 21231-1000; **Phone:** 410-955-8847; **Board Cert:** Internal Medicine 1976; Medical Oncology 1977; **Med School:** Univ Louisville Sch Med 1967; **Resid:** Internal Medicine, Mayo Grad Schl 1971; **Fellow:** Medical Oncology, Johns Hopkins Hosp 1975; **Fac Appt:** Prof Med, Johns Hopkins Univ

Fanucchi, Michael P MD [Onc] - **Spec Exp:** Sarcoma; Aerodigestive Tract Cancer; Lung Cancer; **Hospital:** St Vincent Cath Med Ctrs - Manhattan; **Address:** 325 W 15th St, New York, NY 10011; **Phone:** 212-604-6011; **Board Cert:** Internal Medicine 1980; Medical Oncology 1985; **Med School:** Columbia P&S 1977; **Resid:** Internal Medicine, Bronx Muni Hosp Ctr 1981; **Fellow:** Medical Oncology, Meml Sloan-Kettering Cancer Ctr 1984; **Fac Appt:** Assoc Prof Med, Emory Univ

Fine, Howard Alan MD [Onc] - **Spec Exp:** Brain Tumors; **Hospital:** Natl Inst of Hlth - Clin Ctr; **Address:** NIH/NCI/NOB, Bloch Building, Rm 225 MSC 8202, 9030 Old Georgetown Rd, Bethesda, MD 20892-0001; **Phone:** 301-402-6298; **Board Cert:** Internal Medicine 1987; Medical Oncology 1989; **Med School:** Mount Sinai Sch Med 1984; **Resid:** Internal Medicine, Hosp Univ Penn 1987; **Fellow:** Medical Oncology, Dana Farber Cancer Ctr 1990

Fine, Robert MD [Onc] - **Spec Exp:** Pancreatic Cancer; Drug Development; Brain Tumors; Clinical Trials; **Hospital:** NY-Presby Hosp (page 79); **Address:** Columbia Univ Comprehensive Cancer Ctr, 650 W 168th St, rm BB 20-05, New York, NY 10032; **Phone:** 212-305-1168; **Board Cert:** Internal Medicine 1983; Medical Oncology 1985; **Med School:** Univ Chicago-Pritzker Sch Med 1979; **Resid:** Internal Medicine, Stanford Univ Med Ctr 1982; **Fellow:** Medical Oncology, National Cancer Inst 1988; **Fac Appt:** Assoc Prof Med, Columbia P&S

Fisher, Richard I MD [Onc] - **Spec Exp:** Lymphoma; Hodgkin's Disease; **Hospital:** Univ of Rochester Strong Meml Hosp; **Address:** James P Wilmot Cancer Ctr, 601 Elmwood Ave, Box 704, Rochester, NY 14642; **Phone:** 585-275-5823; **Board Cert:** Internal Medicine 1973; Medical Oncology 1977; **Med School:** Harvard Med Sch 1970; **Resid:** Internal Medicine, Mass Genl Hosp 1972; **Fac Appt:** Prof Med, Univ Rochester

Flomenberg, Neal MD [Onc] - **Spec Exp:** Bone Marrow Transplant; Stem Cell Transplant; Leukemia & lymphoma; **Hospital:** Thomas Jefferson Univ Hosp (page 82); **Address:** Thomas Jefferson Univ Hosp, 125 S 9th St, Ste 801, Philadelphia, PA 19107; **Phone:** 215-955-0356; **Board Cert:** Internal Medicine 1979; Medical Oncology 1981; Hematology 1982; **Med School:** Jefferson Med Coll 1976; **Resid:** Internal Medicine, Montefiore Med Ctr 1979; **Fellow:** Hematology & Oncology, Meml Sloan Kettering Cancer Ctr 1982; **Fac Appt:** Clin Prof Med, Thomas Jefferson Univ

Forastiere, Arlene A MD [Onc] - Spec Exp: Esophageal Cancer; Head & Neck Cancer; **Hospital:** Johns Hopkins Hosp - Baltimore; **Address:** Bunting Blaustein Cancer Research Bldg, 1650 Orleans St, rm G90, Baltimore, MD 21231; **Phone:** 410-955-8964; **Board Cert:** Internal Medicine 1978; Medical Oncology 1981; **Med School:** NY Med Coll 1975; **Resid:** Internal Medicine, Albert Einstein Med Ctr 1977; Internal Medicine, Univ Conn Health Ctr 1978; **Fellow:** Medical Oncology, Meml Sloan Kettering Cancer Ctr 1980; **Fac Appt:** Prof Med, NY Med Coll

Fox, Kevin R MD [Onc] - Spec Exp: Breast Cancer; **Hospital:** Hosp Univ Penn - UPHS (page 84); **Address:** 3400 Spruce St, 14 Penn Tower, Philadelphia, PA 19104; **Phone:** 215-662-7469; **Board Cert:** Internal Medicine 1985; Medical Oncology 1987; **Med School:** Johns Hopkins Univ 1981; **Resid:** Internal Medicine, Johns Hopkins Hosp 1984; **Fellow:** Hematology & Oncology, Hosp Univ Penn 1987; **Fac Appt:** Prof Med, Univ Pennsylvania

Gabrilove, Janice MD [Onc] - Spec Exp: Myelodysplastic Syndromes; Leukemia; **Hospital:** Mount Sinai Med Ctr (page 77); **Address:** Mount Sinai Med Ctr, Box 1129, One Gustave Levy Pl, New York, NY 10029-6574; **Phone:** 212-241-9650; **Board Cert:** Internal Medicine 1980; Medical Oncology 1983; **Med School:** Mount Sinai Sch Med 1977; **Resid:** Internal Medicine, Columbia-Presby Med Ctr 1980; **Fellow:** Hematology & Oncology, Meml Sloan-Kettering Cancer Ctr 1983; **Fac Appt:** Prof Med, Mount Sinai Sch Med

Gelmann, Edward P MD [Onc] - Spec Exp: Prostate Cancer; Testicular Cancer; **Hospital:** Georgetown Univ Hosp; **Address:** Lombardi Cancer Ctr, Podium A, 3800 Reservoir Rd NW, Washington, DC 20007; **Phone:** 202-444-7303; **Board Cert:** Internal Medicine 1979; Medical Oncology 1981; **Med School:** Stanford Univ 1976; **Resid:** Internal Medicine, Univ Chicago Hosps 1978; **Fellow:** Medical Oncology, National Cancer Inst 1981; **Fac Appt:** Prof Med, Georgetown Univ

Geyer Jr, Charles E MD [Onc] - Spec Exp: Breast Cancer; **Hospital:** Allegheny General Hosp; **Address:** Allegheny Cancer Ctr, 320 E North Ave Fl 5, Pittsburgh, PA 15212; **Phone:** 412-359-6147; **Board Cert:** Internal Medicine 1983; Medical Oncology 1987; **Med School:** Texas Tech Univ 1980; **Resid:** Internal Medicine, Baylor Affil Hosps 1983; **Fellow:** Medical Oncology, Baylor Affil Hosps 1985

Glick, John H MD [Onc] - Spec Exp: Breast Cancer; Hodgkin's Disease; Lymphoma, Non-Hodgkin's; **Hospital:** Hosp Univ Penn - UPHS (page 84); **Address:** Abramson Cancer Ctr of Univ Penn, 3400 Spruce St, 1218 Penn Tower, Philadelphia, PA 19104; **Phone:** 215-662-6334; **Board Cert:** Internal Medicine 1973; Medical Oncology 1975; **Med School:** Columbia P&S 1969; **Resid:** Internal Medicine, Presbyterian Hosp 1971; **Fellow:** Medical Oncology, Natl Cancer Inst 1973; Medical Oncology, Stanford Univ 1974; **Fac Appt:** Prof Med, Univ Pennsylvania

Goldstein, Lori J MD [Onc] - Spec Exp: Breast Cancer; **Hospital:** Fox Chase Cancer Ctr (page 73); **Address:** Fox Chase Cancer Ctr, Dept Med Oncology, 333 Cottman Ave, Philadelphia, PA 19111; **Phone:** 215-728-2689; **Board Cert:** Internal Medicine 1985; Medical Oncology 2002; **Med School:** SUNY Upstate Med Univ 1982; **Resid:** Internal Medicine, Presby Univ Hosp 1985; **Fellow:** Medical Oncology, Natl Cancer Inst/NIH 1990

Grana, Generosa MD [Onc] - **Spec Exp:** Breast Cancer; Cancer Genetics; Cancer Prevention; **Hospital:** Cooper Univ Hosp, Virtua West Jersey Hosp - Voorhees (page 73); **Address:** 900 Centennial Blvd, Ste M, Voorhees, NJ 08043; **Phone:** 856-325-6740; **Board Cert:** Internal Medicine 1988; Medical Oncology 2001; **Med School:** Northwestern Univ 1985; **Resid:** Internal Medicine, Temple Univ Hosp 1988; **Fellow:** Hematology & Oncology, Fox Chase Cancer Ctr 1992; **Fac Appt:** Assoc Prof Med, UMDNJ-RW Johnson Med Sch

Grossbard, Michael L MD [Onc] - **Spec Exp:** Lymphoma; Breast Cancer; Gastrointestinal Cancer; **Hospital:** St Luke's - Roosevelt Hosp Ctr - Roosevelt Div (page 72), Beth Israel Med Ctr - Petrie Division (page 72); **Address:** 1000 10th Ave Fl 11 - Ste C02, New York, NY 10019; **Phone:** 212-523-5419; **Board Cert:** Internal Medicine 1989; Medical Oncology 2001; **Med School:** Yale Univ 1986; **Resid:** Internal Medicine, Mass Genl Hosp 1989; **Fellow:** Medical Oncology, Dana Farber Cancer Inst 1991; **Fac Appt:** Assoc Clin Prof Med, Columbia P&S

Grossman, Stuart MD [Onc] - **Spec Exp:** Brain Tumors; Neuro-Oncology; Pain-Cancer; **Hospital:** Johns Hopkins Hosp - Baltimore; **Address:** 550 N Broadway, Ste 1001, Baltimore, MD 21205; **Phone:** 410-955-8837; **Board Cert:** Internal Medicine 1976; Medical Oncology 1983; **Med School:** Univ Rochester 1973; **Resid:** Internal Medicine, Strong Meml Hosp 1976; **Fellow:** Medical Oncology, Johns Hopkins Hosp 1981; **Fac Appt:** Prof Med, Johns Hopkins Univ

Haas, Naomi S Balzer MD [Onc] - **Spec Exp:** Melanoma; Genitourinary Cancer; Kidney Cancer; Clinical Trials; **Hospital:** Fox Chase Cancer Ctr (page 73); **Address:** Fox Chase Cancer Ctr, 333 Cottman Ave, Philadelphia, PA 19111; **Phone:** 215-728-2974; **Board Cert:** Internal Medicine 1988; Medical Oncology 2005; **Med School:** NE Ohio Univ 1985; **Resid:** Internal Medicine, Abington Meml Hosp 1988; **Fellow:** Hematology & Oncology, Fox Chase Cancer Ctr 1989

Hait, William MD/PhD [Onc] - **Spec Exp:** Breast Cancer; **Hospital:** Robert Wood Johnson Univ Hosp - New Brunswick; **Address:** Cancer Inst of NJ, 195 Little Albany St, New Brunswick, NJ 08901-1914; **Phone:** 732-235-8064; **Board Cert:** Internal Medicine 1982; Medical Oncology 1987; **Med School:** Med Coll PA 1978; **Resid:** Internal Medicine, Yale-New Haven Hosp 1982; **Fellow:** Medical Oncology, Yale-New Haven Hosp 1983; **Fac Appt:** Prof Med, UMDNJ-RW Johnson Med Sch

Haller, Daniel G MD [Onc] - **Spec Exp:** Gastrointestinal Cancer; Colon & Rectal Cancer; Cancer Prevention; **Hospital:** Hosp Univ Penn - UPHS (page 84); **Address:** Hosp Univ Penn, Div Hematology/Oncology, 3400 Spruce St, 12 Penn Tower, Philadelphia, PA 19104; **Phone:** 215-662-7666; **Board Cert:** Internal Medicine 1976; Medical Oncology 1979; **Med School:** Univ Pittsburgh 1973; **Resid:** Internal Medicine, Georgetown Univ Hosp 1976; **Fellow:** Medical Oncology, Georgetown Univ Hosp 1978; **Fac Appt:** Prof Med, Univ Pennsylvania

Hesdorffer, Charles MD [Onc] - **Spec Exp:** Stem Cell Transplant; Immunotherapy; Melanoma; Sarcoma; **Hospital:** Johns Hopkins Hosp - Baltimore; **Address:** Johns Hopkins Univ Hosp, 720 Rutland Ave, rm 1025, Baltimore, MD 21205; **Phone:** 410-502-7004; **Board Cert:** Internal Medicine 1995; Medical Oncology 1997; **Med School:** South Africa 1978; **Resid:** Internal Medicine, Univ Wittwatersrand Hosp 1984; **Fellow:** Hematology & Oncology, Columbia-Presby Hosp 1988; **Fac Appt:** Prof Med, Johns Hopkins Univ

Hochster, Howard S MD [Onc] - Spec Exp: Gastrointestinal Cancer; Gynecologic Cancer; Colon & Rectal Cancer; **Hospital:** NYU Med Ctr (page 80); **Address:** NYU Cancer Institute, 160 E 34 St Fl 9, New York, NY 10016; **Phone:** 212-731-5100; **Board Cert:** Internal Medicine 1983; Medical Oncology 1985; Hematology 1986; **Med School:** Yale Univ 1980; **Resid:** Internal Medicine, NYU Med Ctr 1983; **Fellow:** Hematology & Oncology, NYU Med Ctr 1985; Medical Oncology, Jules Bordet Inst 1986; **Fac Appt:** Prof Med, NYU Sch Med

Holland, James F MD [Onc] - Spec Exp: Breast Cancer; Colon Cancer; Lung Cancer; **Hospital:** Mount Sinai Med Ctr (page 77); **Address:** Ruttenberg Cancer Ctr, Div Med Oncology, 1 Gustave L Levy Pl, Box 1129, New York, NY 10029-6500; **Phone:** 212-241-4495; **Board Cert:** Internal Medicine 1955; **Med School:** Columbia P&S 1947; **Resid:** Internal Medicine, Columbia-Presby Hosp 1949; **Fellow:** Medical Oncology, Francis Delafield Hosp 1953; **Fac Appt:** Prof Med, Mount Sinai Sch Med

Hudes, Gary R MD [Onc] - Spec Exp: Prostate Cancer; Genitourinary Cancer; Kidney Cancer; **Hospital:** Fox Chase Cancer Ctr (page 73); **Address:** Fox Chase Cancer Ctr, 333 Cottman Ave, rm C307, Philadelphia, PA 19111; **Phone:** 215-728-3889; **Board Cert:** Internal Medicine 1982; Hematology 1984; Medical Oncology 1985; **Med School:** SUNY Downstate 1979; **Resid:** Internal Medicine, Graduate Hosp 1982; **Fellow:** Hematology & Oncology, Presby-Univ Penn Med Ctr 1985

Hudis, Clifford A MD [Onc] - Spec Exp: Breast Cancer; **Hospital:** Meml Sloan Kettering Cancer Ctr (page 76); **Address:** Meml Sloan Kettering Cancer Ctr, 205 E 64th St, New York, NY 10021; **Phone:** 212-639-5449; **Board Cert:** Internal Medicine 1986; Medical Oncology 2001; **Med School:** Med Coll PA Hahnemann 1983; **Resid:** Internal Medicine, Hosp Med Coll Penn 1986; **Fellow:** Medical Oncology, Meml Sloan Kettering Cancer Ctr 1991; **Fac Appt:** Assoc Prof Med, Cornell Univ-Weill Med Coll

Ilson, David H MD [Onc] - Spec Exp: Esophageal Cancer; Colon & Rectal Cancer; Gastrointestinal Cancer; Mesothelioma; **Hospital:** Meml Sloan Kettering Cancer Ctr (page 76); **Address:** Meml Sloan-Kettering Cancer Ctr, 1275 York Ave, New York, NY 10021; **Phone:** 212-639-8306; **Board Cert:** Internal Medicine 1989; Medical Oncology 2002; **Med School:** NYU Sch Med 1986; **Resid:** Internal Medicine, Bellevue-NYU Sch Med 1989; **Fellow:** Medical Oncology, Meml Sloan Kettering Hosp 1992; **Fac Appt:** Assoc Prof Med, Cornell Univ-Weill Med Coll

Isaacs, Claudine J MD [Onc] - Spec Exp: Breast Cancer; Breast Cancer Risk Assessment; **Hospital:** Georgetown Univ Hosp; **Address:** Lombardi Cancer Ctr, Podium B, 3800 Reservoir Rd NW, Washington, DC 20007; **Phone:** 202-444-3677; **Board Cert:** Internal Medicine 2002; Medical Oncology 2003; **Med School:** McGill Univ 1987; **Resid:** Internal Medicine, Montreal General Hosp 1990; Hematology & Oncology, McGill Univ Hosp 1992; **Fellow:** Medical Oncology, Georgetown Univ Med Ctr 1993; **Fac Appt:** Assoc Prof Med, Georgetown Univ

Jurcic, Joseph G MD [Onc] - Spec Exp: Leukemia; Myelodysplastic Syndromes; Clinical Trials; **Hospital:** Meml Sloan Kettering Cancer Ctr (page 76); **Address:** Memorial Sloan Kettering Cancer Ctr, 1275 York Ave, New York, NY 10021; **Phone:** 212-639-2955; **Board Cert:** Internal Medicine 2001; Medical Oncology 2005; Hematology 1998; **Med School:** Univ Pennsylvania 1988; **Resid:** Internal Medicine, Barnes Hosp 1991; **Fellow:** Hematology & Oncology, Meml Sloan Kettering Cancer Ctr 1994; **Fac Appt:** Assoc Prof Med, Cornell Univ-Weill Med Coll

Karp, Judith MD [Onc] - Spec Exp: Leukemia; Clinical Trials; Myelodysplastic Syndromes; **Hospital:** Johns Hopkins Hosp - Baltimore; **Address:** 1650 Orleans St, rm 289, Baltimore, MD 21231; **Phone:** 410-502-7726; **Board Cert:** Internal Medicine 1976; **Med School:** Stanford Univ 1971; **Resid:** Internal Medicine, John Hopkins Hosp 1974; **Fellow:** Medical Oncology, John Hopkins Hosp 1977; **Fac Appt:** Prof Med, Johns Hopkins Univ

Kelsen, David MD [Onc] - Spec Exp: Gastrointestinal Cancer; Neuroendocrine Tumors; Unknown Primary Cancer; Merkel Cell Carcinoma; **Hospital:** Meml Sloan Kettering Cancer Ctr (page 76); **Address:** Gastrointestinal Oncology Svc, 1275 York Ave Howard Bldg Fl 9 - rm 918, New York, NY 10021; **Phone:** 212-639-8470; **Board Cert:** Internal Medicine 1976; Medical Oncology 1979; **Med School:** Hahnemann Univ 1972; **Resid:** Internal Medicine, Temple Univ Hosp 1976; **Fellow:** Medical Oncology, Meml Sloan Kettering Cancer Ctr 1978; **Fac Appt:** Prof Med, Cornell Univ-Weill Med Coll

Kemeny, Nancy MD [Onc] - Spec Exp: Colon Cancer; Rectal Cancer; Liver Cancer; **Hospital:** Meml Sloan Kettering Cancer Ctr (page 76); **Address:** Meml Sloan Kettering Cancer Ctr, 1275 York Ave, Ste Howard 916, New York, NY 10021; **Phone:** 212-639-8068; **Board Cert:** Internal Medicine 1974; Medical Oncology 1981; **Med School:** UMDNJ-NJ Med Sch, Newark 1971; **Resid:** Internal Medicine, St Luke's Hosp 1974; **Fellow:** Medical Oncology, Mem Sloan Kettering Cancer Ctr 1976; **Fac Appt:** Prof Med, Cornell Univ-Weill Med Coll

Kirkwood, John M MD [Onc] - Spec Exp: Melanoma; Immunotherapy; **Hospital:** UPMC Presby, Pittsburgh, UPMC Shadyside; **Address:** Hillman Cancer Research Pavilion, 5117 Centre Ave, Ste 1.32, Pittsburgh, PA 15213-1862; **Phone:** 412-623-7707; **Board Cert:** Internal Medicine 1976; Medical Oncology 1981; **Med School:** Yale Univ 1973; **Resid:** Internal Medicine, Yale-New Haven Hosp 1976; **Fellow:** Medical Oncology, Dana Farber Cancer Inst 1979; **Fac Appt:** Prof Med, Univ Pittsburgh

Kris, Mark G MD [Onc] - Spec Exp: Lung Cancer; Mediastinal Tumors; Thymoma; Thoracic Cancers; **Hospital:** Meml Sloan Kettering Cancer Ctr (page 76); **Address:** Memorial Sloan Kettering Cancer Ctr, 1275 York Ave, Howard H1018, New York, NY 10021; **Phone:** 212-639-7590; **Board Cert:** Internal Medicine 1980; Medical Oncology 1983; **Med School:** Cornell Univ-Weill Med Coll 1977; **Resid:** Internal Medicine, New York Hosp 1980; **Fellow:** Medical Oncology, Meml Sloan Kettering Cancer Ctr 1983; **Fac Appt:** Prof Med, Cornell Univ-Weill Med Coll

Langer, Corey J MD [Onc] - Spec Exp: Lung Cancer; Head & Neck Cancer; Mesothelioma; **Hospital:** Fox Chase Cancer Ctr (page 73); **Address:** Fox Chase Cancer Ctr, 333 Cottman Ave, Philadelphia, PA 19111-2412; **Phone:** 215-728-2985; **Board Cert:** Internal Medicine 1984; Hematology 1986; Medical Oncology 1987; **Med School:** Boston Univ 1981; **Resid:** Internal Medicine, Graduate Hosp 1984; Hematology & Oncology, Presby Hosp 1986; **Fellow:** Medical Oncology, Fox Chase Cancer Ctr 1987; **Fac Appt:** Assoc Prof Med, Temple Univ

Levine, Ellis MD [Onc] - Spec Exp: Breast Cancer; Urologic Cancer; **Hospital:** Roswell Park Cancer Inst; **Address:** Roswell Park Cancer Inst, Elm & Carlton St, Buffalo, NY 14263-0001; **Phone:** 716-845-8547; **Board Cert:** Internal Medicine 1982; Medical Oncology 1985; **Med School:** Univ Pittsburgh 1979; **Resid:** Internal Medicine, Univ Minn Hosps 1982; **Fellow:** Medical Oncology, Univ Minn Hosps 1984; **Fac Appt:** Assoc Prof Med, SUNY Buffalo

Levy, Michael H MD/PhD [Onc] - **Spec Exp:** Pain Management; Palliative Care; Pain-Cancer; Ethics; **Hospital:** Fox Chase Cancer Ctr (page 73); **Address:** Fox Chase Cancer Ctr, Dept Medical Oncology, 333 Cottman Ave, Ste C307, Philadelphia, PA 19111; **Phone:** 215-728-3637; **Board Cert:** Internal Medicine 1979; Medical Oncology 1981; **Med School:** Jefferson Med Coll 1976; **Resid:** Internal Medicine, Mt Sinai Med Ctr 1978; Internal Medicine, Hosp Univ Penn 1979; **Fellow:** Hematology & Oncology, Hosp Univ Penn 1981

Livingston, Philip MD [Onc] - **Spec Exp:** Melanoma; Vaccine Therapy; Immunotherapy; **Hospital:** Meml Sloan Kettering Cancer Ctr (page 76); **Address:** 1275 York Ave, New York, NY 10021-6007; **Phone:** 646-888-2376; **Board Cert:** Internal Medicine 1980; Allergy & Immunology 1974; Rheumatology 1974; Medical Oncology 1981; **Med School:** Harvard Med Sch 1969; **Resid:** Internal Medicine, N Shore Hosp-Cornell Med Ctr 1971; **Fellow:** Immunology, NYU Med Ctr 1973; Medical Oncology, Meml Sloan Kettering Cancer Inst 1977; **Fac Appt:** Prof Med, Cornell Univ-Weill Med Coll

Lyman, Gary H MD [Onc] - **Spec Exp:** Breast Cancer; **Hospital:** Univ of Rochester Strong Meml Hosp; **Address:** Univ of Rochester Strong Meml Hosp, 601 Elmwood Ave, Box 704, Rochester, NY 14642-8704; **Phone:** 585-275-3335; **Board Cert:** Internal Medicine 1987; Medical Oncology 1977; Hematology 1979; **Med School:** SUNY Buffalo 1972; **Resid:** Internal Medicine, Univ North Carolina Hosp 1974; **Fellow:** Medical Oncology, Roswell Park Meml Inst 1976; Biostatistics, Harvard Med Sch 1982; **Fac Appt:** Prof Med, Univ Rochester

Macdonald, John S MD [Onc] - **Spec Exp:** Colon Cancer; Gastrointestinal Cancer; Pancreatic Cancer; **Hospital:** St Vincent Cath Med Ctrs - Manhattan; **Address:** 325 W 15th St, New York, NY 10011-5903; **Phone:** 212-604-6011; **Board Cert:** Internal Medicine 1973; Medical Oncology 1975; **Med School:** Harvard Med Sch 1969; **Resid:** Internal Medicine, Beth Israel Hosp 1971; **Fellow:** Hematology & Oncology, Natl Cancer Inst 1974; **Fac Appt:** Prof Med, NY Med Coll

Marks, Stanley M MD [Onc] - **Spec Exp:** Leukemia; Lymphoma; **Hospital:** UPMC Shadyside; **Address:** 5115 Centre Ave, Fl 3, Pittsburgh, PA 15232; **Phone:** 412-235-1020; **Board Cert:** Internal Medicine 1976; Hematology 1978; **Med School:** Univ Pittsburgh 1973; **Resid:** Internal Medicine, Presby Univ Hosp 1976; **Fellow:** Hematology, Peter Bent Brigham Hosp 1978; **Fac Appt:** Assoc Clin Prof Med, Drexel Univ Coll Med

Marshall, John L MD [Onc] - **Spec Exp:** Gastrointestinal Cancer; Drug Development; **Hospital:** Georgetown Univ Hosp; **Address:** Lombardi Cancer Ctr, Podium A, 3800 Reservoir Rd NW, Washington, DC 20007; **Phone:** 202-444-7064; **Board Cert:** Internal Medicine 2001; Medical Oncology 2003; **Med School:** Univ Louisville Sch Med 1988; **Resid:** Internal Medicine, Georgetown Univ Hosp 1991; **Fellow:** Medical Oncology, Georgetown Univ Hosp 1993; **Fac Appt:** Assoc Prof Med, Georgetown Univ

Maslak, Peter G MD [Onc] - **Spec Exp:** Leukemia; Stem Cell Transplant; Myelodysplastic Syndromes; Clinical Trials; **Hospital:** Meml Sloan Kettering Cancer Ctr (page 76); **Address:** Meml Sloan Kettering Cancer Ctr, 1275 York Ave, New York, NY 10021-6007; **Phone:** 212-639-5518; **Board Cert:** Internal Medicine 1987; Hematology 2000; Medical Oncology 1989; **Med School:** Mount Sinai Sch Med 1984; **Resid:** Internal Medicine, Univ Michigan Med Ctr 1987; **Fellow:** Hematology & Oncology, Meml Sloan Kettering Cancer Ctr 1990

Masters, Gregory A MD [Onc] - Spec Exp: Lung Cancer; Esophageal Cancer; Thoracic Cancers; **Hospital:** Christiana Hospital; **Address:** Med Onc-Hem Consultants, Graham Cancer Ctr, 4701 Ogletown-Stanton Rd, Ste 2200, Newark, DE 19713; **Phone:** 302-366-1200; **Board Cert:** Internal Medicine 2003; Medical Oncology 2005; **Med School:** Northwestern Univ 1990; **Resid:** Internal Medicine, Hosp Univ Penn 1993; **Fellow:** Medical Oncology, Univ Chicago Hosps 1995; **Fac Appt:** Assoc Prof Med, Thomas Jefferson Univ

McGuire III, William P MD [Onc] - Spec Exp: Gynecologic Cancer; Ovarian Cancer; Breast Cancer; **Hospital:** Franklin Square Hosp; **Address:** Harry & Jeanette Weinberg Cancer Inst, 9103 Franklin Square Drive, Ste 2200, Baltimore, MD 21287; **Phone:** 443-777-7826; **Board Cert:** Internal Medicine 1974; Medical Oncology 1981; **Med School:** Baylor Coll Med 1971; **Resid:** Internal Medicine, Yale-New Haven Hosp 1973; **Fac Appt:** Clin Prof Med, Univ MD Sch Med

Meropol, Neal J MD [Onc] - Spec Exp: Gastrointestinal Cancer; **Hospital:** Fox Chase Cancer Ctr (page 73); **Address:** Fox Chase Cancer Ctr, Medical Oncology, 333 Cottman Ave, Philadelphia, PA 19111; **Phone:** 215-728-2450; **Board Cert:** Internal Medicine 1988; Medical Oncology 2001; **Med School:** Vanderbilt Univ 1985; **Resid:** Internal Medicine, Univ Hosps/Case West Res 1988; **Fellow:** Hematology & Oncology, Hosp Univ Penn 1992; **Fac Appt:** Prof Med, Temple Univ

Mintzer, David M MD [Onc] - Spec Exp: Breast Cancer; Gastrointestinal Cancer; Head & Neck Cancer; **Hospital:** Pennsylvania Hosp (page 84); **Address:** 230 W Washington Square Fl 2, Philadelphia, PA 19106; **Phone:** 215-829-6088; **Board Cert:** Internal Medicine 1980; Hematology 1982; Medical Oncology 1983; **Med School:** Jefferson Med Coll 1977; **Resid:** Internal Medicine, Pennsylvania Hosp 1980; **Fellow:** Hematology, Jefferson Med Coll 1982; Medical Oncology, Meml Sloan Kettering Cancer Ctr 1984; **Fac Appt:** Assoc Clin Prof Med, Univ Pennsylvania

Moore, Anne MD [Onc] - Spec Exp: Breast Cancer; **Hospital:** NY-Presby Hosp (page 79); **Address:** New York Presbyterian Hosp, 428 E 72nd St, Ste 300, New York, NY 10021-4873; **Phone:** 212-746-2085; **Board Cert:** Internal Medicine 1973; Hematology 1976; Medical Oncology 1977; **Med School:** Columbia P&S 1969; **Resid:** Internal Medicine, Cornell Univ Med Ctr 1973; **Fellow:** Medical Oncology, Rockefeller Univ 1973; **Fac Appt:** Prof Med, Cornell Univ-Weill Med Coll

Motzer, Robert J MD [Onc] - Spec Exp: Kidney Cancer; Testicular Cancer; Prostate Cancer; **Hospital:** Meml Sloan Kettering Cancer Ctr (page 76); **Address:** 1275 York Ave, Box 239, New York, NY 10021; **Phone:** 646-422-4312; **Board Cert:** Internal Medicine 1984; Medical Oncology 1987; **Med School:** Univ Mich Med Sch 1981; **Resid:** Internal Medicine, Meml Sloan Kettering Cancer Ctr 1984; **Fellow:** Medical Oncology, Meml Sloan Kettering Cancer Ctr 1987; **Fac Appt:** Assoc Prof Med, Cornell Univ-Weill Med Coll

Muggia, Franco MD [Onc] - Spec Exp: Breast Cancer; Gynecologic Cancer; **Hospital:** NYU Med Ctr (page 80); **Address:** NYU Clinical Cancer Ctr, 160 E 34th St Fl 8, New York, NY 10016; **Phone:** 212-731-5433; **Board Cert:** Internal Medicine 1968; Hematology 1974; Medical Oncology 1973; **Med School:** Cornell Univ-Weill Med Coll 1961; **Resid:** Internal Medicine, Hartford Hosp 1964; Internal Medicine, Francis A Delafield Hosp 1966; **Fac Appt:** Prof Med, NYU Sch Med

Medical Oncology

Nissenblatt, Michael MD [Onc] - **Spec Exp:** Breast Cancer; Colon Cancer; Hereditary Cancer; Familial Cancer; **Hospital:** Robert Wood Johnson Univ Hosp - New Brunswick, St Peter's Univ Hosp; **Address:** 205 Easton Ave, New Brunswick, NJ 08901-1722; **Phone:** 732-828-9570; **Board Cert:** Internal Medicine 1976; Medical Oncology 1979; **Med School:** Columbia P&S 1973; **Resid:** Internal Medicine, Johns Hopkins Hosp 1976; **Fellow:** Medical Oncology, Johns Hopkins Hosp 1978; **Fac Appt:** Clin Prof Med, Robert W Johnson Med Sch

Norton, Larry MD [Onc] - **Spec Exp:** Breast Cancer; **Hospital:** Meml Sloan Kettering Cancer Ctr (page 76); **Address:** 205 E 64th St, New York, NY 10021; **Phone:** 212-639-5438; **Board Cert:** Internal Medicine 1975; Medical Oncology 1977; **Med School:** Columbia P&S 1972; **Resid:** Internal Medicine, Bronx Muni Hosp 1974; **Fac Appt:** Prof Med, Cornell Univ-Weill Med Coll

O'Reilly, Eileen M MD [Onc] - **Spec Exp:** Pancreatic Cancer; Clinical Trials; Biliary Cancer; Neuroendocrine Tumors; **Hospital:** Meml Sloan Kettering Cancer Ctr (page 76); **Address:** 1275 York Ave, Box 324, New York, NY 10021; **Phone:** 212-639-6672; **Med School:** Ireland 1990; **Resid:** Internal Medicine, St Vincent's Hosp 1994; **Fellow:** Hematology, St Vincent's Hosp 1995; Medical Oncology, Memorial-Sloan Kettering Cancer Ctr 1997; **Fac Appt:** Asst Prof Med, Cornell Univ-Weill Med Coll

Offit, Kenneth MD [Onc] - **Spec Exp:** Cancer Genetics; Breast Cancer; Lymphoma; **Hospital:** Meml Sloan Kettering Cancer Ctr (page 76); **Address:** 1275 York Ave, Box 295, New York, NY 10021-6094; **Phone:** 212-434-5149; **Board Cert:** Internal Medicine 1985; Medical Oncology 1987; **Med School:** Harvard Med Sch 1982; **Resid:** Internal Medicine, Lenox Hill Hosp 1985; **Fellow:** Hematology & Oncology, Meml Sloan Kettering Cancer Ctr 1988; **Fac Appt:** Prof Med, Cornell Univ-Weill Med Coll

Oster, Martin W MD [Onc] - **Spec Exp:** Breast Cancer; Gastrointestinal Cancer; Lung Cancer; **Hospital:** NY-Presby Hosp (page 79); **Address:** NY Presby Hosp-Columbia Presby Med Ctr, 161 Fort Washington Ave, New York, NY 10032-3713; **Phone:** 212-305-8231; **Board Cert:** Internal Medicine 1974; Medical Oncology 1975; **Med School:** Columbia P&S 1971; **Resid:** Internal Medicine, Mass Genl Hosp 1973; **Fellow:** Medical Oncology, Natl Cancer Inst/NIH 1976; **Fac Appt:** Assoc Clin Prof Med, Columbia P&S

Ozols, Robert R MD/PhD [Onc] - **Spec Exp:** Ovarian Cancer; **Hospital:** Fox Chase Cancer Ctr (page 73); **Address:** Fox Chase Cancer Ctr, 333 Cottman Ave, rm P 2051, Philadelphia, PA 19111; **Phone:** 215-728-2570; **Board Cert:** Internal Medicine 1977; Medical Oncology 1979; **Med School:** Univ Rochester 1974; **Resid:** Internal Medicine, Dartmouth-Hitchcock Hosp 1976; **Fellow:** Medical Oncology, Natl Cancer Inst 1979; **Fac Appt:** Prof Med, Temple Univ

Pasmantier, Mark MD [Onc] - **Spec Exp:** Lung Cancer; Ovarian Cancer; **Hospital:** NY-Presby Hosp (page 79); **Address:** 407 E 70th St, FL 3, New York, NY 10021-5302; **Phone:** 212-517-5900; **Board Cert:** Internal Medicine 1972; Hematology 1974; Medical Oncology 1975; **Med School:** NYU Sch Med 1966; **Resid:** Internal Medicine, Harlem Hosp 1970; **Fellow:** Hematology, Montefiore Hosp Med Ctr 1971; Medical Oncology, New York Hosp 1972; **Fac Appt:** Clin Prof Med, Cornell Univ-Weill Med Coll

Pecora, Andrew L MD [Onc] - **Spec Exp:** Stem Cell Transplant; Myelodysplastic Syndromes; Melanoma; Immunotherapy; **Hospital:** Hackensack Univ Med Ctr (page 74); **Address:** The Cancer Ctr at Hackensack Univ Med Ctr, 20 Prospect Ave, Ste 400, Hackensack, NJ 07601; **Phone:** 201-996-5900; **Board Cert:** Internal Medicine 1986; Hematology 1988; Medical Oncology 1989; **Med School:** UMDNJ-NJ Med Sch, Newark 1983; **Resid:** Internal Medicine, New York Hosp-Cornell Med Ctr 1986; **Fellow:** Hematology & Oncology, Meml Sloan Kettering Cancer Ctr 1988; **Fac Appt:** Prof Med, UMDNJ-NJ Med Sch, Newark

Petrylak, Daniel P MD [Onc] - **Spec Exp:** Genitourinary Cancer; Prostate Cancer; Bladder Cancer; **Hospital:** NY-Presby Hosp (page 79); **Address:** 161 Fort Washington Ave, New York, NY 10032-3713; **Phone:** 212-305-1731; **Board Cert:** Internal Medicine 2001; Medical Oncology 2003; **Med School:** Case West Res Univ 1985; **Resid:** Internal Medicine, Jacobi Med Ctr 1988; **Fellow:** Oncology, Meml-Sloan Kettering Cancer Ctr 1991; **Fac Appt:** Assoc Prof Med, Columbia P&S

Pfister, David G MD [Onc] - **Spec Exp:** Head & Neck Cancer; Laryngeal Cancer; Thyroid Cancer; **Hospital:** Meml Sloan Kettering Cancer Ctr (page 76); **Address:** Memorial Sloan Kettering Cancer Ctr, 1275 York Ave, Box 188, New York, NY 10021; **Phone:** 212-639-8235; **Board Cert:** Internal Medicine 1985; Medical Oncology 1989; **Med School:** Univ Pennsylvania 1982; **Resid:** Internal Medicine, Hosp Univ Penn 1985; **Fellow:** Epidemiology, Yale New Haven Hosp 1987; Hematology & Oncology, Meml Sloan Kettering Cancer Ctr 1989; **Fac Appt:** Prof Med, Cornell Univ-Weill Med Coll

Saltz, Leonard B MD [Onc] - **Spec Exp:** Colon & Rectal Cancer; Gastrointestinal Cancer & Rare Tumors; Liver Cancer; Neuroendocrine Tumors; **Hospital:** Meml Sloan Kettering Cancer Ctr (page 76); **Address:** Memorial Sloan Kettering Cancer Ctr, 1275 York Ave, Howard 917, New York, NY 10021; **Phone:** 212-639-2501; **Board Cert:** Internal Medicine 1986; Hematology 1988; Medical Oncology 1989; **Med School:** Yale Univ 1983; **Resid:** Internal Medicine, New York Hosp-Cornell Med Ctr 1986; **Fellow:** Hematology & Oncology, New York Hosp-Cornell Med Ctr/Rockefeller Univ 1987; **Fac Appt:** Prof Med, Cornell Univ-Weill Med Coll

Scheinberg, David MD/PhD [Onc] - **Spec Exp:** Leukemia; Immunotherapy; Vaccine Therapy; **Hospital:** Meml Sloan Kettering Cancer Ctr (page 76); **Address:** 1275 York Ave, New York, NY 10021-6007; **Phone:** 646 888-2668; **Board Cert:** Internal Medicine 1986; Medical Oncology 1995; **Med School:** Johns Hopkins Univ 1983; **Resid:** Internal Medicine, New York Hosp/Cornell 1985; **Fellow:** Medical Oncology, Meml Sloan Kettering Cancer Ctr 1987; **Fac Appt:** Prof Med, Cornell Univ-Weill Med Coll

Scher, Howard MD [Onc] - **Spec Exp:** Genitourinary Cancer; Prostate Cancer; Bladder Cancer; **Hospital:** Meml Sloan Kettering Cancer Ctr (page 76); **Address:** 1275 York Ave, New York, NY 10021; **Phone:** 646-422-4330; **Board Cert:** Internal Medicine 1979; Medical Oncology 1985; **Med School:** NYU Sch Med 1976; **Resid:** Internal Medicine, Bellevue Hosp 1980; **Fellow:** Medical Oncology, Meml Sloan Kettering Cancer Ctr 1983; **Fac Appt:** Prof Med, Cornell Univ-Weill Med Coll

Schilder, Russell J MD [Onc] - **Spec Exp:** Gynecologic Cancer; Hematologic Malignancies; Drug Development; Clinical Trials; **Hospital:** Fox Chase Cancer Ctr (page 73); **Address:** Fox Chase Cancer Center, 333 Cottman Ave, Philadelphia, PA 19111; **Phone:** 215-728-4300; **Board Cert:** Internal Medicine 1986; Hematology 1988; Medical Oncology 1989; **Med School:** Univ Miami Sch Med 1983; **Resid:** Internal Medicine, Temple Univ Hosp 1986; **Fellow:** Hematology & Oncology, Fox Chase Cancer Ctr 1989; **Fac Appt:** Prof Med, Temple Univ

Schuchter, Lynn M MD [Onc] - **Spec Exp:** Melanoma; Breast Cancer; Clinical Trials; **Hospital:** Hosp Univ Penn - UPHS (page 84); **Address:** Univ Penn/Abramson Cancer Ctr, 3400 Spruce St, 12 Penn Tower, Philadelphia, PA 19104; **Phone:** 215-662-7907; **Board Cert:** Internal Medicine 1985; Medical Oncology 1989; **Med School:** Ros Franklin Univ/Chicago Med Sch 1982; **Resid:** Internal Medicine, Michael Reese Hosp 1985; **Fellow:** Medical Oncology, Johns Hopkins Hosp 1989; **Fac Appt:** Assoc Prof Med, Univ Pennsylvania

Shields, Peter G MD [Onc] - **Spec Exp:** Lung Cancer; Hematologic Malignancies; **Hospital:** Georgetown Univ Hosp; **Address:** Lombardi Cancer Ctr, 3800 Reservoir Rd NW, Lower Level, Washington, DC 20057; **Phone:** 202-444-9495; **Board Cert:** Internal Medicine 1986; Medical Oncology 1989; Hematology 1990; **Med School:** Mount Sinai Sch Med 1983; **Resid:** Internal Medicine, George Washington Univ Hosp 1986; **Fellow:** Hematology & Oncology, George Washington Univ Hosp 1990; **Fac Appt:** Prof Med, Georgetown Univ

Sidransky, David MD [Onc] - **Spec Exp:** Head & Neck Cancer; **Hospital:** Johns Hopkins Hosp - Baltimore; **Address:** Johns Hopkins Hospital, 1550 Orleans St, rm 5-N03, Baltimore, MD 21231; **Phone:** 410-502-5153; **Board Cert:** Internal Medicine 1988; **Med School:** Baylor Coll Med 1984; **Resid:** Internal Medicine, Baylor Coll Medicine 1988; **Fellow:** Medical Oncology, Johns Hopkins Hosp 1992; **Fac Appt:** Prof Oto, Johns Hopkins Univ

Smith, Mitchell R MD/PhD [Onc] - **Spec Exp:** Lymphoma; Leukemia; Multiple Myeloma; Hematologic Malignancies; **Hospital:** Fox Chase Cancer Ctr (page 73); **Address:** Fox Chase Cancer Center, 333 Cottman Ave, Ste C307, Philadelphia, PA 19111; **Phone:** 215-728-2570; **Board Cert:** Internal Medicine 1985; Hematology 1988; Medical Oncology 1987; **Med School:** Case West Res Univ 1979; **Resid:** Pathology, Barnes Jewish Hosp 1983; Internal Medicine, Barnes Jewish Hosp 1984; **Fellow:** Medical Oncology, Meml Sloan-Ketter Cancer Ctr 1988

Speyer, James MD [Onc] - **Spec Exp:** Ovarian Cancer; Breast Cancer; Cardiac Toxicity in Cancer Therapy; **Hospital:** NYU Med Ctr (page 80); **Address:** NYU Clinical Cancer Center, 160 E 34th St, New York, NY 10016-4750; **Phone:** 212-731-5432; **Board Cert:** Internal Medicine 1977; Hematology 1978; Medical Oncology 1979; **Med School:** Johns Hopkins Univ 1974; **Resid:** Internal Medicine, Columbia-Presby Med Ctr 1976; Hematology, Columbia-Presby Med Ctr 1977; **Fellow:** Medical Oncology, Natl Cancer Inst 1979; **Fac Appt:** Clin Prof Med, NYU Sch Med

Spriggs, David MD [Onc] - **Spec Exp:** Ovarian Cancer; Drug Development; Uterine Cancer; **Hospital:** Meml Sloan Kettering Cancer Ctr (page 76); **Address:** 1275 York Ave, Box 67, New York, NY 10021-6007; **Phone:** 212-639-2203; **Board Cert:** Internal Medicine 1981; Medical Oncology 1985; **Med School:** Univ Wisc 1977; **Resid:** Internal Medicine, Columbia-Presby Hosp 1981; **Fellow:** Medical Oncology, Dana-Farber Cancer Inst 1985; **Fac Appt:** Prof Med, Cornell Univ-Weill Med Coll

Stadtmauer, Edward A MD [Onc] - **Spec Exp:** Bone Marrow & Stem Cell Transplant; Leukemia; Multiple Myeloma; **Hospital:** Hosp Univ Penn - UPHS (page 84); **Address:** Univ Penn Cancer Ctr, 3400 Spruce St, 16 Penn Tower, Philadelphia, PA 19104; **Phone:** 215-662-7909; **Board Cert:** Internal Medicine 1986; Hematology 1988; Medical Oncology 1989; **Med School:** Univ Pennsylvania 1983; **Resid:** Internal Medicine, Bronx Muni Hosp 1986; **Fellow:** Hematology & Oncology, Hosp Univ Penn 1989; **Fac Appt:** Assoc Prof Med, Univ Pennsylvania

Stoopler, Mark MD [Onc] - **Spec Exp:** Lung Cancer; Esophageal Cancer; Unknown Primary Cancer; **Hospital:** NY-Presby Hosp (page 79); **Address:** 161 Fort Washington Ave, Ste 936, New York, NY 10032-3713; **Phone:** 212-305-8230; **Board Cert:** Internal Medicine 1978; Medical Oncology 1981; **Med School:** Cornell Univ-Weill Med Coll 1975; **Resid:** Internal Medicine, North Shore Univ Hosp 1978; Internal Medicine, Memorial Hosp 1978; **Fellow:** Medical Oncology, Meml-Sloan Kettering Cancer Ctr 1980; **Fac Appt:** Assoc Clin Prof Med, Columbia P&S

Straus, David J MD [Onc] - **Spec Exp:** Lymphoma; Multiple Myeloma; **Hospital:** Meml Sloan Kettering Cancer Ctr (page 76); **Address:** 1275 York Ave, New York, NY 10021-6007; **Phone:** 212-639-8365; **Board Cert:** Internal Medicine 1972; Hematology 1976; Medical Oncology 1977; **Med School:** Marquette Sch Med 1969; **Resid:** Internal Medicine, Montefiore Med Ctr 1972; Medical Oncology, Meml Sloan Kettering Cancer Ctr 1977; **Fellow:** Hematology, Beth Israel Hosp 1973; **Fac Appt:** Prof Med, Cornell Univ-Weill Med Coll

Tkaczuk, Katherine H MD [Onc] - **Spec Exp:** Breast Cancer; **Hospital:** Univ of MD Med Sys; **Address:** Univ MD Cancer Ctr, 22 S Greene St, rm S9D12, Baltimore, MD 21201; **Phone:** 410-328-7904; **Board Cert:** Internal Medicine 1989; Medical Oncology 2001; **Med School:** Poland 1984; **Resid:** Internal Medicine, St Agnes Hosp 1989; **Fellow:** Hematology & Oncology, Univ Maryland Cancer Ctr 1992; **Fac Appt:** Assoc Prof Med, Univ MD Sch Med

Trump, Donald MD [Onc] - **Spec Exp:** Prostate Cancer; Genitourinary Cancer; Drug Discovery & Development; **Hospital:** Roswell Park Cancer Inst; **Address:** Elm & Carlton St, Buffalo, NY 14263; **Phone:** 716-845-3499; **Board Cert:** Internal Medicine 1973; Medical Oncology 1977; **Med School:** Johns Hopkins Univ 1970; **Resid:** Internal Medicine, Johns Hopkins Hosp 1975; **Fellow:** Medical Oncology, Johns Hopkins Hosp 1974

Vogel, Victor G MD [Onc] - **Spec Exp:** Breast Cancer; Cancer Genetics; Drug Development; Clinical Trials; **Hospital:** Magee-Womens Hosp - UPMC; **Address:** Magee-Womens Hosp, Breast Cancer Prevention, 300 Halket St, rm 3524, Pittsburgh, PA 15213-3180; **Phone:** 412-641-6500; **Board Cert:** Internal Medicine 1984; Medical Oncology 2003; Public Health & Genl Preventive Med 1993; **Med School:** Temple Univ 1978; **Resid:** Internal Medicine, Baltimore City Hosp 1981; **Fellow:** Medical Oncology, Johns Hopkins Hosp 1986; Epidemiology, Johns Hopkins Hosp 1986; **Fac Appt:** Prof Med, Univ Pittsburgh

Weiner, Louis M MD [Onc] - **Spec Exp:** Gastrointestinal Cancer; Immunotherapy; Thoracic Cancers; **Hospital:** Fox Chase Cancer Ctr (page 73), Jeanes Hosp; **Address:** Fox Chase Cancer Ctr, 333 Cottman Ave, rm C315, Philadelphia, PA 19111; **Phone:** 215-728-2480; **Board Cert:** Internal Medicine 1980; Medical Oncology 1985; **Med School:** Mount Sinai Sch Med 1977; **Resid:** Internal Medicine, Med Ctr Hosp Vermont 1981; **Fellow:** Hematology & Oncology, New England Med Ctr 1984; **Fac Appt:** Prof Med, Temple Univ

Wolff, Antonio C MD [Onc] - **Spec Exp:** Breast Cancer; Drug Development; **Hospital:** Johns Hopkins Hosp - Baltimore; **Address:** 1650 Orleans St, rm 189, Baltimore, MD 21231; **Phone:** 410-614-4192; **Board Cert:** Internal Medicine 2000; Medical Oncology 2000; **Med School:** Brazil 1986; **Resid:** Internal Medicine, Mt Sinai Med Ctr 1991; **Fellow:** Hematology & Oncology, Washington Univ Med Ctr 1992; Medical Oncology, Johns Hopkins Hosp 1995; **Fac Appt:** Assoc Prof Med, Johns Hopkins Univ

Zelenetz, Andrew D MD/PhD [Onc] - **Spec Exp:** Lymphoma; **Hospital:** Meml Sloan Kettering Cancer Ctr (page 76); **Address:** Meml Sloan-Kettering Cancer Ctr, 1275 York Ave, New York, NY 10021; **Phone:** 212-639-2656; **Board Cert:** Internal Medicine 1992; Medical Oncology 1993; **Med School:** Harvard Med Sch 1984; **Resid:** Internal Medicine, Stanford Univ Med Ctr 1986; **Fellow:** Medical Oncology, Stanford Univ Med Ctr 1991; **Fac Appt:** Asst Prof Med, Cornell Univ-Weill Med Coll

Southeast

Antonia, Scott J MD/PhD [Onc] - **Spec Exp:** Kidney Cancer; Lung Cancer; **Hospital:** H Lee Moffitt Cancer Ctr & Research Inst; **Address:** H Lee Moffitt Cancer Ctr, 12902 Magnolia Drive, Tampa, FL 33612; **Phone:** 813-979-3883; **Board Cert:** Internal Medicine 2002; Medical Oncology 1995; **Med School:** Univ Conn 1989; **Resid:** Internal Medicine, Yale-New Haven Hosp 1991; **Fellow:** Medical Oncology, Yale-New Haven Hosp 1994; **Fac Appt:** Assoc Prof Med, Univ S Fla Coll Med

Arteaga, Carlos L MD [Onc] - **Spec Exp:** Breast Cancer; **Hospital:** Vanderbilt Univ Med Ctr; **Address:** Vanderbilt-Ingram Cancer Ctr-Medicine & Cancer Biology, 777 Preston Research Bldg, Nashville, TN 37232-6838; **Phone:** 615-936-3524; **Board Cert:** Internal Medicine 1984; Medical Oncology 1989; **Med School:** Ecuador 1980; **Resid:** Internal Medicine, Grady Meml Hosp 1984; **Fellow:** Hematology & Oncology, Univ Texas Hlth Sci Ctr 1987; **Fac Appt:** Prof Med, Vanderbilt Univ

Balducci, Lodovico MD [Onc] - **Spec Exp:** Genitourinary Cancer; Breast Cancer; **Hospital:** H Lee Moffitt Cancer Ctr & Research Inst, Tampa Genl Hosp; **Address:** H Lee Moffitt Cancer Ctr, 12902 Magnolia Drive, Tampa, FL 33612; **Phone:** 813-745-8658; **Board Cert:** Internal Medicine 1987; Hematology 1978; Medical Oncology 1979; **Med School:** Italy 1968; **Resid:** Internal Medicine, Univ Miss Med Ctr 1976; Hematology & Oncology, Univ Miss Med Ctr 1979; **Fellow:** Internal Medicine, A Gemelli Genl Hosp 1970; **Fac Appt:** Prof Med, Univ S Fla Coll Med

Benedetto, Pasquale W MD [Onc] - **Spec Exp:** Genitourinary Cancer; Bladder Cancer; Kidney Cancer; Pancreatic Cancer; **Hospital:** Univ of Miami Hosp & Clins/Sylvester Comp Canc Ctr, Jackson Meml Hosp; **Address:** Sylvester Comp Cancer Ctr, Med Oncology, 1475 NW 12th Ave, Ste 3310, Locator D8-4, Miami, FL 33136; **Phone:** 305-243-4909; **Board Cert:** Internal Medicine 1979; Medical Oncology 1981; Hematology 1982; **Med School:** Cornell Univ-Weill Med Coll 1976; **Resid:** Internal Medicine, Johns Hopkins Hosp 1979; **Fellow:** Medical Oncology, Meml Sloan Kettering Cancer Ctr 1981; **Fac Appt:** Prof Med, Univ Miami Sch Med

Berlin, Jordan MD [Onc] - Spec Exp: Gastrointestinal Cancer; Pancreatic Cancer; Liver Cancer; **Hospital:** Vanderbilt Univ Med Ctr; **Address:** 777 Preston Research Building, Nashville, TN 37232-6307; **Phone:** 615-322-6053; **Board Cert:** Internal Medicine 2002; Medical Oncology 2005; **Med School:** Univ IL Coll Med 1989; **Resid:** Internal Medicine, Univ Cincinnati 1992; **Fellow:** Medical Oncology, Univ Wisconsin 1995; **Fac Appt:** Assoc Prof Med, Vanderbilt Univ

Bernard, Stephen MD [Onc] - Spec Exp: Gastrointestinal Cancer; Palliative Care; Clinical Trials; **Hospital:** Univ NC Hosps; **Address:** Univ North Carolina Sch Med, 3009 Old Clinic, CB 7305, Chapel Hill, NC 27599; **Phone:** 919-966-4431; **Board Cert:** Internal Medicine 1987; Medical Oncology 1979; Hospice & Palliative Medicine 2004; **Med School:** Univ NC Sch Med 1973; **Resid:** Internal Medicine, Columbia-Presby Med Ctr 1976; **Fellow:** Hematology & Oncology, Wash Univ Hosps 1978; **Fac Appt:** Prof Med, Univ NC Sch Med

Bolger, Graeme B MD [Onc] - Spec Exp: Prostate Cancer; Testicular Cancer; **Hospital:** Univ of Ala Hosp at Birmingham; **Address:** 1530 3rd Ave S, Ste FOT-1105, Birmingham, AL 35294; **Phone:** 205-975-0088; **Board Cert:** Internal Medicine 1984; Medical Oncology 2000; **Med School:** McGill Univ 1980; **Resid:** Internal Medicine, Johns Hopkins Hosp 1984; **Fellow:** Medical Oncology, Fred Hutchinson Cancer Rsch 1985; Oncology, Meml Sloan-Kettering Cancer Ctr 1992; **Fac Appt:** Assoc Prof Med, Univ Ala

Boston, Barry MD [Onc] - Spec Exp: Gastrointestinal Cancer; Genitourinary Cancer; Prostate Cancer; **Hospital:** St Francis Hosp - Memphis, Methodist Univ Hosp - Memphis; **Address:** Univ of Tennessee Cancer Inst, 7945 Wolf River Blvd, Ste 300, Germantown, TN 38138; **Phone:** 901-752-6131; **Board Cert:** Internal Medicine 1974; Medical Oncology 1977; **Med School:** Louisiana State Univ 1971; **Resid:** Internal Medicine, Univ Tenn Hosp-VA Hosp 1973; Hematology, Univ Tenn Hosp-VA Hosp 1973; **Fellow:** Medical Oncology, Yale-New Haven Hosp 1975; **Fac Appt:** Assoc Prof Med, Univ Tenn Coll Med, Memphis

Brawley, Otis W MD [Onc] - Spec Exp: Breast Cancer; Prostate Cancer; **Hospital:** Emory Univ Hosp, Grady Hlth Sys; **Address:** Winship Cancer Inst, 1365 Clifton Rd NE, Atlanta, GA 30322; **Phone:** 404-778-1900; **Board Cert:** Internal Medicine 1988; Medical Oncology 2003; **Med School:** Univ Chicago-Pritzker Sch Med 1985; **Resid:** Internal Medicine, Univ Hosp Cleveland 1988; **Fellow:** Oncology, Natl Cancer Inst 1990; **Fac Appt:** Prof Med, Emory Univ

Brescia, Frank J MD [Onc] - Spec Exp: Palliative Care; Breast Cancer; Gastrointestinal Cancer; Ethics; **Hospital:** MUSC Med Ctr; **Address:** Med Univ South Carolina, Div Hem/Onc, 96 Jonathan Lucas St, Ste 903, Box 250635, Charleston, SC 29425; **Phone:** 843-792-4271; **Board Cert:** Internal Medicine 1974; Medical Oncology 1975; **Med School:** UMDNJ-NJ Med Sch, Newark 1975; **Resid:** Internal Medicine, North Shore Univ Hosp 1970; **Fellow:** Medical Oncology, Meml Sloan Kettering Cancer Ctr 1974; **Fac Appt:** Prof Med, Med Univ SC

Burris III, Howard A MD [Onc] - Spec Exp: Drug Development; Drug Discovery; Breast Cancer; **Hospital:** Centennial Med Ctr, Baptist Hosp - Nashville; **Address:** 250 25th Ave N Bldg Atrium - Ste 100, Nashville, TN 37203; **Phone:** 615-329-7276; **Board Cert:** Internal Medicine 1988; Medical Oncology 2001; **Med School:** Univ S Ala Coll Med 1985; **Resid:** Internal Medicine, Brooke Army Med Ctr 1988; **Fellow:** Medical Oncology, Brooke Army Med Ctr 1991

Butler, William M MD [Onc] - **Spec Exp:** Hyperbaric Medicine in Breast Cancer; Breast Cancer; Prostate Cancer; Lung Cancer; **Hospital:** Palmetto Richland Mem Hosp; **Address:** SC Oncology Associates, 166 Stoneridge St, Columbia, SC 29210; **Phone:** 803-461-3000; **Board Cert:** Internal Medicine 1975; Hematology 1980; Medical Oncology 1979; **Med School:** Tulane Univ 1972; **Resid:** Internal Medicine, Charity Hosp 1975; **Fellow:** Hematology, Walter Reed AMC 1980; **Fac Appt:** Clin Prof Med, Univ SC Sch Med

Carbone, David MD [Onc] - **Spec Exp:** Lung Cancer; **Hospital:** Vanderbilt Univ Med Ctr; **Address:** Vanderbilt-Ingram Cancer Ctr, 685 Preston Rsch Bldg, 2200 Pierce Ave, Nashville, TN 37232-6838; **Phone:** 615-936-3524; **Board Cert:** Internal Medicine 1988; Medical Oncology 2001; **Med School:** Johns Hopkins Univ 1985; **Resid:** Internal Medicine, Johns Hopkins Hosp 1988; **Fellow:** Oncology, Natl Cancer Inst 1991; **Fac Appt:** Prof Med, Vanderbilt Univ

Carey, Lisa A MD [Onc] - **Spec Exp:** Breast Cancer; **Hospital:** Univ NC Hosps; **Address:** Univ North Carolina - Div Hem/Onc, Campus Box 7305, 3009 Old Clinic Bldg, Chapel Hill, NC 27599; **Phone:** 919-966-4431; **Board Cert:** Internal Medicine 2003; Medical Oncology 2003; **Med School:** Johns Hopkins Univ 1990; **Resid:** Internal Medicine, Johns Hopkins Hosp 1993; **Fellow:** Oncology, Johns Hopkins Hosp 1996; **Fac Appt:** Asst Prof Med, Univ NC Sch Med

Carpenter Jr, John MD [Onc] - **Spec Exp:** Breast Cancer; **Hospital:** Univ of Ala Hosp at Birmingham; **Address:** 1530 3rd Ave S, Birmingham, AL 35294; **Phone:** 205-934-2084; **Board Cert:** Internal Medicine 1972; Hematology 1981; Medical Oncology 1975; **Med School:** Tulane Univ 1968; **Resid:** Internal Medicine, Grady Meml Hosp 1971; **Fellow:** Hematology & Oncology, Emory Univ 1973; **Fac Appt:** Prof Med, Univ Ala

Chao, Nelson Jen An MD [Onc] - **Spec Exp:** Bone Marrow Transplant; Lymphoma; Leukemia; **Hospital:** Duke Univ Med Ctr; **Address:** Duke Univ Med Ctr, Box 3961, Durham, NC 27710; **Phone:** 919-668-1002; **Board Cert:** Internal Medicine 1984; Medical Oncology 1987; **Med School:** Yale Univ 1981; **Resid:** Internal Medicine, Stanford Univ Med Ctr 1984; **Fellow:** Oncology, Stanford Univ Med Ctr 1987; **Fac Appt:** Prof Med, Duke Univ

Chingos, James C MD [Onc] - **Spec Exp:** Breast Cancer; Prostate Cancer; Lung Cancer; **Hospital:** Shands Jacksonville; **Address:** 655 W 8th St, 4th Fl Pavilion North, Jacksonville, FL 32209; **Phone:** 904-244-3273; **Board Cert:** Internal Medicine 1976; Medical Oncology 1981; **Med School:** Albany Med Coll 1973; **Resid:** Internal Medicine, New England Med Ctr 1975; Internal Medicine, Meml Sloan-Kettering Cancer Ctr 1976; **Fellow:** Medical Oncology, New England Med Ctr 1977; **Fac Appt:** Assoc Prof Med, Univ Fla Coll Med

Colon-Otero, Gerardo MD [Onc] - **Spec Exp:** Ovarian Cancer; Breast Cancer; Hematologic Malignancies; **Hospital:** Mayo - Jacksonville, St Luke's Hosp - Jacksonville; **Address:** Mayo Clinic Jacksonville, 4500 San Pablo Rd S, Jacksonville, FL 32224-1865; **Phone:** 904-953-2000; **Board Cert:** Internal Medicine 1982; Hematology 1984; Medical Oncology 1985; **Med School:** Puerto Rico 1979; **Resid:** Internal Medicine, Mayo Clinic 1982; **Fellow:** Hematology, Mayo Clinic 1984; Medical Oncology, Univ Va Med Ctr 1986; **Fac Appt:** Assoc Prof Med, Mayo Med Sch

Conry, Robert M MD [Onc] - **Spec Exp:** Melanoma; Lung Cancer; Colon & Rectal Cancer; Sarcoma; **Hospital:** Univ of Ala Hosp at Birmingham; **Address:** The Kirkin Clinic At Acton Rd, 2145 Bonner Way, Birmingham, AL 35243; **Phone:** 205-978-0250; **Board Cert:** Medical Oncology 1997; Hematology 2001; **Med School:** Univ Ala 1987; **Resid:** Internal Medicine, Univ Alabama Hosp 1990; **Fellow:** Medical Oncology, Univ Alabama Hosp 1993; **Fac Appt:** Assoc Prof Med, Univ Ala

Crawford, Jeffrey MD [Onc] - **Spec Exp:** Lung Cancer; **Hospital:** Duke Univ Med Ctr; **Address:** Duke Univ Med Ctr, Box 3476, 400 Trent Drive 25167A Bldg, Morris Cancer Bldg, Durham, NC 27710-0001; **Phone:** 919-668-6688; **Board Cert:** Internal Medicine 1977; Hematology 1980; Medical Oncology 1981; **Med School:** Ohio State Univ 1974; **Resid:** Internal Medicine, Duke Univ Med Ctr 1977; **Fellow:** Hematology & Oncology, Duke Univ Med Ctr 1981; **Fac Appt:** Prof Med, Duke Univ

Daud, Adil I MD [Onc] - **Spec Exp:** Melanoma; Skin Cancer; Drug Development; **Hospital:** H Lee Moffitt Cancer Ctr & Research Inst; **Address:** H Lee Moffitt Cancer Ctr & Rsch Inst, 12902 Magnolia Drive, Tampa, FL 33612; **Phone:** 813-745-8581; **Board Cert:** Internal Medicine 1997; Hematology 2000; Medical Oncology 2000; **Med School:** India 1987; **Resid:** Internal Medicine, Indiana Univ; **Fellow:** Hematology & Oncology, Meml Sloan Kettering Cancer Ctr

De Simone, Philip MD [Onc] - **Spec Exp:** Colon Cancer; Pancreatic Cancer; **Hospital:** Univ of Kentucky Chandler Hosp; **Address:** UKMC Markey Cancer Ctr, CC-160, 800 Rose St, Lexington, KY 40536; **Phone:** 859-323-6448; **Board Cert:** Internal Medicine 1972; Hematology 1974; **Med School:** Univ VT Coll Med 1967; **Resid:** Internal Medicine, Univ Kentucky Hosp 1972; **Fellow:** Hematology & Oncology, Univ Kentucky Hosp 1974; **Fac Appt:** Prof Med, Univ KY Coll Med

Dunphy, Frank R MD [Onc] - **Spec Exp:** Lung Cancer; Head & Neck Cancer; **Hospital:** Duke Univ Med Ctr; **Address:** Duke Univ, Morris Cancer Bldg, 400 Trent Drive 25167A Bldg, Durham, NC 27710; **Phone:** 919-668-6688; **Board Cert:** Internal Medicine 1984; Hematology 1986; Medical Oncology 1989; **Med School:** Louisiana State Univ 1979; **Resid:** Internal Medicine, Lousiana St Univ Hosp 1983; **Fellow:** Hematology & Oncology, Louisiana St Univ Hosp 1985; **Fac Appt:** Assoc Prof Med, Duke Univ

Flinn, Ian MD/PhD [Onc] - **Spec Exp:** Hematologic Malignancies; Lymphoma; Bone Marrow Transplant; Clinical Trials; **Hospital:** Centennial Med Ctr; **Address:** Tennessee Oncology, 250 25th Ave N, Ste 110, Nashville, TN 37203; **Phone:** 615-320-5090; **Board Cert:** Hematology 1996; Medical Oncology 1997; **Med School:** Johns Hopkins Univ 1990; **Resid:** Internal Medicine, Univ Michigan Med Ctr 1993; **Fellow:** Medical Oncology, Johns Hopkins Univ Hosps 1993

Garst, Jennifer L MD [Onc] - **Spec Exp:** Lung Cancer; **Hospital:** Duke Univ Med Ctr; **Address:** Duke Univ Med Ctr, 25176 Morris Bldg, Box 3198, Durham, NC 27710; **Phone:** 919-668-6688; **Board Cert:** Medical Oncology 1997; **Med School:** Med Coll GA 1990; **Resid:** Internal Medicine, Univ Texas Hosp 1993; **Fellow:** Hematology & Oncology, Duke Univ Med Ctr 1996; **Fac Appt:** Prof Med, Duke Univ

Gockerman, Jon Paul MD [Onc] - **Spec Exp:** Leukemia; Lymphoma; **Hospital:** Duke Univ Med Ctr; **Address:** Duke Univ Med Ctr, 1 Trent Drive, rm 25153, Box 3872, Morris Bldg, Durham, NC 27710; **Phone:** 919-684-8964; **Board Cert:** Internal Medicine 1972; Hematology 1974; Medical Oncology 1973; **Med School:** Univ Chicago-Pritzker Sch Med 1967; **Resid:** Internal Medicine, Duke Univ Med Ctr 1969; **Fellow:** Hematology & Oncology, Duke Univ Med Ctr 1971

Goldberg, Richard M MD [Onc] - **Spec Exp:** Stomach Cancer; Esophageal Cancer; Colon & Rectal Cancer; Pancreatic Cancer; **Hospital:** Univ NC Hosps; **Address:** Division of Hematology/Oncology, CB 7305, 3009 Old Clinic Bldg SW, Chapel Hill, NC 27599-0001; **Phone:** 919-843-7711; **Board Cert:** Internal Medicine 1982; Medical Oncology 1985; **Med School:** SUNY Upstate Med Univ 1979; **Resid:** Internal Medicine, Emory Univ Med Ctr 1982; **Fellow:** Medical Oncology, Georgetown Univ Med Ctr 1984; **Fac Appt:** Prof Med, Univ NC Sch Med

Graham, Mark MD [Onc] - **Spec Exp:** Breast Cancer; Breast Cancer Genetics; **Hospital:** WakeMed Cary; **Address:** Waverly Hematology/Oncology, 300 Ashville Ave, Ste 310, Cary, NC 27511; **Phone:** 919-233-8585; **Board Cert:** Internal Medicine 1989; **Med School:** Mayo Med Sch 1982; **Resid:** Internal Medicine, Duke Univ Med Ctr 1985; **Fellow:** Medical Oncology, Univ CO Hlth Sci Ctr 1990; Medical Oncology, Mayo Clinic; **Fac Appt:** Assoc Clin Prof Med, Univ NC Sch Med

Greco, F Anthony MD [Onc] - **Spec Exp:** Lung Cancer; Unknown Primary Cancer; **Hospital:** Centennial Med Ctr; **Address:** Sarah Cannon Research Inst, 250 25th Ave N Atrium Bldg - Ste 100, Nashville, TN 37203; **Phone:** 615-320-5090; **Board Cert:** Internal Medicine 1975; Medical Oncology 1977; **Med School:** W VA Univ 1972; **Resid:** Internal Medicine, Univ West Virginia Hosp 1974; **Fellow:** Medical Oncology, Natl Cancer Inst 1976

Grosh, William W MD [Onc] - **Spec Exp:** Melanoma; Sarcoma; Neuroendocrine Tumors; **Hospital:** Univ Virginia Med Ctr; **Address:** UVA Health System, Div Hem/Oncology, PO Box 800716, Charlottesville, VA 22908; **Phone:** 434-924-1904; **Board Cert:** Internal Medicine 1978; Medical Oncology 1985; **Med School:** Columbia P&S 1974; **Resid:** Internal Medicine, Vanderbilt Univ Med Ctr 1977; **Fellow:** Medical Oncology, Vanderbilt Univ Med Ctr 1983; **Fac Appt:** Assoc Prof Med, Univ VA Sch Med

Hande, Kenneth MD [Onc] - **Spec Exp:** Drug Discovery; Sarcoma; Carcinoid Tumors; **Hospital:** Vanderbilt Univ Med Ctr, VA Med Ctr - Nashville; **Address:** Vanderbilt Univ Med Ctr, 777 Preston Research Building, Nashville, TN 37232-6307; **Phone:** 615-322-4967; **Board Cert:** Internal Medicine 1975; Medical Oncology 1977; **Med School:** Johns Hopkins Univ 1972; **Resid:** Internal Medicine, Barnes Hosp 1974; **Fellow:** Medical Oncology, Natl Cancer Inst 1977; **Fac Appt:** Prof Med, Vanderbilt Univ

Hurd, David MD [Onc] - **Spec Exp:** Lymphoma; Leukemia; Bone Marrow Transplant; **Hospital:** Wake Forest Univ Baptist Med Ctr (page 85); **Address:** Wake Forest Sch Med, Comp Cancer Ctr, Medical Center Boulevard, Winston-Salem, NC 27157-1082; **Phone:** 336-713-5440; **Board Cert:** Internal Medicine 1977; Medical Oncology 1981; **Med School:** Univ IL Coll Med 1974; **Resid:** Internal Medicine, Univ Minn Hosp 1977; **Fellow:** Medical Oncology, Univ Minn Hosp 1979; **Fac Appt:** Prof Med, Wake Forest Univ

Jahanzeb, Mohammad MD [Onc] - **Spec Exp:** Breast Cancer; Lung Cancer; **Hospital:** Methodist Univ Hosp - Memphis, St Francis Hosp - Memphis; **Address:** Univ Tennessee Coll Med, Div Hem/Onc, 1331 Union Ave, Ste 800, Memphis, TN 38104; **Phone:** 901-722-0532; **Board Cert:** Medical Oncology 2003; Hematology 2005; **Med School:** Pakistan 1986; **Resid:** Internal Medicine, New Britain Genl Hosp 1990; **Fellow:** Hematology & Oncology, Washington Univ 1993; **Fac Appt:** Prof Med, Univ Tenn Coll Med, Memphis

Jillella, Anand MD [Onc] - **Spec Exp:** Bone Marrow Transplant; Leukemia; Lymphoma; Multiple Myeloma; **Hospital:** Med Coll of GA Hosp and Clin; **Address:** Med Coll Ga - BMT Program, 1120 15th St, BAA 5407, Augusta, GA 30912-3125; **Phone:** 706-721-2505; **Board Cert:** Internal Medicine 1992; Medical Oncology 1997; **Med School:** India 1985; **Resid:** Internal Medicine, Med Coll Georgia 1992; **Fellow:** Medical Oncology, Yale-New Haven Hosp 1996; **Fac Appt:** Prof Med, Med Coll GA

Johnson, David H MD [Onc] - **Spec Exp:** Lung Cancer; Breast Cancer; Drug Development; **Hospital:** Vanderbilt Univ Med Ctr; **Address:** Vanderbilt Univ Med Ctr, Div Med Onc, 2220 Pierce Ave, 777 PRB, Nashville, TN 37232; **Phone:** 615-322-6053; **Board Cert:** Internal Medicine 1979; Medical Oncology 1983; **Med School:** Med Coll GA 1976; **Resid:** Internal Medicine, Univ South Alabama Med Ctr 1979; Internal Medicine, Med Coll Georgia Hosps 1980; **Fellow:** Medical Oncology, Vanderbilt Univ Med Ctr 1983; **Fac Appt:** Prof Med, Vanderbilt Univ

Kraft, Andrew S MD [Onc] - **Spec Exp:** Prostate Cancer; Sarcoma; Drug Development; Clinical Trials; **Hospital:** MUSC Med Ctr; **Address:** 86 Jonathan Lucas St, PO BOX 250955, Charleston, SC 29425; **Phone:** 843-792-8284; **Board Cert:** Internal Medicine 1980; Medical Oncology 1985; **Med School:** Univ Pennsylvania 1975; **Resid:** Internal Medicine, Mt Sinai Hosp 1979; **Fellow:** Medical Oncology, Natl Cancer Inst 1983; **Fac Appt:** Prof Med, Med Univ SC

Kvols, Larry K MD [Onc] - **Spec Exp:** Gastrointestinal Cancer; Carcinoid Tumors; Neuroendocrine Tumors; **Hospital:** H Lee Moffitt Cancer Ctr & Research Inst; **Address:** H Lee Moffitt Cancer Ctr & Research Inst, 12902 Magnolia Drive, Ste WCBIGI, Tampa, FL 33612-9497; **Phone:** 813-972-8324; **Board Cert:** Internal Medicine 1976; Medical Oncology 1977; **Med School:** Baylor Coll Med 1970; **Resid:** Internal Medicine, Johns Hopkins Hosp 1972; **Fellow:** Hematology & Oncology, Johns Hopkins Hosp 1973; **Fac Appt:** Prof Med, Mayo Med Sch

Lawson, David H MD [Onc] - **Spec Exp:** Melanoma; **Hospital:** Emory Univ Hosp; **Address:** Winship Cancer Institute, 1365 Clifton Rd NE, Atlanta, GA 30322; **Phone:** 404-778-1900; **Board Cert:** Internal Medicine 1977; Medical Oncology 1979; **Med School:** Emory Univ 1974; **Resid:** Internal Medicine, Emory Univ Hosps 1977; **Fellow:** Medical Oncology, Emory Univ Hosps 1979; **Fac Appt:** Assoc Prof Med, Emory Univ

Lesser, Glenn J MD [Onc] - **Spec Exp:** Neuro-Oncology; Brain Tumors; **Hospital:** Wake Forest Univ Baptist Med Ctr (page 8.5); **Address:** Wake Forest University Div of Hem/Onc, Medical Center Blvd, Winston-Salem, NC 27157-1082; **Phone:** 336-716-9527; **Board Cert:** Internal Medicine 1990; Medical Oncology 1993; **Med School:** Penn State Univ-Hershey Med Ctr 1987; **Resid:** Internal Medicine, NC Bapt Hosp/Bowman Gray Sch Med 1991; **Fellow:** Medical Oncology, Johns Hopkins Oncology Ctr 1994; **Fac Appt:** Assoc Prof Med, Wake Forest Univ

Limentani, Steven A MD [Onc] - **Spec Exp:** Breast Cancer; Multiple Myeloma; Clinical Trials; **Hospital:** Carolinas Med Ctr; **Address:** 1100 S Tryon St, Ste 400, Charlotte, NC 28203; **Phone:** 704-446-9046; **Board Cert:** Internal Medicine 1989; Hematology 2002; Medical Oncology 2001; **Med School:** Tufts Univ 1986; **Resid:** Internal Medicine, New England Deaconess Hosp 1989; **Fellow:** Hematology & Oncology, New England Med Ctr 1992; **Fac Appt:** Clin Prof Med, Univ NC Sch Med

Lossos, Izidore MD [Onc] - **Spec Exp:** Lymphoma; Hodgkin's Disease; Leukemia; **Hospital:** Univ of Miami Hosp & Clins/Sylvester Comp Canc Ctr, Jackson Meml Hosp; **Address:** Univ Miami - Sylvester Comp Cancer Ctr, 1475 NW 12th Ave, D8-4, Miami, FL 33136; **Phone:** 305-243-4785; **Med School:** Israel 1987; **Resid:** Internal Medicine, Hadassah Univ Hosp 1995; **Fellow:** Hematology & Oncology, Hadassah Univ Hosp 1997; Medical Oncology, Stanford Univ 2001; **Fac Appt:** Assoc Prof Med, Univ Miami Sch Med

Lyckholm, Laurel Jean MD [Onc] - **Spec Exp:** Neuro-Oncology; **Hospital:** Med Coll of VA Hosp; **Address:** Med Coll of VA, Div Hem/Onc, PO Box 980230, Richmond, VA 23298; **Phone:** 804-828-9723; **Board Cert:** Internal Medicine 1989; Medical Oncology 1993; Hematology 1994; **Med School:** Creighton Univ 1985; **Resid:** Internal Medicine, Creighton Univ 1989; **Fellow:** Hematology & Oncology, Univ IA Coll Med 1992; **Fac Appt:** Assoc Prof Med, Med Coll VA

Lynch Jr, James W MD [Onc] - **Spec Exp:** Lymphoma; Immunotherapy; Lung Cancer; **Hospital:** Shands Hlthcre at Univ of FL; **Address:** Shands Hlthcare, Div Hematology/Oncology, PO Box 100277, Gainesville, FL 32610-0277; **Phone:** 352-392-3000; **Board Cert:** Internal Medicine 1987; Medical Oncology 2001; **Med School:** Eastern VA Med Sch 1984; **Resid:** Internal Medicine, Univ Florida 1987; **Fellow:** Medical Oncology, Natl Cancer Inst 1991; **Fac Appt:** Prof Med, Univ Fla Coll Med

Marcom, Paul K MD [Onc] - **Spec Exp:** Breast Cancer; Clinical Trials; Cancer Genetics; **Hospital:** Duke Univ Med Ctr; **Address:** Duke Univ Med Ctr, Morris Cancer Bldg, rm 25167, Box 3115, Durham, NC 27710; **Phone:** 919-684-3877; **Board Cert:** Internal Medicine 2003; Medical Oncology 2005; **Med School:** Baylor Coll Med 1989; **Resid:** Internal Medicine, Duke Univ Med Ctr 1992; Hematology & Oncology, Duke Univ Med Ctr 1995; **Fac Appt:** Assoc Prof Med, Duke Univ

Miller, Donald M MD/PhD [Onc] - **Spec Exp:** Melanoma; Lung Cancer; **Hospital:** Univ of Louisville Hosp; **Address:** 529 S Jackson St, Louisville, KY 40202; **Phone:** 502-562-4790; **Board Cert:** Internal Medicine 1979; **Med School:** Duke Univ 1973; **Resid:** Internal Medicine, Peter Bent Brigham Hosp 1975; **Fellow:** Internal Medicine, Harvard Univ Hosp 1978; Medical Oncology, Natl Cancer Inst 1979; **Fac Appt:** Prof Med, Univ Louisville Sch Med

Moore, Joseph O MD [Onc] - **Spec Exp:** Leukemia; Hodgkin's Disease; Lymphoma, Non-Hodgkin's; Neuroendocrine Tumors; **Hospital:** Duke Univ Med Ctr; **Address:** Duke Univ Med Ctr, Box 3872, Durham, NC 27710; **Phone:** 919-684-8964; **Board Cert:** Internal Medicine 1975; Medical Oncology 1977; **Med School:** Johns Hopkins Univ 1970; **Resid:** Internal Medicine, Johns Hopkins Hosp 1975; **Fellow:** Hematology & Oncology, Duke Univ 1977; **Fac Appt:** Prof Med, Duke Univ

Nabell, Lisle M MD [Onc] - **Spec Exp:** Breast Cancer; Head & Neck Cancer; **Hospital:** Univ of Ala Hosp at Birmingham; **Address:** Univ of Alabama, 1530 3rd Ave S, Ste WTI237, Birmingham, AL 35294; **Phone:** 205-934-3061; **Board Cert:** Internal Medicine 2000; Medical Oncology 2000; **Med School:** Univ NC Sch Med 1987; **Resid:** Internal Medicine, Univ Alabama Hosp 1990; **Fellow:** Hematology & Oncology, Univ Alabama Hosp 1992; **Fac Appt:** Assoc Prof Med, Univ Ala

O'Regan, Ruth M MD [Onc] - Spec Exp: Breast Cancer; Breast Cancer Risk Assessment; Cancer Prevention; Clinical Trials; **Hospital:** Emory Univ Hosp; **Address:** Emory Univ Winship Cancer Inst, 1365 Clifton Rd C Bldg - Ste 4005, Atlanta, GA 30322; **Phone:** 404-778-1900; **Board Cert:** Internal Medicine 1999; Medical Oncology 2000; **Med School:** Ireland 1988; **Resid:** Internal Medicine, Med Coll Wisc 1995; Medical Oncology, Northwestern Univ Hosp 1999; **Fellow:** Medical Oncology, Northwestern Univ Hosp 1998; **Fac Appt:** Asst Prof Med, Emory Univ

Orlowski, Robert Z MD/PhD [Onc] - Spec Exp: Multiple Myeloma; Lymphoma, Non-Hodgkin's; Leukemia; Clinical Trials; **Hospital:** Univ NC Hosps; **Address:** UNC Cancer Hosp, M0041 Gravely Bldg, Campus Box 7218, 101 Manning Drive, Chapel Hill, NC 27599; **Phone:** 919-966-7782; **Board Cert:** Medical Oncology 1997; **Med School:** Yale Univ 1991; **Resid:** Internal Medicine, Barnes Hosp/Wash Univ 1994; **Fellow:** Hematology & Oncology, Johns Hopkins Hosp 1998; **Fac Appt:** Assoc Prof Med, Univ NC Sch Med

Perez, Edith A MD [Onc] - Spec Exp: Breast Cancer; Breast Cancer Risk Assessment; Clinical Trials; **Hospital:** Mayo - Jacksonville; **Address:** Mayo Clinic, 4500 San Pablo Rd Davis Bldg Fl 8, Jacksonville, FL 32224; **Phone:** 904-953-7283; **Board Cert:** Internal Medicine 1983; Hematology 1986; Medical Oncology 1987; **Med School:** Univ Puerto Rico 1979; **Resid:** Internal Medicine, Loma Linda Univ Med Ctr 1982; **Fellow:** Hematology & Oncology, Martinez VA Hosp/UC Davis 1987; **Fac Appt:** Prof Med, Mayo Med Sch

Posey III, James A MD [Onc] - Spec Exp: Gastrointestinal Cancer; Colon Cancer; Liver Cancer; Biliary Cancer; **Hospital:** Univ of Ala Hosp at Birmingham; **Address:** Wallace Tumor Institute, 24 6th Ave S, rm 263A, Birmingham, AL 35294-3300; **Phone:** 205-934-0916; **Board Cert:** Medical Oncology 1997; **Med School:** Howard Univ 1991; **Resid:** Internal Medicine, Georgetown Univ Med Ctr 1994; **Fellow:** Hematology & Oncology, Georgetown Univ Med Ctr 1997; **Fac Appt:** Assoc Prof Med, Univ Ala

Robert, Nicholas J MD [Onc] - Spec Exp: Breast Cancer; **Hospital:** Inova Fairfax Hosp; **Address:** 8503 Arlington Blvd, Ste 400, Fairfax, VA 22031; **Phone:** 703-280-5390; **Board Cert:** Internal Medicine 1978; Anatomic Pathology 1979; Medical Oncology 1981; Hematology 1984; **Med School:** McGill Univ 1974; **Resid:** Internal Medicine, Royal Victoria Hosp 1976; Pathology, Mass Genl Hosp 1979; **Fellow:** Hematology, Peter Bent Brigham Hosp 1980; Medical Oncology, Dana Farber Cancer Inst 1981

Robert-Vizcarrondo, Francisco MD [Onc] - Spec Exp: Lung Cancer; Mesothelioma; Drug Development; Clinical Trials; **Hospital:** Univ of Ala Hosp at Birmingham; **Address:** 1824 6th Ave S, Room NT-CC-2555D, Birmingham, AL 35294; **Phone:** 205-934-5077; **Board Cert:** Internal Medicine 1973; Hematology 1976; Medical Oncology 1975; **Med School:** Puerto Rico 1969; **Resid:** Internal Medicine, U PR Hosp 1972; Hematology, U PR Hosp 1974; **Fellow:** Medical Oncology, Univ Ala Hosp at Birmingham 1976; **Fac Appt:** Prof Med, Univ Ala

Romond, Edward H MD [Onc] - Spec Exp: Breast Cancer; **Hospital:** Univ of Kentucky Chandler Hosp; **Address:** Univ Kentucky Med Ctr, Div Hematology/Oncology, CC413 Roach Facility Markey Ctr 0093 St, Lexington, KY 40536-0093; **Phone:** 859-323-8043; **Board Cert:** Internal Medicine 1980; Hematology 1984; Medical Oncology 1983; **Med School:** Univ KY Coll Med 1977; **Resid:** Internal Medicine, Michigan State Univ Hosps 1980; **Fellow:** Hematology & Oncology, Michigan State Univ 1983; **Fac Appt:** Prof Med, Univ KY Coll Med

Roth, Bruce J MD [Onc] - Spec Exp: Prostate Cancer; Bladder Cancer; Testicular Cancer; **Hospital:** Vanderbilt Univ Med Ctr; **Address:** Vanderbilt Ingram Cancer Center, 777 Preston Research Bldg, Nashville, TN 37232-6307; **Phone:** 615-343-4070; **Board Cert:** Internal Medicine 1983; Medical Oncology 1985; **Med School:** St Louis Univ 1980; **Resid:** Internal Medicine, Indiana Univ Med Ctr 1983; **Fellow:** Hematology & Oncology, Indiana Univ Med Ctr 1986; **Fac Appt:** Prof Med, Vanderbilt Univ

Rothenberg, Mace MD [Onc] - Spec Exp: Pancreatic Cancer; Colon & Rectal Cancer; Clinical Trials; **Hospital:** Vanderbilt Univ Med Ctr; **Address:** Vanderbilt Ingram Cancer Center, 777 Preston Research Bldg, Nashville, TN 37232-6307; **Phone:** 615-322-4967; **Board Cert:** Internal Medicine 1985; Medical Oncology 1987; **Med School:** NYU Sch Med 1982; **Resid:** Internal Medicine, Vanderbilt Univ Med Ctr 1985; **Fellow:** Medical Oncology, Natl Cancer Inst 1988; **Fac Appt:** Prof Med, Vanderbilt Univ

Sandler, Alan MD [Onc] - Spec Exp: Lung Cancer; Sarcoma; **Hospital:** Vanderbilt Univ Med Ctr; **Address:** Vanderbilt Univ Med Ctr-Thoracic Onc, 777 Preston Research Bldg, Nashville, TN 37232-0021; **Phone:** 615-343-4070; **Med School:** Rush Med Coll 1987; **Resid:** Internal Medicine, Yale-New Haven Hosp 1990; **Fellow:** Medical Oncology, Yale Univ 1993; **Fac Appt:** Assoc Prof Med, Vanderbilt Univ

Schwartz, Michael A MD [Onc] - Spec Exp: Breast Cancer; Lymphoma; Colon Cancer; **Hospital:** Mount Sinai Med Ctr - Miami, Miami Heart Inst; **Address:** Oncology Hematology Associates, 4306 Alton Rd Fl 3, Miami Beach, FL 33140; **Phone:** 305-535-3310; **Board Cert:** Internal Medicine 1989; Medical Oncology 2004; Hematology 2004; **Med School:** UMDNJ-RW Johnson Med Sch 1986; **Resid:** Internal Medicine, Mt Sinai Medical Ctr 1989; **Fellow:** Hematology & Oncology, Meml Sloan Kettering Cancer Ctr 1992; **Fac Appt:** Asst Clin Prof Med, Univ Miami Sch Med

Seewaldt, Victoria L MD [Onc] - Spec Exp: Breast Cancer; Clinical Trials; **Hospital:** Duke Univ Med Ctr; **Address:** Duke Univ Med Ctr, 25167A Morris Cancer Bldg, Durham, NC 27710; **Phone:** 919-668-6688; **Board Cert:** Internal Medicine 1995; **Med School:** UC Davis 1989; **Resid:** Obstetrics & Gynecology, Univ Wash Med Ctr 1990; Internal Medicine, Univ Wash Med Ctr 1992; **Fellow:** Medical Oncology, Fred Hutchinson Cancer Ctr 1995; Breast Cancer, Fred Hutchinson Cancer Ctr 1998; **Fac Appt:** Assoc Prof Med, Duke Univ

Serody, Jonathan S MD [Onc] - Spec Exp: Breast Cancer Vaccine Therapy; Clinical Trials; Lymphoma; **Hospital:** Univ NC Hosps; **Address:** Lineberger Comprehensive Cancer Ctr, Univ NC Sch Medicine CB# 7295, Chapel Hill, NC 27599-7295; **Phone:** 919-966-8644; **Board Cert:** Internal Medicine 1989; Hematology 1996; **Med School:** Univ VA Sch Med 1986; **Resid:** Internal Medicine, Univ NC Med Ctr 1989; **Fellow:** Hematology, Univ NC Med Ctr 1992; Bone Marrow Transplant, Fred Hutchinson Transplant Program; **Fac Appt:** Assoc Prof Med, Univ NC Sch Med

Shea, Thomas MD [Onc] - Spec Exp: Bone Marrow Transplant; Lymphoma; Leukemia; **Hospital:** Univ NC Hosps; **Address:** Univ N Carolina, Dept Medicine, 3009 Old Clinic Bldg , Box 7305, Chapel Hill, NC 27599; **Phone:** 919-966-7746; **Board Cert:** Internal Medicine 1982; Hematology 1984; Medical Oncology 1985; **Med School:** Univ NC Sch Med 1978; **Resid:** Internal Medicine, Beth Israel Deaconess Med Ctr 1982; **Fellow:** Hematology & Oncology, Beth Israel Deaconess Med Ctr 1985; Bone Marrow Transplant, Dana Farber Cancer Inst 1988; **Fac Appt:** Prof Med, Univ NC Sch Med

Shin, Dong Moon MD [Onc] - **Spec Exp:** Head & Neck Cancer; Cancer Prevention; Mesothelioma; Thymoma; **Hospital:** Emory Univ Hosp; **Address:** Emory Winship Cancer Inst, 1365 C Clifton Rd NE, Ste 3090, Atlanta, GA 30322; **Phone:** 404-778-5990; **Board Cert:** Internal Medicine 1985; Medical Oncology 1989; **Med School:** South Korea 1975; **Resid:** Internal Medicine, Cook Co Hosp 1985; **Fellow:** Medical Oncology, Univ Texas MD Anderson Cancer Ctr 1986; **Fac Appt:** Prof Med, Emory Univ

Smith, Thomas Joseph MD [Onc] - **Spec Exp:** Breast Cancer; Palliative Care; **Hospital:** Med Coll of VA Hosp; **Address:** Med Coll Va, Div Hem/Onc, PO Box 980230, Richmond, VA 23298-0230; **Phone:** 804-828-9992; **Board Cert:** Internal Medicine 1982; Medical Oncology 1987; **Med School:** Yale Univ 1979; **Resid:** Internal Medicine, Hosp Univ Penn 1982; **Fellow:** Medical Oncology, Med Coll Virginia 1987; **Fac Appt:** Prof Med, Med Coll VA

Socinski, Mark A MD [Onc] - **Spec Exp:** Lung Cancer; **Hospital:** Univ NC Hosps; **Address:** UNC Chapel Hill, Div Hem/Onc, 3009 Old Clinic Bldg, Campus Box 7305, Chapel Hill, NC 27599-7305; **Phone:** 919-966-4431; **Board Cert:** Internal Medicine 1988; Medical Oncology 1991; **Med School:** Univ VT Coll Med 1984; **Resid:** Internal Medicine, Beth Israel Hosp 1986; **Fellow:** Medical Oncology, Dana-Farber Cancer Inst 1989; **Fac Appt:** Assoc Prof Med, Univ NC Sch Med

Sosman, Jeffrey MD [Onc] - **Spec Exp:** Kidney Cancer; Melanoma; Drug Discovery; **Hospital:** Vanderbilt Univ Med Ctr; **Address:** Vanderbilt Ingram Cancer Ctr, 777 Preston Research Bldg, Nashville, TN 37232-6307; **Phone:** 615-322-4967; **Board Cert:** Anatomic Pathology 1985; Internal Medicine 1987; Medical Oncology 1989; **Med School:** Albert Einstein Coll Med 1981; **Resid:** Anatomic Pathology, Univ Chicago Hosps 1985; Internal Medicine, Univ Wisconsin Hosp 1986; **Fellow:** Medical Oncology, Univ Wisconsin 1989; **Fac Appt:** Clin Prof Med, Vanderbilt Univ

Sotomayor, Eduardo M MD [Onc] - **Spec Exp:** Lymphoma; Gene Therapy; Vaccine Therapy; Clinical Trials; **Hospital:** H Lee Moffitt Cancer Ctr & Research Inst; **Address:** H Lee Moffitt Cancer Inst, 12902 Magnolia Drive, rm 3056, Tampa, FL 33612; **Phone:** 813-745-1387; **Board Cert:** Internal Medicine 1996; Medical Oncology 1997; **Med School:** Peru 1988; **Resid:** Internal Medicine, Univ Miami Sch Med 1995; **Fellow:** Immunology, Univ Miami Sch Med 1989; Oncology, Johns Hopkins Hosp 1998; **Fac Appt:** Assoc Prof Med, Univ S Fla Coll Med

Stone, Joel MD [Onc] - **Spec Exp:** Lung Cancer; Breast Cancer; **Hospital:** St Vincent's Med Ctr - Jacksonville; **Address:** St Vincent's Med Ctr, 1801 Barrs St, Ste 800, Jacksonville, FL 32204; **Phone:** 904-388-2619; **Board Cert:** Internal Medicine 1977; Medical Oncology 1979; **Med School:** Univ VA Sch Med 1974; **Resid:** Internal Medicine, Univ KY Med Ctr 1977; **Fellow:** Hematology & Oncology, Emory Univ 1979

Sutton, Linda Marie MD [Onc] - **Spec Exp:** Breast Cancer; Palliative Care; **Hospital:** Duke Univ Med Ctr; **Address:** Duke Univ Med Ctr, 3100 Tower Blvd, Ste 600, Durham, NC 27707; **Phone:** 919-419-5005; **Board Cert:** Internal Medicine 2002; Medical Oncology 2003; **Med School:** Univ Mass Sch Med 1987; **Resid:** Internal Medicine, Montefiore Med Ctr 1990; **Fellow:** Hematology & Oncology, Duke Univ Med Ctr 1993

Thigpen, James Tate MD [Onc] - **Spec Exp:** Gynecologic Cancer; Breast Cancer; Lung Cancer; **Hospital:** Univ Hosps & Clins - Jackson; **Address:** Univ Mississippi Med Ctr, Div Med Onc, 2500 N State St, Jackson, MS 39216; **Phone:** 601-984-5590; **Board Cert:** Internal Medicine 1972; Hematology 1974; Medical Oncology 1975; **Med School:** Univ Miss 1973; **Resid:** Internal Medicine, Univ Miss Med Ctr 1971; **Fellow:** Hematology & Oncology, Univ Miss Med Ctr 1973; **Fac Appt:** Prof Med, Univ Miss

Medical Oncology

Torti, Frank M MD [Onc] - **Spec Exp:** Prostate Cancer; Urologic Cancer; **Hospital:** Wake Forest Univ Baptist Med Ctr (page 85); **Address:** Wake Forest Med Ctr-Comp Cancer Ctr, Medical Center Blvd, Winston-Salem, NC 27157-1082; **Phone:** 336-716-7971; **Board Cert:** Internal Medicine 1976; Medical Oncology 1978; **Med School:** Harvard Med Sch 1974; **Resid:** Internal Medicine, Beth Israel Hosp 1976; **Fellow:** Medical Oncology, Stanford Univ Med Ctr 1979; **Fac Appt:** Prof Med, Wake Forest Univ

Troner, Michael MD [Onc] - **Spec Exp:** Head & Neck Cancer; Urologic Cancer; **Hospital:** Baptist Hosp of Miami; **Address:** 8940 N Kendall Drive, Ste 300, East Tower, Miami, FL 33176-2132; **Phone:** 305-595-2141; **Board Cert:** Internal Medicine 1972; Medical Oncology 1973; **Med School:** SUNY Downstate 1968; **Resid:** Internal Medicine, Univ Maryland Hosp 1971; **Fellow:** Medical Oncology, Univ Miami Med Ctr 1973; **Fac Appt:** Assoc Clin Prof Med, Univ Miami Sch Med

Vance, Ralph MD [Onc] - **Spec Exp:** Lung Cancer; **Hospital:** Univ Hosps & Clins - Jackson; **Address:** Univ Mississippi Med Ctr, Div Med Onc, 2500 N State St, Jackson, MS 39216; **Phone:** 601-984-5590; **Med School:** Univ Miss 1972; **Resid:** Internal Medicine, Univ Hosp; **Fellow:** Hematology & Oncology, Univ Hosp; **Fac Appt:** Prof Med, Univ Miss

Vaughan, William Perry MD [Onc] - **Spec Exp:** Bone Marrow Transplant; Breast Cancer; **Hospital:** Univ of Ala Hosp at Birmingham; **Address:** Univ Ala Birmingham, 1900 Univ Blvd, rm 541, Tinsley Harrison Twr, Birmingham, AL 35294; **Phone:** 205-934-1908; **Board Cert:** Internal Medicine 1975; Medical Oncology 1979; **Med School:** Univ Conn 1972; **Resid:** Internal Medicine, Univ Chicago Hosps 1975; **Fellow:** Oncology, Johns Hopkins Hosp 1977; **Fac Appt:** Prof Med, Univ Ala

Weiss, Geoffrey R MD [Onc] - **Spec Exp:** Gastrointestinal Cancer; Genitourinary Cancer; Melanoma; **Hospital:** Univ Virginia Med Ctr; **Address:** Univ Virginia Hlth System, Div Hem/Onc, PO Box 800716, Charlottesville, VA 22908-0716; **Phone:** 434-243-0066; **Board Cert:** Internal Medicine 1977; Medical Oncology 1981; **Med School:** St Louis Univ 1974; **Resid:** Internal Medicine, Temple Univ Hosp 1978; **Fellow:** Medical Oncology, Dana Farber Cancer Inst 1982; **Fac Appt:** Prof Med, Univ VA Sch Med

Williams, Michael MD [Onc] - **Spec Exp:** Lymphoma; Multiple Myeloma; Leukemia; **Hospital:** Univ Virginia Med Ctr; **Address:** UVA Hlth System, Div Hem/Oncology, PO Box 800716, Charlottesville, VA 22908-0716; **Phone:** 434-924-9637; **Board Cert:** Internal Medicine 1982; Medical Oncology 1987; Hematology 1988; **Med School:** Univ Cincinnati 1979; **Resid:** Internal Medicine, Univ Virginia Med Ctr 1983; **Fellow:** Hematology & Oncology, Univ Virginia Med Ctr 1986; **Fac Appt:** Prof Med, Univ VA Sch Med

Wingard, John R MD [Onc] - **Spec Exp:** Bone Marrow Transplant; Leukemia; Multiple Myeloma; **Hospital:** Shands Hlthcre at Univ of FL; **Address:** 1376 Mowry Rd, Ste 145, Box 103633, Gainesville, FL 32610; **Phone:** 352-273-8010; **Board Cert:** Internal Medicine 1977; Medical Oncology 1981; **Med School:** Johns Hopkins Univ 1973; **Resid:** Internal Medicine, Memphis City Hosps 1976; Internal Medicine, VA Hosp 1977; **Fellow:** Medical Oncology, Johns Hopkins Hosp 1979; **Fac Appt:** Prof Med, Univ Fla Coll Med

Yunus, Furhan MD [Onc] - **Spec Exp:** Multiple Myeloma; Lymphoma; **Hospital:** Methodist Univ Hosp - Memphis, St Jude Children's Research Hosp; **Address:** Univ TN Cancer Inst, 1331 Union Ave, Ste 800, Memphis, TN 38104; **Phone:** 901-722-0561; **Board Cert:** Internal Medicine 1993; Medical Oncology 1995; **Med School:** Pakistan 1986; **Resid:** Internal Medicine, Methodist Hosp 1993; **Fellow:** Hematology & Oncology, Univ Ariz Coll Med 1995; **Fac Appt:** Asst Prof Med, Univ Tenn Coll Med, Memphis

Midwest

Albain, Kathy MD [Onc] - **Spec Exp:** Breast Cancer; Lung Cancer; Cancer Survivors-Late Effects of Therapy; **Hospital:** Loyola Univ Med Ctr; **Address:** Loyola Univ Med Ctr, 2160 S First Ave, Bldg 112 - Ste 109, Maywood, IL 60153-5590; **Phone:** 708-327-3102; **Board Cert:** Internal Medicine 1981; Medical Oncology 1983; **Med School:** Univ Mich Med Sch 1978; **Resid:** Internal Medicine, Univ Illinois Med Ctr 1981; **Fellow:** Hematology & Oncology, Univ Chicago Hosps 1984; **Fac Appt:** Prof Med, Loyola Univ-Stritch Sch Med

Anderson, Joseph M MD [Onc] - **Spec Exp:** Breast Cancer; Palliative Care; Neuro-Oncology; **Hospital:** Henry Ford Hosp; **Address:** 2799 W Grand Blvd, Ste K13, Detroit, MI 48202; **Phone:** 313-916-1854; **Board Cert:** Internal Medicine 1985; Medical Oncology 1989; **Med School:** Univ Mich Med Sch 1982; **Resid:** Internal Medicine, Henry Ford Hosp 1986; **Fellow:** Medical Oncology, Henry Ford Hosp 1988

Benson III, Al B MD [Onc] - **Spec Exp:** Colon Cancer; Carcinoid Tumors; Pancreatic Cancer; **Hospital:** Northwestern Meml Hosp, Jesse A Brown VA Med Ctr; **Address:** 675 N St Clair, Ste 21-100, Chicago, IL 60611; **Phone:** 312-695-0990; **Board Cert:** Internal Medicine 1979; Medical Oncology 1983; **Med School:** SUNY Buffalo 1976; **Resid:** Internal Medicine, Univ Wisc Hosps 1979; **Fellow:** Medical Oncology, Univ Wisc Hosps 1984; **Fac Appt:** Prof Med, Northwestern Univ

Bitran, Jacob MD [Onc] - **Spec Exp:** Breast Cancer; Bone Marrow Transplant; Lung Cancer; **Hospital:** Adv Luth Genl Hosp, Rush N Shore Med Ctr; **Address:** Lutheran Genl Cancer Care Specialists, 1700 Luther Lane, Park Ridge, IL 60068-1270; **Phone:** 847-268-8200; **Board Cert:** Internal Medicine 1974; Hematology 1986; Medical Oncology 1977; **Med School:** Univ IL Coll Med 1971; **Resid:** Pathology, Rush Presby St Luke's Hosp 1973; Internal Medicine, Michael Reese Hosp 1973; **Fellow:** Hematology & Oncology, Univ Chicago Hosps 1977; **Fac Appt:** Prof Med, Ros Franklin Univ/Chicago Med Sch

Bolwell, Brian J MD [Onc] - **Spec Exp:** Bone Marrow Transplant; Hematologic Malignancies; **Hospital:** Cleveland Clin Fdn (page 71); **Address:** Cleveland Clinic Fdn, 9500 Euclid Ave, rm R32, Cleveland, OH 44195; **Phone:** 216-444-6922; **Board Cert:** Internal Medicine 1985; Medical Oncology 1987; **Med School:** Case West Res Univ 1981; **Resid:** Internal Medicine, Univ Hosp 1984; **Fellow:** Hematology & Oncology, Hosp Univ Penn 1987; **Fac Appt:** Prof Med, Cleveland Cl Coll Med/Case West Res

Bonomi, Philip MD [Onc] - **Spec Exp:** Lung Cancer; Thymoma; Mesothelioma; **Hospital:** Rush Univ Med Ctr; **Address:** 1725 W Harrison St, Ste 821, Chicago, IL 60612; **Phone:** 312-942-3312; **Board Cert:** Internal Medicine 1975; Medical Oncology 1977; **Med School:** Univ IL Coll Med 1970; **Resid:** Internal Medicine, Geisinger Med Ctr 1972; Internal Medicine, Geisinger Med Ctr 1975; **Fellow:** Medical Oncology, Rush Presby-St Luke's Med Ctr 1977; **Fac Appt:** Prof Med, Rush Med Coll

Borden, Ernest C MD [Onc] - **Spec Exp:** Melanoma; Immunotherapy; Sarcoma; Vaccine Therapy; **Hospital:** Cleveland Clin Fdn (page 71); **Address:** Cleveland Clinic Fdn, Desk R40, 9500 Euclid Ave, Cleveland, OH 44195; **Phone:** 216-444-8183; **Board Cert:** Internal Medicine 1973; Medical Oncology 1975; **Med School:** Duke Univ 1966; **Resid:** Internal Medicine, Hosp Univ Penn 1968; **Fellow:** Medical Oncology, Johns Hopkins Hosp 1973; **Fac Appt:** Prof Med, Cleveland Cl Coll Med/Case West Res

Bricker, Leslie J MD [Onc] - **Spec Exp:** Palliative Care; **Hospital:** Henry Ford Hosp; **Address:** Henry Ford Hospital, 2799 W Grand Blvd, CFP 5, Detroit, MI 48202; **Phone:** 313-916-1859; **Board Cert:** Internal Medicine 1980; Hematology 1982; Medical Oncology 1983; **Med School:** Wayne State Univ 1977; **Resid:** Internal Medicine, Sinai Hosp 1980; **Fellow:** Hematology & Oncology, Univ Mich Hosp 1983; **Fac Appt:** Assoc Prof Med, Wayne State Univ

Brockstein, Bruce E MD [Onc] - **Spec Exp:** Head & Neck Cancer; Sarcoma; Melanoma; **Hospital:** Evanston Hosp, Highland Park Hosp; **Address:** Evanston Northwestern Healthcare, Div Hem/Onc, 2650 Ridge Ave, rm 5134, Evanston, IL 60201; **Phone:** 847-570-2515; **Board Cert:** Internal Medicine 2003; Medical Oncology 2005; **Med School:** Univ Chicago-Pritzker Sch Med 1990; **Resid:** Internal Medicine, Hosp Univ Penn 1993; **Fellow:** Hematology & Oncology, Univ Chicago Hosps 1996; **Fac Appt:** Assoc Prof Med, Northwestern Univ

Buckner, Jan Craig MD [Onc] - **Spec Exp:** Brain Tumors; Neuro-Oncology; **Hospital:** Mayo Med Ctr & Clin - Rochester; **Address:** Mayo Clinic, 200 First St SW, Rochester, MN 55905; **Phone:** 507-284-4320; **Board Cert:** Internal Medicine 1983; Medical Oncology 1985; **Med School:** Univ NC Sch Med 1980; **Resid:** Internal Medicine, Butterworth Hosp 1983; **Fellow:** Medical Oncology, Mayo Clinic 1985; **Fac Appt:** Prof Med, Mayo Med Sch

Budd, George T MD [Onc] - **Spec Exp:** Breast Cancer; **Hospital:** Cleveland Clin Fdn (page 71); **Address:** Cleveland Clinic, Taussig Cancer Ctr, 9500 Euclid Ave, Desk R35, Cleveland, OH 44195; **Phone:** 216-444-6480; **Board Cert:** Internal Medicine 1980; Medical Oncology 1983; **Med School:** Univ Kans 1976; **Resid:** Internal Medicine, Cleveland Clinic 1980; **Fellow:** Hematology & Oncology, Cleveland Clinic 1982

Bukowski, Ronald M MD [Onc] - **Spec Exp:** Kidney Cancer; **Hospital:** Cleveland Clin Fdn (page 71); **Address:** Cleveland Clinic, Taussig Cancer Ctr, 9500 Euclid Ave, Desk R35, Cleveland, OH 44195-0001; **Phone:** 216-444-6825; **Board Cert:** Internal Medicine 1974; Medical Oncology 1975; Hematology 1976; **Med School:** Northwestern Univ 1967; **Resid:** Internal Medicine, Cleveland Clin Fdn 1969; Internal Medicine, Cleveland Clin Fdn 1973; **Fellow:** Hematology, Cleveland Clin Fdn 1975; **Fac Appt:** Prof Med, Cleveland Cl Coll Med/Case West Res

Burt, Richard K MD [Onc] - **Spec Exp:** Autoimmune Disease; **Hospital:** Northwestern Meml Hosp; **Address:** Northwestern Univ, 750 N Lakeshore Drive, Ste 649, Chicago, IL 60611; **Phone:** 312-908-0059; **Board Cert:** Internal Medicine 1989; Medical Oncology 1993; **Med School:** St Louis Univ 1984; **Resid:** Internal Medicine, Baylor Coll Med 1988; **Fellow:** Medical Oncology, Natl Inst Hlth Clin Ctr 1991; Hematology, Nat Inst Hlth Clin Ctr 1993; **Fac Appt:** Assoc Prof Med, Northwestern Univ

Byrd, John C MD [Onc] - **Spec Exp:** Leukemia-Chronic Lymphocytic; **Hospital:** Arthur G James Cancer Hosp & Research Inst; **Address:** BI02 Starling-Loving Hall, 320 W 10th Ave, Columbus, OH 43210; **Phone:** 614-293-3196; **Board Cert:** Medical Oncology 1997; **Med School:** Univ Ark 1991; **Resid:** Internal Medicine, Walter Reed AMC 1994; **Fellow:** Hematology & Oncology, Walter Reed AMC 1997; **Fac Appt:** Assoc Prof Med, Ohio State Univ

Chapman, Robert A MD [Onc] - **Spec Exp:** Lung Cancer; **Hospital:** Henry Ford Hosp; **Address:** 2799 W Grand Blvd, Detroit, MI 48202; **Phone:** 313-916-1841; **Board Cert:** Internal Medicine 1985; Medical Oncology 1989; **Med School:** Cornell Univ-Weill Med Coll 1976; **Resid:** Internal Medicine, Henry Ford Hosp 1979; **Fellow:** Medical Oncology, Meml Sloan Kettering Cancer Ctr 1981

Chitambar, Christopher R MD [Onc] - **Spec Exp:** Lymphoma; Leukemia; Breast Cancer; **Hospital:** Froedtert Meml Lutheran Hosp; **Address:** Med Coll Wisconsin, Div Neoplastic Disease, 9200 W Wisconsin Ave, Milwaukee, WI 53226-3522; **Phone:** 414-805-4600; **Board Cert:** Internal Medicine 1980; Hematology 1982; Medical Oncology 1983; **Med School:** India 1977; **Resid:** Internal Medicine, Brackenridge Hosp 1980; **Fellow:** Hematology & Oncology, Univ Colo Hlth Sci Ctr 1983; **Fac Appt:** Prof Med, Med Coll Wisc

Clamon, Gerald MD [Onc] - **Spec Exp:** Lung Cancer; Drug Development; **Hospital:** Univ Iowa Hosp & Clinics; **Address:** Univ Iowa Hosps & Clins, Dept Internal Med, 200 Hawkins Drive, rm 5970 JPP, Iowa City, IA 52242; **Phone:** 319-356-1932; **Board Cert:** Internal Medicine 1976; Medical Oncology 1979; **Med School:** Washington Univ, St Louis 1971; **Resid:** Internal Medicine, Barnes Hosp 1976; **Fellow:** Natl Cancer Inst 1974; Medical Oncology, Univ Iowa Hosp & Clinics 1977; **Fac Appt:** Prof Med, Univ Iowa Coll Med

Clark, Joseph I MD [Onc] - **Spec Exp:** Kidney Cancer; Melanoma; Head & Neck Cancer; **Hospital:** Loyola Univ Med Ctr, Hines VA Hosp; **Address:** Cardinal Bernardin Canc Ctr, Loyola Univ Med Ctr, 2160 S 1st Ave, rm 343, Maywood, IL 60153; **Phone:** 708-327-3236; **Board Cert:** Internal Medicine 2002; Medical Oncology 2006; **Med School:** Loyola Univ-Stritch Sch Med 1989; **Resid:** Internal Medicine, Loyola Univ Med Ctr/Hines VA Hosp 1992; **Fellow:** Hematology & Oncology, Fox Chase Cancer Ctr/Temple Univ Hosp 1995; **Fac Appt:** Assoc Prof Med, Loyola Univ-Stritch Sch Med

Cleary, James F MD [Onc] - **Spec Exp:** Palliative Care; Head & Neck Cancer; **Hospital:** Univ WI Hosp & Clins; **Address:** K6/518 CSC, 600 Highland Ave, Madison, WI 53792; **Phone:** 608-263-8090; **Med School:** Australia 1984; **Resid:** Internal Medicine, Royal Adelaide Hosp 1987; **Fellow:** Medical Oncology, Royal Adelaide Hosp 1990; **Fac Appt:** Assoc Prof Med, Univ Wisc

Clinton, Steven MD/PhD [Onc] - **Spec Exp:** Genitourinary Cancer; Prostate Cancer; Nutrition & Cancer Prevention/Control; **Hospital:** Ohio St Univ Med Ctr; **Address:** A434 Starling Loving Hall, 320 W 10th Ave, Columbus, OH 43210; **Phone:** 614-293-7560; **Board Cert:** Internal Medicine 1987; Medical Oncology 1991; **Med School:** Univ IL Coll Med 1984; **Resid:** Internal Medicine, Univ Chicago Hosps 1987; **Fellow:** Medical Oncology, Dana Farber Cancer Inst/Harvard 1991; **Fac Appt:** Assoc Prof Med, Ohio State Univ

Cobleigh, Melody A MD [Onc] - **Spec Exp:** Breast Cancer; **Hospital:** Rush Univ Med Ctr; **Address:** Rush Univ Med Ctr, 1725 W Harrison St, Ste 855, Chicago, IL 60612-3828; **Phone:** 312-942-5904; **Board Cert:** Internal Medicine 1979; Medical Oncology 1981; **Med School:** Rush Med Coll 1976; **Resid:** Internal Medicine, Rush Presby-St Lukes Med Ctr 1979; **Fellow:** Medical Oncology, Indiana Univ 1981; **Fac Appt:** Prof Med, Rush Med Coll

Daugherty, Christopher K MD [Onc] - **Spec Exp:** Leukemia & Lymphoma; Stem Cell Transplant; **Hospital:** Univ of Chicago Hosps; **Address:** University of Chicago Hospspitals, 5841 S Maryland Ave, MC 2115, Chicago, IL 60637; **Phone:** 773-702-6149; **Board Cert:** Medical Oncology 1997; **Med School:** Indiana Univ 1989; **Resid:** Internal Medicine, Indiana Univ 1993; **Fellow:** Hematology & Oncology, Univ Chicago Hosps 1997; Medical Ethics, Univ Chicago Hosps

Davis, Mellar MD [Onc] - **Spec Exp:** Palliative Care; Lung Cancer (advanced); **Hospital:** Cleveland Clin Fdn (page 71); **Address:** Cleveland Clin Fdn, 9500 Euclid Ave, Desk R35, Cleveland, OH 44195; **Phone:** 216-445-4622; **Board Cert:** Internal Medicine 1980; Hematology 1982; Medical Oncology 1983; **Med School:** Ohio State Univ 1977; **Resid:** Internal Medicine, Riverside Meth Hosp 1979; **Fellow:** Hematology, Mayo Clinic 1981; Medical Oncology, Mayo Clinic 1982

Di Persio, John MD/PhD [Onc] - Spec Exp: Bone Marrow Transplant; Hematologic Malignancies; Leukemia; **Hospital:** Barnes-Jewish Hosp; **Address:** Wash Univ Sch Med, Sect BMT & Leukemia, 660 S Euclid Ave, Box 8007, St Louis, MO 63110; **Phone:** 314-454-8306; **Board Cert:** Internal Medicine 1984; Medical Oncology 1987; Hematology 1988; **Med School:** Univ Rochester 1980; **Resid:** Internal Medicine, Parkland Meml Hosp 1984; **Fellow:** Hematology & Oncology, UCLA Sch Med 1987; **Fac Appt:** Prof Med, Washington Univ, St Louis

Dreicer, Robert MD [Onc] - Spec Exp: Breast Cancer; Prostate Cancer; **Hospital:** Cleveland Clin Fdn (page 71); **Address:** Cleveland Clinic, Taussig Cancer Ctr, 9500 Euclid Ave, Desk R35, Cleveland, OH 44195; **Phone:** 216-445-4623; **Board Cert:** Internal Medicine 1986; Medical Oncology 1989; **Med School:** Univ Tex, Houston 1983; **Resid:** Internal Medicine, Ind Univ Med Ctr 1986; **Fellow:** Medical Oncology, Univ Wisconsin Hosp & Clins 1989

Einhorn, Lawrence MD [Onc] - Spec Exp: Testicular Cancer; Lung Cancer; Urologic Cancer; **Hospital:** Indiana Univ Hosp (page 70); **Address:** 535 Barnhill Drive, rm 473, Indianapolis, IN 46202; **Phone:** 317-274-0920; **Board Cert:** Internal Medicine 1972; Medical Oncology 1975; **Med School:** UCLA 1967; **Resid:** Internal Medicine, Indiana Univ Hosp 1969; **Fellow:** Medical Oncology, Indiana Univ Hosp 1972; **Fac Appt:** Prof Med, Indiana Univ

Eng, Charis MD [Onc] - Spec Exp: Breast Cancer; Ovarian Cancer; Cancer Genetics; **Hospital:** Cleveland Clin Fdn (page 71); **Address:** Cleveland Clinic Foundation, 9500 Euclid Ave, MC NE50, Cleveland, OH 44195; **Phone:** 216-444-3440; **Board Cert:** Internal Medicine 1991; Medical Oncology 1997; **Med School:** Univ Chicago-Pritzker Sch Med 1988; **Resid:** Internal Medicine, Beth Israel Hosp 1991; **Fellow:** Medical Oncology, Dana-Farber Cancer Inst 1995

Ensminger, William D MD/PhD [Onc] - Spec Exp: Gastrointestinal Cancer; Liver Cancer; Clinical Trials; **Hospital:** Univ Michigan Hlth Sys; **Address:** Upjohn Center, rm 3709, 1310 E Catherine, Ann Arbor, MI 48109-0504; **Phone:** 734-764-5468; **Board Cert:** Internal Medicine 1976; Medical Oncology 1979; **Med School:** Harvard Med Sch 1973; **Resid:** Internal Medicine, Beth Israel Hosp 1975; **Fellow:** Medical Oncology, Dana Farber Cancer Inst 1977; **Fac Appt:** Prof Med, Univ Mich Med Sch

Fleming, Gini F MD [Onc] - Spec Exp: Breast Cancer; Gynecologic Cancer; **Hospital:** Univ of Chicago Hosps; **Address:** Univ Chicago Hospitals, 5841 S Maryland MC2115, Chicago, IL 60637-1470; **Phone:** 773-702-6149; **Board Cert:** Internal Medicine 1988; Medical Oncology 2001; Hematology 2002; **Med School:** Univ IL Coll Med 1985; **Resid:** Internal Medicine, Univ Chicago-Pritzker Sch Med 1988; **Fellow:** Hematology & Oncology, Univ Chicago-Pritzker Sch Med 1992; **Fac Appt:** Prof Med, Univ Chicago-Pritzker Sch Med

Fracasso, Paula M MD/PhD [Onc] - Spec Exp: Ovarian Cancer; Gynecologic Cancer; Breast Cancer; **Hospital:** Barnes-Jewish Hosp; **Address:** Washington Univ Sch Med, 660 N Euclid, Box 8056, St Louis, MO 63110-1002; **Phone:** 314-454-8817; **Board Cert:** Internal Medicine 1987; Medical Oncology 2003; **Med School:** Yale Univ 1984; **Resid:** Internal Medicine, Beth Israel Hosp 1987; **Fellow:** Cancer Research, Mass Inst Tech 1989; Hematology & Oncology, Tufts-New England Med Ctr 1991; **Fac Appt:** Assoc Prof Med, Washington Univ, St Louis

Gerson, Stanton MD [Onc] - **Spec Exp:** Leukemia; Lymphoma, Non-Hodgkin's; Stem Cell Transplant; **Hospital:** Univ Hosps Case Med Ctr; **Address:** Case Comprehensive Cancer Ctr, 11000 Euclid Ave, 1 WEARN 151, Cleveland, OH 44106-5065; **Phone:** 216-844-8562; **Board Cert:** Internal Medicine 1980; Medical Oncology 1983; Hematology 1982; **Med School:** Harvard Med Sch 1977; **Resid:** Internal Medicine, Hosp Univ Penn 1980; **Fellow:** Hematology & Oncology, Hosp Univ Penn 1983; **Fac Appt:** Prof Med, Case West Res Univ

Golomb, Harvey MD [Onc] - **Spec Exp:** Lung Cancer; Leukemia; Lymphoma; **Hospital:** Univ of Chicago Hosps; **Address:** Univ of Chicago Hospital, 5758 S Maryland Ave, MC 9015, Chicago, IL 60637-1463; **Phone:** 773-702-6115; **Board Cert:** Internal Medicine 1975; Medical Oncology 1979; **Med School:** Univ Pittsburgh 1968; **Resid:** Internal Medicine, Johns Hopkins Hosp 1972; Clinical Genetics, Johns Hopkins Hosp 1973; **Fellow:** Hematology & Oncology, Univ Chicago Hosps 1975; **Fac Appt:** Prof Med, Univ Chicago-Pritzker Sch Med

Gradishar, William J MD [Onc] - **Spec Exp:** Breast Cancer; **Hospital:** Northwestern Meml Hosp; **Address:** 676 N St Claire St, Ste 21-100, Chicago, IL 60611; **Phone:** 312-695-0990; **Board Cert:** Internal Medicine 1985; Medical Oncology 1989; **Med School:** Univ IL Coll Med 1982; **Resid:** Internal Medicine, Michael Reese Hosp 1985; **Fellow:** Hematology & Oncology, Univ Chicago Hosps 1990; **Fac Appt:** Prof Med, Northwestern Univ

Gruber, Stephen B MD/PhD [Onc] - **Spec Exp:** Cancer Genetics; Colon & Rectal Cancer; Melanoma; **Hospital:** Univ Michigan Hlth Sys; **Address:** 1524 BSRB, 109 Zina Pitcher Pl, Ann Arbor, MI 48109-2200; **Phone:** 734-647-8906; **Board Cert:** Internal Medicine 1995; Medical Oncology 1998; **Med School:** Univ Pennsylvania 1992; **Resid:** Internal Medicine, Hosp Univ Penn 1994; **Fellow:** Medical Oncology, Johns Hopkins Hosp 1997; Clinical Genetics, Univ Michigan Hlth Sys 1999; **Fac Appt:** Assoc Prof Med, Univ Mich Med Sch

Hartmann, Lynn Carol MD [Onc] - **Spec Exp:** Breast Cancer; Ovarian Cancer; **Hospital:** Mayo Med Ctr & Clin - Rochester; **Address:** Mayo Clinic Gonda 10 South, 200 First St SW, Rochester, MN 55905; **Phone:** 507-284-3903; **Board Cert:** Internal Medicine 1986; Medical Oncology 1989; **Med School:** Northwestern Univ 1983; **Resid:** Internal Medicine, Univ Ia Hosps/Clinics 1986; **Fellow:** Medical Oncology, Mayo Clinic 1989; **Fac Appt:** Prof Med, Mayo Med Sch

Hayes, Daniel F MD [Onc] - **Spec Exp:** Breast Cancer; **Hospital:** Univ Michigan Hlth Sys; **Address:** Univ Michigan Comprehensive Cancer Ctr, 1500 E Med Ctr Drive, rm 6312, Box 0942, Ann Arbor, MI 48109-0942; **Phone:** 734-615-6725; **Board Cert:** Internal Medicine 1982; Medical Oncology 1985; **Med School:** Indiana Univ 1979; **Resid:** Internal Medicine, Parkland Meml Hosp 1982; **Fellow:** Medical Oncology, Dana Farber Cancer Inst 1985; **Fac Appt:** Prof Med, Univ Mich Med Sch

Hoffman, Philip C MD [Onc] - **Spec Exp:** Lung Cancer; Breast Cancer; Esophageal Cancer; **Hospital:** Univ of Chicago Hosps, Little Company of Mary Hosp & Hlth Care Ctrs; **Address:** 5841 S Maryland Ave, MC 2115, Chicago, IL 60637-1463; **Phone:** 773-834-7424; **Board Cert:** Internal Medicine 1975; Hematology 1980; Medical Oncology 1981; **Med School:** Jefferson Med Coll 1972; **Resid:** Internal Medicine, Hosp Univ Penn 1975; **Fellow:** Hematology & Oncology, Univ Chicago Hosps 1980; **Fac Appt:** Prof Med, Univ Chicago-Pritzker Sch Med

Medical Oncology

Hussain, Maha H MD [Onc] - **Spec Exp:** Prostate Cancer; Bladder Cancer; Testicular Cancer; **Hospital:** Univ Michigan Hlth Sys; **Address:** University of Michigan Cancer Ctr, 1500 E Medical Drive, Ann Arbor, MI 48109; **Phone:** 734-936-8906; **Board Cert:** Internal Medicine 1986; Medical Oncology 1989; **Med School:** Iraq 1980; **Resid:** Internal Medicine, Wayne State Univ Affil Hosps 1986; **Fellow:** Medical Oncology, Wayne State Univ Affil Hosps 1989; **Fac Appt:** Prof Med, Univ Mich Med Sch

Ingle, James N MD [Onc] - **Spec Exp:** Breast Cancer; **Hospital:** Rochester Meth Hosp; **Address:** Mayo Clinic, 200 First St SW, 12 East, Rochester, MN 55905; **Phone:** 507-284-8432; **Board Cert:** Internal Medicine 1974; Medical Oncology 1975; **Med School:** Johns Hopkins Univ 1971; **Resid:** Internal Medicine, Johns Hopkins Hosp 1976; Medical Oncology, Natl Cancer Inst 1975; **Fac Appt:** Prof Med, Mayo Med Sch

Kalaycio, Matt E MD [Onc] - **Spec Exp:** Leukemia; **Hospital:** Cleveland Clin Fdn (page 71); **Address:** Taussig Cancer Ctr, 9500 Euclid Ave, Desk R35, Cleveland, OH 44195; **Phone:** 216-444-3705; **Board Cert:** Internal Medicine 2002; Hematology 2004; Medical Oncology 1995; **Med School:** W VA Univ 1988; **Resid:** Internal Medicine, Mercy Hosp 1991; **Fellow:** Hematology & Oncology, Cleveland Clinic 1994; **Fac Appt:** Assoc Prof Med, Cleveland Cl Coll Med/Case West Res

Kalemkerian, Gregory MD [Onc] - **Spec Exp:** Lung Cancer; Mesothelioma; Thymoma; **Hospital:** Univ Michigan Hlth Sys; **Address:** 1500 E Medical Center Dr, C350MIB, Ann Arbor, MI 48109-0848; **Phone:** 734-936-5281; **Board Cert:** Internal Medicine 1988; Medical Oncology 2001; **Med School:** Northwestern Univ 1985; **Resid:** Internal Medicine, Northwestern Meml Hosp 1988; **Fac Appt:** Assoc Clin Prof Med, Univ Mich Med Sch

Kaminski, Mark S MD [Onc] - **Spec Exp:** Lymphoma; Bone Marrow Transplant; Drug Development; Clinical Trials; **Hospital:** Univ Michigan Hlth Sys; **Address:** Univ Michigan Cancer Ctr, 1500 E Medical Ctr Drive, rm 4316, Ann Arbor, MI 48109-0936; **Phone:** 734-936-5310; **Board Cert:** Internal Medicine 1981; Medical Oncology 1983; **Med School:** Stanford Univ 1978; **Resid:** Internal Medicine, Barnes Hosp 1981; **Fellow:** Medical Oncology, Stanford Univ Med Ctr 1985; **Fac Appt:** Prof Med, Univ Mich Med Sch

Kindler, Hedy Lee MD [Onc] - **Spec Exp:** Mesothelioma; Pancreatic Cancer; Colon & Rectal Cancer; **Hospital:** Univ of Chicago Hosps; **Address:** Univ of Chicago Hospital, 5758 S Maryland Ave, MC 9015, Chicago, IL 60637; **Phone:** 773-834-7424; **Board Cert:** Internal Medicine 2002; Medical Oncology 1995; **Med School:** SUNY Buffalo 1985; **Resid:** Internal Medicine, UCLA Med Ctr; **Fellow:** Medical Oncology, Meml Sloan Kettering Cancer Ctr; **Fac Appt:** Asst Prof Med, Univ Chicago-Pritzker Sch Med

Kosova, Leonard MD [Onc] - **Spec Exp:** Breast Cancer; Lymphoma; Lung Cancer; **Hospital:** Adv Luth Genl Hosp; **Address:** 8915 W Golf Rd, Ste 3, Niles, IL 60714-5825; **Phone:** 847-827-9060; **Board Cert:** Internal Medicine 1974; Hematology 1972; Medical Oncology 1975; **Med School:** Univ IL Coll Med 1961; **Resid:** Internal Medicine, Hines VA Hosp 1964; **Fellow:** Hematology & Oncology, Hektoen Inst-Cook Cty Hosp 1965

Lippman, Marc E MD [Onc] - **Spec Exp:** Breast Cancer; **Hospital:** Univ Michigan Hlth Sys; **Address:** Univ Mich Health System, 3101 Taubman Ctr, 1500 E Medical Ctr Dr, Ann Arbor, MI 48109-0368; **Phone:** 734-936-4495; **Board Cert:** Internal Medicine 1987; Endocrinology 1975; Medical Oncology 1977; **Med School:** Yale Univ 1968; **Resid:** Internal Medicine, Johns Hopkins Hosp 1970; **Fellow:** Medical Oncology, Natl Cancer Inst 1973; Endocrinology, Yale-New Haven Hosp 1974; **Fac Appt:** Prof Med, Univ Mich Med Sch

Locker, Gershon Y MD [Onc] - **Spec Exp:** Gastrointestinal Cancer; Ovarian Cancer; Breast Cancer; Cancer Genetics; **Hospital:** Evanston Hosp, Northwestern Meml Hosp; **Address:** Evanston Hospital-Kellog Cancer Ctr, 2650 Ridge Ave, rm 5134, Evanston, IL 60201-1781; **Phone:** 847-570-2515; **Board Cert:** Internal Medicine 1976; Medical Oncology 1977; **Med School:** Harvard Med Sch 1973; **Resid:** Internal Medicine, Univ Chicago Hosps 1975; **Fellow:** Medical Oncology, Natl Cancer Inst 1978; **Fac Appt:** Prof Med, Northwestern Univ

Loehrer, Patrick J MD [Onc] - **Spec Exp:** Gastrointestinal Cancer; Thymoma; Genitourinary Cancer; **Hospital:** Indiana Univ Hosp (page 70); **Address:** Indiana Cancer Pavilion, 535 Barnhill Drive, rm 473, Indianapolis, IN 46202-5112; **Phone:** 317-278-7418; **Board Cert:** Internal Medicine 1981; Medical Oncology 2006; **Med School:** Rush Med Coll 1978; **Resid:** Internal Medicine, Rush-Presby-St Lukes Hosp 1981; **Fellow:** Medical Oncology, Indiana Univ 1983; **Fac Appt:** Prof Med, Indiana Univ

Loprinzi, Charles L MD [Onc] - **Spec Exp:** Breast Cancer; **Hospital:** Mayo Med Ctr & Clin - Rochester; **Address:** Mayo Clinic, Dept Med Oncology, 200 First St SW, Rochester, MN 55905-0001; **Phone:** 507-284-4137; **Board Cert:** Internal Medicine 1982; Medical Oncology 1985; **Med School:** Oregon Hlth Sci Univ 1979; **Resid:** Internal Medicine, Maricopa Co Hosp 1982; **Fellow:** Medical Oncology, Univ Wisconsin Med Ctr 1984; **Fac Appt:** Prof Med, Mayo Med Sch

Markowitz, Sanford D MD [Onc] - **Spec Exp:** Colon & Rectal Cancer; Hereditary Cancer; **Hospital:** Univ Hosps Case Med Ctr; **Address:** Ireland Cancer Ctr, 11000 Euclid Ave Fl 6, Cleveland, OH 44106; **Phone:** 216-844-3127; **Board Cert:** Internal Medicine 1984; Medical Oncology 1987; **Med School:** Yale Univ 1980; **Resid:** Internal Medicine, Univ Chicago Hosp 1984; **Fellow:** Medical Oncology, Natl Cancer Inst 1986; **Fac Appt:** Prof Med, Case West Res Univ

Olopade, Olufunmilayo I F MD [Onc] - **Spec Exp:** Breast Cancer; Hereditary Cancer; Cancer Genetics; **Hospital:** Univ of Chicago Hosps; **Address:** Univ Chicago Hospital, 5758 S Maryland Ave, MC 9015, Chicago, IL 60637-1470; **Phone:** 773-702-6149; **Board Cert:** Internal Medicine 1986; Hematology 2001; Medical Oncology 1989; **Med School:** Nigeria 1980; **Resid:** Internal Medicine, Cook Co Hosp 1986; **Fellow:** Hematology & Oncology, Univ Chicago Hosps 1991; **Fac Appt:** Prof Med, Univ Chicago-Pritzker Sch Med

Perry, Michael MD [Onc] - **Spec Exp:** Lung Cancer; Breast Cancer; **Hospital:** Univ of Missouri Hosp & Clins; **Address:** Ellis Fischel Cancer Ctr, 115 Business Loop 70 W, DC 116.71, rm 524, Columbia, MO 65203-3299; **Phone:** 573-882-4979; **Board Cert:** Internal Medicine 1987; Hematology 1974; Medical Oncology 1975; **Med School:** Wayne State Univ 1970; **Resid:** Internal Medicine, Mayo Grad Sch 1972; **Fellow:** Hematology, Mayo Grad Sch 1974; Medical Oncology, Mayo Grad Sch 1975; **Fac Appt:** Prof Med, Univ MO-Columbia Sch Med

Peterson, Bruce MD [Onc] - **Spec Exp:** Lymphoma; Leukemia; **Hospital:** Univ Minn Med Ctr, Fairview - Univ Campus; **Address:** Division Medical Oncology, MMC 286, Univ of Minnesota, Minneapolis, MN 55455; **Phone:** 612-624-5631; **Board Cert:** Internal Medicine 1974; Medical Oncology 1977; **Med School:** Univ Minn 1971; **Resid:** Internal Medicine, Fletcher Allen Hlthcare 1973; Internal Medicine, Fairview-Univ Med Ctr 1974; **Fellow:** Medical Oncology, Fairview-Univ Med Ctr 1977; **Fac Appt:** Prof Med, Univ Minn

Picus, Joel MD [Onc] - **Spec Exp:** Pancreatic Cancer; Prostate Cancer; Colon Cancer; **Hospital:** Barnes-Jewish Hosp; **Address:** Washington University School of Medicine-Dept Medicine, 660 S Euclid Ave, Box Campus 8056, St Louis, MO 63110; **Phone:** 314-362-5737; **Board Cert:** Internal Medicine 1987; Medical Oncology 1989; Hematology 1990; **Med School:** Harvard Med Sch 1984; **Resid:** Internal Medicine, Duke Univ Med Ctr 1987; **Fellow:** Hematology & Oncology, UCSF Med Ctr 1991; **Fac Appt:** Assoc Prof Med, Washington Univ, St Louis

Pienta, Kenneth J MD [Onc] - **Spec Exp:** Prostate Cancer; **Hospital:** Univ Michigan Hlth Sys; **Address:** Cancer Center/Geriatrics Center, 1500 E Medical Center Drive, rm 7303 CCGC, Ann Arbor, MI 48109-0946; **Phone:** 734-647-3421; **Board Cert:** Internal Medicine 2001; Medical Oncology 2001; **Med School:** Johns Hopkins Univ 1986; **Resid:** Internal Medicine, Univ Chicago Hosps 1988; **Fellow:** Medical Oncology, Johns Hopkins Hosp 1991; **Fac Appt:** Prof Med, Univ Mich Med Sch

Raghavan, Derek MD/PhD [Onc] - **Spec Exp:** Prostate Cancer; Testicular Cancer; Bladder Cancer; **Hospital:** Cleveland Clin Fdn (page 71); **Address:** Cleveland Clinic Taussig Cancer Ctr, 9500 Euclid Ave, MC R35, Cleveland, OH 44195; **Phone:** 216-445-6888; **Med School:** Australia 1974; **Resid:** Internal Medicine, Royal Prince Alfred Hosp 1977; **Fellow:** Medical Oncology, Royal Prince Alfred Hosp 1979; Medical Oncology, Royal Marsden Hosp; **Fac Appt:** Prof Med, Cleveland Cl Coll Med/Case West Res

Ratain, Mark J MD [Onc] - **Spec Exp:** Solid Tumors; Drug Discovery & Development; **Hospital:** Univ of Chicago Hosps; **Address:** 5841 S Maryland Ave, MC 2115, Chicago, IL 60637; **Phone:** 773-702-6149; **Board Cert:** Internal Medicine 1983; Hematology 1986; Medical Oncology 1985; **Med School:** Yale Univ 1980; **Resid:** Internal Medicine, Johns Hopkins Hosp 1983; **Fellow:** Hematology & Oncology, Univ Chicago 1986; **Fac Appt:** Prof Med, Univ Chicago-Pritzker Sch Med

Remick, Scot C MD [Onc] - **Spec Exp:** AIDS Related Cancers; Clinical Trials; Drug Development; **Hospital:** Univ Hosps Case Med Ctr; **Address:** Univ Hosp Case Med Ctr, Div Hem/Oncology, 11100 Euclid Ave, BHC-6, LKSD 1236, Cleveland, OH 44106; **Phone:** 216-844-3951; **Board Cert:** Internal Medicine 1985; Medical Oncology 1987; **Med School:** NY Med Coll 1982; **Resid:** Internal Medicine, Johns Hopkins Hosp 1985; **Fellow:** Medical Oncology, Univ Wisconsin Clin Cancer Ctr 1988; **Fac Appt:** Prof Med, Case West Res Univ

Richards, Jon MD/PhD [Onc] - **Spec Exp:** Testicular Cancer; Prostate Cancer; Melanoma; **Hospital:** Adv Luth Genl Hosp, Rush N Shore Med Ctr; **Address:** Cancer Care Ctr, 1700 Luther Ln Fl 2, Park Ridge, IL 60068; **Phone:** 847-268-8200; **Board Cert:** Internal Medicine 1998; **Med School:** Cornell Univ-Weill Med Coll 1983; **Resid:** Internal Medicine, Univ Chicago Hosp 1985; **Fellow:** Hematology & Oncology, Univ Chicago Hosp 1988; **Fac Appt:** Asst Prof Med, Univ IL Coll Med

Rosen, Steven T MD [Onc] - **Spec Exp:** Hematologic Malignancies; Breast Cancer; Lymphoma; **Hospital:** Northwestern Meml Hosp; **Address:** Northwestern Univ, 303 E Chicago Ave, Lurie 3-125, Chicago, IL 60611-3013; **Phone:** 312-695-1153; **Board Cert:** Internal Medicine 1979; Medical Oncology 1981; Hematology 1984; **Med School:** Northwestern Univ 1976; **Resid:** Internal Medicine, Northwestern Univ Hosp 1979; **Fellow:** Medical Oncology, Natl Cancer Inst 1981; **Fac Appt:** Prof Med, Northwestern Univ

Ruckdeschel, John C MD [Onc] - **Spec Exp:** Lung Cancer; Mesothelioma; **Hospital:** Karmanos Cancer Inst; **Address:** Karmanos Cancer Inst-Executive Offices, 4100 John R Fl 2, Detroit, MI 48201; **Phone:** 313-526-8621; **Board Cert:** Internal Medicine 1976; Medical Oncology 1977; **Med School:** Albany Med Coll 1971; **Resid:** Internal Medicine, Johns Hopkins Hosp 1972; Internal Medicine, Beth Israel Hosp 1976; **Fellow:** Medical Oncology, Natl Cancer Inst 1975; **Fac Appt:** Prof Med, Wayne State Univ

Salgia, Ravi MD/PhD [Onc] - **Spec Exp:** Lung Cancer; Mesothelioma; Thoracic Cancers; **Hospital:** Univ of Chicago Hosps; **Address:** University of Chicago Hospitals, 5841 S Maryland Ave, MC 2115, Chicago, IL 60637; **Phone:** 773-702-6149; **Board Cert:** Medical Oncology 2006; **Med School:** Loyola Univ-Stritch Sch Med 1987; **Resid:** Internal Medicine, Johns Hopkins Hospital 1990; **Fellow:** Medical Oncology, Dana-Farber Cancer Inst 1993; **Fac Appt:** Assoc Prof Med, Univ IL Coll Med

Saroja, Kurubarahalli MD [Onc] - **Spec Exp:** Neutron Therapy for Advanced Cancer; Head & Neck Cancer; Sarcoma; Prostate Cancer; **Hospital:** Delnor - Comm Hosp, Central DuPage Hosp; **Address:** Raymond G Scott Cancer Care Center, 304 Randall, Geneva, IL 60134; **Phone:** 630-262-8554; **Board Cert:** Pediatrics 1978; Radiation Oncology 1987; Neonatal-Perinatal Medicine 1981; **Med School:** India 1967; **Resid:** Pediatrics, Cook Co Hosp 1976; Radiation Oncology, Rush-Presby St Lukes 1985; **Fellow:** Neonatal-Perinatal Medicine, Milwaukee Co Med Comp 1978

Schiffer, Charles A MD [Onc] - **Spec Exp:** Leukemia; Lymphoma; Multiple Myeloma; **Hospital:** Karmanos Cancer Inst, Harper Univ Hosp; **Address:** Karmanos Cancer Inst, Cancer Research Ctr, 4100 John R, 4-Hudson Webber, Detroit, MI 48201; **Phone:** 313-576-8737; **Board Cert:** Internal Medicine 1972; Medical Oncology 1973; **Med School:** NYU Sch Med 1968; **Resid:** Internal Medicine, Bellevue-NY VA Hosp-NYU 1972; **Fellow:** Medical Oncology, Natl Cancer Inst 1974; **Fac Appt:** Prof Med, Wayne State Univ

Schilsky, Richard MD [Onc] - **Spec Exp:** Gastrointestinal Cancer; Pancreatic Cancer; Drug Development; **Hospital:** Univ of Chicago Hosps; **Address:** Univ Chicago- Bio Sciences Div, 5841 S Maryland Ave, MC 7132, Chicago, IL 60637; **Phone:** 773-834-3914; **Board Cert:** Internal Medicine 1978; Medical Oncology 1979; **Med School:** Univ Chicago-Pritzker Sch Med 1975; **Resid:** Internal Medicine, Univ Texas 1977; **Fac Appt:** Prof Med, Univ Chicago-Pritzker Sch Med

Schwartz, Burton S MD [Onc] - **Spec Exp:** Lymphoma; Breast Cancer; **Hospital:** Abbott - Northwestern Hosp; **Address:** 800 E 28th St, Piper Bldg, Ste 405, Minneapolis, MN 55407; **Phone:** 612-863-8585; **Board Cert:** Internal Medicine 1980; Hematology 1976; Medical Oncology 1977; **Med School:** Meharry Med Coll 1968; **Resid:** Internal Medicine, Michael Reese Hosp 1971; **Fellow:** Hematology, Univ Minn Hosp 1976; **Fac Appt:** Clin Prof Med, Univ Minn

Shapiro, Charles L MD [Onc] - **Spec Exp:** Breast Cancer; **Hospital:** Arthur G James Cancer Hosp & Research Inst; **Address:** Starling Loving Hall, rm B405, 320 W 10th Ave, Columbus, OH 43210; **Phone:** 614-293-6401; **Board Cert:** Internal Medicine 1987; Medical Oncology 2005; **Med School:** SUNY Buffalo 1984; **Resid:** Internal Medicine, Temple Univ Hosp 1987; **Fellow:** Medical Oncology, Dana Farber Cancer Inst 1991; **Fac Appt:** Assoc Prof Med, Ohio State Univ

Medical Oncology

Silverman, Paula MD [Onc] - **Spec Exp:** Breast Cancer; **Hospital:** Univ Hosps Case Med Ctr; **Address:** Univ Hosp Cleveland, Ireland Cancer Ctr, 11100 Euclid Ave, Cleveland, OH 44106; **Phone:** 216-844-8510; **Board Cert:** Internal Medicine 1984; Medical Oncology 1989; **Med School:** Case West Res Univ 1981; **Resid:** Internal Medicine, Univ Hosps 1984; **Fellow:** Hematology & Oncology, Case Western Reserve Univ 1987; **Fac Appt:** Assoc Prof Med, Case West Res Univ

Sledge Jr, George W MD [Onc] - **Spec Exp:** Breast Cancer; **Hospital:** Indiana Univ Hosp (page 70); **Address:** 535 Barnhill Drive, rm 473, Indianapolis, IN 46202; **Phone:** 317-274-0920; **Board Cert:** Internal Medicine 1980; Medical Oncology 1983; **Med School:** Tulane Univ 1977; **Resid:** Internal Medicine, St Louis Univ 1980; **Fellow:** Medical Oncology, Univ Texas 1983; **Fac Appt:** Prof Med, Indiana Univ

Stadler, Walter M MD [Onc] - **Spec Exp:** Kidney Cancer; Prostate Cancer; Bladder Cancer; **Hospital:** Univ of Chicago Hosps; **Address:** Univ Chicago Hosps, Div Hem/Onc, 5758 S Maryland Ave, MC 9015, Chicago, IL 60637; **Phone:** 773-834-7424; **Board Cert:** Internal Medicine 2002; Medical Oncology 2003; **Med School:** Yale Univ 1988; **Resid:** Internal Medicine, Michael Reese Hosp 1991; **Fellow:** Medical Oncology, Univ Chicago Hosps 1994; **Fac Appt:** Prof Med, Univ Chicago-Pritzker Sch Med

Todd III, Robert F MD/PhD [Onc] - **Spec Exp:** Gastrointestinal Cancer; Lung Cancer; **Hospital:** Univ Michigan Hlth Sys; **Address:** Univ Michigan Cancer Ctr, 7216CCGC, 1500 E Med Ctr Dr, Box 0948, Ann Arbor, MI 48109; **Phone:** 734-647-8903; **Board Cert:** Internal Medicine 1979; Medical Oncology 1981; **Med School:** Duke Univ 1976; **Resid:** Internal Medicine, Peter Bent Brigham Hosp 1978; **Fellow:** Medical Oncology, Dana Farber Cancer Inst 1981; **Fac Appt:** Prof Med, Univ Mich Med Sch

Urba, Susan G MD [Onc] - **Spec Exp:** Head & Neck Cancer; **Hospital:** Univ Michigan Hlth Sys; **Address:** Comp Cancer Ctr & Geriatrics Ctr, 1500 E Med Ctr Drive, rm 4214, Ann Arbor, MI 48109-0922; **Phone:** 734-647-8902; **Board Cert:** Internal Medicine 1986; Medical Oncology 1991; **Med School:** Univ Mich Med Sch 1983; **Resid:** Internal Medicine, Univ Mich Med Ctr 1986; **Fellow:** Hematology & Oncology, Univ Mich Med Ctr 1988; **Fac Appt:** Assoc Prof Med, Univ Mich Med Sch

Vokes, Everett E MD [Onc] - **Spec Exp:** Lung Cancer; Head & Neck Cancer; Esophageal Cancer; **Hospital:** Univ of Chicago Hosps; **Address:** Univ Chicago Hosps, 5841 S Maryland Ave, MC 2115, Chicago, IL 60637-1470; **Phone:** 773-834-3093; **Board Cert:** Internal Medicine 1983; Medical Oncology 1985; **Med School:** Germany 1980; **Resid:** Internal Medicine, Ravenswood Hosp-Univ Illinois 1982; Internal Medicine, USC Med Ctr 1983; **Fellow:** Medical Oncology, Univ Chicago 1986; **Fac Appt:** Prof Med, Univ Chicago-Pritzker Sch Med

Von Roenn, Jamie H MD [Onc] - **Spec Exp:** Palliative Care; AIDS Related Cancers; Breast Cancer; **Hospital:** Northwestern Meml Hosp; **Address:** Northwestern Memorial Hosp, 675 N St Clair Fl 21 - Ste 100, Chicago, IL 60611; **Phone:** 312-695-0990; **Board Cert:** Internal Medicine 1983; Medical Oncology 1985; **Med School:** Rush Med Coll 1980; **Resid:** Internal Medicine, Rush-Presby-St Lukes Hosp 1983; **Fellow:** Medical Oncology, Rush-Presby-St Lukes Hosp 1985; **Fac Appt:** Prof Med, Northwestern Univ

Wade, James C MD [Onc] - **Spec Exp:** Infections in Cancer Patients; Bone Marrow Transplant; Leukemia; **Hospital:** Froedtert Meml Lutheran Hosp; **Address:** 9200 W Wisconsin Ave, FEC 3963A, Milwauke, WI 53226; **Phone:** 414-805-6800; **Board Cert:** Internal Medicine 1977; Infectious Disease 1982; Medical Oncology 1981; **Med School:** Univ Utah 1974; **Resid:** Internal Medicine, Johns Hopkins Hosp 1977; **Fellow:** Medical Oncology, Natl Cancer Inst/NIH 1979; Infectious Disease, Univ Wash/Fred Hutchinson Cancer Rsch Ctr 1982; **Fac Appt:** Prof Med, Med Coll Wisc

Walsh, T Declan MD [Onc] - **Spec Exp:** Palliative Care; Pain-Cancer; **Hospital:** Cleveland Clin Fdn (page 71); **Address:** 9500 Euclid Ave, MC M76, Cleveland, OH 44195; **Phone:** 216-444-7793; **Board Cert:** Internal Medicine 1986; Medical Oncology 1987; **Med School:** Ireland 1971; **Resid:** Internal Medicine, Bridgeport Hosp; **Fellow:** Medical Oncology, Meml Sloan Kettering Cancer Ctr 1987; St Christophers Hospice

Weiner, George J MD [Onc] - **Spec Exp:** Lymphoma; Leukemia; Immunotherapy; **Hospital:** Univ Iowa Hosp & Clinics; **Address:** Holden Comprehensive Cancer Center, 200 Hawkins Drive Bldg 5970JPP, Iowa City, IA 52242; **Phone:** 319-356-1932; **Board Cert:** Internal Medicine 1985; Hematology 1988; Medical Oncology 1987; **Med School:** Ohio State Univ 1981; **Resid:** Medical Oncology, Med Coll Ohio 1984; **Fellow:** Hematology & Oncology, Univ Mich Med Ctr 1987; **Fac Appt:** Prof Med, Univ Iowa Coll Med

Weissman, David E MD [Onc] - **Spec Exp:** Palliative Care; Pain-Cancer; **Hospital:** Froedtert Meml Lutheran Hosp; **Address:** Med Coll Wisc, Dept Hem/Onc, 9200 W Wisconsin Ave, Milwaukee, WI 53226-3596; **Phone:** 414-805-6633; **Board Cert:** Internal Medicine 1983; Medical Oncology 1985; **Med School:** UCSD 1980; **Resid:** Internal Medicine, UCSD Univ Hosp 1983; **Fellow:** Medical Oncology, Johns Hopkins Hosp 1985; **Fac Appt:** Prof Med, Univ Wisc

Wicha, Max S MD [Onc] - **Spec Exp:** Breast Cancer; Stem Cell Transplant; **Hospital:** Univ Michigan Hlth Sys; **Address:** Comp Cancer Ctr & Geriatrics Ctr, 1500 E Med Ctr Dr, rm 6302 CCGC, Box 0942, Ann Arbor, MI 48109-0942; **Phone:** 734-936-1831; **Board Cert:** Internal Medicine 1977; Medical Oncology 1983; **Med School:** Stanford Univ 1974; **Resid:** Internal Medicine, Univ Chicago Hosp 1977; **Fellow:** Medical Oncology, Natl Inst Hlth 1980; **Fac Appt:** Prof Med, Univ Mich Med Sch

Wilding, George MD [Onc] - **Spec Exp:** Prostate Cancer; Kidney Cancer; Genitourinary Cancer; Drug Discovery & Development; **Hospital:** Univ WI Hosp & Clins; **Address:** UWCCC, Clinical Science Ctr, K4-614, 600 Highland Ave, MC 6164, Madison, WI 53792; **Phone:** 608-263-8610; **Board Cert:** Internal Medicine 1983; Medical Oncology 1985; **Med School:** Univ Mass Sch Med 1980; **Resid:** Internal Medicine, Univ Mass Med Ctr 1983; **Fellow:** Medical Oncology, Natl Cancer Inst 1985

Williams, Stephen D MD [Onc] - **Spec Exp:** Testicular Cancer; Gynecologic Cancer; Genitourinary Cancer; **Hospital:** Indiana Univ Hosp (page 70); **Address:** Indiana University Cancer Ctr, 535 Barnhill Drive, rm 473, Inianapolis, IN 46202; **Phone:** 317-274-0920; **Board Cert:** Internal Medicine 1976; Medical Oncology 1979; **Med School:** Indiana Univ 1971; **Resid:** Internal Medicine, Indiana Univ Hosp 1975; **Fellow:** Medical Oncology, Indiana Univ Hosp 1978; **Fac Appt:** Prof Med, Indiana Univ

Worden, Francis P MD [Onc] - **Spec Exp:** Head & Neck Cancer; Palliative Care; Clinical Trials; **Hospital:** Univ Michigan Hlth Sys; **Address:** Cancer Center & Geriatric Center, 1500 E Medical Center Drive, rm 4214, Ann Arbor, MI 48109; **Phone:** 734-647-8902; **Board Cert:** Internal Medicine 1997; Medical Oncology 2000; **Med School:** Indiana Univ 1993; **Resid:** Internal Medicine & Pediatrics, Detroit Med Ctr 1997; **Fellow:** Medical Oncology, Detroit Med Ctr 1920; **Fac Appt:** Asst Clin Prof Med, Univ Mich Med Sch

Medical Oncology

Yee, Douglas MD [Onc] - **Spec Exp:** Breast Cancer; **Hospital:** Univ Minn Med Ctr, Fairview - Univ Campus; **Address:** Univ Minnesota Cancer Ctr, 420 Delaware St SE, MMC 88, Minneapolis, MN 55455; **Phone:** 612-625-5411; **Board Cert:** Internal Medicine 1984; Medical Oncology 1987; **Med School:** Univ Chicago-Pritzker Sch Med 1981; **Resid:** Internal Medicine, Univ NC Med Ctr; **Fellow:** Medical Oncology, NIH-Clin Ctr; **Fac Appt:** Prof Med, Univ Minn

Great Plains and Mountains

Akerley, Wallace MD [Onc] - **Spec Exp:** Lung Cancer; Clinical Trials; **Hospital:** Univ Utah Hosps and Clins; **Address:** Huntsman Cancer Inst, 2000 Circle of Hope, rm 2165, Salt Lake City, UT 84112; **Phone:** 801-585-0100; **Board Cert:** Internal Medicine 1984; Medical Oncology 1987; Hematology 1988; **Med School:** Brown Univ 1981; **Resid:** Internal Medicine, USC Medical Ctr 1985; **Fellow:** Medical Oncology, USC Medical Ctr 1986; Hematology, Norris Cotton Cancer Ctr/Dartmouth 1988; **Fac Appt:** Prof Med, Univ Utah

Armitage, James MD [Onc] - **Spec Exp:** Lymphoma; Bone Marrow Transplant; **Hospital:** Nebraska Med Ctr; **Address:** 987680 Nebraska Medical Center, Omaha, NE 68198-7680; **Phone:** 402-559-7290; **Board Cert:** Internal Medicine 1976; Medical Oncology 1977; Hematology 1984; **Med School:** Univ Nebr Coll Med 1973; **Resid:** Internal Medicine, Univ Nebraska Med Ctr 1975; **Fellow:** Hematology & Oncology, Univ Iowa Hosp 1977; **Fac Appt:** Prof Med, Univ Nebr Coll Med

Beatty, Patrick G MD [Onc] - **Spec Exp:** Hematologic Malignancies; Lymphoma; **Hospital:** St Patrick Hospital - Missoula; **Address:** PO Box 7877, Missoula, MT 59807; **Phone:** 406-728-2539; **Board Cert:** Internal Medicine 1980; Medical Oncology 1985; **Resid:** Internal Medicine, Vanderbilt Univ Med Ctr 1979; **Fellow:** Oncology, Univ Washington Hosps 1982

Bierman, Philip J MD [Onc] - **Spec Exp:** Lymphoma; Bone Marrow Transplant; **Hospital:** Nebraska Med Ctr; **Address:** Nebraska Medical Ctr, Dept Hem/Oncology, 987680 Nebraska Medical Ctr, Omaha, NE 68198-7680; **Phone:** 402-559-5520; **Board Cert:** Internal Medicine 1982; Hematology 1986; Medical Oncology 1985; **Med School:** Univ MO-Kansas City 1979; **Resid:** Internal Medicine, Univ Nebraska Med Ctr 1983; **Fellow:** Medical Oncology, Univ Nebraska Med Ctr 1985; Hematology, City of Hope Natl Med Ctr 1986; **Fac Appt:** Assoc Prof Med, Univ Nebr Coll Med

Bunn Jr, Paul MD [Onc] - **Spec Exp:** Lung Cancer; Lymphoma; **Hospital:** Univ Colorado Hosp; **Address:** Univ Colorado Cancer Ctr, Box 6510, MS F-704, Aurora, CO 80045-0510; **Phone:** 720-848-0300; **Board Cert:** Internal Medicine 1974; Medical Oncology 1975; **Med School:** Cornell Univ-Weill Med Coll 1971; **Resid:** Internal Medicine, Moffitt Hosp/ UCSF Med Ctr 1973; **Fellow:** Medical Oncology, Natl Cancer Inst 1976; **Fac Appt:** Prof Med, Univ Colorado

Buys, Saundra S MD [Onc] - **Spec Exp:** Breast Cancer; Breast Cancer Risk Assessment; Breast Cancer Genetics; **Hospital:** Univ Utah Hosps and Clins; **Address:** Huntsman Cancer Institute, 2000 Circle of Hope, Ste 210, Salt Lake City, UT 84112; **Phone:** 801-585-3525; **Board Cert:** Internal Medicine 1982; Medical Oncology 1985; Hematology 1984; **Med School:** Tufts Univ 1979; **Resid:** Internal Medicine, Univ of Utah Hosps and Clinics 1982; **Fellow:** Hematology & Oncology, Univ Utah Hosps and Clinics 1985; **Fac Appt:** Prof Med, Univ Utah

Cowan, Kenneth H MD/PhD [Onc] - **Spec Exp:** Breast Cancer; **Hospital:** Nebraska Med Ctr; **Address:** Eppley Cancer Center, 986805 Nebraska Medical Ctr, Omaha, NE 68198-6805; **Phone:** 402-559-4238; **Board Cert:** Internal Medicine 1978; Medical Oncology 1981; **Med School:** Case West Res Univ 1974; **Resid:** Internal Medicine, Parkland Meml Hosp 1977

Dakhil, Shaker MD [Onc] - **Spec Exp:** Leukemia; Mesothelioma; Lymphoma; **Hospital:** Univ of Kansas Hosp; **Address:** Cancer Center Kansas, 818 N Emporia, Ste 403, Wichita, KS 67214; **Phone:** 316-262-4467; **Board Cert:** Internal Medicine 1978; Medical Oncology 1981; **Med School:** Lebanon 1976; **Resid:** Internal Medicine, Wayne State Univ Hosp 1978; **Fellow:** Hematology & Oncology, Univ Michigan Sch Med 1981; **Fac Appt:** Assoc Clin Prof Med, Univ Kans

Ebbert, Larry P MD [Onc] - **Spec Exp:** Breast Cancer; Mesothelioma; **Hospital:** Rapid City Reg Hosp; **Address:** Rapid City Regional Hosp, Dept Med Oncology, 353 Fairmont Blvd, Rapid City, SD 57701; **Phone:** 605-719-2301; **Board Cert:** Internal Medicine 1973; Hematology 1974; Medical Oncology 1975; **Med School:** Ohio State Univ 1969; **Resid:** Internal Medicine, Univ Missouri Med Ctr 1971; **Fellow:** Hematology & Oncology, Duke Univ Med Ctr 1973; **Fac Appt:** Asst Clin Prof Med, Univ SD Sch Med

Eckhardt, S Gail MD [Onc] - **Spec Exp:** Gastrointestinal Cancer; Drug Development; **Hospital:** Univ Colorado Hosp; **Address:** Univ Colorado Hospital, Box 6510, MS F-704, Aurora, CO 80045-0510; **Phone:** 720-848-0300; **Board Cert:** Internal Medicine 1988; Medical Oncology 1993; **Med School:** Univ Tex Med Br, Galveston 1985; **Resid:** Internal Medicine, Univ Virginia Med Ctr 1988; **Fellow:** Research, Scripps Clinic 1989; Medical Oncology, UCSD Med Ctr 1992; **Fac Appt:** Prof Med, Univ Colorado

Fabian, Carol J MD [Onc] - **Spec Exp:** Breast Cancer; Breast Cancer Risk Assessment; **Hospital:** Univ of Kansas Hosp; **Address:** Univ Kansas Med Ctr, Div Clinical Oncology, 3901 Rainbow Blvd, Ste 1347 Bell, Kansas City, KS 66160-7418; **Phone:** 913-588-7791; **Board Cert:** Internal Medicine 1976; Medical Oncology 1977; **Med School:** Univ Kans 1972; **Resid:** Internal Medicine, Wesley Med Ctr 1975; **Fellow:** Medical Oncology, Univ Kansas Med Ctr 1977; **Fac Appt:** Prof Med, Univ Kans

Glode, L Michael MD [Onc] - **Spec Exp:** Prostate Cancer; Genitourinary Cancer; **Hospital:** Univ Colorado Hosp; **Address:** U Colo Hlth Scis Ctr, Div Med Oncology, PO Box 6510, MS F710, Aurora, CO 80045-0510; **Phone:** 720-848-0170; **Board Cert:** Internal Medicine 1975; Medical Oncology 1981; **Med School:** Washington Univ, St Louis 1972; **Resid:** Internal Medicine, Univ Texas SW Med Sch 1973; Immunology, Natl Inst Hlth 1976; **Fellow:** Medical Oncology, Dana Farber Cancer Inst 1978; **Fac Appt:** Prof Med, Univ Colorado

Grem, Jean L MD [Onc] - **Spec Exp:** Colon & Rectal Cancer; Pancreatic Cancer; Stomach Cancer; Esophageal Cancer; **Hospital:** Nebraska Med Ctr; **Address:** 987680 Nebraska Medical Ctr, Omaha, NE 68198-7680; **Phone:** 402-559-6210; **Board Cert:** Internal Medicine 1983; Medical Oncology 1985; **Med School:** Jefferson Med Coll 1980; **Resid:** Internal Medicine, Univ Iowa Hosps & Clinics 1983; **Fellow:** Medical Oncology, Univ Wisc Clin Cancer Ctr 1986; **Fac Appt:** Prof Med, Univ Nebr Coll Med

Hauke, Ralph J MD [Onc] - **Spec Exp:** Urologic Cancer; Vaccine Therapy; Clinical Trials; **Hospital:** Nebraska Med Ctr, VA Medical Ctr - Omaha; **Address:** Peggy D Cowdery Patient Care Ctr, 987835 Nebraska Med Ctr, Omaha, NE 68198-7835; **Phone:** 402-559-6210; **Board Cert:** Internal Medicine 1996; Medical Oncology 2001; **Med School:** Panama 1990; **Resid:** Internal Medicine, Univ Nebraska Coll Med 1996; **Fellow:** Medical Oncology, Univ Nebraska Med Ctr 2001; **Fac Appt:** Assoc Prof Med, Univ Nebr Coll Med

Medical Oncology

Kane, Madeleine A MD/PhD [Onc] - **Spec Exp:** Head & Neck Cancer; Gastrointestinal Cancer; Neuroendocrine Tumors; **Hospital:** Univ Colorado Hosp, VA Med Ctr; **Address:** Univ Colorado Cancer Ctr, 1665 N Ursula St Cancer Bldg, Box 6510, MS F704, Aurora, CO 80045; **Phone:** 720-848-0300; **Board Cert:** Internal Medicine 1981; Medical Oncology 1983; Hematology 1986; **Med School:** Univ Miami Sch Med 1978; **Resid:** Internal Medicine, Stanford Univ Med Ctr 1981; **Fellow:** Hematology & Oncology, Univ Colo Hlth Sci Ctr 1984; **Fac Appt:** Prof Med, Univ Colorado

Kelly, Karen Lee MD [Onc] - **Spec Exp:** Lung Cancer; **Hospital:** Univ of Kansas Hosp; **Address:** Univ Kansas Hospital Cancer Ctr, 3901 Rainbow Blvd, Kansas City, KS 66160; **Phone:** 913-588-4761; **Board Cert:** Internal Medicine 1987; Medical Oncology 2003; **Med School:** Univ Kans 1984; **Resid:** Internal Medicine, Univ Colo Hlth Sci Ctr 1987; **Fellow:** Medical Oncology, Univ Colo Hlth Sci Ctr 1990; **Fac Appt:** Assoc Prof Med, Univ Colorado

Samlowski, Wolfram E MD [Onc] - **Spec Exp:** Kidney Cancer; Melanoma; Immunotherapy; **Hospital:** Univ Utah Hosps and Clins; **Address:** Huntsman Cancer Inst, 2000 Circle of Hope Drive, Ste 2100, Salt Lake City, UT 84112; **Phone:** 801-585-0255; **Board Cert:** Internal Medicine 1981; Medical Oncology 1985; **Med School:** Ohio State Univ 1978; **Resid:** Internal Medicine, Wayne State Univ 1981; **Fellow:** Hematology & Oncology, Univ Utah 1984; **Fac Appt:** Prof Med, Univ Utah

Samuels, Brian L MD [Onc] - **Spec Exp:** Sarcoma; **Hospital:** Kootenai Med Ctr; **Address:** North Idaho Cancer Center, 700 W Ironwood Drive, Ste 103, Coeur D'Alene, ID 83814; **Phone:** 208-666-3800; **Board Cert:** Internal Medicine 1984; Medical Oncology 1987; **Med School:** Zimbabwe 1976; **Resid:** Internal Medicine, Albert Einstein Med Ctr 1981; Internal Medicine, Albert Einstein Med Ctr 1984; **Fellow:** Hematology & Oncology, Univ Chicago Hosps 1988

Tschetter, Loren K MD [Onc] - **Spec Exp:** Lung Cancer; Esophageal Cancer; Unknown Primary Cancer; Clinical Trials; **Hospital:** Sioux Valley Hosp; **Address:** Sioux Valley Cancer Ctr, 1020 W 18th St, Sioux Falls, SD 57104; **Phone:** 605-328-8000; **Board Cert:** Internal Medicine 1972; Hematology 1980; **Med School:** Univ Kans 1968; **Resid:** Internal Medicine, Mayo Clinic 1972; **Fellow:** Hematology, Mayo Clinic 1980; **Fac Appt:** Clin Prof Med, Univ SD Sch Med

Ward, John H MD [Onc] - **Spec Exp:** Breast Cancer; Gastrointestinal Cancer; **Hospital:** Univ Utah Hosps and Clins; **Address:** Huntsman Cancer Inst, 2000 Circle of Hope, Ste 2100, Salt Lake City, UT 84112-5550; **Phone:** 801-585-0255; **Board Cert:** Internal Medicine 1979; Medical Oncology 1981; Hematology 1982; **Med School:** Univ Utah 1976; **Resid:** Internal Medicine, Duke Univ Med Ctr 1979; **Fellow:** Hematology & Oncology, Univ Utah 1982; **Fac Appt:** Prof Med, Univ Utah

Southwest

Abbruzzese, James L MD [Onc] - **Spec Exp:** Gastrointestinal Cancer; Pancreatic Cancer; Clinical Trials; **Hospital:** UT MD Anderson Cancer Ctr (page 81); **Address:** Univ Tex MD Anderson Cancer Ctr, 1515 Holcombe Blvd, Unit 426, Houston, TX 77030; **Phone:** 713-792-2828; **Board Cert:** Internal Medicine 1981; Medical Oncology 1983; **Med School:** Univ Chicago-Pritzker Sch Med 1978; **Resid:** Internal Medicine, Johns Hopkins Hosp 1981; **Fellow:** Medical Oncology, Dana-Farber Cancer Inst 1983; **Fac Appt:** Assoc Prof Med, Univ Tex, Houston

Ahmann, Frederick R MD [Onc] - **Spec Exp:** Prostate Cancer; Testicular Cancer; Bladder Cancer; **Hospital:** Univ Med Ctr - Tucson; **Address:** Arizona Cancer Ctr, 1515 N Campbell Ave, Box 245024, Tucson, AZ 85724; **Phone:** 520-694-2873; **Board Cert:** Internal Medicine 1977; Medical Oncology 1981; **Med School:** Univ MO-Columbia Sch Med 1974; **Resid:** Internal Medicine, Georgetown Univ Med Ctr 1977; **Fellow:** Medical Oncology, Univ Med Ctr 1980; **Fac Appt:** Prof Med, Univ Ariz Coll Med

Ajani, Jaffer A MD [Onc] - **Spec Exp:** Gastrointestinal Cancer; Esophageal Cancer; Stomach Cancer; Neuroendocrine Tumors; **Hospital:** UT MD Anderson Cancer Ctr (page 81); **Address:** Univ Tex MD Anderson Cancer Ctr, Faculty Ctr Unit 426, Box 301402, Houston, TX 77230; **Phone:** 713-792-2828; **Board Cert:** Internal Medicine 1979; Medical Oncology 1983; **Med School:** India 1971; **Resid:** Family Medicine, Penn Stae Univ-Altoona 1977; Internal Medicine, Tulane Univ Sch Med 1980; **Fellow:** Medical Oncology, MD Anderson Cancer Ctr 1983; **Fac Appt:** Prof Med, Univ Tex, Houston

Alberts, David S MD [Onc] - **Spec Exp:** Cancer Prevention; Ovarian Cancer; **Hospital:** Univ Med Ctr - Tucson; **Address:** Arizona Cancer Center, 1515N Campbell Ave, PO Box 245024, Tucson, AZ 85724; **Phone:** 520-626-7685; **Board Cert:** Internal Medicine 1973; Medical Oncology 1973; **Med School:** Univ VA Sch Med 1966; **Resid:** Medical Oncology, Natl Cancer Inst-NIH 1969; Internal Medicine, Univ Minn Hosps 1971; **Fellow:** Clinical Pharmacology, UC San Francisco 1974; **Fac Appt:** Prof Med, Univ Ariz Coll Med

Anthony, Lowell B MD [Onc] - **Spec Exp:** Gastrointestinal Cancer; Carcinoid Tumors; Neuroendocrine Tumors; **Hospital:** Med Ctr LA @ New Orleans (Univ Hosp); **Address:** 3600 Prytania St, Ste 35, New Orleans, LA 70115; **Phone:** 504-895-5748; **Board Cert:** Internal Medicine 1983; Medical Oncology 1989; **Med School:** Vanderbilt Univ 1979; **Resid:** Internal Medicine, Vanderbilt Univ Med Ctr 1982; **Fellow:** Medical Oncology, Vanderbilt Univ Med Ctr 1985; **Fac Appt:** Assoc Prof Med, Louisiana State Univ

Arun, Banu K MD [Onc] - **Spec Exp:** Breast Cancer; Cancer Prevention; Clinical Trials; **Hospital:** UT MD Anderson Cancer Ctr (page 81); **Address:** 1155 Pressler, Unit 1354, Houston, TX 77030; **Phone:** 713-792-2817; **Med School:** Turkey 1990; **Resid:** Internal Medicine, Univ Istanbul 1994; **Fellow:** Hematology & Oncology, Lombardi Cancer Ctr-Georgetown Univ 1997; **Fac Appt:** Assoc Prof Med, Univ Tex, Houston

Benjamin, Robert S MD [Onc] - **Spec Exp:** Sarcoma; **Hospital:** UT MD Anderson Cancer Ctr (page 81); **Address:** UT MD Anderson Cancer Ctr, 1515 Holcombe Blvd, Unit 450, Houston, TX 77030; **Phone:** 713-792-3626; **Board Cert:** Internal Medicine 1973; Medical Oncology 1973; **Med School:** NYU Sch Med 1968; **Resid:** Internal Medicine, Bellevue Hosp Ctr-NYU 1970; **Fellow:** Medical Oncology, Baltimore Cancer Rsch Ctr 1972; **Fac Appt:** Prof Med, Univ Tex, Houston

Bruera, Eduardo MD [Onc] - **Spec Exp:** Palliative Care; **Hospital:** UT MD Anderson Cancer Ctr (page 81); **Address:** 1515 Holcombe Ave, Unit 8, Houston, TX 77030; **Phone:** 713-792-6085; **Med School:** Argentina ; **Resid:** Internal Medicine, Hospital Privado; **Fellow:** Medical Oncology, Cross Cancer Inst; **Fac Appt:** Prof Med, Univ Tex, Houston

Buzdar, Aman U MD [Onc] - **Spec Exp:** Breast Cancer; **Hospital:** UT MD Anderson Cancer Ctr (page 81); **Address:** UT MD Anderson Canc Ctr, 1155 Pressler St, Unit 1354, Houston, TX 77030-4009; **Phone:** 713-792-2817; **Board Cert:** Internal Medicine 1975; Medical Oncology 1979; **Med School:** Pakistan 1967; **Resid:** Internal Medicine, Norwalk Hosp 1973; Internal Medicine, Lakewood Hosp 1971; **Fellow:** Hematology, Norwalk Hosp 1974; Oncology, MD Anderson Cancer Ctr 1975; **Fac Appt:** Prof Med, Univ Tex, Houston

Medical Oncology

Camoriano, John MD [Onc] - **Spec Exp:** Lymphoma; Breast Cancer; Bone Marrow Transplant; Myeloproliferative Disorders; **Hospital:** Mayo Clin Hosp - Scottsdale; **Address:** 13400 E Shea, Scottsdale, AZ 85259; **Phone:** 480-301-8335; **Board Cert:** Internal Medicine 1985; Medical Oncology 1989; Hematology 1988; **Med School:** Univ Nebr Coll Med 1982; **Resid:** Internal Medicine, Univ OK 1985; **Fellow:** Hematology & Oncology, Mayo Grad Sch Med 1989; **Fac Appt:** Asst Prof Med, Mayo Med Sch

Chang, Jenny C N MD [Onc] - **Spec Exp:** Breast Cancer; Clinical Trials; **Hospital:** Methodist Hosp - Houston; **Address:** One Baylor Plaza, MS BCM600, Houston, TX 77030; **Phone:** 713-798-1609; **Med School:** England 1989; **Resid:** Internal Medicine 1993; **Fellow:** Medical Oncology, Royal Marsden Hosp 1997; **Fac Appt:** Assoc Prof Med, Baylor Coll Med

Estey, Elihu MD [Onc] - **Spec Exp:** Leukemia; Myelodysplastic Syndromes; Clinical Trials; **Hospital:** UT MD Anderson Cancer Ctr (page 81); **Address:** 1515 Holcolmbe Blvd, Box 61, Houston, TX 77030; **Phone:** 713-792-7544; **Board Cert:** Internal Medicine 1975; Medical Oncology 1981; **Med School:** Johns Hopkins Univ 1972; **Resid:** Internal Medicine, Bellevue Hosp Ctr 1975; **Fellow:** Medical Oncology, MD Anderson Cancer Ctr 1978

Fay, Joseph W MD [Onc] - **Spec Exp:** Bone Marrow Transplant; Melanoma; Leukemia & Lymphoma; **Hospital:** Baylor Univ Medical Ctr; **Address:** 3409 Worth St, Sammons Tower, Suite 600, Dallas, TX 75246; **Phone:** 214-370-1500; **Board Cert:** Internal Medicine 1975; Medical Oncology 1977; Hematology 1978; **Med School:** Ohio State Univ 1972; **Resid:** Internal Medicine, Duke Med Ctr 1974; Oncology, Natl Cancer Institute 1976; **Fellow:** Hematology, Duke Med Ctr 1977; **Fac Appt:** Clin Prof Med, Univ Tex SW, Dallas

Fitch, Tom R MD [Onc] - **Spec Exp:** Breast Cancer; Sarcoma; Cancer Prevention; Palliative Care; **Hospital:** Mayo Clin Hosp - Scottsdale; **Address:** Mayo Clinic - Scottsdale, 13400 E Shea Blvd, Scottsdale, AZ 85259; **Phone:** 480-301-8335; **Board Cert:** Internal Medicine 1985; Hematology 1988; Medical Oncology 1987; **Med School:** Univ Kans 1982; **Resid:** Internal Medicine, Univ Michigan Med Ctr 1985; **Fellow:** Hematology & Oncology, Mayo Clinic 1988; **Fac Appt:** Asst Prof Med, Mayo Med Sch

Fossella, Frank V MD [Onc] - **Spec Exp:** Lung Cancer; **Hospital:** UT MD Anderson Cancer Ctr (page 81); **Address:** Dept Thoracic Head/Neck Med Oncol, Unit 432, Box 301402, Houston, TX 77230-1402; **Phone:** 713-792-6363; **Board Cert:** Internal Medicine 1985; Medical Oncology 1987; **Med School:** Baylor Coll Med 1982; **Resid:** Internal Medicine, Baylor Coll Med 1985; **Fellow:** Medical Oncology, Baylor Coll Med 1987; **Fac Appt:** Prof Med, Univ Tex, Houston

Glisson, Bonnie S MD [Onc] - **Spec Exp:** Head & Neck Cancer; Lung Cancer; **Hospital:** UT MD Anderson Cancer Ctr (page 81); **Address:** 1515 Holcombe Blvd, Unit 432, Houston, TX 77030; **Phone:** 713-792-6363; **Board Cert:** Internal Medicine 1982; Medical Oncology 1985; **Med School:** Ohio State Univ 1979; **Resid:** Internal Medicine, Univ Va Med Ctr 1982; **Fellow:** Medical Oncology, Univ Fla Health Sci Ctr 1985; **Fac Appt:** Prof Med, Univ Tex, Houston

Haley, Barbara MD [Onc] - **Spec Exp:** Breast Cancer; **Hospital:** UT Southwestern Med Ctr - Dallas; **Address:** UTSW Med Ctr, 5323 Harry Hines Blvd, Dallas, TX 75390-8852; **Phone:** 214-648-4180; **Board Cert:** Internal Medicine 1979; Hematology 1984; **Med School:** Univ Tex SW, Dallas 1976; **Resid:** Internal Medicine, Parkland Meml Hosp 1979; **Fellow:** Hematology & Oncology, Parkland Meml Hosp 1981; **Fac Appt:** Prof Med, Univ Tex SW, Dallas

Herbst, Roy S MD/PhD [Onc] - Spec Exp: Lung Cancer; Head & Neck Cancer; Breast Cancer; Drug Development; **Hospital:** UT MD Anderson Cancer Ctr (page 81); **Address:** Thoracic/Head & Neck Med Onc - Unit 432, UT MD Anderson Cancer Ctr, PO Box 301402, Houston, TX 77230-1402; **Phone:** 713-792-6363; **Board Cert:** Internal Medicine 1994; Medical Oncology 1997; **Med School:** Cornell Univ-Weill Med Coll 1991; **Resid:** Internal Medicine, Brigham & Women's Hosp 1994; **Fellow:** Medical Oncology, Dana Farber Cancer Inst 1996; **Fac Appt:** Assoc Prof Med, Univ Tex, Houston

Hong, Waun Ki MD [Onc] - Spec Exp: Lung Cancer; Head & Neck Cancer; Thoracic Cancers; **Hospital:** UT MD Anderson Cancer Ctr (page 81); **Address:** 1515 Holcombe Blvd, Unit 421, Houston, TX 77030; **Phone:** 713-745-6791; **Board Cert:** Internal Medicine 1976; Medical Oncology 1979; **Med School:** South Korea 1967; **Resid:** Internal Medicine, Boston VA Hosp 1973; **Fellow:** Medical Oncology, Meml Sloan-Kettering Cancer Ctr 1975; **Fac Appt:** Prof Med, Univ Tex, Houston

Hortobagyi, Gabriel N MD [Onc] - Spec Exp: Breast Cancer; **Hospital:** UT MD Anderson Cancer Ctr (page 81); **Address:** UT MD Anderson Cancer Ctr, Dept Breast Oncology, PO Box 301429, Unit 1354, Houston, TX 77030-1439; **Phone:** 713-792-2817; **Board Cert:** Internal Medicine 1975; Medical Oncology 1977; **Med School:** Colombia 1970; **Resid:** Internal Medicine, St Lukes Hosp 1974; **Fellow:** Medical Oncology, MD Anderson Cancer Ctr 1976; **Fac Appt:** Prof Med, Univ Tex, Houston

Hutchins, Laura MD [Onc] - Spec Exp: Breast Cancer; Melanoma; **Hospital:** UAMS Med Ctr; **Address:** Univ Arkansas Med Scis, Dept Hem/Onc, 4301 W Markham St, MS 508, Little Rock, AR 72205-7101; **Phone:** 501-686-8511; **Board Cert:** Internal Medicine 1980; Hematology 1984; Medical Oncology 1987; **Med School:** Univ Ark 1977; **Resid:** Internal Medicine, Univ Ark Med Scis 1980; **Fellow:** Hematology & Oncology, Univ Ark Med Scis 1983; **Fac Appt:** Prof Med, Univ Ark

Jones, Stephen E MD [Onc] - Spec Exp: Breast Cancer; **Hospital:** Baylor Univ Medical Ctr; **Address:** Baylor-Sammons Cancer Ctr, 3535 Worth St, Ste 600, Dallas, TX 75246; **Phone:** 214-370-1000; **Board Cert:** Internal Medicine 1972; Medical Oncology 1973; **Med School:** Case West Res Univ 1966; **Resid:** Internal Medicine, Stanford Univ Hosp 1968; **Fellow:** Medical Oncology, Stanford Univ Hosp 1972; **Fac Appt:** Prof Med, Baylor Coll Med

Karp, Daniel D MD [Onc] - Spec Exp: Lung Cancer; **Hospital:** UT MD Anderson Cancer Ctr (page 81); **Address:** 1515 Holcombe Blvd, Unit 432, Houston, TX 77030-4009; **Phone:** 713-792-6363; **Board Cert:** Internal Medicine 1976; Hematology 1980; Medical Oncology 1981; **Med School:** Duke Univ 1973; **Resid:** Internal Medicine, Dartmouth-Hitchcock Med Ctr 1976; **Fellow:** Hematology, Dartmouth-Hitchcock Med Ctr 1978; Medical Oncology, Dana Farber Cancer Inst 1979; **Fac Appt:** Prof Med, Univ Tex, Houston

Kies, Merrill S MD [Onc] - Spec Exp: Head & Neck Cancer; Lung Cancer; **Hospital:** UT MD Anderson Cancer Ctr (page 81); **Address:** Dept Thoracic, Head & Neck Oncology, 1515 Holcombe Blvd, Unit 432, Houston, TX 77030; **Phone:** 713-792-6363; **Board Cert:** Internal Medicine 1976; Medical Oncology 1979; **Med School:** Loyola Univ-Stritch Sch Med 1973; **Resid:** Internal Medicine, Walter Reed AMC 1976; **Fellow:** Medical Oncology, Brooke AMC 1978; **Fac Appt:** Prof Med, Univ Tex, Houston

Medical Oncology

Kwak, Larry W MD/PhD [Onc] - **Spec Exp:** Lymphoma; Multiple Myeloma; Vaccine Therapy; Immunotherapy; **Hospital:** UT MD Anderson Cancer Ctr (page 81); **Address:** MD Anderson Cancer Ctr, Dept Lymphoma/Myeloma, 1515 Holcombe Blvd, Ste 429, Houston, TX 77030; **Phone:** 713-745-4244; **Board Cert:** Internal Medicine 1987; Medical Oncology 1989; **Med School:** Northwestern Univ 1982; **Resid:** Internal Medicine, Stanford Univ Hosp 1987; **Fellow:** Oncology, Stanford Univ Hosp 1989

Legha, Sewa Singh MD [Onc] - **Spec Exp:** Melanoma; Breast Cancer; Endocrine Cancers; Sarcoma; **Hospital:** St Luke's Episcopal Hosp - Houston, Methodist Hosp - Houston; **Address:** 6624 Fannin, Ste 1440, Houston, TX 77030; **Phone:** 713-797-9711; **Board Cert:** Internal Medicine 1987; Medical Oncology 1977; **Med School:** India 1970; **Resid:** Internal Medicine, Milwaukee Co Genl Hosp/Med Coll Wisc 1974; Medical Oncology, Natl Cancer Inst 1976; **Fellow:** Medical Oncology, MD Anderson Hosp 1977; **Fac Appt:** Clin Prof Med, Baylor Coll Med

Lippman, Scott M MD [Onc] - **Spec Exp:** Cancer Prevention; Lung Cancer; Head & Neck Cancer; **Hospital:** UT MD Anderson Cancer Ctr (page 81); **Address:** UTMD Anderson Cancer Ctr, Unit 432, 1515 Holcombe Blvd, P.O.Box 301439, Houston, TX 77230-1439; **Phone:** 713-745-5439; **Board Cert:** Internal Medicine 1987; Hematology 1988; Medical Oncology 1989; **Med School:** Johns Hopkins Univ 1981; **Resid:** Internal Medicine, Harbor-UCLA Med Ctr 1983; **Fellow:** Hematology, Stanford Univ Med Ctr 1985; Hematology & Oncology, Univ Ariz Hlth Scis Ctr 1987; **Fac Appt:** Prof Med, Univ Tex, Houston

Livingston, Robert B MD [Onc] - **Spec Exp:** Bone Marrow Transplant; Breast Cancer; Lung Cancer; **Hospital:** Univ Med Ctr - Tucson; **Address:** University Medical Center, 3838 N Campbell Ave, Tucson, AZ 85724; **Phone:** 520-694-2873; **Board Cert:** Internal Medicine 1972; Medical Oncology 1973; **Med School:** Univ Okla Coll Med 1965; **Resid:** Internal Medicine, Univ Oklahoma Med Ctr 1971; **Fellow:** Medical Oncology, Univ Texas Cancer Ctr 1973; **Fac Appt:** Prof Med, Univ Wash

Logothetis, Christopher J MD [Onc] - **Spec Exp:** Prostate Cancer; Bladder Cancer; **Hospital:** UT MD Anderson Cancer Ctr (page 81); **Address:** UT MD Anderson Cancer Ctr, Dept GU Onc, Unit 1374, Box 301439, Houston, TX 77230-1439; **Phone:** 713-792-2830; **Board Cert:** Internal Medicine 1978; Medical Oncology 1981; **Med School:** Greece 1974; **Resid:** Internal Medicine, Univ Texas 1979; **Fellow:** Hematology & Oncology, Univ Tex-MD Anderson Cancer Ctr 1981; **Fac Appt:** Prof Med, Univ Tex, Houston

Markman, Maurie MD [Onc] - **Spec Exp:** Ovarian Cancer; Gynecologic Cancer; Drug Development; Palliative Care; **Hospital:** UT MD Anderson Cancer Ctr (page 81); **Address:** Univ Texas MD Anderson Cancer Ctr, 1515 Holcombe Blvd, Box 121, Houston, TX 77030-4009; **Phone:** 713-745-7140; **Board Cert:** Internal Medicine 1977; Hematology 1982; Medical Oncology 1981; **Med School:** NYU Sch Med 1974; **Resid:** Internal Medicine, Bellevue Hosp Ctr 1978; **Fellow:** Medical Oncology, Johns Hopkins Hosp 1980; **Fac Appt:** Prof Med, Univ Tex, Houston

Miller, Thomas P MD [Onc] - **Spec Exp:** Lymphoma; **Hospital:** Univ Med Ctr - Tucson; **Address:** Arizona Cancer Ctr, 1515 N Campbell Ave, PO Box 245024, Tucson, AZ 85724; **Phone:** 520-626-2667; **Board Cert:** Internal Medicine 1977; Medical Oncology 1981; **Med School:** Univ IL Coll Med 1972; **Resid:** Internal Medicine, Univ Illinois Hosps 1977; **Fellow:** Hematology & Oncology, Univ Med Ctr 1980; **Fac Appt:** Prof Med, Univ Ariz Coll Med

Millikan, Randall MD/PhD [Onc] - **Spec Exp:** Bladder Cancer; Genitourinary Cancer; Clinical Trials; **Hospital:** UT MD Anderson Cancer Ctr (page 81); **Address:** 1155 Pressler Ln, Box 1374, Bellaire, TX 77030; **Phone:** 713-792-2830; **Board Cert:** Internal Medicine 1991; Medical Oncology 1995; **Med School:** Univ Miami Sch Med 1988; **Resid:** Internal Medicine, Mayo Clinic 1991; **Fellow:** Medical Oncology, Mayo Clinic 1994; **Fac Appt:** Assoc Prof Med, Univ Tex, Houston

Nemunaitis, John G MD [Onc] - **Spec Exp:** Cancer Genetics; Vaccine Therapy; Lung Cancer; **Hospital:** Baylor Univ Medical Ctr; **Address:** Mary Crowley Med Rsch Ctr, 3535 Worth St, Ste 302, Dallas, TX 75246; **Phone:** 214-370-1870; **Board Cert:** Internal Medicine 1987; **Med School:** Case West Res Univ 1982; **Resid:** Internal Medicine, Boston City Hosp 1985; **Fellow:** Hematology & Oncology, Fred Hutchinson Cancer Rsch Ctr 1989

Northfelt, Donald W MD [Onc] - **Spec Exp:** Breast Cancer; Colon & Rectal Cancer; Lung Cancer; **Hospital:** Mayo Clin Hosp - Scottsdale; **Address:** Mayo Clinic Scottsdale, 13400 E Shea Blvd, Scottsdale, AZ 85259; **Phone:** 480-301-8335; **Board Cert:** Internal Medicine 1988; Medical Oncology 2001; **Med School:** Univ Minn 1985; **Resid:** Internal Medicine, UCLA Med Ctr 1988; **Fellow:** Hematology & Oncology, UCSF 1991; **Fac Appt:** Assoc Prof Med, Mayo Med Sch

O'Brien, Susan M MD [Onc] - **Spec Exp:** Leukemia; Lymphoma; **Hospital:** UT MD Anderson Cancer Ctr (page 81); **Address:** Univ Texas MD Anderson Cancer Ctr, Dept Leukemia, Unit 428, Box 301439, Houston, TX 77230; **Phone:** 713-792-7305; **Board Cert:** Internal Medicine 1983; Medical Oncology 1987; **Med School:** UMDNJ-NJ Med Sch, Newark 1980; **Resid:** Internal Medicine, UMDNJ Med Ctr 1983; **Fellow:** Medical Oncology, Univ TX MD Anderson Med Ctr 1987; **Fac Appt:** Prof Med, Univ Tex, Houston

O'Shaughnessy, Joyce A MD [Onc] - **Spec Exp:** Breast Cancer; **Hospital:** Baylor Univ Medical Ctr; **Address:** US Oncology, 3535 Worth St, Ste 600, Dallas, TX 75246; **Phone:** 214-370-1000; **Board Cert:** Internal Medicine 1985; Medical Oncology 1987; **Med School:** Yale Univ 1982; **Resid:** Internal Medicine, Mass Genl Hosp 1985; **Fellow:** Medical Oncology, National Cancer Inst 1988

Osborne, Charles K MD [Onc] - **Spec Exp:** Breast Cancer; **Hospital:** Methodist Hosp - Houston; **Address:** 1 Baylor Plaza, MS BCM600, Houston, TX 77030; **Phone:** 713-798-1641; **Board Cert:** Internal Medicine 1975; Medical Oncology 1977; **Med School:** Univ MO-Columbia Sch Med 1972; **Resid:** Internal Medicine, Johns Hopkins Hosp 1974; **Fellow:** Medical Oncology, Natl Cancer Inst 1977; **Fac Appt:** Prof Med, Baylor Coll Med

Papadopoulos, Nicholas E MD [Onc] - **Spec Exp:** Melanoma; **Hospital:** UT MD Anderson Cancer Ctr (page 81); **Address:** 1515 Holcombe Blvd, Unit 430, Houston, TX 77030; **Phone:** 713-792-2821; **Med School:** Greece 1966; **Resid:** Internal Medicine, Baylor Coll Med 1976; **Fellow:** Medical Oncology, MD Anderson Cancer Ctr 1978; **Fac Appt:** Assoc Prof Med, Univ Tex, Houston

Patt, Yehuda Z MD [Onc] - **Spec Exp:** Liver Cancer; Biliary Cancer; Colon & Rectal Cancer; **Hospital:** Univ NM Hlth & Sci Ctr; **Address:** Univ New Mexico CRTC, Div Hem/Onc, 900 Camino de Salud NE, MSC 084630, Albuquerque, NM 87131-0001; **Phone:** 505-272-5837; **Board Cert:** Internal Medicine 1982; Medical Oncology 1987; **Med School:** Israel 1967; **Resid:** Internal Medicine, Tel Aviv-Sheba Med Ctr 1974; **Fellow:** Medical Oncology, UT MD Anderson Cancer Ctr 1977; **Fac Appt:** Prof Med, Univ New Mexico

Pisters, Katherine M W MD [Onc] - **Spec Exp:** Lung Cancer; **Hospital:** UT MD Anderson Cancer Ctr (page 81); **Address:** UT MD Anderson Cancer Ctr, PO Box 301402 Unit 432, Houston, TX 77030-1402; **Phone:** 713-792-6363; **Board Cert:** Internal Medicine 1988; Medical Oncology 2002; **Med School:** Univ Western Ontario 1985; **Resid:** Internal Medicine, N Shore Univ Hosp 1988; **Fellow:** Medical Oncology, Meml Sloan Kettering Cancer Ctr 1991; **Fac Appt:** Prof Med, Univ Tex, Houston

Saiki, John H MD [Onc] - **Hospital:** Univ NM Hlth & Sci Ctr; **Address:** Univ of New Mexico Cancer Ctr, 900 Camino de Salud NE, MSC 084630, Albuquerque, NM 87131-0001; **Phone:** 505-272-5837; **Board Cert:** Internal Medicine 1970; Medical Oncology 1973; **Med School:** McGill Univ 1961; **Resid:** Internal Medicine, Univ New Mexico 1968; Hematology, Univ New Mexico 1969; **Fellow:** Medical Oncology, MD Anderson Hosp 1970; **Fac Appt:** Prof Med, Univ New Mexico

Salem, Philip A MD [Onc] - **Spec Exp:** Breast Cancer; Lymphoma; Lung Cancer; **Hospital:** St Luke's Episcopal Hosp - Houston; **Address:** 6624 Fannin St, Ste 1630, Houston, TX 77030; **Phone:** 713-796-1221; **Med School:** Lebanon 1965; **Resid:** Medical Oncology, Meml Sloan Kettering Cancer Ctr 1970; **Fellow:** Oncology Research, MD Anderson Cancer Ctr 1972; **Fac Appt:** Clin Prof Med, Univ Tex, Houston

Schiller, Joan H MD [Onc] - **Spec Exp:** Lung Cancer; **Hospital:** UT Southwestern Med Ctr - Dallas; **Address:** Univ Texas SW, 5323 Harry Hines Blvd, Dallas, TX 75390-8852; **Phone:** 214-648-4180; **Board Cert:** Internal Medicine 1983; Medical Oncology 1987; **Med School:** Univ IL Coll Med 1980; **Resid:** Internal Medicine, Northwestern Meml Hosp 1983; **Fellow:** Medical Oncology, Univ Wisconsin Hosp 1986; **Fac Appt:** Prof Med, Univ Wisc

Stopeck, Alison MD [Onc] - **Spec Exp:** Breast Cancer; Breast Cancer Risk Assessment; **Hospital:** Univ Med Ctr - Tucson; **Address:** 1515 N Campbell Ave, P.O. Box 245024, Tucson, AZ 85724; **Phone:** 520-694-2816; **Board Cert:** Internal Medicine 1988; Medical Oncology 2002; Hematology 2002; **Med School:** Columbia P&S 1985; **Resid:** Internal Medicine, Columbia-Presbyterian Med Ctr 1988; **Fellow:** Hematology & Oncology, New York Hospital 1991; **Fac Appt:** Assoc Prof Med, Univ Ariz Coll Med

Takimoto, Chris Hidemi M MD/PhD [Onc] - **Spec Exp:** Gastrointestinal Cancer; **Hospital:** Univ Hlth Sys - Univ Hosp; **Address:** Inst for Drug Dvlpmt-Cancer Rsch Ctr, 7979 Wurzbach Rd Zeller Bldg Fl 4, San Antonio, TX 78229; **Phone:** 210-562-1725; **Board Cert:** Internal Medicine 1989; Medical Oncology 2005; **Med School:** Yale Univ 1986; **Resid:** Internal Medicine, UCSF Med Ctr 1989; **Fac Appt:** Assoc Prof Med, Univ Tex, San Antonio

Tripathy, Debasish MD [Onc] - **Spec Exp:** Breast Cancer; Clinical Trials; **Hospital:** UT Southwestern Med Ctr - Dallas; **Address:** Univ Texas SW Med Ctr, 5323 Harry Hines Blvd, Dallas, TX 75390-8852; **Phone:** 214-648-4180; **Board Cert:** Internal Medicine 1988; Medical Oncology 2001; **Med School:** Duke Univ 1985; **Resid:** Internal Medicine, Duke Univ Med Ctr 1988; **Fellow:** Hematology & Oncology, USCF Med Ctr 1991; **Fac Appt:** Prof Med, Univ Tex SW, Dallas

Valero, Vicente MD [Onc] - **Spec Exp:** Breast Cancer; **Hospital:** UT MD Anderson Cancer Ctr (page 81), LBJ General Hosp; **Address:** Univ Texas MD Anderson Cancer Ctr, 1515 Holcombe Blvd, Unit 1354, Houston, TX 77030; **Phone:** 713-792-2817; **Board Cert:** Internal Medicine 1985; Hematology 1988; Medical Oncology 1987; **Med School:** Mexico 1980; **Resid:** Internal Medicine, Univ Cincinnati Med Ctr 1985; Hematology & Oncology, Univ Cincinnati Med Ctr 1987; **Fellow:** Hematology & Oncology, Univ Texas Med Br 1988; **Fac Appt:** Prof Med, Univ Tex, Houston

Verschraegen, Claire F MD [Onc] - **Spec Exp:** Ovarian Cancer; Drug Discovery; Mesothelioma; **Hospital:** Univ NM Hlth & Sci Ctr; **Address:** UNM Cancer Research & Treatment Ctr, 900 Camino de Salud NE, rm MS C084630, Albuquerque, NM 87131-0001; **Phone:** 505-272-6760; **Board Cert:** Internal Medicine 2000; Medical Oncology 2000; **Med School:** Belgium 1982; **Resid:** Internal Medicine, Bordet 1985; Internal Medicine, Univ Texas 1991; **Fellow:** Cancer Research, Stehlin Fdn for Cancer Research 1988; Oncology, MD Anderson Cancer Ctr 1994; **Fac Appt:** Prof Med, Univ New Mexico

Von Hoff, Daniel D MD [Onc] - **Spec Exp:** Pancreatic Cancer; Breast Cancer; Drug Discovery; **Hospital:** Scottsdale Hlthcare - Shea; **Address:** Translational Genomics Research Institute, 445 N 5th St, Ste 600, Phoenix, AZ 85004; **Phone:** 602-343-8492; **Board Cert:** Internal Medicine 1976; Medical Oncology 1979; **Med School:** Columbia P&S 1973; **Resid:** Internal Medicine, UCSF Med Ctr 1975; **Fac Appt:** Prof Med, Univ Ariz Coll Med

Willson, James KV MD [Onc] - **Spec Exp:** Gastrointestinal Cancer; Colon Cancer; Pancreatic Cancer; **Hospital:** UT Southwestern Med Ctr - Dallas; **Address:** UTSW Med Ctr, NB2.308, 5323 Harry Hines Blvd, Dallas, TX 75390-8590; **Phone:** 214-648-7070; **Board Cert:** Internal Medicine 1980; Medical Oncology 1981; **Med School:** Univ Ala 1976; **Resid:** Internal Medicine, Johns Hopkins Hosp 1978; **Fellow:** Medical Oncology, Natl Cancer Inst-NIH 1980; **Fac Appt:** Prof Med, Univ Tex SW, Dallas

West Coast and Pacific

Abrams, Donald I MD [Onc] - **Spec Exp:** AIDS Related Cancers; **Hospital:** San Francisco Genl Hosp; **Address:** Positive Hlth Program-SF Genl Hosp, 995 Potrero Ave, Bldg 80, Ward 84, San Francisco, CA 94110; **Phone:** 415-476-4082 x444; **Board Cert:** Internal Medicine 1980; Medical Oncology 1983; **Med School:** Stanford Univ 1977; **Resid:** Internal Medicine, Kaiser Fdn Hosp 1980; **Fellow:** Medical Oncology, UCSF Cancer Rsch 1982; **Fac Appt:** Clin Prof Med, UCSF

Appelbaum, Frederick R MD [Onc] - **Spec Exp:** Bone Marrow Transplant; Leukemia; **Hospital:** Univ Wash Med Ctr; **Address:** 1100 Fairview Ave N, rm D5-310, PO Box 19024, Seattle, WA 98109; **Phone:** 206-288-1024; **Board Cert:** Internal Medicine 1975; Medical Oncology 1977; **Med School:** Tufts Univ 1972; **Resid:** Internal Medicine, Univ Michigan Med Ctr 1974; **Fellow:** Medical Oncology, Natl Cancer Inst 1976; **Fac Appt:** Prof Med, Univ Wash

Ball, Edward D MD [Onc] - **Spec Exp:** Bone Marrow & Stem Cell Transplant; Leukemia & Lymphoma; Multiple Myeloma; **Hospital:** UCSD Med Ctr; **Address:** 3855 Health Sciences Dr, #0960, La Jolla, CA 92093; **Phone:** 858-822-6600; **Board Cert:** Internal Medicine 1979; Medical Oncology 1983; Hematology 2000; **Med School:** Case West Res Univ 1976; **Resid:** Internal Medicine, Hartford Hosp 1979; **Fellow:** Hematology & Oncology, Univ Hosps Cleveland 1981; Hematology & Oncology, Dartmouth-Hitchcock Hosp 1982; **Fac Appt:** Prof Med, UCSD

Beer, Tomasz MD [Onc] - **Spec Exp:** Prostate Cancer; **Hospital:** OR Hlth & Sci Univ; **Address:** 3303 SW Bond Ave, CH7M, Portland, OR 97239; **Phone:** 503-494-6594; **Board Cert:** Internal Medicine 1995; Medical Oncology 2000; **Med School:** Johns Hopkins Univ 1991; **Resid:** Internal Medicine, Oreg Hlth Scis Univ 1994; Internal Medicine, Oreg Hlth Scis Univ 1996; **Fellow:** Hematology & Oncology, Oreg Hlth Scis Univ 1999; **Fac Appt:** Assoc Prof Med, Oregon Hlth Sci Univ

Bensinger, William I MD [Onc] - Spec Exp: Multiple Myeloma; Stem Cell Transplant; **Hospital:** Univ Wash Med Ctr; **Address:** Fred Hutchinson Cancer Research Ctr, 825 Eastlake Ave E, MS E5-390, Seattle, WA 98109-1024; **Phone:** 206-288-1024; **Board Cert:** Internal Medicine 1978; Medical Oncology 1979; **Med School:** Northwestern Univ 1973; **Resid:** Internal Medicine, Univ Wash Hosps 1978; **Fellow:** Medical Oncology, Univ Wash Hosps 1979; **Fac Appt:** Assoc Prof Med, Univ Wash

Blanke, Charles D MD [Onc] - Spec Exp: Colon & Rectal Cancer; Gastrointestinal Cancer; **Hospital:** OR Hlth & Sci Univ; **Address:** Oregon Health Science Ctr, 3303 SW Bond Ave, MC PV240, Portland, OR 97239; **Phone:** 503-494-8469; **Board Cert:** Internal Medicine 1991; Medical Oncology 1995; **Med School:** Northwestern Univ 1988; **Resid:** Internal Medicine, LaCrosse Lutheran Hosp 1991; **Fellow:** Medical Oncology, Clarian-Indiana Univ 1994; **Fac Appt:** Assoc Prof Med, Oregon Hlth Sci Univ

Carlson, Robert Wells MD [Onc] - Spec Exp: Breast Cancer; **Hospital:** Stanford Univ Med Ctr; **Address:** Dept Medicine, 875 Blake Wilbur Drive, Stanford, CA 94305; **Phone:** 650-723-7621; **Board Cert:** Internal Medicine 1981; Medical Oncology 1983; **Med School:** Stanford Univ 1978; **Resid:** Internal Medicine, Barnes Hosp Group 1980; Internal Medicine, Stanford Univ Hosp 1981; **Fellow:** Medical Oncology, Stanford Univ Hosp 1983; **Fac Appt:** Prof Med, Stanford Univ

Chap, Linnea MD [Onc] - Spec Exp: Breast Cancer; **Hospital:** St John's Regional Med Ctr, Santa Monica - UCLA Med Ctr; **Address:** Premier Oncology, 2020 Santa Monica Blvd, Ste 510, Santa Monica, CA 90404-2023; **Phone:** 310-633-8400; **Board Cert:** Internal Medicine 1991; Hematology 1994; Medical Oncology 1995; **Med School:** Univ Chicago-Pritzker Sch Med 1988; **Resid:** Internal Medicine, Northwestern Meml Hosp 1991; **Fellow:** Hematology & Oncology, UCLA Med Ctr 1992

Chlebowski, Rowan T MD/PhD [Onc] - Spec Exp: Breast Cancer; **Hospital:** LAC - Harbor - UCLA Med Ctr; **Address:** 1124 W Carson St J3 Bldg, Torrance, CA 90502; **Phone:** 310-222-2218; **Board Cert:** Internal Medicine 1980; Medical Oncology 1981; **Med School:** Case West Res Univ 1974; **Resid:** Internal Medicine, MetroHealth Med Ctr 1976; Medical Oncology, LAC-USC Med Ctr 1979; **Fac Appt:** Prof Med, UCLA

Chow, Warren Allen MD [Onc] - Spec Exp: Sarcoma; Bone Cancer; **Hospital:** City of Hope Natl Med Ctr & Beckman Rsch (page 69); **Address:** 1500 E Duarte Rd, Duarte, CA 91010; **Phone:** 626-359-8111; **Board Cert:** Hematology 2004; Medical Oncology 2003; **Med School:** Ros Franklin Univ/Chicago Med Sch 1986; **Resid:** Internal Medicine, Cedars-Sinai Med Ctr 1990; **Fellow:** Hematology & Oncology, City of Hope 1992; Molecular Genetics, City of Hope 1994; **Fac Appt:** Assoc Prof Med

Deeg, H. Joachim MD [Onc] - Spec Exp: Bone Marrow Failure Disorders; Hematologic Malignancies; **Hospital:** Univ Wash Med Ctr; **Address:** Fred Hutchinson Cancer Research Center, 1100 Fairview Avenue N, D1-100, Box 19024, Seattle, WA 98109-1024; **Phone:** 206-667-5985; **Board Cert:** Internal Medicine 1976; Medical Oncology 1979; **Med School:** Germany 1972; **Fac Appt:** Prof Med, Univ Wash

Disis, Mary Lenora MD [Onc] - Spec Exp: Breast Cancer; Ovarian Cancer; Clinical Trials; **Hospital:** Univ Wash Med Ctr; **Address:** Univ Washington, Ctr Translational Medicine Women's Hlth, 815 Mercer St Fl 2, Seattle, WA 98109; **Phone:** 206-616-1823; **Board Cert:** Internal Medicine 1989; Medical Oncology 1997; **Med School:** Univ Nebr Coll Med 1986; **Resid:** Internal Medicine, Univ Illinois Med Ctr 1990; **Fellow:** Medical Oncology, Fred Hutchinson Cancer Ctr 1993; **Fac Appt:** Assoc Prof Med, Univ Wash

Druker, Brian MD [Onc] - **Spec Exp:** Leukemia; **Hospital:** OR Hlth & Sci Univ; **Address:** 3181 SW Sam Jackson Park Rd, MC L592, Portland, OR 97239-3098; **Phone:** 503-494-5058; **Board Cert:** Internal Medicine 1984; Medical Oncology 1987; **Med School:** UCSD 1981; **Resid:** Internal Medicine, Barnes Jewish Hosp 1984; **Fellow:** Medical Oncology, Dana-Farber Cancer Inst 1987; **Fac Appt:** Prof Med, Oregon Hlth Sci Univ

Ellis, Georgiana K MD [Onc] - **Spec Exp:** Breast Cancer; Clinical Trials; **Hospital:** Univ Wash Med Ctr; **Address:** Univ Washington Med Ctr, 1959 NE Pacific St, Seattle, WA 98195-6043; **Phone:** 206-288-2048; **Board Cert:** Internal Medicine 1985; Medical Oncology 1987; **Med School:** Univ Wash 1982; **Resid:** Internal Medicine, Univ Washington 1985; **Fellow:** Medical Oncology, Univ Washington 1988; **Fac Appt:** Assoc Prof Med, Univ Wash

Figlin, Robert A MD [Onc] - **Spec Exp:** Urologic Cancer; Kidney Cancer; Immunotherapy; **Hospital:** City of Hope Natl Med Ctr & Beckman Rsch (page 69), UCLA Med Ctr (page 83); **Address:** City of Hope Natl Med Ctr, Med Oncology & Therapeutics Research, 1500 E Duarte Rd, Duarte, CA 91010; **Phone:** 626-256-4673; **Board Cert:** Internal Medicine 1979; Medical Oncology 1983; **Med School:** Med Coll PA Hahnemann 1976; **Resid:** Internal Medicine, Cedars Sinai Med Ctr 1980; **Fellow:** Hematology & Oncology, UCLA Ctr Hlth Sci 1982; **Fac Appt:** Prof Med, UCLA

Ford, James M MD [Onc] - **Spec Exp:** Gastrointestinal Cancer; Colon & Rectal Cancer; Cancer Genetics; **Hospital:** Stanford Univ Med Ctr; **Address:** Stanford Comp Cancer Ctr, 875 Blake Wilbur Drive, Ste Clinic B, Stanford, CA 94305-5820; **Phone:** 650-723-7621; **Board Cert:** Internal Medicine 1996; Medical Oncology 2005; **Med School:** Yale Univ 1989; **Resid:** Internal Medicine, Stanford Univ Med Ctr 1991; **Fellow:** Medical Oncology, Stanford Univ Med Ctr 1994; **Fac Appt:** Assoc Prof Med, Stanford Univ

Forscher, Charles A MD [Onc] - **Spec Exp:** Bone Tumors; Sarcoma-Soft Tissue; **Hospital:** Cedars-Sinai Med Ctr, UCLA Med Ctr (page 83); **Address:** Outpatient Cancer Ctr, Lower Level, 8700 Beverly Blvd, Los Angeles, CA 90048; **Phone:** 310-423-8045; **Board Cert:** Internal Medicine 1981; Hematology 1986; Medical Oncology 1987; **Med School:** Albert Einstein Coll Med 1978; **Resid:** Internal Medicine, Montefiore Med Ctr 1981; **Fellow:** Hematology, Montefiore Med Ctr 1983; Neoplastic Diseases, Mt Sinai Med Ctr 1985; **Fac Appt:** Clin Prof Med, UCLA

Gandara, David R MD [Onc] - **Spec Exp:** Lung Cancer; **Hospital:** UC Davis Med Ctr; **Address:** UC Davis Cancer Ctr, 4501 X St, Ste 3016, Sacramento, CA 95817; **Phone:** 916-734-5959; **Board Cert:** Internal Medicine 1976; Medical Oncology 1979; **Med School:** Univ Tex Med Br, Galveston 1973; **Resid:** Internal Medicine, Madigan Med Ctr 1976; **Fellow:** Hematology & Oncology, Letterman AMC 1978; **Fac Appt:** Asst Prof Med, UC Davis

Ganz, Patricia A MD [Onc] - **Spec Exp:** Breast Cancer; **Hospital:** UCLA Med Ctr (page 83); **Address:** UCLA, Cancer Prev/Control Rsch, A2-125 CHS, 650 Charles Young Drive S, Box 956900, Los Angeles, CA 90095-6900; **Phone:** 310-206-1404; **Board Cert:** Internal Medicine 1976; Medical Oncology 1979; **Med School:** UCLA 1973; **Resid:** Internal Medicine, UCLA Med Ctr 1976; **Fellow:** Hematology, UCLA Med Ctr 1978; **Fac Appt:** Prof Med, UCLA

Glaspy, John A MD [Onc] - **Spec Exp:** Breast Cancer; Melanoma; Lymphoma; **Hospital:** UCLA Med Ctr (page 83); **Address:** 100 UCLA Medical Plaza Plaza, Ste 550, Los Angeles, CA 90095; **Phone:** 310-794-4955; **Board Cert:** Internal Medicine 1982; Medical Oncology 1985; Hematology 1986; **Med School:** UCLA 1979; **Resid:** Internal Medicine, UCLA Med Ctr 1982; **Fellow:** Hematology & Oncology, UCLA Med Ctr 1984; **Fac Appt:** Prof Med, UCLA

Gralow, Julie MD [Onc] - **Spec Exp:** Breast Cancer; **Hospital:** Univ Wash Med Ctr; **Address:** Seattle Cancer Care Alliance-UW, 825 Eastlake Ave E, Box 358081, MS G4-83, Seattle, WA 98109; **Phone:** 206-288-7722; **Board Cert:** Medical Oncology 2005; **Med School:** USC Sch Med 1988; **Resid:** Internal Medicine, Brigham & Women's Hosp 1991; **Fellow:** Oncology, Univ Wash Med Ctr 1994; **Fac Appt:** Assoc Prof Med, Univ Wash

Horning, Sandra J MD [Onc] - **Spec Exp:** Hodgkin's Disease; Bone Marrow & Stem Cell Transplant; Lymphoma; **Hospital:** Stanford Univ Med Ctr; **Address:** Stanford Cancer Center, 875 Blake Wilbur Drive, Stanford, CA 94305; **Phone:** 650-723-7621; **Board Cert:** Internal Medicine 1978; Medical Oncology 1981; **Med School:** Univ Iowa Coll Med 1975; **Resid:** Internal Medicine, Strong Meml Hosp 1978; **Fellow:** Medical Oncology, Stanford Univ 1980; **Fac Appt:** Prof Med, Stanford Univ

Jacobs, Charlotte D MD [Onc] - **Spec Exp:** Sarcoma; Unknown Primary Cancer; **Hospital:** Stanford Univ Med Ctr; **Address:** 875 Blake Wilbur Drive, Stanford, CA 94305; **Phone:** 650-723-7621 x2; **Board Cert:** Internal Medicine 1975; Medical Oncology 1977; **Med School:** Washington Univ, St Louis 1972; **Resid:** Internal Medicine, Barnes Hosp 1974; Internal Medicine, UCSF Med Ctr 1975; **Fellow:** Medical Oncology, Stanford Univ 1977; **Fac Appt:** Prof Med, Stanford Univ

Jahan, Thierry Marie MD [Onc] - **Spec Exp:** Endocrine Tumors; Lung Cancer; Mesothelioma; Thyroid Cancer; **Hospital:** UCSF Med Ctr; **Address:** UCSF Comprehensive Cancer Center, 1600 Divisadero St, San Francisco, CA 94115; **Phone:** 415-353-9888; **Board Cert:** Hematology 1994; Medical Oncology 1995; Internal Medicine 1990; **Med School:** Geo Wash Univ 1987; **Resid:** Internal Medicine, Cedars-Sinai Med Ctr 1990; **Fac Appt:** Asst Clin Prof Med, UCSF

Kaplan, Lawrence D MD [Onc] - **Spec Exp:** AIDS Related Cancers; Lymphoma; **Hospital:** UCSF Med Ctr; **Address:** UCSF Medical Center, 400 Parnassus Ave, rm A502, San Francisco, CA 94143-0324; **Phone:** 415-353-2737; **Board Cert:** Internal Medicine 1983; Medical Oncology 1985; **Med School:** UCLA 1980; **Resid:** Internal Medicine, Boston City Hosp 1983; **Fellow:** Hematology & Oncology, UCSF Med Ctr 1985; **Fac Appt:** Clin Prof Med, UCSF

Koczywas, Marianna MD [Onc] - **Spec Exp:** Lung Cancer; **Hospital:** City of Hope Natl Med Ctr & Beckman Rsch (page 69); **Address:** City of Hope National Medical Center, 1500 E Duarte Rd, Duarte, CA 91010; **Phone:** 626-359-8111; **Board Cert:** Internal Medicine 1997; Hematology 2000; Medical Oncology 2001; **Med School:** Poland 1984; **Resid:** Internal Medicine, Troczewski City Hosp 1988; Internal Medicine, St. Francis Med Ctr 1997; **Fellow:** Hematology & Oncology, City of Hope Natl Med Ctr 2000

Maloney, David G MD/PhD [Onc] - **Spec Exp:** Lymphoma; Bone Marrow & Stem Cell Transplant; Vaccine Therapy; **Hospital:** Univ Wash Med Ctr; **Address:** FHCRC-MS D1-100, 1100 Fairview Ave N, Box 19024, Seattle, WA 98109-1024; **Phone:** 206-667-5616; **Board Cert:** Internal Medicine 1988; Medical Oncology 2005; **Med School:** Stanford Univ 1985; **Resid:** Internal Medicine, Brigham & Women's Hosp 1988; **Fellow:** Medical Oncology, Stanford Univ Med Ctr 1994; **Fac Appt:** Prof Med, Univ Wash

Margolin, Kim Allyson MD [Onc] - **Spec Exp:** Melanoma; Kidney Cancer; Germ Cell Tumors; **Hospital:** City of Hope Natl Med Ctr & Beckman Rsch (page 69); **Address:** City of Hope Comprehensive Cancer Ctr, 1500 E Duarte Rd, Duarte, CA 91010-3012; **Phone:** 626-359-8111 x62307; **Board Cert:** Internal Medicine 1982; Hematology 1986; Medical Oncology 1985; **Med School:** Stanford Univ 1979; **Resid:** Internal Medicine, Yale-New Haven Hosp 1982; **Fellow:** Hematology & Oncology, UC San Diego Med Ctr 1983; Hematology & Oncology, City of Hope Med Ctr 1985

Martins, Renato G MD [Onc] - **Spec Exp:** Head & Neck Cancer; Lung Cancer; Mesothelioma; Salivary Gland Tumors; **Hospital:** Univ Wash Med Ctr; **Address:** Fred Hutchinson Cancer Rsch Ctr, 825 Eastlake Ave E, MS G4-830, Seattle, WA 98109; **Phone:** 206-288-2048; **Board Cert:** Internal Medicine 1995; Medical Oncology 1998; **Med School:** Brazil 1992; **Resid:** Internal Medicine, Gunderson Clinic 1995; **Fellow:** Medical Oncology, Mass Genl Hosp 1998

Meyskens, Frank MD [Onc] - **Spec Exp:** Cancer Prevention; Melanoma; Sarcoma; **Hospital:** UC Irvine Med Ctr; **Address:** UC Urvine Cancer Ctr, 101 The City Drive Bldg 56 - rm 215, Orange, CA 92868; **Phone:** 714-456-6310; **Board Cert:** Internal Medicine 1975; Medical Oncology 1981; **Med School:** UCSF 1972; **Resid:** Internal Medicine, Moffit-Calif Hosps 1974; **Fellow:** Hematology & Oncology, NCI 1977; **Fac Appt:** Prof Med, UC Irvine

Mitchell, Beverly MD [Onc] - **Spec Exp:** Hematologic Malignancies; Leukemia; Lymphoma; **Hospital:** Stanford Univ Med Ctr; **Address:** Stanford Cancer Center, 800 Welch Rd, Stanford, CA 94305-5402; **Phone:** 650-725-9621; **Board Cert:** Internal Medicine 1973; Hematology 1978; **Med School:** Harvard Med Sch 1969; **Resid:** Internal Medicine, Univ Washington Med Ctr 1972; **Fellow:** Metabolism, Univ Zurich 1975; Hematology & Oncology, Univ Michigan 1977; **Fac Appt:** Prof Med, Stanford Univ

Mortimer, Joanne MD [Onc] - **Spec Exp:** Breast Cancer; Clinical Trials; **Hospital:** UCSD Med Ctr; **Address:** Moores UCSD Cancer Ctr, 3855 Health Sciences Drive, MC 0987, La Jolla, CA 92093-1503; **Phone:** 858-822-6135; **Board Cert:** Internal Medicine 1980; Medical Oncology 1983; **Med School:** Loyola Univ-Stritch Sch Med 1977; **Resid:** Internal Medicine, Cleveland Clinic 1980; **Fellow:** Medical Oncology, Cleveland Clinic 1982; **Fac Appt:** Prof Med, UCSD

Natale, Ronald B MD [Onc] - **Spec Exp:** Lung Cancer; **Hospital:** Cedars-Sinai Med Ctr; **Address:** Cedars-Sinai Comp Cancer Ctr, 8700 Beverly Blvd, Ste C2000, Los Angeles, CA 90048; **Phone:** 310-423-1101; **Board Cert:** Internal Medicine 1977; Medical Oncology 1979; **Med School:** Wayne State Univ 1974; **Resid:** Internal Medicine, Wayne State Univ 1977; **Fellow:** Hematology & Oncology, Meml Sloan Kettering 1980; **Fac Appt:** Prof Med, Univ Mich Med Sch

Nichols, Craig R MD [Onc] - **Spec Exp:** Testicular Cancer; Hodgkin's Disease; Lymphoma; **Hospital:** OR Hlth & Sci Univ; **Address:** Oregon Cancer Center, 3303 SW Bond Ave Fl 7th, MC CH7M, Portland, OR 97239-3098; **Phone:** 503-494-6594; **Board Cert:** Internal Medicine 1981; Medical Oncology 1985; **Med School:** Oregon Hlth Sci Univ 1978; **Resid:** Internal Medicine, Oschner Foundation Hosp 1981; **Fellow:** Medical Oncology, Indiana Univ 1985; **Fac Appt:** Prof Med, Oregon Hlth Sci Univ

Medical Oncology

O'Day, Steven J MD [Onc] - **Spec Exp:** Melanoma; Melanoma-Advanced; **Hospital:** St John's Hlth Ctr, Santa Monica; **Address:** The Angeles Clinic & Research Inst, 11818 Wilshire Blvd, Ste 200, Los Angeles, CA 90025; **Phone:** 310-231-2178; **Board Cert:** Internal Medicine 1991; Medical Oncology 1993; **Med School:** Johns Hopkins Univ 1988; **Resid:** Internal Medicine, Johns Hopkins Hosp 1991; **Fellow:** Medical Oncology, Dana Farber Cancer Inst 1992; **Fac Appt:** Assoc Clin Prof Med, USC-Keck School of Medicine

Pegram, Mark D MD [Onc] - **Spec Exp:** Breast Cancer; Ovarian Cancer; **Hospital:** UCLA Med Ctr (page 83); **Address:** 2336 Santa Monica Blvd, Ste 301, Santa Monica, CA 90404; **Phone:** 310-829-5471; **Board Cert:** Internal Medicine 1989; Hematology 1996; Medical Oncology 2003; **Med School:** Univ NC Sch Med 1986; **Resid:** Internal Medicine, Dallas County Hosp 1989; **Fellow:** Hematology & Oncology, UCLA Med Ctr 1993; **Fac Appt:** Prof Med, UCLA

Petersdorf, Stephen MD [Onc] - **Spec Exp:** Lymphoma; Myelodysplastic Syndromes; Leukemia; **Hospital:** Univ Wash Med Ctr; **Address:** Fred Hutchinson Cancer Research Ctr, 825 Eastlake Ave E, MS G6800, Seattle, WA 98109-1023; **Phone:** 206-288-1024; **Board Cert:** Internal Medicine 1986; Hematology 2001; Medical Oncology 2001; **Med School:** Brown Univ 1983; **Resid:** Internal Medicine, Univ Washington Med Ctr 1986; **Fellow:** Hematology & Oncology, Univ Washington Med Ctr 1989; **Fac Appt:** Assoc Prof Med, Univ Wash

Picozzi Jr, Vincent J MD [Onc] - **Spec Exp:** Pancreatic Cancer; **Hospital:** Virginia Mason Med Ctr; **Address:** Virginia Mason Med Ctr, Div Hem/Onc, MS C2-Hem, Seattle, WA 98111; **Phone:** 206-223-6193; **Board Cert:** Internal Medicine 1981; Hematology 1986; Medical Oncology 1987; **Med School:** Stanford Univ 1978; **Resid:** Internal Medicine, Peter Bent Brigham Med Ctr 1981; **Fellow:** Hematology, Stanford Univ Med Ctr 1983; Medical Oncology, Stanford Univ MEd Ctr 1984; **Fac Appt:** Clin Prof Med, Univ Wash

Pinto, Harlan Andrew MD [Onc] - **Spec Exp:** Head & Neck Cancer; Clinical Trials; **Hospital:** Stanford Univ Med Ctr, VA Hlth Care Sys - Palo Alto; **Address:** Stanford Med Ctr Oncol Div, 875 Blake Wilbur Drive, Stanford, CA 94305; **Phone:** 650-723-7621; **Board Cert:** Internal Medicine 1986; Medical Oncology 2002; **Med School:** Yale Univ 1983; **Resid:** Internal Medicine, Mass Genl Hosp 1986; **Fellow:** Medical Oncology, Stanford Univ Med Sch 1991; **Fac Appt:** Assoc Prof Med, Stanford Univ

Prados, Michael MD [Onc] - **Spec Exp:** Neuro-Oncology; Brain Tumors; **Hospital:** UCSF Med Ctr; **Address:** UCSF Med Ctr, Div Neuro-Oncology, 400 Parnassus Ave, rm A-808, San Francisco, CA 94143; **Phone:** 415-353-2966; **Board Cert:** Internal Medicine 1977; **Med School:** Louisiana State Univ 1974; **Resid:** Internal Medicine, Earl K Long Hosp 1977; **Fac Appt:** Prof NS, UCSF

Press, Oliver W MD/PhD [Onc] - **Spec Exp:** Lymphoma; Bone Marrow Transplant; **Hospital:** Univ Wash Med Ctr; **Address:** 1100 Fairview Ave N, MS D3-190, Seattle, WA 98109; **Phone:** 206-667-1864; **Board Cert:** Internal Medicine 1982; Medical Oncology 1985; **Med School:** Univ Wash 1979; **Resid:** Internal Medicine, Mass Genl Hosp 1982; Internal Medicine, Univ Hosp 1983; **Fellow:** Medical Oncology, Univ Washington 1985; **Fac Appt:** Prof Med, Univ Wash

Quinn, David MD/PhD [Onc] - **Spec Exp:** Testicular Cancer; Prostate Cancer; Kidney Cancer; **Hospital:** USC Norris Comp Cancer Ctr; **Address:** 1441 Eastlake Ave, Ste 3440, Los Angeles, CA 90033; **Phone:** 323-865-3956; **Med School:** Australia 1987; **Resid:** Internal Medicine, St Vincent's Hosp 1992; **Fellow:** Medical Oncology, St Vincent's Hosp 1995; **Fac Appt:** Asst Prof Med, USC Sch Med

Ross, Helen Jane MD [Onc] - **Spec Exp:** Lung Cancer; Esophageal Cancer; Chest Wall Tumors; Clinical Trials; **Hospital:** Providence Portland Med Ctr; **Address:** Oregon Clinic-Cardiothoracic Surgery, 1111 NE 99th Ave, Ste 201, Portland, OR 97220; **Phone:** 503-215-5696; **Board Cert:** Internal Medicine 1987; Medical Oncology 1989; **Med School:** UCLA 1984; **Resid:** Internal Medicine, Cedars Sinai Med Ctr 1987; **Fellow:** Medical Oncology, UCLA Med Ctr 1989; **Fac Appt:** Assoc Prof Med, Oregon Hlth Sci Univ

Rugo, Hope S MD [Onc] - **Spec Exp:** Breast Cancer; Complementary Medicine; **Hospital:** UCSF Med Ctr; **Address:** UCSF Comp Cancer Ctr-Breast Care Ctr, 1600 Divisadero St Fl 2, San Francisco, CA 94115; **Phone:** 415-353-7070; **Board Cert:** Internal Medicine 1987; Medical Oncology 1989; **Med School:** Univ Pennsylvania 1984; **Resid:** Internal Medicine, UCSF Med Ctr 1987; **Fellow:** Hematology & Oncology, UCSF Med Ctr 1989; **Fac Appt:** Assoc Clin Prof Med, UCSF

Russell, Christy A MD [Onc] - **Spec Exp:** Breast Cancer; **Hospital:** USC Univ Hosp - R K Eamer Med Plz; **Address:** Norris Cancer Ctr, The Breast Ctr, 1441 Eastlake Ave, Los Angeles, CA 90033; **Phone:** 323-865-3371; **Board Cert:** Internal Medicine 1983; Medical Oncology 1985; **Med School:** Med Coll PA Hahnemann 1980; **Fac Appt:** Assoc Prof Med, USC Sch Med

Shibata, Stephen I MD [Onc] - **Spec Exp:** Gastrointestinal Cancer; Clinical Trials; **Hospital:** City of Hope Natl Med Ctr & Beckman Rsch (page 69); **Address:** City of Hope Cancer Ctr, 1500 E Duarte Rd, Duarte, CA 91010; **Phone:** 626-471-9200 x7; **Board Cert:** Internal Medicine 1988; Medical Oncology 1991; **Med School:** UC Irvine 1985; **Resid:** Internal Medicine, St Mary Med Ctr 1988; **Fellow:** Medical Oncology, City of Hope Cancer Ctr 1990; Bone Marrow Transplant, City of Hope Cancer Ctr 1991; **Fac Appt:** Assoc Prof Med

Sikic, Branimir I MD [Onc] - **Spec Exp:** Unknown Primary Cancer; Clinical Trials; **Hospital:** Stanford Univ Med Ctr; **Address:** Stanford Comp Cancer Ctr, Med Oncology, 875 Blake Wilbur Drive, Stanford, CA 94305; **Phone:** 650-723-7621; **Board Cert:** Internal Medicine 1975; Medical Oncology 1979; **Med School:** Ros Franklin Univ/Chicago Med Sch 1972; **Resid:** Internal Medicine, Georgetown Univ Hosp 1975; **Fellow:** Medical Oncology, Natl Cancer Inst 1978; Medical Oncology, Georgetown Univ Hosp 1979; **Fac Appt:** Prof Med, Stanford Univ

Small, Eric J MD [Onc] - **Spec Exp:** Prostate Cancer; Vaccine Therapy; Genitourinary Cancer; **Hospital:** UCSF Med Ctr; **Address:** UCSF Urologic Oncology Practice, 1600 Divisadero St, San Francisco, CA 94115; **Phone:** 415-353-7171; **Board Cert:** Internal Medicine 1988; Medical Oncology 2001; **Med School:** Case West Res Univ 1985; **Resid:** Internal Medicine, Beth Israel Hosp 1988; **Fellow:** Hematology & Oncology, Cancer Research Inst/UCSF 1991; **Fac Appt:** Prof Med, UCSF

Stewart, Forrest Marc MD [Onc] - **Spec Exp:** Unknown Primary Cancer; Sarcoma; **Hospital:** Univ Wash Med Ctr; **Address:** Fred Hutchinson Cancer Rsch Ctr, 825 Eastlake Ave E, Box 19023, Seattle, WA 98109; **Phone:** 206-288-7222; **Board Cert:** Internal Medicine 1980; Hematology 1982; Medical Oncology 1985; **Med School:** Indiana Univ 1977; **Resid:** Internal Medicine, Indiana Univ Med Ctr 1980; Medical Oncology, Indiana Univ Med Ctr 1981; **Fellow:** Hematology, Univ Virginia Med Ctr 1983; **Fac Appt:** Prof Med, Univ Wash

Stockdale, Frank E MD/PhD [Onc] - **Spec Exp:** Breast Cancer; **Hospital:** Stanford Univ Med Ctr; **Address:** Stanford University Medical Ctr, 875 Lake Wilbur Drive, Stanford, CA 94305-5826; **Phone:** 650-723-6449; **Med School:** Univ Pennsylvania 1963; **Resid:** Internal Medicine, Stanford Univ Med Ctr 1967; **Fellow:** Hematology & Oncology, Natl Inst Hlth; **Fac Appt:** Prof Emeritus Med, Stanford Univ

Tempero, Margaret MD [Onc] - **Spec Exp:** Pancreatic Cancer; Gastrointestinal Cancer; **Hospital:** UCSF Med Ctr; **Address:** UCSF, Multi-Disciplinary Practice, 1600 Divisadero St, Box 1705, San Francisco, CA 94115; **Phone:** 415-353-9888; **Board Cert:** Internal Medicine 1980; Hematology 1984; Medical Oncology 1983; **Med School:** Univ Nebr Coll Med 1977; **Resid:** Internal Medicine, Univ Nebraska Hosp 1980; **Fellow:** Medical Oncology, Univ Nebraska 1982

Thompson, John A MD [Onc] - **Spec Exp:** Melanoma; **Hospital:** Univ Wash Med Ctr; **Address:** Univ Wash Med Ctr, Cancer Ctr PO Box 19023, MS G4100, Seattle, WA 98195; **Phone:** 206-288-7222; **Board Cert:** Internal Medicine 1982; Medical Oncology 1985; **Med School:** Univ Ala 1979; **Resid:** Internal Medicine, Univ Wash Med Ctr 1982; **Fellow:** Medical Oncology, Univ Washington 1985

Urba, Walter J MD [Onc] - **Spec Exp:** Breast Cancer; **Hospital:** Providence Portland Med Ctr; **Address:** Oregon Clinic, Div of Medical Oncology, 5050 NE Hoyt, Ste 611, Portland, OR 97213; **Phone:** 503-215-5696; **Board Cert:** Internal Medicine 1985; Medical Oncology 1987; **Med School:** Univ Miami Sch Med 1981; **Resid:** Internal Medicine, Morristown Meml Hosp 1983; **Fellow:** Medical Oncology, Natl Cancer Inst 1986; **Fac Appt:** Assoc Clin Prof Med, Oregon Hlth Sci Univ

Venook, Alan P MD [Onc] - **Spec Exp:** Gastrointestinal Cancer; Colon & Rectal Cancer; Liver Cancer; **Hospital:** UCSF Med Ctr; **Address:** UCSF Comprehensive Cancer Ctr, Multi Disciplinary Practice, 1600 Divisadero St Fl 4, Box 1705, San Francisco, CA 94115; **Phone:** 415-353-9888; **Board Cert:** Internal Medicine 1985; Medical Oncology 1987; Hematology 1988; **Med School:** UCSF 1980; **Resid:** Internal Medicine, UC Davis Med Ctr 1985; **Fellow:** Hematology & Oncology, UCSF Med Ctr 1987; **Fac Appt:** Prof Med

Vescio, Robert A MD [Onc] - **Spec Exp:** Multiple Myeloma; **Hospital:** Cedars-Sinai Med Ctr; **Address:** Cedars Sinai Med Ctr, Dept Hem/Oncology, 8700 Beverly Blvd, Los Angeles, CA 90048; **Phone:** 310-423-1825; **Board Cert:** Internal Medicine 1989; Hematology 2004; Medical Oncology 2003; **Med School:** UCSD 1986; **Resid:** Internal Medicine, UCSD Med Ctr 1989; **Fellow:** Hematology & Oncology, UCLA Med Ctr 1993; **Fac Appt:** Assoc Prof Med, UCLA

Vogelzang, Nicholas MD [Onc] - **Spec Exp:** Prostate Cancer; Mesothelioma; Kidney Cancer; **Hospital:** Univ Med Ctr - Las Vegas, Summerlin Hosp Med Ctr; **Address:** Nevada Cancer Institute, One Breakthrough Way, Las Vegas, NV 89135; **Phone:** 702-822-5100; **Board Cert:** Internal Medicine 1978; Medical Oncology 1981; **Med School:** Univ IL Coll Med 1974; **Resid:** Internal Medicine, Rush-Presby St Luke's Med Ctr 1978; **Fellow:** Medical Oncology, Univ Minn Med Ctr 1981; **Fac Appt:** Prof Med, Univ Nevada

Volberding, Paul Arthur MD [Onc] - **Spec Exp:** AIDS Related Cancers; **Hospital:** UCSF Med Ctr; **Address:** 4150 Clemens St, VAMC 111, San Francisco, CA 94121; **Phone:** 415-750-2203; **Board Cert:** Internal Medicine 1978; Medical Oncology 1981; **Med School:** Univ Minn 1975; **Resid:** Internal Medicine, Univ Utah Med Ctr 1978; **Fellow:** Medical Oncology, UCSF Med Ctr 1981; **Fac Appt:** Prof Med, UCSF

Weber, Jeffrey S MD/PhD [Onc] - **Spec Exp:** Kidney Cancer; Melanoma; Breast Cancer; **Hospital:** USC Norris Comp Cancer Ctr; **Address:** USC/ Norris Cancer Ctr, 1441 Eastlake Ave, Ste 3440, Los Angeles, CA 90033-1048; **Phone:** 323-865-3962; **Board Cert:** Internal Medicine 1983; Medical Oncology 1987; **Med School:** NYU Sch Med 1980; **Resid:** Internal Medicine, UCSD Med Ctr 1983; **Fellow:** Medical Oncology, Natl Cancer Inst 1990; **Fac Appt:** Assoc Prof Med, USC Sch Med

Yen, Yun MD [Onc] - **Spec Exp:** Liver Cancer; Biliary Cancer; **Hospital:** City of Hope Natl Med Ctr & Beckman Rsch (page 69); **Address:** City of Hope Comprehensive Cancer Ctr, 1500 E Duarte Rd, Duarte, CA 91010; **Phone:** 626-359-8111 x62307; **Board Cert:** Internal Medicine 1990; Medical Oncology 2003; **Med School:** Taiwan 1982; **Resid:** Internal Medicine, St Luke's Hosp 1990; **Fellow:** Hematology & Oncology, Yale-New Haven Hosp 1993; **Fac Appt:** Prof Med, USC Sch Med

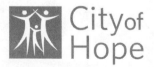

Cleveland Clinic

Taussig Cancer Center

The Taussig Cancer Center logs more than 180,000 patient visits annually. A team of 250 cancer specialists cares for patients with breast, lung, urologic, endocrine, gastrointestinal, gynecologic, head and neck, musculoskeletal and ophthalmic cancers; cancers of the brain and spinal cord; skin cancer and melanoma; and hematologic malignancies. They also have a world-renowned palliative care program. The quality and innovation of our programs has led to a ranking as one of the nation's top cancer centers by *U.S.News & World Report*.

State-of-the-art patient care is provided in the context of major clinical and translational research programs. Bench-to-bedside research allows patients with resistant cancers to have access to experimental therapies, if indicated.

Our Bone Marrow Transplant program consistently achieves excellent outcomes. We have one of the most experienced teams in the nation, having performed over 2,900 bone marrow transplant procedures since 1977.

In our multidisciplinary clinics, subspecialists bring their expertise to bear on specific tumor types and aspects of treatment and recovery. Medical, surgical and radiation oncologists collaborate closely with pathologists, radiologists, oncology nurses and social workers. These interactions enhance effective communication and optimize the options for individual patients with complex problems.

In 2006, Taussig Cancer Center introduced a Late Effects Clinic for cancer survivors. This multidisciplinary clinic helps to address health problems that can arise as late effects of successful cancer treatment.

The center also is one of just a few hospitals in the region to offer different technologies for administering stereotactic radiosurgery. Image-guided radiation therapy is used for extracranial lesions, and the Gamma Knife is used to treat primary and metastatic brain tumors.

To stay at the forefront of cancer research, Cleveland Clinic continues to recruit world-renowned investigators, maintaining a focus on discovery and innovation.

To schedule an appointment or for more information about the Cleveland Clinic Taussig Cancer Center, call 800.890.2467 or visit www.clevelandclinic.org/cancertopdocs.

Taussig Cancer Center | 9500 Euclid Avenue / W14 | Cleveland OH 44195

Cancer Genetics at the Center for Personalized Genetic Healthcare

It has long been recognized that people in some families are prone to developing cancer. The last few decades of genetic research have provided us with the ability to identify some of the genetic risk factors that underlie this predisposition. At the Cleveland Clinic's Center for Personalized Genetic Healthcare, we specialize in the evaluation and management of high risk families. Our goal is to prevent cancer by identifying individuals at high-risk for developing cancer, and offering personalized medical management to them and their family members. For more information or to schedule an appointment, call 800.998.4785.

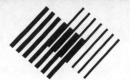

Maimonides Cancer Center offers a fully integrated approach to cancer care that includes prevention, education, screening, diagnostics, treatment, palliative care and clinical research – all in one location. Staffed by a multidisciplinary team of leading oncologists, nurses, social workers and treatment specialists, the Maimonides Cancer Center provides compassionate, patient-centered, state-of-the-art care that is both accessible and comfortable. This freestanding, 50,000 square foot facility contains the following specialty centers:

Radiation Oncology Center: equipped with state-of-the art imaging and treatment delivery technologies; offers patients the most precise treatments available, yet does so in an airy, life-affirming environment.

Medical Oncology Center: provides oral drug therapies, intravenous chemotherapy infusions, transfusions, intravenous hydration, and antibiotics.

Pediatric Oncology Center: treats children with cancer in a child-friendly environment, and features special areas set aside for parent conferences.

Surgical Oncology Center: provides a convenient location for minor surgical procedures relating to cancer, including biopsies; and pre- and post-surgical care for the most complex cases.

Women's Center: provides mammography, sonography, computerized interpretation, biopsy procedures, same-day reading of results, treatment plans tailored for each patient.

Resource Center: offers access to integrative (complementary) oncology services, a library with Internet resources, social services, and dietary advice.

Research Center: conducts clinical trials that not only help advance science but also offer appropriately screened patients, who wish to volunteer, new therapies and medications.

Passionate about medicine. Compassionate about people.

Sponsorship: Private, Non-Profit
Beds: 432
Accreditation: Awarded Accreditation from the Joint Commission on
Accreditation of Healthcare Organizations (JCAHO).

SUB-SPECIALIZED CLINICAL EXPERTISE

At Memorial Sloan-Kettering, the sole focus is cancer. Our physicians provide expert care in the hundreds of different subtypes of cancer. For patients, this specialization means a singular level of medical expertise, superb patient care, and an often dramatic effect on a patient's chances for a cure or control of his or her disease.

Our Disease Management Program features medical teams, defined by cancer type (breast, lung, etc.) whose members work together to guide each patient through every aspect of their care—diagnosis, treatment and recovery. These teams have a depth and breadth of experience that is unsurpassed. Using this approach, the treatment plans reflect the combined expertise of many medical professionals, including surgeons, medical oncologists, radiologists, radiation oncologists, pathologists, psychologists and social workers. This approach also ensures that patients who need several different therapies to treat their cancer will receive the best combination for them.

RESEARCH AND EDUCATION

One of Memorial Sloan-Kettering's great strengths is the close relationship between scientists and clinicians. The constant collaboration between our doctors and research scientists means that new drugs and therapies developed in the laboratory can be moved quickly to the bedside, offering patients improved treatment options. The Center's renowned training programs prepare today's physicians, scientists, nurses and other health professionals for tomorrow's leadership roles in science and medicine, especially as it relates to cancer.

SUPPORTING OUR PATIENTS

At Memorial Sloan-Kettering, we have long understood that cancer is not solely a physical disease. For more than 50 years, we have provided expert assistance in dealing with cancer-related distress, and have developed a range of comprehensive programs and services to help patients, families and caregivers manage the unique set of changes that often accompany illness. Many of our programs now serve as models for other cancer centers around the world.

Access to Tomorrow's Cancer Treatments Today

Access to clinical breakthroughs, innovative techniques, leading-edge technologies, the safest and most effective treatment options, and a wide-range of diagnostic, therapeutic, and support services for all types of cancer, including the following specialties:

Head and Neck

Thoracic
(including lung, esophagus)

Gynecologic Oncology

Hematological Malignancies
(including bone marrow transplantation)

Brain Tumors

Radiation Oncology

Prostate/Bladder/Kidney

Medical Oncology

When you're battling cancer, fight smart.

Another day, another breakthrough.

1-800-MD-SINAI
www.mountsinai.org
The Mount Sinai Medical Center
New York, New York

NewYork-Presbyterian
The University Hospital of Columbia and Cornell
NewYork-Presbyterian Cancer Centers

Affiliated with Columbia University College of Physicians and Surgeons and Weill Medical College of Cornell University

Herbert Irving Comprehensive Cancer Center	Weill Cornell Cancer Center
At NewYork-Presbyterian Hospital	At NewYork-Presbyterian Hospital
Columbia University Medical Center	Weill Cornell Medical Center
161 Fort Washington Avenue	525 East 68th Street
New York, NY 10032	New York, NY 10021

OVERVIEW:

NewYork-Presbyterian Cancer Centers are dedicated to reducing cancer morbidity and mortality by providing

- a full continuum of multidisciplinary, state-of-the-art screening, diagnostic, treatment and support services for all phases of the disease process;
- cutting-edge basic, clinical, and public health research;
- full range of cancer-related educational programs and resources to clinicians, scientists, patients and survivors, families, and the cancer prevention community.

The Cancer Centers, which treat over 6,000 new patients annually, draw on the innovation and excellence of the NCI- designated Herbert Irving Comprehensive Cancer Center at NewYork-Presbyterian Hospital/Columbia University Medical Center and oncology services at NewYork-Presbyterian Hospital/Weill Cornell Medical Center. Programs include:

- AIDS-related Malignancies
- Bone Marrow Transplant
- Breast Cancer
- Dermatologic/Skin Cancer
- Gastrointestinal Cancers
- Genitourinary Cancers
- Gynecologic Cancers
- Head and Neck Cancers
- Hematologic Malignancies, such as lymphoma, myeloma and leukemias
- Lung Cancer
- Neurologic Cancer
- Ophthalmic Cancer
- Pediatric Hematology/Oncology
- Urologic Cancers, including bladder, kidney and prostate cancer
- Sarcomas and Mesotheiliomas

The Centers are frequent recipients of major grants and gifts to support research programs. Recent highlights include:

- Avon Products Foundation $10 million award to NewYork-Presbyterian Hospital/Columbia University Medical Center and Columbia University for establishment of the Avon Products Breast Center to support basic, clinical and public health research in breast cancer;
- The Leukemia and Lymphoma Society five-year $7.5 million grant to NewYork-Presbyterian Hospital/Weill Cornell Medical Center to study fundamental causes of multiple myeloma.

Physician Referral: For a physician referral call toll free **1-877-NYP-WELL** (1-877-697-9355) to learn more about our Cancer Centers visit our website at **www.nypcancer.org**

COMPREHENSIVE SERVICES INCLUDE:

- Access to over 400 clinical trials supported by the National Institutes of Health and many prominent pharmaceutical companies.

- Bone marrow and blood stem cell transplant, including New York State approval to perform transplants using unrelated donors for patients with hematologic malignancies.

- CT screening for early lung cancer detection.

- Sentinel node biopsy to assess spread of breast cancer.

- Skin-sparing mastectomy and reconstruction.

- Laparoscopic surgery for colon cancer.

- Intraoperative brachytherapy for GI, prostate and other cancers.

- Stereotactic biopsies for breast cancer and brain cancer.

- Stereotactic gamma radiation for brain tumors.

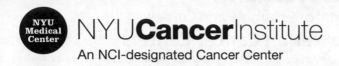

NYU**Cancer**Institute
An NCI-designated Cancer Center

Looking for information on our expert physicians?
1-212-731-5000

NYU Clinical Cancer Center
160 East 34th Street
New York, New York 10016
www.nyuci.org/atcd

NYU Medical Center
550 First Avenue
(at 31st Street)
New York, New York 10016
www.nyumc.org/atcd

**Stephen D. Hassenfeld
Children's Center
for Cancer and Blood
Disorders**
160 East 32nd Street
New York, New York 10016
www.nyumc.org/hassenfeld

A Collaborative Approach
The NYU Cancer Institute, an NCI designated center, is a "matrix cancer center" without walls operating within the larger NYU Medical Center. With over 200 members and a research funding base of over $81 million, this structure strengthens our capabilities to forge collaborations across medical and scientific disciplines, which translates to comprehensive care for our patients and discoveries that will influence the future of this disease.

Renowned Expertise
Our highly skilled Magnet™ nursing team not only plays a pivotal role in coordinating direct patient care, but is also a source of invaluable patient education. Team members' compassion and expertise help patients better manage the symptoms of their disease as well as their special needs.

A Patient-Focused Setting
The NYU Clinical Cancer Center, with over 70 faculty members from various disciplines at the New York University School of Medicine, is the principal outpatient facility of the Cancer Institute and serves as home for our patients and their caregivers. The center and its multidisciplinary team of experts provide access to the latest treatment options and clinical trials along with a variety of programs in cancer prevention, screening, diagnostics, genetic counseling, and supportive services. When it comes to kids and cancer, the Stephen D. Hassenfeld Children's Center for Cancer and Blood Disorders offers not just innovation but insight. As a leading member of the NCI-sponsored Children's Oncology Group, our physicians are known for developing new ways to treat childhood cancer. Our affiliation with Bellevue Hospital, the oldest public hospital in the country, affords clinically distinctive opportunities to learn and care for patients with cancer by observing its presentation and behavior in a variety of patient groups.

THE UNIVERSITY OF TEXAS
MD ANDERSON CANCER CENTER

Making Cancer History®

**The University of Texas
M. D. Anderson Cancer Center**

1515 Holcombe Blvd.
Houston, Texas 77030-4095
Tel. 713-792-6161
Toll Free 877-MDA-6789
http://www.mdanderson.org

LYMPHOMA & MYELOMA CENTER

Cancers that affect the blood cells require specialized treatment. At M. D. Anderson, we have specialized expertise in diagnosing, treating and managing lymphomas and myelomas. Ours is one of the largest multidisciplinary programs for hematology in the nation. Lymphomas treated include Hodgkin's and non-Hodgkin's; B-cell and T-cell, follicular cell, small cleaved-cell, Mantle Cell and cutaneous T-cell, along with Multiple Myeloma and Waldenstrom's macroglobulinemia.

The Lymphoma and Myeloma Center offers many novel treatment options, including the use of monoclonal antibodies, cytokine therapy, vaccine therapy, and liposomal drug delivery.

LEUKEMIA CENTER

The Leukemia Center treats all leukemias (acute and chronic), myelodysplastic syndromes, aplastic and other anemias, myeloproliferative syndromes and other related hematologic malignancies. We also provide biological therapeutics and immunotherapeutic approaches to a wide variety of hematologic and solid tumor diseases.

STEM CELL TRANSPLANTATION

We are one of the largest centers in the world for stem cell transplants, performing more than 600 procedures for adults and children each year, more than any other center in the nation. Our program is recognized by the National Marrow Donor Program (NMDP) as a specialized center for matched unrelated donor transplants, and maintains an advanced cell processing laboratory that is dedicated to preparing safe and effective hematologic tissues for transplantation. The stem cell collection unit is one of the most active facilities in the world, performing over 1,000 blood stem cell collections annually.

MORE INFORMATION

For more information or to make an appointment, call 877-MDA-6789, or visit us online at http://www.mdanderson.org.

At M. D. Anderson Cancer Center, our mission is simple – to eliminate cancer. Achieving that goal begins with integrated programs in cancer treatment, clinical trials, education programs and cancer prevention.

We focus exclusively on cancer and have seen cases of every kind. That means you receive expert care no matter what your diagnosis.

Choosing the right partner for cancer care really does make a difference. The fact is, people who choose M. D. Anderson over other hospitals and clinics often have better results. That is how we've been making cancer history for over sixty years.

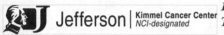

HEMATOLOGY/MEDICAL ONCOLOGY PROGRAM

UCLA Health System

1-800-UCLA-MD1 (825-2631)
www.uclahealth.org

The UCLA Hematology/Oncology Program provides both investigative and standard-of-care therapy for adults and children with hematologic and oncology diseases.

Cancer researchers have long believed that the future of treatment rests in targeted therapies — "smart" drugs that, unlike the non-discriminating chemotherapy approach, take aim at the proteins, enzymes and pathways unique to cancer. Six drugs that utilize this strategy gained U.S. Food & Drug Administration approval after years of laboratory and clinical research at UCLA, including Herceptin, Avastin, Tarceva, Iressa, Gleevec and Sutent for lung, breast, kidney and colorectal cancers as well as chronic myelogenous leukemia and gastrointestinal stromal tumors.

UCLA researchers are breaking new ground in cutting-edge gene therapy and with angiogenesis inhibitors, a class of drugs that attempt to fight cancer by cutting off the blood supply to tumors. And state-of-the-art molecular genetics provide the foundation for UCLA's Brain Tumor Program.

UCLA's Jonsson Cancer Center

Designated by the National Cancer Institute as one of only 39 comprehensive cancer centers in the United States, UCLA's Jonsson Cancer Center has earned an international reputation for developing new cancer therapies, providing the best in experimental and traditional treatments, and expertly guiding and training the next generation of medical researchers. The center's 250 physicians and scientists treat upwards of 20,000 patient visits per year and offer hundreds of clinical trials that provide the latest in experimental cancer treatments (www.cancer.mednet.ucla.edu). The center also offers patients and families complete psychological and support services.

UCLA's Jonsson Cancer Center has been ranked the best cancer center in California by *U.S. News & World Report*'s Annual Best Hospitals survey for the seventh year. UCLA Medical Center, of which the Cancer Center is a part, has ranked best in the West for the past 17 years.

Call 1-800 UCLA-MD1 (825-2631)
for a referral to a UCLA doctor.

THE UCLA HEMATOLOGY/ ONCOLOGY PROGRAM OFFERS TREATMENTS FOR:

Advanced malignancies

Breast cancer

Bone marrow/stem cell transplantation

Gastrointestinal oncology

Genitourinary oncology

Head and neck cancers

Leukemia

Lymphomas

Melanoma

Multiple myeloma

Neuro-oncology

Thoracic oncology

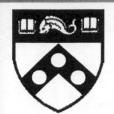

Penn Cancer Services
University of Pennsylvania Health System
Philadelphia, PA
1-800-789-PENN (7366)
pennhealth.com/cancer

Leader in Cancer Care: Abramson Cancer Center of the University of Pennsylvania

The Abramson Cancer Center is one of a select group of cancer centers in the country awarded the prestigious designation of *Comprehensive Cancer Center*. This status reflects our outstanding research, clinical services, education and information services and community outreach.

The Cancer Center has established a variety of interdisciplinary centers dedicated to specific cancers. Each center offers patients a complete evaluation and treatment options by a team of doctors with recognized expertise in that type of cancer.

What Sets Abramson Apart?

More than 300 full-time Penn faculty are actively involved in the diagnosis and treatment of patients with cancer
Patients benefit from having a dedicated multidisciplinary team working with them throughout their cancer experience
Emphasis on patient education to empower our patients to be active participants in their care.
The Cancer Risk Evaluation Program for women concerned about their risk for breast and ovarian cancer.
One of the foremost cancer research centers in the country
Comprehensive medical care for patients with other medical conditions such diabetes, pregnancy or heart disease.
Penn's cancer specialists work closely with a patient's personal physician.
Full range of support services to compliment medical care including nutritional counseling, support groups, cancer rehabilitation, complementary and alternative therapies and pain and symptom management.
Cancer Network of select community hospitals in Pennsylvania and New Jersey who collaborate with the Cancer Center

The Raymond and Ruth Perelman Center for Advanced Medicine

Opening in 2008, the will encompass the Abramson Cancer Center, blending outstanding medical practitioners with state-of-the-art technology to offer the most advanced cancer treatment options available.

The Roberts Proton Therapy Center

Opening in 2009, **the Center will be the largest proton therapy treatment facility in the world facilitating scientific research to measure and improve this innovative therapy.**

Overview

The University of Pennsylvania Health System is one of the leading health care providers in the country, known for its innovative approaches to cancer diagnosis and treatment as well as the care and compassion of its staff. United in its commitment to clinical excellence and advanced research, the Health System is dedicated to improving the chances for recovery and enhancing the quality of life for its patients.

Locations
Hospital of the University of Pennsylvania
Penn Presbyterian Medical Center
Pennsylvania Hospital
Penn Medicine at Radnor
Penn Medicine at Cherry Hill

B44

Wake Forest University Baptist
MEDICAL CENTER ®
Comprehensive Cancer Center

Medical Center Boulevard • Winston-Salem, NC 27157
PAL® (Physician-to-physician calls) 1-800-277-7654
Health On-Call® (Patient access) 1-800-446-2255
www.wfubmc.edu/cancer/

TOP RANKINGS
The Comprehensive Cancer Center of Wake Forest University Baptist Medical is among an elite group of only 39 U.S. cancer centers designated by the National Cancer Institute as comprehensive, indicating excellence in research, patient care and education. The comprehensive designation was renewed for an additional five years in late 2006.

RESEARCH ADVANTAGES
Wake Forest Baptist offers more cancer-related clinical trials than any other hospital in western N.C. From gene therapy to vitamin and nutrition studies to new surgical and radiological treatments, patients benefit from the leading edge of cancer knowledge and care. Innovative basic science, public health and clinical research promote new discovery about prevention, detection and treatment of cancers. Wake Forest scientists were first in the world to discover cancer resistant cells in mice.

TECHNOLOGY AND TREATMENT STRENGTHS
Wake Forest University Baptist Medical Center is home to North Carolina's first Gamma Knife, a non-invasive, stereotactic radiosurgical tool used to treat malignant and benign brain tumors once considered inoperable. Operated by one of the nation's most experienced treatment teams, the Gamma Knife painlessly bombards tumors with precisely focused beams of gamma energy – sparing normal tissue -- and is performed on an outpatient basis. Extracranial body stereotactic radiosurgery offers new options for other types of cancers.

Wake Forest Baptist offers an integrated brachytherapy unit (IBU) and highly targeted Intensity Modulated Radiation Therapy (IMRT) for treatment of prostate, brain, lung, head and neck, and gynecological cancers. Other treatment innovations include IPHC (intraperitoneal hyperthermic chemotherapy) for abdominal cavity cancers and radiofrequency ablation for liver malignancies.

MULTIDISCIPLINARY EXPERTISE
Expert, subspecialized oncology teams provide patients a consensus opinion on treatment. Multidisciplinary centers include the Thoracic Oncology Program, the Breast Care Center, the Brain Tumor Clinic and the Head and Neck Cancers Multidisciplinary Clinic.

**To make an appointment or find a specialist, call Health On-Call®
at 1-800-446-2255.**

HIGHLIGHTS OF EXCELLENCE

- Western North Carolina's only NCI-designated Comprehensive Cancer Center offers the convenience and comfort of a state-of-the-art Outpatient Cancer Center. The nation's first Cancer Patient Support Group was developed here.

- The Cancer Center's Blood and Marrow Transplant Program operates the nation's second-largest collection site.

- The Breast Cancer Risk Assessment Clinic and the Hereditary Cancer Clinic help patients understand their risk profile.

- Minimally invasive treatments include high dose rate (HDR) brachytherapy for prostate cancer. Lymph node mapping increases chance for lymph-sparing breast surgery.

- Clinical trials testing new methods of drug delivery offer patients with brain tumors potentially more effective treatment while minimizing effects on healthy tissue.

KNOWLEDGE MAKES ALL THE DIFFERENCE.

Neurological Surgery

A neurological surgeon provides the operative and non-operative management (i.e., prevention, diagnosis, evaluation, treatment, critical care and rehabilitation) of disorders of the central, peripheral and autonomic nervous systems, including their supporting structures and vascular supply; the evaluation and treatment of pathological processes which modify function or activity of the nervous system; and the operative and non-operative management of pain. A neurological surgeon treats patients with disorders of the nervous system; disorders of the brain, meninges, skull and their blood supply, including the extracranial carotid and vertebral arteries; disorders of the pituitary gland; disorders of the spinal cord, meninges and vertebral column, including those which may require treatment by spinal fusion or instrumentation; and disorders of the cranial and spinal nerves throughout their distribution.

Training Required: Seven years (including general surgery)

Pediatric Neurological Surgery: The American Board of Pediatric Neurological Surgery (ABPNS) is not a recognized ABMS subspecialty. However, this designation has been included because the certification process is meaningful and rigorous. It is awarded to those doctors who hold a current ABMS certification in Neurological Surgery, have completed a fully accredited one year, post-graduate fellowship in pediatric neurological surgery, and have submitted surgical logs indicating a practice of pediatric neurological surgery for one year, followed by a written examination.

Neurological Surgery

New England

Black, Peter MD/PhD [NS] - Spec Exp: Brain Tumors; Pituitary Tumors; Hospital: Brigham & Women's Hosp, Children's Hospital - Boston; Address: Brigham & Women's Hosp, Dept Neurosurg, 75 Francis St, Boston, MA 02115; Phone: 617-732-6810; Board Cert: Neurological Surgery 1984; Med School: McGill Univ 1970; Resid: Surgery, Mass Genl Hosp 1972; Neurological Surgery, Mass Genl Hosp 1980; Fellow: Neurosurgical Oncology, Mass Genl Hosp 1976; Fac Appt: Prof NS, Harvard Med Sch

Borges, Lawrence F MD [NS] - Spec Exp: Spinal Surgery; Spinal Tumors; Hospital: Mass Genl Hosp; Address: Mass Genl Hosp, Div Neurosurg, 32 Fruit St, Boston, MA 02114-2620; Phone: 617-726-6156; Board Cert: Neurological Surgery 1986; Med School: Johns Hopkins Univ 1977; Resid: Neurological Surgery, Mass Genl Hosp 1983; Fac Appt: Assoc Prof S, Harvard Med Sch

Chapman, Paul H MD [NS] - Spec Exp: Pediatric Neurosurgery; Brain & Spinal Tumors-Pediatric; Hospital: Mass Genl Hosp; Address: MGH Gray 5, 55 Fruit St, rm GRB-502, Boston, MA 02114-2622; Phone: 617-726-3887; Board Cert: Neurological Surgery 1976; Pediatric Neurological Surgery 1996; Med School: Harvard Med Sch 1964; Resid: Surgery, Mass Genl Hosp 1966; Neurological Surgery, Mass Genl Hosp 1972; Fellow: Neurological Surgery, Hosp Sick Chldn; Fac Appt: Prof S, Harvard Med Sch

Cosgrove, G Rees MD [NS] - Spec Exp: Brain Tumors; Hospital: Lahey Clin, Emerson Hosp; Address: Lahey Clinic, 41 Mall Rd, Burlington, MA 01805; Phone: 781-744-1990; Board Cert: Neurological Surgery 1989; Med School: Queens Univ 1980; Resid: Neurological Surgery, Montreal Neur Inst 1986; Fac Appt: Prof NS, Tufts Univ

David, Carlos MD [NS] - Spec Exp: Cerebrovascular Surgery; Skull Base Tumors & Surgery; Hospital: Lahey Clin, Emerson Hosp; Address: Lahey Clinic, Dept Neurosurgery, 41 Mall Rd, Burlington, MA 01805; Phone: 781-744-8643; Board Cert: Neurological Surgery 2001; Med School: Univ Miami Sch Med 1990; Resid: Neurological Surgery, Jackson Memorial Hosp 1995; Fellow: Cerebrovascular & Skull Base Surgery, Barrow Neuro Inst 1997; Fac Appt: Assoc Clin Prof NS, Tufts Univ

Day, Arthur L MD [NS] - Spec Exp: Orbital Tumors/Cancer; Brain Tumors; Hospital: Brigham & Women's Hosp, St Elizabeth's Med Ctr; Address: Brigham & Womens Hosp, Dept Neurosurgery, 75 Francis St, Boston, MA 02115; Phone: 617-525-7777; Board Cert: Neurological Surgery 1980; Med School: Louisiana State Univ 1972; Resid: Neurological Surgery, Shands-Univ Florida Hosp 1977; Fellow: Neurological Pathology, Shands-Univ Florida Hosp 1978; Fac Appt: Prof NS, Harvard Med Sch

Duhaime, Ann Christine MD [NS] - Spec Exp: Pediatric Neurosurgery; Brain Tumors; Hospital: Dartmouth - Hitchcock Med Ctr; Address: Chldns Hosp at Dartmouth-Hitchcock Med Ctr, One Medical Center Drive, Lebanon, NH 03756; Phone: 603-653-9880; Board Cert: Neurological Surgery 1990; Pediatric Neurological Surgery 1996; Med School: Univ Pennsylvania 1981; Resid: Neurological Surgery, Hosp Univ Penn 1987; Fellow: Pediatric Neurological Surgery, Chldns Hosp 1987; Fac Appt: Prof S, Dartmouth Med Sch

Goumnerova, Liliana MD [NS] - **Spec Exp:** Pediatric Neurosurgery; Brain Tumors; **Hospital:** Children's Hospital - Boston, Dana-Farber Cancer Inst; **Address:** Chldns Hosp, 300 Longwood Ave, Hunniwell Fl 2, Boston, MA 02115; **Phone:** 617-355-6364; **Board Cert:** Neurological Surgery 1992; Pediatric Neurological Surgery 1997; **Med School:** Canada 1980; **Resid:** Neurological Surgery, Univ Ottawa 1986; **Fellow:** Pediatric Neurological Surgery, Hosp for Sick Chldn 1988; Neurological Science, Univ Penn 1990; **Fac Appt:** Assoc Prof S, Harvard Med Sch

Martuza, Robert L MD [NS] - **Spec Exp:** Brain Tumors; Skull Base Surgery; **Hospital:** Mass Genl Hosp; **Address:** Mass General Hosp, 55 Fruit St, White Bldg, rm 502, Boston, MA 02114; **Phone:** 617-726-8581; **Board Cert:** Neurological Surgery 1983; **Med School:** Harvard Med Sch 1973; **Resid:** Neurological Surgery, Mass Genl Hosp 1980; **Fac Appt:** Prof NS, Harvard Med Sch

Penar, Paul MD [NS] - **Spec Exp:** Brain & Spinal Tumors; Stereotactic Radiosurgery; Pain-Chronic; **Hospital:** FAHC - Med Ctr Campus; **Address:** Div Neurosurgery, Fletcher 5, 111 Colchester Ave, Burlington, VT 05401; **Phone:** 802-847-3072; **Board Cert:** Neurological Surgery 1989; **Med School:** Univ Mich Med Sch 1981; **Resid:** Neurological Surgery, Yale-New Haven Hosp 1987

Piepmeier, Joseph MD [NS] - **Spec Exp:** Neuro-Oncology; Brain & Spinal Cord Tumors; **Hospital:** Yale - New Haven Hosp; **Address:** Yale Sch Med, Dept Neurosurgery, 333 Cedar St Fl TMP-410, New Haven, CT 06520; **Phone:** 203-785-2791; **Board Cert:** Neurological Surgery 1984; **Med School:** Univ Tenn Coll Med, Memphis 1975; **Resid:** Neurological Surgery, Yale-New Haven Hosp 1982; **Fac Appt:** Prof NS, Yale Univ

Mid Atlantic

Andrews, David MD [NS] - **Spec Exp:** Brain Tumors; Stereotactic Radiosurgery; **Hospital:** Thomas Jefferson Univ Hosp (page 82); **Address:** Thom Jefferson Univ Hosp, Dept Neurosurg, 909 Walnut St Fl 2, Philadelphia, PA 19107-5109; **Phone:** 215-503-7005; **Board Cert:** Neurological Surgery 1992; **Med School:** Univ Colorado 1983; **Resid:** Neurological Surgery, NY Presby Hos-Cornell Med Ctr 1989; **Fellow:** Neuro-Oncology, Meml Sloan Kettering Cancer Ctr 1987; **Fac Appt:** Prof NS, Thomas Jefferson Univ

Bilsky, Mark H MD [NS] - **Spec Exp:** Spinal Tumors; Skull Base Tumors; Brain Tumors; **Hospital:** Meml Sloan Kettering Cancer Ctr (page 76), NY-Presby Hosp (page 79); **Address:** Memorial Sloan Kettering Cancer Ctr, 1275 York Ave, rm C705, New York, NY 10021; **Phone:** 212-639-8526; **Board Cert:** Neurological Surgery 1999; **Med School:** Emory Univ 1988; **Resid:** Neurological Surgery, NY Hosp-Cornell Med Ctr 1994; **Fellow:** Neuro-Oncology, Louisville Univ Med Ctr 1995; **Fac Appt:** Assoc Prof NS, Cornell Univ-Weill Med Coll

Neurological Surgery

Brem, Henry MD [NS] - **Spec Exp:** Brain & Spinal Cord Tumors; Skull Base Tumors; Pituitary Tumors; **Hospital:** Johns Hopkins Hosp - Baltimore, Johns Hopkins Bayview Med Ctr; **Address:** Johns Hopkins Med Ctr-Dept NeuroSurgery, 600 N Wolfe St Bldg Meyer 7-113, Baltimore, MD 21287; **Phone:** 410-955-2248; **Board Cert:** Neurological Surgery 1986; **Med School:** Harvard Med Sch 1978; **Resid:** Neurological Surgery, Columbia-Presby Med Ctr 1984; **Fellow:** Neurological Surgery, Johns Hopkins Hosp 1980; **Fac Appt:** Prof NS, Johns Hopkins Univ

Bruce, Jeffrey MD [NS] - **Spec Exp:** Brain Tumors; Pituitary Tumors; Skull Base Surgery; **Hospital:** NY-Presby Hosp (page 79); **Address:** NY Presby Hosp, Dept Neurosurgery, 710 W 168th St N1 Bldg Fl 4 - rm 434, New York, NY 10032; **Phone:** 212-305-7346; **Board Cert:** Neurological Surgery 1993; **Med School:** UMDNJ-RW Johnson Med Sch 1983; **Resid:** Neurological Surgery, Columbia-Presby Med Ctr 1990; **Fellow:** Neurological Surgery, Nat Inst Health 1985; **Fac Appt:** Prof NS, Columbia P&S

Camins, Martin B MD [NS] - **Spec Exp:** Spinal Surgery; Brain Tumors; Microsurgery; **Hospital:** Mount Sinai Med Ctr (page 77), Lenox Hill Hosp; **Address:** 205 E 68th St, Ste T1C, New York, NY 10021-5735; **Phone:** 212-570-0100; **Board Cert:** Neurological Surgery 1980; **Med School:** Ros Franklin Univ/Chicago Med Sch 1969; **Resid:** Neurology, Neuro Inst-Columbia-Presby Med Ctr 1971; Neurological Surgery, Neuro Inst-Columbia Presb Med Ctry 1975; **Fellow:** Neurological Surgery, National Hosp 1974; Neurological Surgery, NYU Med Ctr 1978; **Fac Appt:** Clin Prof NS, Mount Sinai Sch Med

Carmel, Peter MD [NS] - **Spec Exp:** Brain Tumors-Pediatric; Skull Base Surgery; Pediatric Neurosurgery; **Hospital:** UMDNJ-Univ Hosp-Newark; **Address:** 90 Bergen St, Ste 8100, Newark, NJ 07104; **Phone:** 973-972-2323; **Board Cert:** Neurological Surgery 1969; Pediatric Neurological Surgery 1996; **Med School:** NYU Sch Med 1960; **Resid:** Neurological Surgery, Neuro Inst/Columbia Presby Med Ctr 1967; **Fac Appt:** Prof NS, UMDNJ-NJ Med Sch, Newark

Carson, Benjamin S MD [NS] - **Spec Exp:** Brain & Spinal Cord Tumors; Pediatric Neurosurgery; **Hospital:** Johns Hopkins Hosp - Baltimore; **Address:** 600 N Wolfe St, Harvey 811, Baltimore, MD 21287-8811; **Phone:** 410-955-7888; **Board Cert:** Neurological Surgery 1988; Pediatric Neurological Surgery ; **Med School:** Univ Mich Med Sch 1977; **Resid:** Neurological Surgery, Johns Hopkins Hosp 1983; **Fellow:** Pediatric Neurological Surgery, Queen Elizabeth II Med Ctr 1984; **Fac Appt:** Assoc Prof NS, Johns Hopkins Univ

de Lotbiniere, Alain MD [NS] - **Spec Exp:** Pain Management; Brain Tumors; Pituitary Tumors; **Hospital:** Northern Westchester Hosp; **Address:** Brain & Spine Surgeons of New York, 244 Westchester Ave, Ste 310, White Plains, NY 10603; **Phone:** 914-948-6688; **Board Cert:** Neurological Surgery 1994; **Med School:** McGill Univ 1981; **Resid:** Surgery, Royal Victoria Hosp 1983; Neurological Surgery, Royal Victoria Hosp 1988; **Fellow:** Neurological Surgery, Univ of Cambridge 1989

Di Giacinto, George V MD [NS] - **Spec Exp:** Spinal Surgery; Brain Tumors; Pain Management; **Hospital:** St Luke's - Roosevelt Hosp Ctr - Roosevelt Div (page 72); **Address:** 425 W 59th St, Ste 4E, New York, NY 10019; **Phone:** 212-523-8500; **Board Cert:** Neurological Surgery 1981; **Med School:** Harvard Med Sch 1970; **Resid:** Neurological Surgery, Columbia-Presby Hosp 1978

Feldstein, Neil A MD [NS] - **Spec Exp:** Pediatric Neurosurgery; Brain Tumors-Pediatric; Craniofacial Surgery-Pediatric; **Hospital:** NY-Presby Hosp (page 79); **Address:** Neurological Inst, 710 W 168th St Fl 2 - rm 213, New York, NY 10032; **Phone:** 212-305-1396; **Board Cert:** Neurological Surgery 1995; Pediatric Neurological Surgery 1995; **Med School:** NYU Sch Med 1984; **Resid:** Neurological Surgery, Baylor Coll Med 1989; **Fellow:** Pediatric Neurological Surgery, NYU Med Ctr 1991; **Fac Appt:** Asst Prof NS, Columbia P&S

Flamm, Eugene S MD [NS] - **Spec Exp:** Brain Tumors; **Hospital:** Montefiore Med Ctr; **Address:** Montefiore Med Ctr, 111 E 210th St, Bronx, NY 10467-2841; **Phone:** 718-920-2339; **Board Cert:** Neurological Surgery 1973; **Med School:** SUNY Buffalo 1962; **Resid:** Surgery, New York Hosp 1964; Neurological Surgery, NYU Med Ctr 1970; **Fellow:** Neurological Surgery, Univ Zurich 1971; **Fac Appt:** Prof NS, Albert Einstein Coll Med

Goodrich, James T MD [NS] - **Spec Exp:** Craniofacial Surgery/Reconstruction; Brain Tumors-Pediatric; Pediatric Neurosurgery; **Hospital:** Montefiore Med Ctr, Jacobi Med Ctr; **Address:** Montefiore Med Ctr, Dept Ped Neurosurgery, 111 E 210th St, Bronx, NY 10467-2401; **Phone:** 718-920-4197; **Board Cert:** Neurological Surgery 1989; Pediatric Neurological Surgery 1996; **Med School:** Columbia P&S 1980; **Resid:** Neurological Surgery, NY Neurological Inst 1986; **Fac Appt:** Prof NS, Albert Einstein Coll Med

Gutin, Philip MD [NS] - **Spec Exp:** Brain Tumors; Meningioma; **Hospital:** Meml Sloan Kettering Cancer Ctr (page 76), NY-Presby Hosp (page 79); **Address:** Meml Sloan Kettering Cancer Ctr, Dept Neurosurgery, 1275 York Ave, rm C703, New York, NY 10021-6007; **Phone:** 212-639-8556; **Board Cert:** Neurological Surgery 1981; **Med School:** Univ Pennsylvania 1971; **Resid:** Neurological Surgery, UCSF Med Ctr 1979; **Fellow:** Natl Cancer Inst 1976; **Fac Appt:** Prof NS, Cornell Univ-Weill Med Coll

Judy, Kevin MD [NS] - **Spec Exp:** Brain Tumors; **Hospital:** Hosp Univ Penn - UPHS (page 84), Pennsylvania Hosp (page 84); **Address:** Hosp Univ Penn-Dept Neurosurg, 3400 Spruce St, 3 Silverstein, Philadelphia, PA 19104; **Phone:** 215-662-7854; **Board Cert:** Neurological Surgery 1997; **Med School:** Univ Pittsburgh 1984; **Resid:** Surgery, Mercy Hosp 1986; Neurological Surgery, Johns Hopkins Hosp 1992; **Fellow:** Neurological Surgery, Johns Hopkins Hosp 1991; **Fac Appt:** Assoc Prof NS, Univ Pennsylvania

Kassam, Amin MD [NS] - **Spec Exp:** Skull Base Tumors & Surgery; Cerebrovascular Surgery; Endoscopic Surgery; Minimally Invasive Neurosurgery; **Hospital:** UPMC Presby, Pittsburgh; **Address:** Univ Pittsburgh Med Ctr, Dept Neurosurgery, 200 Lothrop St, Ste B400, Pittsburgh, PA 15213; **Phone:** 412-647-3685; **Med School:** Univ Toronto 1991; **Resid:** Neurological Surgery, Univ Ottawa Med Ctr 1997; **Fac Appt:** Assoc Prof NS, Univ Pittsburgh

Kelly, Patrick J MD [NS] - **Spec Exp:** Brain Tumors; Gliomas; **Hospital:** NYU Med Ctr (page 80), Lenox Hill Hosp; **Address:** NYU Med Ctr, Dept Neurological Surgery, 530 1st Ave, Ste 8R, New York, NY 10016; **Phone:** 212-263-8002; **Board Cert:** Neurological Surgery 1978; **Med School:** SUNY Buffalo 1966; **Resid:** Neurological Surgery, Northwestern Univ Hosp 1972; Neurological Surgery, Univ Texas Med Br Hosp 1974; **Fellow:** Neurological Surgery, St Anne Hosp 1977; **Fac Appt:** Prof NS, NYU Sch Med

Kobrine, Arthur MD/PhD [NS] - **Spec Exp:** Brain & Spinal Cord Tumors; **Hospital:** Sibley Mem Hosp, Georgetown Univ Hosp; **Address:** 2440 M St NW, Ste 315, Washington, DC 20037-1404; **Phone:** 202-293-7136; **Board Cert:** Neurological Surgery 1976; **Med School:** Northwestern Univ 1968; **Resid:** Neurological Surgery, Northwestern Univ Hosp 1970; Neurological Surgery, Walter Reed Army Hosp 1973; **Fellow:** Physiology, Geo Wash Univ 1979; **Fac Appt:** Clin Prof NS, Georgetown Univ

Neurological Surgery

Kondziolka, Douglas MD [NS] - **Spec Exp:** Brain Tumors-Adult & Pediatric; Brain Tumors-Metastatic; Gamma Knife Surgery; **Hospital:** UPMC Presby, Pittsburgh, Chldns Hosp of Pittsburgh - UPMC; **Address:** Univ Pittsburgh Med Ctr, Dept Neurological Surgery, 200 Lothrop St, Ste B400, Pittsburgh, PA 15213; **Phone:** 412-647-9990; **Board Cert:** Neurological Surgery 1994; **Med School:** Univ Toronto 1985; **Resid:** Neurological Surgery, Univ Toronto 1991; **Fellow:** Stereo Neurological Surgery, UPMC Presby Med Ctr 1991; **Fac Appt:** Prof NS, Univ Pittsburgh

Lavyne, Michael H MD [NS] - **Spec Exp:** Spinal Tumors; **Hospital:** NY-Presby Hosp (page 79), Hosp For Special Surgery; **Address:** 110 E 55th St Fl 9, New York, NY 10022; **Phone:** 212-486-9100; **Board Cert:** Neurological Surgery 1982; **Med School:** Cornell Univ-Weill Med Coll 1972; **Resid:** Neurological Surgery, Mass Genl Hosp 1979; **Fellow:** Neurology, Beth Israel Hosp 1974; **Fac Appt:** Clin Prof NS, Cornell Univ-Weill Med Coll

Loftus, Christopher M MD [NS] - **Spec Exp:** Cerebrovascular Surgery; Brain Tumors; **Hospital:** Temple Univ Hosp; **Address:** Temple Univ School Med, 3401 N Broad St, Parkinson Pavilion 540, Philadelphia, PA 19140; **Phone:** 215-707-9790; **Board Cert:** Neurological Surgery 1987; **Med School:** SUNY Downstate 1979; **Resid:** Neurological Surgery, Columbia-Presby Med Ctr 1985; **Fac Appt:** Prof NS, Temple Univ

Lunsford, L Dade MD [NS] - **Spec Exp:** Brain Tumors; Stereotactic Radiosurgery; **Hospital:** UPMC Presby, Pittsburgh, Chldns Hosp of Pittsburgh - UPMC; **Address:** UPMC Presbyterian Hosp, 200 Lothrop St, Ste B400, Pittsburgh, PA 15213-2536; **Phone:** 412-647-3685; **Board Cert:** Neurological Surgery 1983; **Med School:** Columbia P&S 1974; **Resid:** Neurological Surgery, Univ Pittsburgh Med Ctr 1980; **Fellow:** Stereo Neurological Surgery, Karolinska Hospital 1981; **Fac Appt:** Prof NS, Univ Pittsburgh

McCormick, Paul C MD [NS] - **Spec Exp:** Spinal Surgery; Spinal Tumors; **Hospital:** NY-Presby Hosp (page 79), Valley Hosp; **Address:** 710 W 168th St, Ste 406, New York, NY 10032-2603; **Phone:** 212-305-7976; **Board Cert:** Neurological Surgery 1993; **Med School:** Columbia P&S 1982; **Resid:** Neurological Surgery, Columbia Presby Med Ctr 1989; **Fellow:** Neurological Surgery, Natl Inst Hlth 1984; Spinal Surgery, Med Coll Wisconsin 1990; **Fac Appt:** Prof NS, Columbia P&S

O'Rourke, Donald MD [NS] - **Spec Exp:** Neuro-Oncology; Brain Tumors; **Hospital:** Hosp Univ Penn - UPHS (page 84); **Address:** Hosp Univ Penn - Dept Neurosurg, 3400 Spruce St, 3 Silverstein, Philadelphia, PA 19104; **Phone:** 215-662-3490; **Board Cert:** Neurological Surgery 1998; **Med School:** Univ Pennsylvania 1987; **Resid:** Neurological Surgery, Hosp Univ Penn 1994; **Fac Appt:** Assoc Prof NS, Univ Pennsylvania

Pollack, Ian MD [NS] - **Spec Exp:** Pediatric Neurosurgery; Brain Tumors; Craniofacial Surgery; **Hospital:** Chldns Hosp of Pittsburgh - UPMC, UPMC Presby, Pittsburgh; **Address:** Chldns Hosp Pittsburgh, Div Neurosurgery, 3705 Fifth Ave, Ste 3670A, Pittsburgh, PA 15213-2524; **Phone:** 412-692-5881; **Board Cert:** Neurological Surgery 1996; Pediatric Neurological Surgery 1997; **Med School:** Johns Hopkins Univ 1984; **Resid:** Neurological Surgery, Univ Pittsburgh Med Ctr 1991; **Fellow:** Pediatric Neurological Surgery, Hosp Sick Chldn 1992; **Fac Appt:** Prof NS, Univ Pittsburgh

Post, Kalmon MD [NS] - **Spec Exp:** Pituitary Tumors; **Hospital:** Mount Sinai Med Ctr (page 77); **Address:** 5 E 98th St, Fl 7, New York, NY 10029-6501; **Phone:** 212-241-0933; **Board Cert:** Neurological Surgery 1978; **Med School:** NYU Sch Med 1967; **Resid:** Surgery, Bellevue Hosp 1969; Neurological Surgery, Bellevue Hosp-NYU 1975; **Fac Appt:** Prof NS, Mount Sinai Sch Med

Rosenwasser, Robert H MD [NS] - **Spec Exp:** Cerebrovascular Surgery; Neuro-Oncology; **Hospital:** Thomas Jefferson Univ Hosp (page 82); **Address:** Thomas Jefferson University Hospital, 909 Walnut St Fl 2, Philadelphia, PA 19107; **Phone:** 215-955-7000; **Board Cert:** Neurological Surgery 1987; **Med School:** Louisiana State Univ 1979; **Resid:** Neurological Surgery, Temple Univ Hosp 1984; **Fellow:** Neurological Vascular Surgery, Univ West Ontarion 1985; Interventional Neuroradiology, NYU Med Ctr 1993; **Fac Appt:** Prof NS, Thomas Jefferson Univ

Sen, Chandranath MD [NS] - **Spec Exp:** Brain Tumors; Skull Base Tumors; Skull Base Surgery; **Hospital:** St Luke's - Roosevelt Hosp Ctr - Roosevelt Div (page 72); **Address:** St Lukes Roosevelt Hosp Ctr, Dept Neurosurgery, 1000 10th Ave, Ste 5G-80, New York, NY 10019; **Phone:** 212-523-6720; **Board Cert:** Neurological Surgery 1989; **Med School:** India 1976; **Resid:** Surgery, Univ Wisconsin Hosps 1980; Neurological Surgery, Univ Wisconsin Hosps 1985; **Fellow:** Microsurgery, Univ Pittsburgh Med Ctr 1986

Stieg, Philip E MD/PhD [NS] - **Spec Exp:** Skull Base Surgery; Meningioma; Chordomas; **Hospital:** NY-Presby Hosp (page 79); **Address:** 525 E 68th St, STARR 651, New York, NY 10021-9800; **Phone:** 212-746-4684; **Board Cert:** Neurological Surgery 1992; **Med School:** Med Coll Wisc 1983; **Resid:** Neurological Surgery, Dallas Chldns Hosp/Parkland Meml Hosp 1988; **Fellow:** Neurological Biology, Karolinska Inst 1988; **Fac Appt:** Prof NS, Cornell Univ-Weill Med Coll

Sutton, Leslie N MD [NS] - **Spec Exp:** Brain Tumors-Pediatric; **Hospital:** Chldns Hosp of Philadelphia, The; **Address:** Childrens Hosp of Phila -Div Neurosurgery, 34th St & Civic Ctr Blvd Wood 6 Bldg, Philadelphia, PA 19104; **Phone:** 215-590-2780; **Board Cert:** Neurological Surgery 1984; Pediatric Neurological Surgery 1996; **Med School:** Univ Pennsylvania 1975; **Resid:** Neurological Surgery, Hosp Univ Penn 1981; **Fac Appt:** Prof NS, Univ Pennsylvania

Turtz, Alan R MD [NS] - **Spec Exp:** Brain Tumors; Pituitary Tumors; Spinal Surgery; **Hospital:** Cooper Univ Hosp; **Address:** 3 Cooper Plaza, Ste 403, Camden, NJ 08103; **Phone:** 856-968-7898; **Board Cert:** Neurological Surgery 1995; **Med School:** Med Coll PA 1986; **Resid:** Neurological Surgery, Med Coll Penn 1992; **Fac Appt:** Asst Prof NS, Jefferson Med Coll

Wisoff, Jeffrey H MD [NS] - **Spec Exp:** Pediatric Neurosurgery; Brain Tumors-Pediatric; **Hospital:** NYU Med Ctr (page 80), Maimonides Med Ctr (page 75); **Address:** 317 E 34th St, Ste 1002, New York, NY 10016-4974; **Phone:** 212-263-6419; **Board Cert:** Neurological Surgery 1990; Pediatric Neurological Surgery 1996; **Med School:** Geo Wash Univ 1978; **Resid:** Neurological Surgery, NYU Med Ctr/Bellevue Hosp 1984; **Fellow:** Pediatric Neurological Surgery, NYU Med Ctr 1985; **Fac Appt:** Assoc Prof NS, NYU Sch Med

Southeast

Asher, Anthony MD [NS] - **Spec Exp:** Brain Tumors; Stereotactic Radiosurgery; **Hospital:** Carolinas Med Ctr, Presby Hosp - Charlotte; **Address:** 225 Baldwin Ave, Charlotte, NC 28204; **Phone:** 704-376-1605; **Board Cert:** Neurological Surgery 1998; **Med School:** Wayne State Univ 1987; **Resid:** Neurological Surgery, Univ Mich Med Ctr 1995; **Fellow:** Surgical Oncology, Natl Cancer Inst 1991

Boop, Frederick A MD [NS] - **Spec Exp:** Pediatric Neurosurgery; Brain Tumors; **Hospital:** Le Bonheur Chldns Med Ctr, Methodist Univ Hosp - Memphis; **Address:** Semmes Murphy Clinic, 1211 Union Ave, Ste 200, Memphis, TN 38104; **Phone:** 901-259-5340; **Board Cert:** Neurological Surgery 1993; **Med School:** Univ Ark 1983; **Resid:** Neurological Surgery, Univ Tex Hlth Sci Ctr 1989; Neurological Surgery, Inst Neur/Hosp Sick Chldn 1987; **Fellow:** Epilepsy, Univ Minn 1989; Pediatric Neurological Surgery, Ark Chldns Hosp 1990; **Fac Appt:** Assoc Prof NS, Univ Tenn Coll Med, Memphis

Brem, Steven MD [NS] - **Spec Exp:** Brain Tumors; Pituitary Tumors; Clinical Trials; **Hospital:** H Lee Moffitt Cancer Ctr & Research Inst; **Address:** H. Lee Moffitt Cancer Ctr/ Neurosurgery, 12902 Magnolia Drive, Tampa, FL 33612-9497; **Phone:** 813-745-3063; **Board Cert:** Neurological Surgery 1983; **Med School:** Harvard Med Sch 1972; **Resid:** Neurological Surgery, Massachusetts Genl Hosp 1981; **Fellow:** Oncology, Natl Cancer Inst 1976; **Fac Appt:** Prof NS, Univ S Fla Coll Med

Ewend, Matthew MD [NS] - **Spec Exp:** Brain Tumors; Pituitary Tumors; Pediatric Neurosurgery; **Hospital:** Univ NC Hosps; **Address:** Univ North Carolina Neurosurgery, 3015 Burnett Womack Bldg, CB# 7060, Chapel Hill, NC 27599; **Phone:** 919-966-1374; **Board Cert:** Neurological Surgery 2001; **Med School:** Johns Hopkins Univ 1990; **Resid:** Neurological Surgery, Johns Hopkins Hospital 1994; **Fellow:** Neuro-Oncology, National Institutes of Health 1996; **Fac Appt:** Asst Prof NS, Univ NC Sch Med

Ferraz, Francisco M MD [NS] - **Spec Exp:** Brain Tumors; **Hospital:** Virginia Hosp Ctr - Arlington, Inova Loudoun Hosp; **Address:** 611 S Carlin Springs Rd, Ste 105, Arlington, VA 22204; **Phone:** 703-845-1552; **Board Cert:** Neurological Surgery 1987; **Med School:** Brazil 1975; **Resid:** Neurological Surgery, Georgetown Univ Affil Hosp 1982; **Fac Appt:** Assoc Prof NS, Georgetown Univ

Friedman, Allan H MD [NS] - **Spec Exp:** Brain Tumors; Skull Base Tumors; **Hospital:** Duke Univ Med Ctr; **Address:** Duke Univ Med Ctr, DUMC 3807, Durham, NC 27710; **Phone:** 919-681-6421; **Board Cert:** Neurological Surgery 1983; **Med School:** Univ IL Coll Med 1974; **Resid:** Neurological Surgery, Duke Univ Med Ctr 1980; **Fellow:** Vascular Surgery, Univ Western Ontario 1981; **Fac Appt:** Prof S, Duke Univ

Fuchs, Herbert E MD/PhD [NS] - **Spec Exp:** Pediatric Neurosurgery; Brain Tumors-Pediatric; **Hospital:** Duke Univ Med Ctr; **Address:** Duke Univ Med Ctr, Box 3272, Durham, NC 27710; **Phone:** 919-681-0894; **Board Cert:** Neurological Surgery 1995; Pediatric Neurological Surgery 1997; **Med School:** Duke Univ 1984; **Resid:** Neurological Surgery, Duke Univ Med Ctr 1991; **Fellow:** Pediatric Neurological Surgery, Chldns Meml Hosp 1992; **Fac Appt:** Assoc Prof S, Duke Univ

Guthrie, Barton L MD [NS] - **Spec Exp:** Brain Tumors; Stereotactic Radiosurgery; **Hospital:** Univ of Ala Hosp at Birmingham; **Address:** Univ Alabama, Div Neurosurg, 510 20th St S, FOT 1038, Birmingham, AL 35294; **Phone:** 205-934-8136; **Board Cert:** Neurological Surgery 1992; **Med School:** Univ Ala 1980; **Resid:** Neurological Surgery, Mayo Clinic 1988; **Fellow:** Neurological Surgery, Stanford Univ Med Ctr 1988; **Fac Appt:** Assoc Prof NS, Univ Ala

Heros, Roberto MD [NS] - **Spec Exp:** Cerebrovascular Surgery; Skull Base Surgery; Brain Tumors; **Hospital:** Jackson Meml Hosp; **Address:** Univ Miami, Dept Neurosurgery, 1095 NW 14th Terrace, Miami, FL 33136; **Phone:** 305-243-4572; **Board Cert:** Neurological Surgery 1979; **Med School:** Univ Tenn Coll Med, Memphis 1968; **Resid:** Surgery, Mass Genl Hosp 1970; Neurological Surgery, Mass Genl Hosp 1976; **Fac Appt:** Prof NS, Univ Miami Sch Med

Markert Jr, James M MD [NS] - **Spec Exp:** Brain Tumors; Gamma Knife Surgery; Clinical Trials; **Hospital:** Univ of Ala Hosp at Birmingham; **Address:** Univ Alabama, Div Neurosurgery, 510 20th St S, FOT 1050, Birmingham, AL 35294; **Phone:** 205-975-6985; **Board Cert:** Neurological Surgery 1999; **Med School:** Columbia P&S 1988; **Resid:** Neurological Surgery, Univ Mich Med Ctr 1995; **Fellow:** Neuro-Oncology, Mass Genl Hosp; **Fac Appt:** Prof NS, Univ Ala

Morrison, Glenn MD [NS] - **Spec Exp:** Pediatric Neurosurgery; Craniofacial Surgery; Spinal Cord Tumors; Brain Tumors-Pediatric; **Hospital:** Miami Children's Hosp, Jackson Meml Hosp; **Address:** Medical Arts Bldg, 3215 SW 62nd Ave, Ste 3109, Miami, FL 33155; **Phone:** 305-662-8386; **Board Cert:** Neurological Surgery 1976; Pediatric Neurological Surgery 1996; **Med School:** Case West Res Univ 1967; **Resid:** Neurological Surgery, Case Western Univ Hosp 1974; **Fac Appt:** Prof NS, Univ Miami Sch Med

Olson, Jeffrey J MD [NS] - **Spec Exp:** Neuro-Oncology; Brain Tumors; Stereotactic Radiosurgery; **Hospital:** Emory Univ Hosp, Crawford Long Hosp of Emory Univ; **Address:** Emory Univ, Dept Neurosurgery, 1365B Clifton Rd NE, Ste 2200, Atlanta, GA 30322; **Phone:** 404-778-5770; **Board Cert:** Neurological Surgery 1989; **Med School:** Univ Minn 1981; **Resid:** Neurological Surgery, Univ Iowa Hosps & Clinics 1987; **Fellow:** Neurological Surgery, Natl Inst Hlth 1990; **Fac Appt:** Prof NS, Emory Univ

Parent, Andrew D MD [NS] - **Spec Exp:** Pediatric Neurosurgery; Neuroendocrine Tumors; Pituitary Tumors; **Hospital:** Univ Hosps & Clins - Jackson; **Address:** Univ Miss Med Ctr- Dept Neurosurgery, 2500 N State St, Jackson, MS 39216-4500; **Phone:** 601-984-5702; **Board Cert:** Neurological Surgery 1981; **Med School:** Univ VT Coll Med 1970; **Resid:** Neurological Surgery, Emory Univ 1978; **Fellow:** Neurological Surgery, Univ Tex Med Br 1974; **Fac Appt:** Prof NS, Univ Miss

Sampson, John H MD/PhD [NS] - **Spec Exp:** Brain Tumors; Clinical Trials; **Hospital:** Duke Univ Med Ctr; **Address:** Duke Univ Med Ctr, Box 3050, Durham, NC 27710; **Phone:** 919-684-9041; **Board Cert:** Neurological Surgery 2002; **Med School:** Univ Manitoba 1990; **Resid:** Neurological Surgery, Duke Univ Med Ctr 1998; **Fellow:** Neurological Intensive Care, Duke Univ Med Ctr; **Fac Appt:** Assoc Prof S, Duke Univ

Sanford, Robert A MD [NS] - **Spec Exp:** Pediatric Neurosurgery; Brain Tumors-Pediatric; **Hospital:** Le Bonheur Chldns Med Ctr, St Jude Children's Research Hosp; **Address:** 6325 Humphreys Blvd, Memphis, TN 38120; **Phone:** 901-522-7762; **Board Cert:** Neurological Surgery 1976; Pediatric Neurological Surgery 1980; **Med School:** Univ Ark 1967; **Resid:** Neurological Surgery, Univ Minneapolis Med Ctr 1973; **Fac Appt:** Prof NS, Univ Tenn Coll Med, Memphis

Shaffrey, Mark E MD [NS] - **Spec Exp:** Brain Tumors; Clinical Trials; Spinal Cord Tumors; Spinal Tumors; **Hospital:** Univ Virginia Med Ctr; **Address:** UVA Health System, Dept Neurosurgery, PO Box 800212, Charlottesville, VA 22908; **Phone:** 434-924-1843; **Board Cert:** Neurological Surgery 2000; **Med School:** Univ VA Sch Med 1987; **Resid:** Neurological Surgery, Univ Virginia Med Ctr 1991; **Fellow:** Microvascular Physiology, NIH 1992, Neurological Pathology, Univ Virginia Med Ctr 1993; **Fac Appt:** Prof NS, Univ VA Sch Med

Sills Jr, Allen MD [NS] - **Spec Exp:** Brain & Spinal Tumors; Gamma Knife Surgery; **Hospital:** Methodist Univ Hosp - Memphis; **Address:** Semmes-Murphey Clinic, 1211 Union Ave, Ste 200, Memphis, TN 38104; **Phone:** 901-259-5340; **Board Cert:** Neurological Surgery 2002; **Med School:** Johns Hopkins Univ 1990; **Resid:** Neurological Surgery, Johns Hopkins Hosp 1994; **Fellow:** Neuro-Oncology, Hunterian Neurosurg Lab/Johns Hopkins 1996; **Fac Appt:** Prof NS, Univ Tenn Coll Med, Memphis

Neurological Surgery

Tatter, Stephen MD/PhD [NS] - **Spec Exp:** Brain Tumors; Pituitary Tumors; Stereotactic Radiosurgery; **Hospital:** Wake Forest Univ Baptist Med Ctr (page 85); **Address:** Wake Forest Univ Sch Med, Dept Neurosurg, Medical Center Blvd, Winston-Salem, NC 27157-1029; **Phone:** 336-716-4047; **Board Cert:** Neurological Surgery 2004; **Med School:** Cornell Univ-Weill Med Coll 1990; **Resid:** Neurological Surgery, Mass Genl Hosp 1996; **Fellow:** Neurological Surgery, Mass Genl Hosp 1997; **Fac Appt:** Assoc Prof NS, Wake Forest Univ

Wharen Jr, Robert E MD [NS] - **Spec Exp:** Brain Tumors; **Hospital:** St Luke's Hosp - Jacksonville; **Address:** Mayo Clinic, Dept Neurosurgery, 4500 San Pablo Rd, Jacksonville, FL 32224-1865; **Phone:** 904-953-2103; **Board Cert:** Neurological Surgery 1988; **Med School:** Penn State Univ-Hershey Med Ctr 1979; **Resid:** Neurological Surgery, Mayo Clinic 1985; **Fac Appt:** Prof NS, Mayo Med Sch

Young, A Byron MD [NS] - **Spec Exp:** Brain Tumors; Stereotactic Radiosurgery; **Hospital:** Univ of Kentucky Chandler Hosp; **Address:** Univ Kentucky Med Ctr, MS 101, Div Neurosurgery, 800 Rose St, Lexington, KY 40536-0298; **Phone:** 859-323-5861; **Board Cert:** Neurological Surgery 1974; **Med School:** Univ KY Coll Med 1965; **Resid:** Surgery, Vanderbilt Hosp 1967; Neurological Surgery, Vanderbilt Hosp 1971; **Fac Appt:** Prof S, Univ KY Coll Med

Midwest

Albright, A Leland MD [NS] - **Spec Exp:** Pediatric Neurosurgery; Brain Tumors; **Hospital:** Univ WI Hosp & Clins; **Address:** UW Hosp & Clinics, 600 Highland Ave, rm K4/836, Madison, WI 53792; **Phone:** 608-263-9651; **Board Cert:** Neurological Surgery 1981; Pediatric Neurological Surgery 1996; **Med School:** Louisiana State Univ 1969; **Resid:** Surgery, Wash Hosps 1971; Neurological Surgery, Univ Pittsburgh Med Ctr 1978; **Fellow:** Neurological Surgery, Natl Inst Hlth 1974; Immunopathology, Univ Pittsburgh Med Ctr 1978; **Fac Appt:** Prof NS, Univ Wisc

Bakay, Roy A. E. MD [NS] - **Spec Exp:** Brain Tumors; **Hospital:** Rush Univ Med Ctr; **Address:** Rush Univ Med Ctr, 1725 W Harrison St, Ste 970, Chicago, IL 60612; **Phone:** 312-942-6644; **Board Cert:** Neurological Surgery 1985; **Med School:** Northwestern Univ 1975; **Resid:** Neurological Surgery, Univ Washington Sch Med 1981; **Fellow:** Neuronal Plasticity, Natl Inst Hlth 1982; **Fac Appt:** Prof NS, Rush Med Coll

Barnett, Gene H MD [NS] - **Spec Exp:** Brain Tumors; Stereotactic Radiosurgery; **Hospital:** Cleveland Clin Fdn (page 71); **Address:** Cleveland Clinic Brain Tumor Inst, 9500 Euclid Ave, Desk R20, Cleveland, OH 44195; **Phone:** 216-444-5381; **Board Cert:** Neurological Surgery 1990; **Med School:** Case West Res Univ 1980; **Resid:** Neurological Surgery, Cleveland Clinic 1986; **Fellow:** Neurology, Cleveland Clinic 1982; Research, Mass Genl Hosp-Harvard 1987; **Fac Appt:** Prof NS, Cleveland Cl Coll Med/Case West Res

Bauer, Jerry MD [NS] - **Spec Exp:** Brain Tumors; Spinal Surgery; Minimally Invasive Spinal Surgery; **Hospital:** Adv Luth Genl Hosp; **Address:** Ctr Brain & Spine Surg-Parkside Ctr, 1875 Dempster St, Ste 605, Park Ridge, IL 60068-1168; **Phone:** 847-698-1088; **Board Cert:** Neurological Surgery 1982; **Med School:** Univ IL Coll Med 1974; **Resid:** Neurological Surgery, Univ Illinios Med Ctr 1979; **Fac Appt:** Asst Clin Prof NS, Univ IL Coll Med

Chandler, William F MD [NS] - **Spec Exp:** Pituitary Surgery; Brain Tumors; **Hospital:** Univ Michigan Hlth Sys; **Address:** 1500 E Med Center Drive, Ste 3470, Tauban Center, Ann Arbor, MI 48109; **Phone:** 734-936-5020; **Board Cert:** Neurological Surgery 1980; **Med School:** Univ Mich Med Sch 1971; **Resid:** Neurological Surgery, Michigan Hosp 1977; **Fac Appt:** Prof NS, Univ Mich Med Sch

Chiocca, E Antonio MD [NS] - **Spec Exp:** Brain Tumors; Spinal Cord Tumors; **Hospital:** Arthur G James Cancer Hosp & Research Inst, Ohio St Univ Med Ctr; **Address:** OSU Med Ctr, Dept Neurosurgery, 410 W 10th Ave, 1021-N Doan Hall, Columbus, OH 43210; **Phone:** 614-293-9312; **Board Cert:** Neurological Surgery 2000; **Med School:** Univ Tex, Houston 1988; **Resid:** Neurological Surgery, Mass Genl Hosp 1995; **Fac Appt:** Prof NS, Ohio State Univ

Cohen, Alan R MD [NS] - **Spec Exp:** Pediatric Neurosurgery; Brain & Spinal Tumors-Pediatric; Minimally Invasive Neurosurgery; **Hospital:** Rainbow Babies & Chldns Hosp, Univ Hosps Case Med Ctr; **Address:** Rainbow Babies & Chldns Hosp, 11100 Euclid Ave, Ste B501, Cleveland, OH 44106; **Phone:** 216-844-5741; **Board Cert:** Neurological Surgery 1991; Pediatric Neurological Surgery 1997; **Med School:** Cornell Univ-Weill Med Coll 1978; **Resid:** Surgery, NYU Medical Ctr 1980; Neurological Surgery, NYU Medical Ctr 1987; **Fellow:** Neurology, Natl Hosp Queen's Square 1982; **Fac Appt:** Prof NS, Case West Res Univ

Dacey Jr, Ralph G MD [NS] - **Spec Exp:** Cerebrovascular Surgery; Brain Tumors; **Hospital:** Barnes-Jewish Hosp, Barnes-Jewish West County Hosp; **Address:** Wash Univ Sch Med, Dept Neurosurgery, 660 S Euclid Ave, Box 8057, St. Louis, MO 63110; **Phone:** 314-362-3577; **Board Cert:** Internal Medicine 1978; Neurological Surgery 1985; **Med School:** Univ VA Sch Med 1974; **Resid:** Internal Medicine, Strong Meml Hosp 1977; Neurological Surgery, Univ Virginia Med Ctr 1983; **Fac Appt:** Prof NS, Washington Univ, St Louis

Frim, David M MD/PhD [NS] - **Spec Exp:** Pediatric Neurosurgery; Brain & Spinal Tumors; **Hospital:** Univ of Chicago Hosps; **Address:** Univ of Chicago Hosps-Pediatric Neurosurgery, 5841 S Maryland Ave, MC 4066, Chicago, IL 60637-1463; **Phone:** 773-702-2475; **Board Cert:** Neurological Surgery 1998; Pediatric Neurological Surgery 1998; **Med School:** Harvard Med Sch 1988; **Resid:** Neurological Surgery, Mass Genl Hosp 1995; **Fellow:** Pediatric Neurological Surgery, Children's Hosp 1996; **Fac Appt:** Assoc Prof S, Univ Chicago-Pritzker Sch Med

Greene Jr, Clarence S MD [NS] - **Spec Exp:** Pediatric Neurosurgery; Brain Tumors; **Hospital:** Chldns Mercy Hosps & Clinics; **Address:** 2401 Gillham Rd, Kansas City, MO 64108; **Phone:** 816-234-3000; **Board Cert:** Neurological Surgery 1984; Pediatric Neurological Surgery 1997; **Med School:** Howard Univ 1974; **Resid:** Neurological Surgery, Chldns Hosp 1981; Neurological Surgery, Peter Bent Brigham Hosp 1981; **Fellow:** Pediatric Neurological Surgery, Chldns Hosp 1985; **Fac Appt:** Assoc Clin Prof NS, UC Irvine

Grubb Jr, Robert L MD [NS] **Spec Exp:** Brain Tumors; Skull Base Tumors; **Hospital:** Barnes-Jewish Hosp, St Louis Chldns Hosp; **Address:** Wash Univ Sch Med, Dept Neurosurgery, 660 S Euclid Ave, Box 8057, St Louis, MO 63110; **Phone:** 314-362-3577; **Board Cert:** Neurological Surgery 1976; **Med School:** Univ NC Sch Med 1965; **Resid:** Surgery, Barnes Jewish Hosp 1967; Neurological Surgery, Barnes Jewish Hosp 1973; **Fellow:** Neurological Surgery, National Inst Health 1969; **Fac Appt:** Prof NS, Washington Univ, St Louis

Gutierrez, Francisco A MD [NS] - **Spec Exp:** Brain Tumors; Cerebrovascular Surgery; Spinal Surgery; **Hospital:** Northwestern Meml Hosp, Resurrection Med Ctr; **Address:** 201 E Huron St, Ste 9-160, Gaulter Pavilion, Chicago, IL 60611; **Phone:** 312-926-3490; **Board Cert:** Neurological Surgery 1976; **Med School:** Colombia 1965; **Resid:** Neurological Surgery, San Juan de Dios Hosp 1967; Neurological Surgery, Northwestern Meml Hosp 1973; **Fac Appt:** Assoc Prof NS, Northwestern Univ

Neurological Surgery

Kaufman, Bruce A MD [NS] - **Spec Exp:** Pediatric Neurosurgery; Brain & Spinal Cord Tumors; **Hospital:** Chldns Hosp - Wisconsin; **Address:** Chldns Hosp, Dept Neurosurg, 999 N 92nd St, Box 310, Milwaukee, WI 53226; **Phone:** 414-266-6435; **Board Cert:** Neurological Surgery 1992; Pediatric Neurological Surgery ; **Med School:** Case West Res Univ 1982; **Resid:** Neurological Surgery, Univ Hosp Cleveland/Case West Res 1988; **Fellow:** Pediatric Neurological Surgery, Chldns Meml Hosp/Northwestern Univ 1989; **Fac Appt:** Prof NS, Med Coll Wisc

Kranzler, Leonard I MD [NS] - **Spec Exp:** Brain Tumors; **Hospital:** Adv Illinois Masonic Med Ctr, Resurrection Hlth Care St Joseph Hosp; **Address:** 3000 N Halstead St, Ste 701, Chicago, IL 60657; **Phone:** 773-296-6666; **Board Cert:** Neurological Surgery 1974; **Med School:** Northwestern Univ 1963; **Resid:** Neurological Surgery, Northwestern Univ 1969; Neurological Surgery, Chldns Meml Hosp 1967; **Fellow:** Neurological Surgery; **Fac Appt:** Assoc Clin Prof NS, Univ Chicago-Pritzker Sch Med

Levy, Robert M MD/PhD [NS] - **Spec Exp:** Stereotactic Radiosurgery; Brain Tumors; Pain-Chronic; **Hospital:** Northwestern Meml Hosp; **Address:** 675 N Saint Clair St, Ste 2210, Gaulter Pavilion, Chicago, IL 60611-2922; **Phone:** 312-695-8143; **Board Cert:** Neurological Surgery 1991; **Med School:** Stanford Univ 1981; **Resid:** Neurological Surgery, UCSF Med Ctr 1987; **Fellow:** Neurological Surgery, UCSF Med Ctr 1986; **Fac Appt:** Prof NS, Northwestern Univ

Link, Michael J MD [NS] - **Spec Exp:** Skull Base Tumors; Brain Tumors; Cerebrovascular Surgery; **Hospital:** Mayo Med Ctr & Clin - Rochester; **Address:** Mayo Clinic, Dept Neurosurgery, 200 First St SW, Rochester, MN 55905; **Phone:** 507-284-8008; **Board Cert:** Neurological Surgery 2000; **Med School:** Mayo Med Sch 1990; **Resid:** Neurological Surgery, Mayo Clinic 1996; **Fellow:** Cerebrovascular & Skull Base Surgery, Univ Cincinnati/Mayfield Clinic 1998; **Fac Appt:** Assoc Prof NS, Mayo Med Sch

Macdonald, R Loch MD/PhD [NS] - **Spec Exp:** Cerebrovascular Surgery; Brain & Spinal Cord Tumors; **Hospital:** Univ of Chicago Hosps; **Address:** Univ Chicago Hospitals, 5841 S Maryland Ave, MC 3026, Chicago, IL 60637; **Phone:** 773-702-2123; **Board Cert:** Neurological Surgery 1995; **Med School:** Canada 1985; **Resid:** Neurological Surgery, Univ Toronto Med Ctr 1993; **Fac Appt:** Prof S, Univ Chicago-Pritzker Sch Med

Malik, Ghaus MD [NS] - **Spec Exp:** Cerebrovascular Surgery; Brain & Spinal Cord Tumors; **Hospital:** Henry Ford Hosp, William Beaumont Hosp; **Address:** Henry Ford Hosp, Dept Neurosurg, 2799 W Grand Blvd, Detroit, MI 48202; **Phone:** 313-916-1093; **Board Cert:** Neurological Surgery 1978; **Med School:** Pakistan 1968; **Resid:** Surgery, Henry Ford Hosp 1971; Neurological Surgery, Henry Ford Hosp 1975

Origitano, Thomas MD/PhD [NS] - **Spec Exp:** Skull Base Tumors & Surgery; Cerebrovascular Surgery; Brain Tumors; **Hospital:** Loyola Univ Med Ctr; **Address:** Loyola Univ Medical Ctr, Dept Neurosurgery, 2160 S First Ave Bldg 105 - rm 1900, Maywood, IL 60153-3304; **Phone:** 708-216-8920; **Board Cert:** Neurological Surgery 1995; **Med School:** Loyola Univ-Stritch Sch Med 1984; **Resid:** Neurological Surgery, Loyola Univ Med Ctr 1990; **Fac Appt:** Prof NS, Loyola Univ-Stritch Sch Med

Park, Tae Sung MD [NS] - **Spec Exp:** Pediatric Neurosurgery; Neuro-Oncology; **Hospital:** St Louis Chldns Hosp; **Address:** St Louis Children's Hospital, 1 Children's Place, Ste 4-S20, St Louis, MO 63110; **Phone:** 314-454-4629; **Board Cert:** Neurological Surgery 1985; Pediatric Neurological Surgery 1988; **Med School:** Korea 1971; **Resid:** Neurological Surgery, Univ Virginia Hosp 1980; **Fellow:** Neuropathology, Mass General; Pediatric Neurological Surgery, Hospital for Sick Children; **Fac Appt:** Prof NS, St Louis Univ

Raffel, Corey MD/PhD [NS] - **Spec Exp:** Pediatric Neurosurgery; Brain Tumors; Medulloblastoma; **Hospital:** Mayo Med Ctr & Clin - Rochester; **Address:** Mayo Clinic, Dept Neurosurgery, 200 1st St SW, Rochester, MN 55905; **Phone:** 507-284-8008; **Board Cert:** Neurological Surgery 1990; Pediatric Neurological Surgery 1996; **Med School:** UCSD 1980; **Resid:** Neurological Surgery, UCSF Med Ctr 1986; **Fellow:** Pediatric Neurological Surgery, Hosp Sick Chldn 1988; **Fac Appt:** Prof NS, Mayo Med Sch

Rich, Keith M MD [NS] - **Spec Exp:** Brain Tumors; Stereotactic Radiosurgery; **Hospital:** Barnes-Jewish Hosp; **Address:** Washington University School of Medicine, 660 S Euclid Ave, Box 8057, St Louis, MO 63110; **Phone:** 314-362-3577; **Board Cert:** Neurological Surgery 1987; **Med School:** Indiana Univ 1977; **Resid:** Neurological Surgery, Barnes Jewish Hosp 1982; **Fellow:** Neurological Pharmacology, Barnes Jewish Hosp 1984; **Fac Appt:** Assoc Prof NS, Washington Univ, St Louis

Rock, Jack P MD [NS] - **Spec Exp:** Neuro-Oncology; Pituitary Surgery; Skull Base Surgery; Brain Tumors; **Hospital:** Henry Ford Hosp, William Beaumont Hosp; **Address:** Henry Ford Hosp, Dept Neurosurg, 2799 W Grand Blvd, Detroit, MI 48202; **Phone:** 313-916-2241; **Board Cert:** Neurological Surgery 1989; **Med School:** Univ Miami Sch Med 1979; **Resid:** Neurological Surgery, NY Hosp-Cornell Med Ctr 1985; **Fellow:** Univ Maryland 1986

Rosenblum, Mark L MD [NS] - **Spec Exp:** Brain Tumors; Spinal Surgery; Neuro-Oncology; **Hospital:** Henry Ford Hosp, William Beaumont Hosp; **Address:** Henry Ford Hospital, K11, 2799 W Grand Blvd, Detroit, MI 48202; **Phone:** 313-916-1340; **Board Cert:** Neurological Surgery 1982; **Med School:** NY Med Coll 1969; **Resid:** Surgery, UCLA Med Ctr 1973; Neurological Surgery, UCSF Med Ctr 1979; **Fellow:** Neuro-Oncology, Natl Cancer Inst 1972; **Fac Appt:** Prof NS, Case West Res Univ

Ruge, John MD [NS] - **Spec Exp:** Pediatric Neurosurgery; Brain Tumors; **Hospital:** Adv Luth Genl Hosp; **Address:** 1875 Dempster St, Ste 605, Park Ridge, IL 60068; **Phone:** 847-698-1088; **Board Cert:** Neurological Surgery 1993; **Med School:** Northwestern Univ 1983; **Resid:** Neurological Surgery, Northwestern Meml Hosp 1989; **Fellow:** Pediatric Neurological Surgery, Childrens Hosp 1990; **Fac Appt:** Asst Prof S, Rush Med Coll

Ryken, Timothy MD [NS] - **Spec Exp:** Brain Tumors; Spinal Surgery; **Hospital:** Univ Iowa Hosp & Clinics; **Address:** Univ Iowa Hosps & Clinics, Div Neurosurg, 200 Hawkins Drive, rm 1844 JPP, Iowa City, IA 52242; **Phone:** 319-356-2237; **Board Cert:** Neurological Surgery 1998; **Med School:** Univ Iowa Coll Med 1988; **Resid:** Neurological Surgery, Univ Iowa 1995; **Fellow:** Cambridge Univ 1996; **Fac Appt:** Assoc Prof NS, Univ Iowa Coll Med

Shapiro, Scott A MD [NS] - **Spec Exp:** Brain Tumors; Pituitary Tumors; **Hospital:** Indiana Univ Hosp (page 70); **Address:** Inidiana Univ, Wishard Memorial Hospital, 1001 W 10th St, Ste EOP323, Indianapolis, IN 46202; **Phone:** 317-630-7625; **Board Cert:** Neurological Surgery 1990; **Med School:** Indiana Univ 1981; **Resid:** Neurological Surgery, Indiana Univ Med Ctr 1987; **Fac Appt:** Prof NS, Indiana Univ

Thompson, B Gregory MD [NS] - **Spec Exp:** Skull Base Tumors & Surgery; **Hospital:** Univ Michigan Hlth Sys; **Address:** Dept Neurosurgery, 3552 Taubman, 1500 E Medical Center Drive, Ann Arbor, MI 48109; **Phone:** 734-936-7493; **Board Cert:** Neurological Surgery 1998; **Med School:** Univ Kans 1986; **Resid:** Neurological Surgery, Univ Pittsburgh 1993; Research, Natl Inst Hlth 1992; **Fellow:** Neurological Surgery, Barrow Neuro Inst 1994; Interventional Radiology, Thomas Jefferson Univ 2005

Tomita, Tadanori MD [NS] - Spec Exp: Pediatric Neurosurgery; Brain Tumors-Pediatric; **Hospital:** Children's Mem Hosp, Northwestern Meml Hosp; **Address:** Chldns Meml Hosp, Div Ped Neurosurg, 2300 Children's Plaza, Box 28, Chicago, IL 60614-3318; **Phone:** 773-880-4373; **Board Cert:** Neurological Surgery 1984; Pediatric Neurological Surgery 1996; **Med School:** Japan 1970; **Resid:** Neurological Surgery, Kobe Univ 1974; Neurological Surgery, Northwestern Meml Hosp 1980; **Fellow:** Surgery, Meml Sloan Kettering Canc Ctr 1981; **Fac Appt:** Prof NS, Northwestern Univ

Warnick, Ronald E MD [NS] - Spec Exp: Neuro-Oncology; Brain Tumors; **Hospital:** Univ Hosp - Cincinnati, Good Samaritan Hosp - Cincinnati; **Address:** 222 Piedmont Ave, Ste 3100, Cincinnati, OH 45219; **Phone:** 513-475-8629; **Board Cert:** Neurological Surgery 1995; **Med School:** Univ Rochester 1982; **Resid:** Neurological Surgery, NYU Med Ctr 1989; **Fellow:** Neuro-Oncology, UCSF Med Ctr 1991; **Fac Appt:** Prof NS, Univ Cincinnati

Great Plains and Mountains

Cherny, W Bruce MD [NS] - Spec Exp: Pediatric Neurosurgery; Brain Tumors; **Hospital:** St. Luke's Reg Med Ctr - Boise; **Address:** 100 E Idaho St, Ste 202, Boise, ID 83712; **Phone:** 208-381-7360; **Board Cert:** Neurological Surgery 2000; **Med School:** Univ Ariz Coll Med 1987; **Resid:** Neurological Surgery, Barrow Neuro Inst/St Joseph's Med Ctr 1994; **Fellow:** Pediatric Neurological Surgery, Primary Chldns Hosp 1995

Couldwell, William MD/PhD [NS] - Spec Exp: Brain Tumors; Pituitary Tumors; **Hospital:** Univ Utah Hosps and Clins; **Address:** Univ Utah, Dept Neurological Surgery, 175 N Medical Drive E, Salt Lake City, UT 84132-2303; **Phone:** 801-581-6908; **Board Cert:** Neurological Surgery 1994; **Med School:** McGill Univ 1984; **Resid:** Neurological Surgery, LAC/USC Med Ctr 1989; **Fellow:** Neurological Immunology, Montreal Neur Inst/McGill Univ 1991; Neurological Surgery, CHUV; **Fac Appt:** Prof NS, Univ Utah

Johnson, Stephen D MD [NS] - Spec Exp: Skull Base Tumors & Surgery; **Hospital:** Presby - St Luke's Med Ctr; **Address:** Western Neurological Group, 1601 E 19th Ave, Ste 4400, Denver, CO 80218; **Phone:** 303-861-2266; **Board Cert:** Neurological Surgery 1988; **Med School:** Univ Tenn Coll Med, Memphis 1974; **Resid:** Neurological Surgery, Virginia Mason Med Ctr; Neurological Surgery, New York Hosp; **Fellow:** Neurological Surgery, Univ Tennessee; **Fac Appt:** Assoc Prof NS, Univ Colorado

Lillehei, Kevin O MD [NS] - Spec Exp: Neuro-Oncology; Pituitary Tumors; **Hospital:** Univ Colorado Hosp, Exempla Lutheran Med Ctr; **Address:** Univ Colo Hlth Sci Ctr, Div Neurosurg, 4200 E 9th Ave, Campus Box C-307, Denver, CO 80262; **Phone:** 303-315-5651; **Board Cert:** Neurological Surgery 1989; **Med School:** Univ Minn 1979; **Resid:** Neurological Surgery, Univ Mich Med Ctr 1985; **Fac Appt:** Prof NS, Univ Colorado

Southwest

Al-Mefty, Ossama MD [NS] - Spec Exp: Skull Base Surgery; Brain Tumors; Cerebrovascular Surgery; **Hospital:** UAMS Med Ctr, Arkansas Chldns Hosp; **Address:** Univ Hosp of Arkansas for Med Scis, 4301 W Markham Slot 507, Little Rock, AR 72205; **Phone:** 501-686-8757; **Board Cert:** Neurological Surgery 1980; **Med School:** Syria 1972; **Resid:** Surgery, Med Coll Ohio 1974; Neurological Surgery, West Va Med Ctr 1978; **Fac Appt:** Prof NS, Univ Ark

De Monte, Franco MD [NS] - **Spec Exp:** Skull Base Tumors & Surgery; Neuro-Oncology; **Hospital:** UT MD Anderson Cancer Ctr (page 81); **Address:** UT MD Anderson Cancer Ctr, Dept Neurosurgery, 1515 Holcombe Blvd, Ste 442, Houston, TX 77030; **Phone:** 713-792-2400; **Board Cert:** Neurological Surgery 1995; **Med School:** Canada 1985; **Resid:** Neurological Surgery, Univ Western Ontario 1991; **Fellow:** Skull Base Surgery, Loyola Univ-Stritch Sch Med 1992

Hankinson, Hal L MD [NS] - **Spec Exp:** Brain Tumors; **Hospital:** Presbyterian Hospital - Albuquerque, Albuquerque Regional Med Ctr; **Address:** New Mexico Neurosurgery, 522 Lomas Blvd NE, Albuquerque, NM 87102; **Phone:** 505-247-4253; **Board Cert:** Neurological Surgery 1977; **Med School:** Tulane Univ 1967; **Resid:** Neurological Surgery, UCSF Med Ctr 1975; **Fac Appt:** Clin Prof NS, Univ New Mexico

Hassenbusch, Samuel J MD/PhD [NS] - **Spec Exp:** Pain Management; Pain-Cancer; Brain Tumors; Stereotactic Radiosurgery; **Hospital:** UT MD Anderson Cancer Ctr (page 81); **Address:** UT MD Anderson Cancer Ctr, PO Box 301402, Houston, TX 77230-1402; **Phone:** 713-563-8706; **Board Cert:** Neurological Surgery 1992; **Med School:** Johns Hopkins Univ 1978; **Resid:** Surgery, Johns Hopkins Univ 1980; Neurological Surgery, Johns Hopkins Univ 1988; **Fellow:** Research, Keck Fdn-UCSF 1986; **Fac Appt:** Prof NS, Univ Tex, Houston

Lang Jr, Frederick F MD [NS] - **Spec Exp:** Brain & Spinal Tumors; Neuro-Oncology; **Hospital:** UT MD Anderson Cancer Ctr (page 81); **Address:** Univ Texas MD Anderson Cancer Ctr, Box 301402, Houston, TX 77230-1402; **Phone:** 713-792-2400; **Board Cert:** Neurological Surgery 2000; **Med School:** Yale Univ 1988; **Resid:** Neurological Surgery, NYU Med Ctr 1995; **Fellow:** Neurosurgical Oncology, MD Anderson Cancer Ctr 1996; **Fac Appt:** Prof NS, Univ Tex, Houston

Mapstone, Timothy MD [NS] - **Spec Exp:** Brain Tumors-Adult & Pediatric; Pediatric Neurosurgery; **Hospital:** OU Med Ctr, Chldns Hosp OU Med Ctr; **Address:** Univ OK Hlth Sci Ctr, Dept Neurosurgery, 1000 N Lincoln Blvd, Ste 400, Oklahoma City, OK 73104; **Phone:** 405-271-4912; **Board Cert:** Neurological Surgery 1985; Pediatric Neurological Surgery 2005; **Med School:** Case West Res Univ 1977; **Resid:** Neurological Surgery, Univ Hosps 1983; **Fellow:** Research, Case West Res; **Fac Appt:** Prof NS, Univ Okla Coll Med

Mickey, Bruce E MD [NS] - **Spec Exp:** Brain Tumors; Skull Base Surgery; **Hospital:** UT Southwestern Med Ctr - Dallas; **Address:** UTSW Med Ctr, Dept Neurosurgery, 5323 Harry Hines Blvd, Dallas, TX 75390-8855; **Phone:** 214-645-2300; **Board Cert:** Neurological Surgery 1987; **Med School:** Univ Tex SW, Dallas 1978; **Resid:** Neurological Surgery, Parkland Meml Hosp 1984; **Fellow:** Research, Righospitalet 1983; **Fac Appt:** Prof NS, Univ Tex SW, Dallas

Sawaya, Raymond MD [NS] - **Spec Exp:** Brain Tumors; **Hospital:** UT MD Anderson Cancer Ctr (page 81); **Address:** MD Anderson Cancer Ctr, 1515 Holcombe Blvd, Unit 442, Houston, TX 77030; **Phone:** 713-563-8749; **Board Cert:** Neurological Surgery 1985; **Med School:** Lebanon 1974; **Resid:** Neurological Surgery, Univ Cincinnati Med Ctr 1980; Neurological Surgery, Johns Hopkins Med Ctr 1981; **Fellow:** Neuro-Oncology, Natl Inst Hlth 1982; **Fac Appt:** Prof NS, Univ Tex, Houston

Spetzler, Robert F MD [NS] - **Spec Exp:** Skull Base Tumors & Surgery; Cerebrovascular Surgery; **Hospital:** St Joseph's Hosp & Med Ctr - Phoenix; **Address:** Barrow Neurosurgical Assocs, 2910 N Third Ave, Phoenix, AZ 85013; **Phone:** 602-406-3489; **Board Cert:** Neurological Surgery 1979; **Med School:** Northwestern Univ 1971; **Resid:** Neurological Surgery, UCSF Med Ctr 1976; **Fac Appt:** Prof S, Univ Ariz Coll Med

Neurological Surgery

Adler Jr, John R MD [NS] - **Spec Exp:** Stereotactic Radiosurgery; Brain Tumors; **Hospital:** Stanford Univ Med Ctr; **Address:** Stanford Univ Med Ctr, Dept Neurosurg, 300 Pasteur Drive, rm R 205, Stanford, CA 94305-5327; **Phone:** 650-723-5573; **Board Cert:** Neurological Surgery 1990; **Med School:** Harvard Med Sch 1980; **Resid:** Neurological Surgery, Chldns Hosp 1987; Neurological Surgery, Mass Genl Hosp 1985; **Fellow:** Cerebrovascular Disease, Karolinska Inst 1986; **Fac Appt:** Prof NS, Stanford Univ

Apuzzo, Michael L J MD [NS] - **Spec Exp:** Brain Tumors; Stereotactic Radiosurgery; **Hospital:** LAC & USC Med Ctr, USC Norris Comp Cancer Ctr; **Address:** 1420 N San Pablo Street, PMBA106, Los Angeles, CA 90033-1029; **Phone:** 323-226-7421; **Board Cert:** Neurological Surgery 1975; **Med School:** Boston Univ 1965; **Resid:** Neurological Surgery, Hartford Hosp; Neurological Surgery, Hartford Hosp 1973; **Fellow:** Neurological Physiology, Yale Univ Hosp; **Fac Appt:** Prof NS, USC Sch Med

Badie, Behnam MD [NS] - **Spec Exp:** Brain Tumors; **Hospital:** City of Hope Natl Med Ctr & Beckman Rsch (page 69); **Address:** 1500 E Duarte Rd, City Of Hope Natl Mem Ctr, Duarte, CA 91010; **Phone:** 626-471-7100; **Board Cert:** Neurological Surgery 1998; **Med School:** UCLA 1989; **Resid:** Neurological Surgery, UCLA Med Ctr 1996; **Fac Appt:** Assoc Prof NS, UCLA

Berger, Mitchel S MD [NS] - **Spec Exp:** Brain & Spinal Cord Tumors; Pituitary Tumors; Neuro-Oncology; Pain Management; **Hospital:** UCSF Med Ctr; **Address:** UCSF Med Ctr, Dept Neurosurgery, 505 Parnassus Avenue, M-786, San Francisco, CA 94143-0112; **Phone:** 415-353-3933; **Board Cert:** Neurological Surgery 1991; **Med School:** Univ Miami Sch Med 1979; **Resid:** Neurological Surgery, UCSF Med Ctr 1984; **Fellow:** Neuro-Oncology, UCSF Med Ctr 1985; Pediatric Neurological Surgery, Hosp Sick Chldn 1986; **Fac Appt:** Prof NS, UCSF

Black, Keith L MD [NS] - **Spec Exp:** Brain Tumors; Pituitary Surgery; **Hospital:** Cedars-Sinai Med Ctr; **Address:** Maxine Dunitz Neurosurgical Inst, 8631 W 3rd St, Ste 800E, Los Angeles, CA 90048; **Phone:** 310-423-7900; **Board Cert:** Neurological Surgery 1990; **Med School:** Univ Mich Med Sch 1981; **Resid:** Neurological Surgery, Univ Michigan Med Ctr 1987; **Fac Appt:** Prof NS, UCLA

Boggan, James E MD [NS] - **Spec Exp:** Skull Base Tumors & Surgery; **Hospital:** UC Davis Med Ctr; **Address:** UC Davis, Dept Neurological Surgery, 4860 Y St, Ste 3740, Sacramento, CA 95817; **Phone:** 916-734-2371; **Board Cert:** Neurological Surgery 1985; **Med School:** Univ Chicago-Pritzker Sch Med 1976; **Resid:** Neurological Surgery, UCSF Med Ctr 1982; **Fac Appt:** Prof NS, UC Davis

Delashaw Jr, Johnny B MD [NS] - **Spec Exp:** Skull Base Tumors & Surgery; Neuro-Oncology; **Hospital:** OR Hlth & Sci Univ; **Address:** Oregon Hlth & Sci Univ, Dept Neurosurgery, 3303 SW Bond Ave, Ste CH8N, Portland, OR 97239; **Phone:** 503-494-4314; **Board Cert:** Neurological Surgery 1993; **Med School:** Univ Wash 1983; **Resid:** Neurological Surgery, Univ Virginia Medical Ctr 1990; **Fac Appt:** Prof NS, Oregon Hlth Sci Univ

Edwards, Michael S MD [NS] - **Spec Exp:** Brain Tumors-Pediatric; Pediatric Neurosurgery; Stereotactic Radiosurgery; **Hospital:** Lucile Packard Chldns Hosp/Stanford Univ Med Ctr; **Address:** Pediatric Neurosurgery, 300 Pasteur Drive, Ste R211, MC 5327, Stanford, CA 94305-5327; **Phone:** 650-497-8775; **Board Cert:** Neurological Surgery 1980; Pediatric Neurological Surgery 2006; **Med School:** Tulane Univ 1970; **Resid:** Neurological Surgery, Oschner Fdn Hosp/Charity Hosp 1977; **Fellow:** Pediatric Neuro-Oncology, UCSF Med Ctr 1978; **Fac Appt:** Prof NS, Stanford Univ

Ellenbogen, Richard MD [NS] - **Spec Exp:** Pediatric Neurosurgery; Brain Tumors; **Hospital:** Chldns Hosp and Regl Med Ctr - Seattle, Univ Wash Med Ctr; **Address:** 4800 Sand Point Way NE, MS W-7729, Seattle, WA 98105; **Phone:** 206-987-2544; **Board Cert:** Neurological Surgery 1992; Pediatric Neurological Surgery 1998; **Med School:** Brown Univ 1983; **Resid:** Neurological Surgery, Brigham Womens Hosp/Childrens Hosp 1989; **Fac Appt:** Prof NS, Univ Wash

Giannotta, Steven L MD [NS] - **Spec Exp:** Skull Base Tumors; **Hospital:** USC Univ Hosp - R K Eamer Med Plz, LAC & USC Med Ctr; **Address:** 1520 San Pablo St, Ste 3800, Los Angeles, CA 90033; **Phone:** 323-442-5720; **Board Cert:** Neurological Surgery 1980; **Med School:** Univ Mich Med Sch 1972; **Resid:** Neurological Surgery, Univ Michigan Med Ctr 1978; **Fac Appt:** Prof NS, USC Sch Med

Harsh IV, Griffith MD [NS] - **Spec Exp:** Brain & Spinal Cord Tumors; Skull Base Tumors; Pituitary Tumors; Endoscopic Surgery; **Hospital:** Stanford Univ Med Ctr; **Address:** Stanford Center for Advanced Medicine, 875 Blake Wilbur Drive, MC 5826, Stanford, CA 94305; **Phone:** 650-736-9976; **Board Cert:** Neurological Surgery 1989; **Med School:** Harvard Med Sch 1980; **Resid:** Neurological Surgery, UCSF Med Ctr 1986; **Fellow:** Neuro-Oncology, UCSF Med Ctr 1987; **Fac Appt:** Prof NS, Stanford Univ

Laws Jr, Edward R MD [NS] - **Spec Exp:** Pituitary Surgery; Brain Tumors; **Hospital:** Stanford Univ Med Ctr, Lucile Packard Chldns Hosp/Stanford Univ Med Ctr; **Address:** Stanford Univ Med Ctr, Dept Neurosurgery, rm CC-2330, MC 5821, Stanford, CA 94305-5821; **Phone:** 650-736-0500; **Board Cert:** Neurological Surgery 1974; **Med School:** Johns Hopkins Univ 1963; **Resid:** Neurological Surgery, Johns Hopkins Hosp 1971; **Fac Appt:** Prof NS, Stanford Univ

Liau, Linda MD/PhD [NS] - **Spec Exp:** Brain Tumors; Neuro-Oncology; **Hospital:** UCLA Med Ctr (page 83); **Address:** CHS 74-145, Box 956901, 10833 Le Conte Ave, Los Angeles, CA 90095-6901; **Phone:** 310-267-2621; **Board Cert:** Neurological Surgery 2002; **Med School:** Stanford Univ 1991; **Resid:** Neurological Surgery, UCLA Med Ctr 1998; **Fellow:** Neuro-Oncology, UCLA Med Ctr 1998; **Fac Appt:** Prof NS, UCLA

Linskey, Mark E MD [NS] - **Spec Exp:** Brain Tumors; Gamma Knife Surgery; Skull Base Surgery; **Hospital:** UC Irvine Med Ctr, Chldns Hosp Orange Co - CHOC; **Address:** UCI Med Ctr, Dept Neurosurgery-Route 81, 101 The City Drive S Bldg 56 - Ste 400, Orange, CA 92868-3298; **Phone:** 714-456-6392; **Board Cert:** Neurological Surgery 1996; **Med School:** Columbia P&S 1986; **Resid:** Neurological Surgery, Univ Pittsburgh Hlth Ctrs 1993; **Fellow:** Neuro Oncology, Ludwig Inst Cancer Rsch/Univ Coll London 1994; Neuro-Oncology, Pittsburgh Cancer Inst/Univ Pittsburgh 1992; **Fac Appt:** Assoc Prof NS, UC Irvine

Mamelak, Adam N MD [NS] - **Spec Exp:** Brain Tumors; Spinal Tumors; **Hospital:** Cedars-Sinai Med Ctr, Huntington Memorial Hosp; **Address:** Maxine Dunitz Neurosurgical Institute, 8631 W Third St, Ste 800-East, Los Angeles, CA 90048; **Phone:** 310-423-7900; **Board Cert:** Neurological Surgery 2000; **Med School:** Harvard Med Sch 1990; **Resid:** Neurological Surgery, UCSF Med Ctr 1994; **Fellow:** Epilepsy, UCSF Epilepsy Research Lab 1995

Mayberg, Marc R MD [NS] - **Spec Exp:** Pituitary Surgery; Skull Base Tumors; **Hospital:** Swedish Med Ctr - Seattle; **Address:** Seattle Neuroscience Inst, 550 17th Ave, Ste 500, Seattle, WA 98122; **Phone:** 206-320-2800; **Board Cert:** Neurological Surgery 1988; **Med School:** Mayo Med Sch 1978; **Resid:** Neurological Surgery, Mass Genl Hosp 1984; **Fellow:** Neurological Surgery, Natl Hosp for Nervous Dis 1985

Neurological Surgery

McDermott, Michael W MD [NS] - **Spec Exp:** Brain Tumors; Meningioma; Gamma Knife Surgery; Skull Base Tumors; **Hospital:** UCSF Med Ctr; **Address:** UCSF Dept Neurosurgery, 400 Parnassus Ave, rm A808, San Francisco, CA 94143; **Phone:** 415-353-7500; **Board Cert:** Neurological Surgery 2003; **Med School:** Univ Toronto 1982; **Resid:** Neurological Surgery, Univ British Columbia 1988; **Fellow:** Neuro-Oncology, UCSF Med Ctr 1990; **Fac Appt:** Prof NS, UCSF

Neuwelt, Edward A MD [NS] - **Spec Exp:** Neuro-Oncology; Brain Tumors; **Hospital:** OR Hlth & Sci Univ; **Address:** Oregon Hlth Sci Univ, Dept NS, 3181 SW Sam Jackson Pk Rd, MC-L603, Portland, OR 97239; **Phone:** 503-494-5626; **Board Cert:** Neurological Surgery 1980; **Med School:** Univ Colorado 1972; **Resid:** Neurological Surgery, Univ Tex SW Med Sch 1978; **Fellow:** Neuro-Oncology, Natl Canc Inst, NIH 1976; **Fac Appt:** Prof NS, Oregon Hlth Sci Univ

Ott, Kenneth H MD [NS] - **Spec Exp:** Brain Tumors; Gamma Knife Surgery; Stereotactic Radiosurgery; **Hospital:** Scripps Meml Hosp - La Jolla; **Address:** Neurosurgical Medical Clinic, 501 Washington St, Ste 700, San Diego, CA 92103-2231; **Phone:** 619-297-4481; **Board Cert:** Neurological Surgery 1980; **Med School:** UCSF 1970; **Resid:** Surgery, Mass Genl Hosp 1972; Neurological Surgery, Mass Genl Hosp 1976; **Fac Appt:** Assoc Clin Prof S, UCSD

Pitts, Lawrence H MD [NS] - **Spec Exp:** Skull Base Surgery; Spinal Surgery; **Hospital:** UCSF Med Ctr; **Address:** UCSF Dept of Neurosurgery, 400 Parnassus Ave, rm A808, San Francisco, CA 94143; **Phone:** 415-353-7500; **Board Cert:** Neurological Surgery 1978; **Med School:** Case West Res Univ 1969; **Resid:** Neurological Surgery, UCSF Med Ctr 1975; **Fac Appt:** Prof NS, UCSF

Sekhar, Laligam N MD [NS] - **Spec Exp:** Brain Tumors; Skull Base Tumors; **Hospital:** Harborview Med Ctr, Univ Wash Med Ctr; **Address:** Harborview Med Ctr, UW Med Dept Neurosurg, 325 Ninth Ave, Box 359766, Seattle, WA 98104-2420; **Phone:** 206-744-9300; **Board Cert:** Neurological Surgery 1986; **Med School:** India 1973; **Resid:** Neurology, Univ Cincinnati Med Ctr 1977; Neurology, Univ Pittsburgh Med Ctr 1982; **Fellow:** Skull Base Surgery, Norstadt Krankenhaus 1983; Cerebrovascular Neurosurgery, Univ Zurich Hospital; **Fac Appt:** Prof NS, Univ Wash

Silbergeld, Daniel MD [NS] - **Spec Exp:** Brain Tumors; Brain Tumors-Metastatic; **Hospital:** Univ Wash Med Ctr; **Address:** Univ Wash Med Ctr, Dept Neurosurg, 1959 NE Pacific, Box 356470, Seattle, WA 98195; **Phone:** 206-598-5637; **Board Cert:** Neurological Surgery 1995; **Med School:** Univ Cincinnati 1984; **Resid:** Neurological Surgery, Univ Wash Med Ctr 1990; Research, Univ Wash Med Ctr 1988; **Fellow:** Neuro-Oncology, Univ Wash Med Ctr 1991; Epilepsy, Univ Wash Med Ctr 1991; **Fac Appt:** Assoc Prof NS, Univ Wash

Weiss, Martin H MD [NS] - **Spec Exp:** Brain Tumors; Spinal Cord Tumors; Pituitary Tumors; **Hospital:** USC Univ Hosp - R K Eamer Med Plz; **Address:** LAC-USC Med Ctr, 1200 N State St, Ste 5046, Los Angeles, CA 90033-1029; **Phone:** 323-442-5720; **Board Cert:** Neurological Surgery 1972; **Med School:** Cornell Univ-Weill Med Coll 1963; **Resid:** Surgery, US Army Hosp 1966; Neurological Surgery, Univ Hosp 1970; **Fellow:** Neurological Surgery, NIH-Univ Hosp 1970; **Fac Appt:** Prof NS, USC Sch Med

Yu, John S MD [NS] - **Spec Exp:** Brain Tumors; Spinal Tumors; Clinical Trials; **Hospital:** Cedars-Sinai Med Ctr; **Address:** Cedars Sinai Medical Ctr, 8631 W 3rd St, Ste 800E, Los Angeles, CA 90048; **Phone:** 310-423-7900; **Board Cert:** Neurological Surgery 2002; **Med School:** Harvard Med Sch 1990; **Resid:** Neurological Surgery, Mass General Hosp 1997

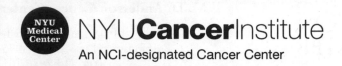

THE UNIVERSITY OF TEXAS
MD ANDERSON
CANCER CENTER
Making Cancer History®

The University of Texas
M. D. Anderson Cancer Center

1515 Holcombe Blvd.
Houston, Texas 77030-4095
Tel. 713-792-6161
Toll Free 877-MDA-6789
http://www.mdanderson.org

BRAIN AND SPINE CENTER

When faced with a tumor involving the brain, spine or skull base, choosing the right treatment center can make a difference in your outcome. With a team approach to personalized care and neurosurgical innovations not available elsewhere, the Brain and Spine Center offers patients with malignant or benign tumors the most effective treatment and best quality of life.

BrainSUITE

BrainSUITE® is an integrated neurosurgery system that allows for more precise treatment of complicated tumors in sensitive areas of the brain. It is the latest advancement in image-guided surgery, providing views of the tumor site using magnetic resonance imaging (iMRI) obtained during surgery. BrainSUITE's imaging systems provide a highly detailed view of the tumor site, enabling the surgeons to get new images at any time to check their work. This allows them to remove as much tumor as possible while protecting critical areas of the brain.

SKULL BASE PROGRAM

M. D. Anderson is one of the few cancer centers in the country with a specialized program for tumors of the skull base. The Skull Base Tumor Program joins together experts from multiple departments to provide each patient with comprehensive, individualized care – all within the M. D. Anderson setting. Surgeons in the Skull Base Tumor Program use both open and minimally invasive diagnostic and surgical approaches, depending on each patient's unique characteristics.

PROTON THERAPY

M. D. Anderson's Proton Therapy Center opened in May 2006 as the largest and most sophisticated center of its type. Proton therapy allows for the most aggressive cancer therapy possible, deriving its advantage over traditional forms of radiation treatment from its ability to deliver targeted radiation doses to the tumor with remarkable precision. Proton therapy radiation avoids the surrounding tissue, generates fewer side effects, and improves tumor control. It is used to treat cancers brain and skull base, head and neck, and eye.

MORE INFORMATION

For more information or to make an appointment, call 877-MDA-6789, or visit us online at http://www.mdanderson.org.

At M. D. Anderson Cancer Center, our mission is simple – to eliminate cancer. Achieving that goal begins with integrated programs in cancer treatment, clinical trials, education programs and cancer prevention.

We focus exclusively on cancer and have seen cases of every kind. That means you receive expert care no matter what your diagnosis.

Choosing the right partner for cancer care really does make a difference. The fact is, people who choose M. D. Anderson over other hospitals and clinics often have better results. That is how we've been making cancer history for over sixty years.

Wake Forest University Baptist
MEDICAL CENTER ®
Comprehensive Cancer Center
Brain Tumor Center of Excellence

Medical Center Boulevard • Winston-Salem, NC 27157
PAL® (Physician-to-physician calls) 1-800-277-7654
Health On-Call® (Patient access) 1-800-446-2255
www.wfubmc.edu/cancer/

OVERVIEW

The Brain Tumor Center of Excellence of Wake Forest University was formed in June 2003. With the goal of being a national leader in patient care and research, the Center has built its program with three basic components: an excellent group of clinicians, a world-renowned researcher to direct the Center, and a mission to grow the clinical and basic research programs to a magnitude that would place Wake Forest among the top brain tumor centers in the United States.

RESEARCH

The Brain Tumor Center of Excellence has three areas of research focus:

- Novel therapeutics – identifying innovative treatments that will improve outcome.

- Bioanatomic imaging – identifying the unique signatures of a cancer through non-invasive imaging of tumor biology, chemistry and physiology, thus allowing individual treatment planning.

- Radiation-induced brain injury – understanding the mechanisms of injury and ways to prevent and treat side effects of brain tumor therapy.

Laboratory researchers are exploring new therapies such as novel chemotherapy drugs, cytotoxins, gene therapy, and radiosensitizers, translating these unique approaches into clinical trials for patients. In addition to studies written and conducted by Comprehensive Cancer Center doctors, clinical trials are also offered from several national Cooperative Groups as well as the pharmaceutical industry. Wake Forest Baptist is one of only nine centers in the country that is part of the New Approaches to Brain Tumor Therapy (NABTT) consortium. In addition, the clinicians and researchers have one of the most extensive laboratory and clinical research programs in the world for the diagnosis, prevention, and treatment of brain injury resulting from a brain tumor and its treatments, particularly radiation therapy.

MULTIDISCIPLINARY CARE

Offering the region's only multidisciplinary clinic for brain tumor treatment, patients are evaluated by a medical oncologist, neurosurgeon, radiation oncologist and other specialists as needed. The entire clinical neuro-oncology team meets regularly to discuss current patients, as well as cases sent in from around the region, southeast, and nationally/internationally. Recommendations for multidisciplinary care are made and communicated to referring physicians and patients.

For patients who receive their brain tumor care at Wake Forest Baptist, the most sophisticated tools in the world are available for diagnosis and treatment. Imaging brain tumor and normal brain anatomy using modalities such as magnetic resonance (MR) imaging, MR spectroscopy, functional MR, and combination computed tomography/positron emission tomography (CT/PET) helps the team plan surgical and radiotherapeutic treatments that have the best chance of cure. Image guided surgery, cortical mapping, awake craniotomy, Leksell® Gamma Knife stereotactic radiosurgery, Gliadel® wafer chemotherapy, convection enhanced drug delivery, and GliaSite® brachytherapy are just some of the leading-edge approaches used for brain tumor patients.

To make an appointment or find a specialist at Wake Forest University Baptist Medical Center, call Health On-Call® 1-800-446-2255

KNOWLEDGE MAKES ALL THE DIFFERENCE.

Neurology

A neurologist specializes in the diagnosis and treatment of all types of disease or impaired function of the brain, spinal cord, peripheral nerves, muscles and autonomic nervous system, as well as the blood vessels that relate to these structures.

Training Required: Four years

Certification in the following subspecialties require additional training and examination.

Child Neurology: A neurologist with special qualifications in child neurology has special skills in the diagnosis and management of neurologic disorders of the neonatal period, infancy, early childhood and adolescence.

Training Required: Four years

Spinal Cord Injury Medicine: A physician who addresses the prevention, diagnosis, treatment and management of traumatic spinal cord injury and non-traumatic etiologies of spinal cord dysfunction by working in an interdisciplinary manner. Care is provided to patients of all ages on a lifelong basis and covers related medical, physical, psychological and vocational disabilities and complications.

Training Required: Four years

Neurology

Mid Atlantic

De Angelis, Lisa MD [N] - **Spec Exp:** Neuro-Oncology; **Hospital:** Meml Sloan Kettering Cancer Ctr (page 76); **Address:** 1275 York Ave, New York, NY 10021-6007; **Phone:** 212-639-7123; **Board Cert:** Neurology 1986; **Med School:** Columbia P&S 1980; **Resid:** Neurology, Neuro Inst-Presby Hosp 1984; **Fellow:** Neuro-Oncology, Neuro Inst-Presby Hosp 1985; Neuro-Oncology, Meml Sloan-Kettering Cancer Ctr 1986; **Fac Appt:** Prof N, Cornell Univ-Weill Med Coll

Glass, Jon MD [N] - **Spec Exp:** Neuro-Oncology; Brain Tumors; Spinal Tumors; **Hospital:** Fox Chase Cancer Ctr (page 73); **Address:** Fox Chase Cancer Ctr, 333 Cottman Ave, Philadelphia, PA 19111; **Phone:** 215-728-3070; **Board Cert:** Neurology 1993; **Med School:** SUNY Downstate 1986; **Resid:** Neurology, Boston Univ 1989; **Fellow:** Neuro-Oncology, Mass Genl Hosp 1991; **Fac Appt:** Asst Prof N, NYU Sch Med

Hiesiger, Emile MD [N] - **Spec Exp:** Pain Management; Neuro-Oncology; **Hospital:** NYU Med Ctr (page 80), VA Med Ctr - Manhattan; **Address:** 530 1st Ave, Ste 5A, New York, NY 10016-6402; **Phone:** 212-263-6123; **Board Cert:** Neurology 1983; **Med School:** NY Med Coll 1978; **Resid:** Neurology, NYU Med Ctr 1982; **Fellow:** Neurology, Meml Sloan-Kettering Cancer Ctr 1984; **Fac Appt:** Assoc Clin Prof N, NYU Sch Med

Laterra, John J MD/PhD [N] - **Spec Exp:** Neuro-Oncology; Brain Tumors; **Hospital:** Johns Hopkins Hosp - Baltimore; **Address:** Johns Hopkins Hosp, Phipps 115, 600 N Wolfe St, Baltimore, MD 21287; **Phone:** 410-614-3853; **Board Cert:** Neurology 1990; **Med School:** Case West Res Univ 1984; **Resid:** Neurology, Univ Mich Hosps 1988; **Fellow:** Research, Johns Hopkins Hosp 1989; **Fac Appt:** Prof N, Johns Hopkins Univ

Posner, Jerome MD [N] - **Spec Exp:** Neuro-Oncology; Brain Tumors; **Hospital:** Meml Sloan Kettering Cancer Ctr (page 76); **Address:** 1275 York Ave, rm C731, New York, NY 10021-6007; **Phone:** 212-639-7047; **Board Cert:** Neurology 1962; **Med School:** Univ Wash 1955; **Resid:** Neurology, Univ WA Affil Hosp 1959; **Fellow:** Biochemistry, Univ WA Affil Hosp 1963; **Fac Appt:** Prof N, Cornell Univ-Weill Med Coll

Rosenfeld, Myrna MD/PhD [N] - **Spec Exp:** Neuro-Oncology; Brain Tumors; **Hospital:** Hosp Univ Penn - UPHS (page 84); **Address:** Hosp Univ Penn, Dept Neurology, 3400 Spruce St, 3W Gates, Philadelphia, PA 19104; **Phone:** 215-746-4707; **Board Cert:** Neurology 1990; **Med School:** Northwestern Univ 1985; **Resid:** Neurology, Northwestern Univ Hosp 1987; Neurology, Univ Hosp Cleveland 1989; **Fellow:** Neuro-Oncology, Meml Sloan Kettering Cancer Ctr; **Fac Appt:** Assoc Prof N, Univ Pennsylvania

Rosenfeld, Steven S MD [N] - **Spec Exp:** Brain Tumors; Gliomas; Neuro-Oncology; **Hospital:** NY-Presby Hosp (page 79); **Address:** Neurological Inst of NY-Brain Tumor Ctr, 710 W 168th St, rm 204, New York, NY 10032; **Phone:** 212-305-1718; **Board Cert:** Neurology 1994; **Med School:** Northwestern Univ 1985; **Resid:** Neurology, Duke Univ Med Ctr 1989; **Fellow:** Neuro-Oncology, Duke Univ Med Ctr 1990; **Fac Appt:** Prof N, Columbia P&S

Southeast

Janss, Anna J MD/PhD [N] - **Spec Exp:** Brain Tumors-Pediatric; Clinical Trials; Cancer Survivors-Late Effects of Therapy; **Hospital:** Chldns Hlthcare Atlanta - Egleston; **Address:** Chldns Hlthcare Atlanta - Egleston, Division Neuro-Oncology, 1405 Clifton Rd NE, Atlanta, GA 30322; **Phone:** 404-785-1200; **Board Cert:** Neurology 1993; **Med School:** Univ Iowa Coll Med 1988; **Resid:** Neurology, Hosp Univ Penn 1992; **Fellow:** Pediatric Neuro-Oncology, Chldns Hosp 1996; **Fac Appt:** Assoc Prof N, Emory Univ

Nabors III, Louis Burt MD [N] - **Spec Exp:** Neuro-Oncology; Brain Tumors; **Hospital:** Univ of Ala Hosp at Birmingham; **Address:** UAB, FOT 1020, 510 20th St S, Birmingham, AL 35294-3410; **Phone:** 205-934-1432; **Board Cert:** Neurology 1999; **Med School:** Univ Tenn Coll Med, Memphis 1991; **Resid:** Neurology, Univ Alabama; **Fellow:** Neuro-Oncology, Univ Alabama; **Fac Appt:** Assoc Prof N, Univ Ala

Patchell, Roy MD [N] - **Spec Exp:** Neuro-Oncology; Brain Tumors; Spinal Tumors; **Hospital:** Univ of Kentucky Chandler Hosp; **Address:** Univ Kentucky Neurosurgery-Chandler Med Ctr, 800 Rose St, MS 105, Lexington, KY 40536; **Phone:** 859-323-5672; **Board Cert:** Neurology 1984; **Med School:** Univ KY Coll Med 1979; **Resid:** Neurology, Johns Hopkins Hosp 1983; **Fellow:** Neuro-Oncology, Meml Sloan-Kettering Canc Ctr 1985; **Fac Appt:** Prof N, Univ KY Coll Med

Phuphanich, Surasak MD [N] - **Spec Exp:** Neuro-Oncology; Brain Tumors; Spinal Tumors; **Hospital:** Emory Univ Hosp; **Address:** Winship Cancer Inst-Emory Univ, 1365 Clifton Rd NE C Bldg Fl 2, Atlanta, GA 30322; **Phone:** 404-778-1900; **Board Cert:** Neurology 1983; **Med School:** Thailand 1975; **Resid:** Neurology, Univ Illinois Med Ctr 1981; **Fellow:** Neuro-Oncology, UCSF Med Ctr 1984; **Fac Appt:** Prof, Emory Univ

Schiff, David MD [N] - **Spec Exp:** Brain Tumors; Spinal Cord Tumors; Neurological Complications of Cancer; Neuro-Oncology; **Hospital:** Univ Virginia Med Ctr; **Address:** Univ VA, Div of Neuro-Oncology, PO Box 800432, Charlottesville, VA 22908; **Phone:** 434-982-4415; **Board Cert:** Neurology 1994; **Med School:** Harvard Med Sch 1988; **Resid:** Neurology, Harvard Longwood 1992; **Fellow:** Neuro-Oncology, Meml Sloan Kettering Cancer Ctr 1993; Mayo Clinic 1994; **Fac Appt:** Assoc Prof NS, Univ VA Sch Med

Schold Jr, S Clifford MD [N] - **Spec Exp:** Brain Tumors; Neuro-Oncology; **Hospital:** H Lee Moffitt Cancer Ctr & Research Inst; **Address:** H Lee Moffitt Cancer Ctr, 12902 Magnolia Dr, MCC VP Admin, Tampa, FL 33612; **Phone:** 813-745-7426; **Board Cert:** Neurology 1980; **Med School:** Univ Ariz Coll Med 1973; **Resid:** Neurology, Colorado Med Ctr 1977; **Fellow:** Neuro-Oncology, Sloan-Kettering Cancer Ctr 1978; **Fac Appt:** Prof N, Univ S Fla Coll Med

Midwest

Barger, Geoffrey R MD [N] - **Spec Exp:** Neuro-Oncology; Brain Tumors; **Hospital:** Harper Univ Hosp; **Address:** Wayne State Univ Hlth Ctr, 4201 St Antoine, Ste 8D-UHC, Detroit, MI 48201; **Phone:** 313-745-4275, **Board Cert:** Neurology 1981; **Med School:** Jefferson Med Coll 1975; **Resid:** Neurology, Penn Hosp 1979; **Fellow:** Neuro-Oncology, Moffitt Hosp & Brain Tumor Ctr/UCSF 1982; **Fac Appt:** Assoc Prof N, Wayne State Univ

Cascino, Terrence L MD [N] - **Spec Exp:** Neuro-Oncology; **Hospital:** Mayo Med Ctr & Clin - Rochester; **Address:** Mayo Clinic, 200 1st St SW, Rochester, MN 55905-0001; **Phone:** 507-284-2576; **Board Cert:** Neurology 1984; **Med School:** Loyola Univ-Stritch Sch Med 1972; **Resid:** Neurology, Mayo Clinic 1980; **Fellow:** Neuro-Oncology, Meml Sloan Kettering Cancer Ctr; **Fac Appt:** Assoc Prof N, Mayo Med Sch

Greenberg, Harry S MD [N] - **Spec Exp:** Neuro-Oncology; Brain Tumors; **Hospital:** Univ Michigan Hlth Sys, Vail Valley Med Ctr; **Address:** Taubman Ctr 1914-0316, 1500 E Med Ctr Dr, Ann Arbor, MI 48109-0316; **Phone:** 734-936-9055; **Board Cert:** Neurology 1980; **Med School:** SUNY Upstate Med Univ 1973; **Resid:** Neurology, Stanford Univ Hosp 1977; **Fellow:** Neuro-Oncology, Sloan Kettering Cancer Ctr 1979; **Fac Appt:** Prof N, Univ Mich Med Sch

Mikkelsen, Tom MD [N] - **Spec Exp:** Brain Tumors; Gliomas; **Hospital:** Henry Ford Hosp, William Beaumont Hosp; **Address:** Henry Ford Hospital, ER 3096, 2799 W Grand Blvd, Detroit, MI 48202; **Phone:** 313-916-8641; **Board Cert:** Neurology 1998; **Med School:** Univ Calgary 1983; **Resid:** Internal Medicine, Calgary General Hosp 1985; Neurology, Montreal Neurological Inst 1988; **Fellow:** Neuro-Oncology, Royal Victoria Hosp 1990; Neuro-Oncology, Ludwig Inst for Cancer Rsch 1992; **Fac Appt:** Assoc Prof N, Case West Res Univ

Newton, Herbert B MD [N] - **Spec Exp:** Neuro-Oncology; Brain & Spinal Tumors; **Hospital:** Ohio St Univ Med Ctr, Arthur G James Cancer Hosp & Research Inst; **Address:** 465 Means Hall, 1654 Upham Dr Fl 4, Columbus, OH 43210; **Phone:** 614-293-8930; **Board Cert:** Neurology 1989; **Med School:** SUNY Buffalo 1984; **Resid:** Neurology, Univ Michigan 1988; **Fellow:** Neuro-Oncology, Meml Sloan-Kettering Cancer Ctr 1990; **Fac Appt:** Prof N, Ohio State Univ

Rogers, Lisa R DO [N] - **Spec Exp:** Neuro-Oncology; Brain Tumors; Brain Radiation Toxicity; **Hospital:** Univ Michigan Hlth Sys; **Address:** Univ Michigan, Dept Neurology, 1914 Taubman Center, Ann Arbor, MI 48109-0316; **Phone:** 734-615-2994; **Board Cert:** Neurology 1982; **Med School:** Kirksville Coll Osteo Med 1976; **Resid:** Neurology, Cleveland Clinic Fdn 1980; **Fellow:** Neuro-Oncology, Meml-Sloan Kettering Cancer Ctr 1982; **Fac Appt:** Prof N, Univ Mich Med Sch

Sagar, Stephen M MD [N] - **Spec Exp:** Neuro-Oncology; Brain Tumors; **Hospital:** Univ Hosps Case Med Ctr; **Address:** Univ Hosp Cleveland, Hanna House, 11100 Euclid Ave Fl 5, Cleveland, OH 44106; **Phone:** 216-844-7510; **Board Cert:** Internal Medicine 1976; Neurology 1979; **Med School:** Harvard Med Sch 1972; **Resid:** Internal Medicine, Peter Bent Brigham Hosp 1974; Neurology, Mass Genl Hosp 1977; **Fellow:** Neurology, Chldns Hosp Med Ctr 1979; **Fac Appt:** Prof N, Case West Res Univ

Vick, Nicholas A MD [N] - **Spec Exp:** Brain Tumors; Neuro-Oncology; **Hospital:** Evanston Hosp; **Address:** Evanston Hosp, Div Neurology, 2650 Ridge Ave, Evanston, IL 60201; **Phone:** 847-570-2570 x11; **Board Cert:** Neurology 1971; **Med School:** Univ Chicago-Pritzker Sch Med 1965; **Resid:** Neurology, Univ Chicago Hosps 1968; **Fellow:** Neurology, Natl Inst Hlth 1970; **Fac Appt:** Prof N, Northwestern Univ

Southwest

Gilbert, Mark R MD [N] - **Spec Exp:** Brain Tumors; Neuro-Oncology; **Hospital:** UT MD Anderson Cancer Ctr (page 81); **Address:** Univ Tex MD Anderson Cancer Ctr, 1515 Holcombe Blvd, Unit 431, Houston, TX 77030; **Phone:** 713-792-6600; **Board Cert:** Internal Medicine 1985; Neurology 1990; **Med School:** Johns Hopkins Univ 1982; **Resid:** Internal Medicine, Johns Hopkins Hosp 1985; Neurology, Johns Hopkins Hosp 1988; **Fellow:** Neuro-Oncology, Johns Hopkins Hosp 1988; **Fac Appt:** Assoc Prof N, Univ Tex, Houston

Levin, Victor A MD [N] - **Spec Exp:** Brain Tumors; Neuro-Oncology; Clinical Trials; **Hospital:** UT MD Anderson Cancer Ctr (page 81); **Address:** 1515 Holcombe Blvd, Unit #431, Houston, TX 77030-4009; **Phone:** 713-792-8297; **Board Cert:** Neurology 1976; **Med School:** Univ Wisc 1966; **Resid:** Neurology, Mass Genl Hosp 1972; **Fac Appt:** Prof Med, Univ Tex, Houston

Shapiro, William R MD [N] - **Spec Exp:** Neuro-Oncology; **Hospital:** St Joseph's Hosp & Med Ctr - Phoenix; **Address:** Barrow Neurology Clinics, 500 W Thomas Rd, Ste 300, Phoenix, AZ 85013; **Phone:** 602-406-6262; **Board Cert:** Neurology 1969; **Med School:** UCSF 1961; **Resid:** Internal Medicine, Univ Wash Hosp 1963; Neurology, NY Hosp-Cornell Med Ctr 1966; **Fellow:** Neuro-Oncology, Natl Inst Hlth 1969; **Fac Appt:** Prof N, Univ Ariz Coll Med

Yung, Wai-Kwan Alfred MD [N] - **Spec Exp:** Neuro-Oncology; Brain Tumors; **Hospital:** UT MD Anderson Cancer Ctr (page 81); **Address:** 1515 Holcombe Blvd, Unit 0431, Houston, TX 77030; **Phone:** 713-794-1285; **Board Cert:** Neurology 1980; **Med School:** Univ Chicago-Pritzker Sch Med 1975; **Resid:** Neurology, UCSD Med Ctr 1978; **Fellow:** Neuro-Oncology, Meml Sloan Kettering Cancer Ctr 1981; **Fac Appt:** Prof N, Univ Tex, Houston

West Coast and Pacific

Cloughesy, Timothy F MD [N] - **Spec Exp:** Neuro-Oncology; Brain Tumors; **Hospital:** UCLA Med Ctr (page 83); **Address:** UCLA Neurological Services, 710 Westwood Plaza, Ste 1-230, Los Angeles, CA 90095; **Phone:** 310-825-5321; **Board Cert:** Neurology 1993; **Med School:** Tulane Univ 1987; **Resid:** Neurology, UCLA Med Ctr 1991; **Fellow:** Neuro-Oncology, Meml Sloan-Kettering Canc Ctr; **Fac Appt:** Clin Prof N, UCLA

Spence, Alexander M MD [N] - **Spec Exp:** Neuro-Oncology; **Hospital:** Univ Wash Med Ctr; **Address:** Univ Wash, Dept Neur, 1959 NE Pacific St, Box 356465, Seattle, WA 98195-0001; **Phone:** 206-543-0252; **Board Cert:** Neurology 1971; **Med School:** Univ Chicago-Pritzker Sch Med 1965; **Resid:** Neurology, Chldns Hosp 1969; Neuropathology, Stanford Univ Med Ctr 1974; **Fac Appt:** Prof N, Univ Wash

Child Neurology

New England

Mandelbaum, David E MD/PhD [ChiN] - **Spec Exp:** Brain Tumors-Pediatric; **Hospital:** Rhode Island Hosp, Women & Infants Hosp - Rhode Island; **Address:** Dept of Neurology, 110 Lockwood St, Ste 342, Providence, RI 02903; **Phone:** 401-444-4345; **Board Cert:** Neurology 1987; Pediatrics 1987; Clinical Neurophysiology 2003; Neurodevelopmental Disabilities 2001; **Med School:** Columbia P&S 1980; **Resid:** Pediatrics, Yale-New Haven Hosp 1982; Neurology, Neuro Inst-Columbia 1983; **Fellow:** Child Neurology, Neuro Inst-Columbia 1985; **Fac Appt:** Prof Ped, Brown Univ

Pomeroy, Scott L MD/PhD [ChiN] - **Spec Exp:** Neuro-Oncology; Brain Tumors; **Hospital:** Children's Hospital - Boston, Dana-Farber Cancer Inst; **Address:** Chldns Hosp, Dept Neurology-Fegan 11, 300 Longwood Ave, Boston, MA 02115; **Phone:** 617-355-6386; **Board Cert:** Pediatrics 2003; Child Neurology 1988; **Med School:** Univ Conn 1982; **Resid:** Pediatrics, Chldns Hosp 1984; Neurology, Barnes Hosp/Washington Univ 1985; **Fellow:** Pediatric Neurology, St Louis Chldns Hosp 1987; Neurological Biology, Washington Univ 1989; **Fac Appt:** Prof N, Harvard Med Sch

Child Neurology

Mid Atlantic

Allen, Jeffrey MD [ChiN] - **Spec Exp:** Neuro-Oncology; Brain Tumors; **Hospital:** NYU Med Ctr (page 80), St Luke's - Roosevelt Hosp Ctr - Roosevelt Div (page 72); **Address:** Hassenfeld Childrens Ctr, 160 E 32nd St, New York, NY 10016; **Phone:** 212-263-6725; **Board Cert:** Child Neurology 1977; **Med School:** Harvard Med Sch 1969; **Resid:** Pediatrics, Montreal Chldns Hosp 1973; Pediatric Neurology, Montreal Neur Inst/McGill 1976; **Fac Appt:** Prof Ped, NYU Sch Med

Duffner, Patricia K MD [ChiN] - **Spec Exp:** Brain Tumors; Cancer Survivors-Late Effects of Therapy; **Hospital:** Women's & Chldn's Hosp of Buffalo, The; **Address:** Women & Chlds Hosp, Dept Neurology, 219 Bryant St, Buffalo, NY 14222-2006; **Phone:** 716-878-7819; **Board Cert:** Pediatrics 1977; Child Neurology 1979; **Med School:** SUNY Buffalo 1972; **Resid:** Pediatrics, Buffalo Chldns Hosp 1975; **Fellow:** Child Neurology, SUNY Buffalo-Buffalo Chldns Hosp 1978; **Fac Appt:** Prof N, SUNY Buffalo

Packer, Roger MD [ChiN] - **Spec Exp:** Brain Tumors; **Hospital:** Chldns Natl Med Ctr; **Address:** Childrens Natl Med Ctr, Dept Neurology, 111 Michigan Ave NW, Washington, DC 20010-2978; **Phone:** 202-884-2120; **Board Cert:** Child Neurology 1982; Pediatrics 1982; **Med School:** Northwestern Univ 1976; **Resid:** Pediatrics, Chldns Med Ctr 1978; Neurology, Chldns Hosp-Univ Penn 1981; **Fac Appt:** Prof N, Geo Wash Univ

Phillips, Peter C MD [ChiN] - **Spec Exp:** Brain Tumors; Neuro-Oncology; **Hospital:** Chldns Hosp of Philadelphia, The; **Address:** Childrens Hosp Philadelphia, 34th St & Civic Center Blvd, Philadelphia, PA 19104; **Phone:** 215-590-3015; **Board Cert:** Pediatrics 1985; Child Neurology 1986; **Med School:** Univ Conn 1978; **Resid:** Pediatrics, Chldns Hosp 1980; Pediatric Neurology, Neuro Inst 1983; **Fellow:** Neuro-Oncology, Meml Sloan Kettering Hosp 1986; **Fac Appt:** Prof N, Univ Pennsylvania

Midwest

Cohen, Bruce H MD [ChiN] - **Spec Exp:** Brain Tumors; Pain Management; **Hospital:** Cleveland Clin Fdn (page 71); **Address:** Cleveland Clinic, 9500 Euclid Ave, Desk S71, Cleveland, OH 44195; **Phone:** 216-444-9182; **Board Cert:** Pediatrics 2004; Child Neurology 1990; **Med School:** Albert Einstein Coll Med 1982; **Resid:** Pediatrics, Chldns Hosp 1984; Child Neurology, Neurologic Inst-Columbia 1987; **Fellow:** Pediatric Neuro-Oncology, Chldns Hosp 1989

West Coast and Pacific

Fisher, Paul G MD [ChiN] - **Spec Exp:** Neuro-Oncology; Brain Tumors; **Hospital:** Lucile Packard Chldns Hosp/Stanford Univ Med Ctr; **Address:** Stanford Cancer Ctr-Dept Neurology, 875 Blake Wilbur Drive, rm 2220, Stanford, CA 94305; **Phone:** 650-725-8630; **Board Cert:** Pediatrics 1995; Child Neurology 1998; **Med School:** UCSF 1989; **Resid:** Pediatrics, Johns Hopkins Univ Hosp 1991; Neurology, Johns Hopkins Univ Hosp 1994; **Fellow:** Neuro-Oncology, Children's Hosp 1994; **Fac Appt:** Assoc Prof Ped, Stanford Univ

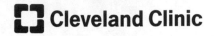

Brain Tumor and Neuro-Oncology Center

Part of the Cleveland Clinic Neurological Institute, the Brain Tumor and Neuro-Oncology Center (BTNC) is a nationally recognized leader in the diagnosis and treatment of primary and metastatic tumors of the brain, spine and nerves, and their effects on the nervous system. Patients have access to the latest advances in surgery, non-invasive radiosurgery, brachytherapy and clinical trials. Innovations in drug therapy and delivery techniques, including blood-brain barrier disruption and convection-enhanced delivery, keep the BTNC at the forefront of brain-tumor treatment and ensure the best patient outcomes. This group of neurosurgeons, neuro-oncologists, medical oncologists, neuroradiologists, radiation oncologists, neuropathologists, advanced practice nurses and nurse practitioners collaborates on individualized treatments to maximize favorable outcomes.

In 2006, BTNC physicians recorded 8,300 outpatient visits and performed more than 900 procedures for brain tumors, including stereotactic radiosurgery (Gamma Knife) and surgery. More than 25 percent of our new patients came from outside of Ohio.

Advances in Metastatic Disease Treatment

The Gamma Knife Center combines sophisticated technology and medical expertise to provide state-of-the-art, non-surgical treatment for patients with a wide range of brain tumors. The most common indication for Gamma Knife radiosurgery is brain metastases, a condition that afflicts nearly a quarter of patients suffering from cancer. Additional treatments are for primary and benign tumors, trigeminal neuralgia and arteriovenous malformations. In 2006, we treated our 2,000th case with Gamma Knife radiosurgery.

We currently are upgrading our equipment to the most technologically advanced model available, the Perfexion, which allows for treatment in a wider range of anatomical structures, offers enhanced planning, uses all imaging modalities, increases patient comfort and reduces treatment time.

To treat metastases to the spine, the BTNC established a Stereotactic Spine Radiosurgery Program that uses the Novalis Shaped-Beam system to deliver a high dose of conformal radiation to spinal tumors.

Research and Clinical Trials

Currently, the BTNC is focusing basic research efforts in the areas of molecular genetics and molecular neuro-oncology, molecular biology of brain tumors, immunology, apoptosis and the blood-brain barrier.

To give patients more therapeutic treatment options, the BTNC offers Phase I, II and III clinical trials of the most promising anti-cancer agents. The center's membership in the New Approaches to Brain Tumor Therapy (NABTT) consortium gives patients additional access to more clinical trials, including some that are conducted at just a few centers across the country. The collaboration of the BTNC with Cleveland Clinic's Taussig Cancer Center provides access to novel anti-cancer agents and biological therapies for patients with primary brain tumors and metastases to the brain from other primary cancer sites.

To schedule an appointment or for more information about Cleveland Clinic, call 800.890.2467 or visit www.clevelandclinic.org/braintumortopdocs.

Brain Tumor and Neuro-Oncology Center | 9500 Euclid Ave. / W14 | Cleveland, Ohio 44195

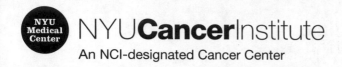

NYUCancer Institute
An NCI-designated Cancer Center

NEURO-ONCOLOGY PROGRAM

UCLA Health System

1-800-UCLA-MD1 (825-2631)
www.uclahealth.org

UCLA's Neuro-oncology Program brings together experts to treat adult and pediatric patients suffering from neuro-oncologic diseases, such as primary malignant brain tumors, primary malignant spinal cord tumors, metastatic brain tumors, carcinomatous meningitis, epidural spinal cord compression, paraneoplastic disorders, and neurologic complications of cancer and its treatment. Team members include specialists in neurology, neurosurgery, medical oncology, radiation oncology, neuropathology, neuroimaging, neuropsychiatry, neuropsychology and social work that meet regularly to review cases and make recommendations.

These experts are leaders not only in defining state-of-the-art care, but are also intimately involved in the design of novel clinical trials, including:

- Antiangiogenesis agents
- Signal transduction inhibitors
- Novel radiation sensitizers
- Immune-based therapies
- Gene therapies
- Biological agents
- Blood-brain barrier delivery systems

High-tech surgical facilities and technologies allow for optimal tumor removal while ensuring maintenance of neurologic function.

UCLA's Jonsson Cancer Center

Designated by the National Cancer Institute as one of only 39 comprehensive cancer centers in the United States, UCLA's Jonsson Cancer Center has earned an international reputation for developing new cancer therapies, providing the best in experimental and traditional treatments, and expertly guiding and training the next generation of medical researchers. The center's 250 physicians and scientists treat upwards of 20,000 patient visits per year and offer hundreds of clinical trials that provide the latest in experimental cancer treatments (www.cancer.mednet.ucla.edu). The center also offers patients and families complete psychological and support services.

UCLA's Jonsson Cancer Center has been ranked the best cancer center in California by *U.S.News & World Report*'s Annual Best Hospitals survey for the seventh year. UCLA Medical Center, of which the Cancer Center is a part, has ranked best in the West for the past 17 years.

Call 1-800-UCLA-MD1 (825-2631)
for a referral to a UCLA doctor.

THE END OF CANCER BEGINS WITH RESEARCH

A vaccine to treat brain cancer shows promising results in research at UCLA's Jonsson Cancer Center. The experimental vaccine, which has been tested at UCLA in adults, stimulates the immune system to target and attack cancer. Researchers are optimistic that targeted approaches to treating brain cancer may hold the key to improving survival and enhancing quality of life in patients.

Volunteers are being recruited now for Phase II studies of the dendritic cell brain cancer vaccine study.

Obstetrics & Gynecology

An obstetrician/gynecologist possesses special knowledge, skills and professional capability in the medical and surgical care of the female reproductive system and associated disorders. This physician serves as a consultant to other physicians and as a primary physician for women.

Training Required: Four years plus two years in clinical practice before certification is complete.

Gynecolgic Oncology: An obstetrician/gynecologist who provides consultation and comprehensive management of patients with gynecologic cancer, including those diagnostic and therapeutic procedures necessary for the total care of the patient with gynecologic cancer and resulting complications.

Training Required: Four years plus two years in clinical practice before certification in obstetrics and gynecology is complete plus additional training and examination in gynecologic oncology.

Reproductive Endocrinology/Infertility: An obstetrician/gynecologist who is capable of managing complex problems relating to reproductive endocrinology and infertility.

Training Required: Four years plus two years in clinical practice before certification in obstetrics and gynecology is complete plus additional training and examination in reproductive endocrinology.

Gynecologic Oncology

New England

Berkowitz, Ross S MD [GO] - **Spec Exp:** Gynecologic Cancer; **Hospital:** Brigham & Women's Hosp, Dana-Farber Cancer Inst; **Address:** Brigham & Women's Hosp, Dept OB/GYN, 75 Francis St, Boston, MA 02115-6110; **Phone:** 617-732-8843; **Board Cert:** Obstetrics & Gynecology 1981; Gynecologic Oncology 1982; **Med School:** Boston Univ 1973; **Resid:** Obstetrics & Gynecology, Boston Hosp for Women 1978; Surgery, Peter Bent Brigham Hosp. 1975; **Fellow:** Gynecologic Oncology, Boston Hosp for Women 1980; **Fac Appt:** Prof ObG, Harvard Med Sch

Brewer, Molly A MD [GO] - **Spec Exp:** Ovarian Cancer; **Hospital:** Univ of Conn Hlth Ctr, John Dempsey Hosp; **Address:** Univ Connecticut Hlth Ctr, Div Gyn Oncology, 263 Farmington Ave, MC2875, Farmington, CT 06032-2875; **Phone:** 860-679-4933; **Board Cert:** Obstetrics & Gynecology 1999; Gynecologic Oncology 2001; **Med School:** SUNY Upstate Med Univ 1991; **Resid:** Obstetrics & Gynecology, Oregon Hlth Scis Univ Hosp 1995; **Fellow:** Gynecologic Oncology, MD Anderson Cancer Ctr 1997

Currie, John L MD [GO] - **Spec Exp:** Gynecologic Cancer; Pelvic Reconstruction; **Hospital:** Hartford Hosp; **Address:** Hartford Hospital, 85 Seymour St Fl 7 - Ste 705, Box 5037, Hartford, CT 06106; **Phone:** 860-545-4341; **Board Cert:** Obstetrics & Gynecology 1991; Gynecologic Oncology 1982; **Med School:** Univ NC Sch Med 1967; **Resid:** Gynecologic Oncology, Hosp Univ Penn 1972; **Fellow:** Gynecologic Oncology, Duke Univ Med Ctr 1980; **Fac Appt:** Prof ObG, Univ Conn

DeMars, Leslie R MD [GO] - **Spec Exp:** Gynecologic Cancer; Laparoscopic Surgery; **Hospital:** Dartmouth - Hitchcock Med Ctr; **Address:** Dartmouth-Hitchcock Med Ctr, Gyn-Oncology, 1 Medical Center Drive, Lebanon, NH 03756; **Phone:** 603-653-3530; **Board Cert:** Obstetrics & Gynecology 2005; Gynecologic Oncology 2005; **Med School:** Univ VT Coll Med 1987; **Resid:** Obstetrics & Gynecology, Univ N Carolina Hosps 1991; **Fellow:** Gynecologic Oncology, Univ N Carolina Hosps 1994; **Fac Appt:** Asst Prof ObG, Dartmouth Med Sch

Goodman, Annekathryn MD [GO] - **Spec Exp:** Gynecologic Cancer; Gynecologic Surgery-Complex; **Hospital:** Mass Genl Hosp; **Address:** 55 Fruit St, Boston, MA 02114; **Phone:** 617-724-4800; **Board Cert:** Obstetrics & Gynecology 2003; Gynecologic Oncology 2003; **Med School:** Tufts Univ 1983; **Resid:** Obstetrics & Gynecology, Tufts New England Med Ctr 1987; **Fellow:** Gynecologic Oncology, Mass Genl Hosp 1990; **Fac Appt:** Assoc Prof ObG, Harvard Med Sch

Muto, Michael G MD [GO] - **Spec Exp:** Ovarian Cancer; Cervical Cancer; Vulva & Vaginal Cancer; **Hospital:** Dana-Farber Cancer Inst; **Address:** Dana Farber Cancer Inst, 44 Binney St Fl 9, Boston, MA 02115; **Phone:** 617-582-7931; **Board Cert:** Gynecologic Oncology 2005; Obstetrics & Gynecology 2005; **Med School:** Univ Mass Sch Med 1983; **Resid:** Obstetrics & Gynecology, Brigham & Women's Hosp 1987; **Fellow:** Gynecologic Oncology, Brigham & Women's Hosp 1990; **Fac Appt:** Assoc Prof ObG, Harvard Med Sch

Rutherford, Thomas MD [GO] - **Spec Exp:** Ovarian Cancer; Uterine Cancer; Ovarian Cancer-Early Detection; Cervical Cancer; **Hospital:** Yale - New Haven Hosp; **Address:** Yale Univ Sch Med Dept Ob-Gyn, 333 Cedar St, Box 208063, New Haven, CT 06520; **Phone:** 203-785-6301; **Board Cert:** Obstetrics & Gynecology 1997; Gynecologic Oncology 2000; **Med School:** Med Coll OH 1989; **Resid:** Obstetrics & Gynecology, Cooper Hosp 1993; **Fellow:** Gynecologic Oncology, Yale-New Haven Hosp 1995; **Fac Appt:** Assoc Prof ObG, Yale Univ

Schwartz, Peter E MD [GO] - **Spec Exp:** Ovarian Cancer; Uterine Cancer; Gynecologic Surgery-Complex; Cervical Cancer; **Hospital:** Yale - New Haven Hosp, Hosp of St Raphael; **Address:** Yale Univ Sch Med, Dept Ob/Gyn, 333 Cedar St, rm FMB-316, New Haven, CT 06510-3289; **Phone:** 203-785-4014; **Board Cert:** Obstetrics & Gynecology 1973; Gynecologic Oncology 1979; **Med School:** Albert Einstein Coll Med 1966; **Resid:** Obstetrics & Gynecology, Yale-New Haven Hosp 1970; **Fellow:** Gynecologic Oncology, MD Anderson Cancer Ctr 1975; **Fac Appt:** Prof ObG, Yale Univ

Tarraza, Hector MD [GO] - **Spec Exp:** Gynecologic Cancer; **Hospital:** Maine Med Ctr; **Address:** 102 Campus Drive, rm 116, Scarborough, ME 04074; **Phone:** 207-883-0069; **Board Cert:** Obstetrics & Gynecology 1998; Gynecologic Oncology 1998; **Med School:** Harvard Med Sch 1981; **Resid:** Obstetrics & Gynecology, Mass Genl Hosp 1985; **Fellow:** Gynecologic Oncology, Mass Genl Hosp 1987; **Fac Appt:** Prof ObG, Univ VT Coll Med

Mid Atlantic

Abu-Rustum, Nadeem R MD [GO] - **Spec Exp:** Ovarian Cancer; Uterine Cancer; Cervical Cancer; Vulvar Disease/Cancer; **Hospital:** Meml Sloan Kettering Cancer Ctr (page 76); **Address:** Meml Sloan Kettering Cancer Ctr, 1275 York Ave, rm H-1308, New York, NY 10021; **Phone:** 212-639-7051; **Board Cert:** Obstetrics & Gynecology 1998; Gynecologic Oncology 2000; **Med School:** Lebanon 1990; **Resid:** Obstetrics & Gynecology, Greater Baltimore Med Ctr 1994; **Fellow:** Gynecologic Oncology, Meml Sloan Kettering Cancer Ctr 1997; **Fac Appt:** Assoc Prof ObG, Cornell Univ-Weill Med Coll

Barakat, Richard MD [GO] - **Spec Exp:** Laparoscopic Surgery; Ovarian Cancer; Uterine Cancer; **Hospital:** Meml Sloan Kettering Cancer Ctr (page 76); **Address:** Memorial Sloan Kettering Cancer Ctr, 1275 York Ave, rm H4135, New York, NY 10021; **Phone:** 212-639-2453; **Board Cert:** Obstetrics & Gynecology 1992; Gynecologic Oncology 1994; **Med School:** SUNY Hlth Sci Ctr 1985; **Resid:** Obstetrics & Gynecology, Bellevue Hosp 1989; **Fellow:** Gynecologic Oncology, Meml Sloan Kettering Cancer Ctr 1991; **Fac Appt:** Assoc Prof ObG, Cornell Univ-Weill Med Coll

Barnes, Willard MD [GO] - **Spec Exp:** Pelvic Tumors; Gynecologic Cancer; **Hospital:** Georgetown Univ Hosp, Virginia Hosp Ctr - Arlington; **Address:** Lombardi Cancer Ctr, Dept Gyn Oncology, 3800 Reservoir Rd NW, Washington, DC 20007-2194; **Phone:** 202-444-2114; **Board Cert:** Obstetrics & Gynecology 1997; Gynecologic Oncology 1997; **Med School:** Univ Miss 1979; **Resid:** Obstetrics & Gynecology, Univ Miss Med Ctr 1983; **Fellow:** Gynecologic Oncology, Georgetown Univ Med Ctr 1985; **Fac Appt:** Assoc Prof ObG, Georgetown Univ

Gynecologic Oncology

Barter, James MD [GO] - Spec Exp: Laparoscopic Surgery; Ovarian Cancer; Gynecologic Cancer; **Hospital:** Suburban Hosp - Bethesda, Holy Cross Hospital - Silver Spring; **Address:** 6301 Executive Blvd, Rockville, MD 20852; **Phone:** 301-770-4967; **Board Cert:** Obstetrics & Gynecology 1997; Gynecologic Oncology 1997; **Med School:** Univ VA Sch Med 1977; **Resid:** Internal Medicine, Univ Kentucky Med Ctr 1979; Obstetrics & Gynecology, Duke Univ Med Ctr 1983; **Fellow:** Gynecologic Oncology, Univ Alabama 1986; **Fac Appt:** Clin Prof ObG, Georgetown Univ

Bristow, Robert E MD [GO] - Spec Exp: Ovarian Cancer; Cervical Cancer; Uterine Cancer; **Hospital:** Johns Hopkins Hosp - Baltimore; **Address:** Johns Hopkins Hosp, 601 Caroline St Fl 8, Baltimore, MD 21287; **Phone:** 410-955-6700; **Board Cert:** Obstetrics & Gynecology 1999; Gynecologic Oncology 2003; **Med School:** USC Sch Med 1991; **Resid:** Obstetrics & Gynecology, Johns Hopkins Hosp 1995; **Fellow:** Gynecologic Oncology, UCLA Med Ctr 1998; **Fac Appt:** Assoc Prof ObG, Johns Hopkins Univ

Caputo, Thomas A MD [GO] - Spec Exp: Cervical Cancer; Ovarian Cancer; Uterine Cancer; **Hospital:** NY-Presby Hosp (page 79); **Address:** 525 E 68th St, Ste J130, New York, NY 10021; **Phone:** 212-746-3179; **Board Cert:** Obstetrics & Gynecology 1993; Gynecologic Oncology 1977; **Med School:** UMDNJ-NJ Med Sch, Newark 1965; **Resid:** Obstetrics & Gynecology, Martland Hosp 1969; **Fellow:** Gynecologic Oncology, Emory Univ Hosp 1974; **Fac Appt:** Clin Prof ObG, Cornell Univ-Weill Med Coll

Carlson, John A MD [GO] - Spec Exp: Gynecologic Cancer; Ovarian Cancer; Gynecologic Surgery-Complex; **Hospital:** St Peter's Univ Hosp; **Address:** St Peter's Univ Hosp, 254 Easton Ave, New Brunswick, NJ 08901; **Phone:** 732-937-6003; **Board Cert:** Obstetrics & Gynecology 1981; Gynecologic Oncology 1982; **Med School:** Georgetown Univ 1974; **Resid:** Obstetrics & Gynecology, Hosp Univ Penn 1978; **Fellow:** Gynecologic Oncology, MD Anderson Hosp 1980; **Fac Appt:** Prof ObG, Drexel Univ Coll Med

Chalas, Eva MD [GO] - Spec Exp: Gynecologic Cancer; Ovarian Cancer; Cervical Cancer; **Hospital:** Stony Brook Univ Med Ctr, Winthrop - Univ Hosp; **Address:** 1077 W Jericho Tpke, Smithtown, NY 11787; **Phone:** 631-864-5440; **Board Cert:** Obstetrics & Gynecology 2006; Gynecologic Oncology 2006; **Med School:** SUNY Stony Brook 1981; **Resid:** Obstetrics & Gynecology, Univ Hosp 1985; **Fellow:** Gynecologic Oncology, Meml Sloan Kettering Cancer Ctr 1987; **Fac Appt:** Prof ObG, SUNY Stony Brook

Cohen, Carmel MD [GO] - Spec Exp: Ovarian Cancer; Cervical Cancer; Pelvic Tumors; **Hospital:** NY-Presby Hosp (page 79); **Address:** Columbia Presby Med Ctr, Div Gyn Oncol, 161 Ft Washington Ave Fl 8th - rm 837, New York, NY 10032; **Phone:** 212-305-3410; **Board Cert:** Obstetrics & Gynecology 2004; Gynecologic Oncology 2004; **Med School:** Tulane Univ 1958; **Resid:** Obstetrics & Gynecology, Mount Sinai Hosp 1964; **Fellow:** Gynecologic Oncology, Mount Sinai Hosp 1965; **Fac Appt:** Prof ObG, Columbia P&S

Coukos, George MD/PhD [GO] - Spec Exp: Ovarian Cancer; Gynecologic Cancer; Vaccine Therapy; Clinical Trials; **Hospital:** Hosp Univ Penn - UPHS (page 84); **Address:** Hosp Univ Penn, 1000 Courtyard Bldg, 3400 Spruce St, Philadelphia, PA 19104; **Phone:** 215-662-3316; **Board Cert:** Obstetrics & Gynecology 2004; Gynecologic Oncology 2004; **Med School:** Italy 1987; **Resid:** Obstetrics & Gynecology, Hosp Univ Penn 1997; **Fellow:** Gynecologic Oncology, Hosp Univ Penn 2000; **Fac Appt:** Assoc Prof ObG, Univ Pennsylvania

Curtin, John P MD [GO] - **Spec Exp:** Uterine Cancer; Ovarian Cancer; Laparoscopic Surgery; **Hospital:** NYU Med Ctr (page 80); **Address:** NYU Clinical Cancer Ctr, 160 E 34th St Fl 4, New York, NY 10016-6402; **Phone:** 212-731-5345; **Board Cert:** Obstetrics & Gynecology 1996; Gynecologic Oncology 1996; **Med School:** Creighton Univ 1979; **Resid:** Obstetrics & Gynecology, Univ Minn Med Ctr 1984; **Fellow:** Gynecologic Oncology, Meml Sloan-Kettering Cancer Ctr 1988; **Fac Appt:** Prof ObG, NYU Sch Med

Dottino, Peter R MD [GO] - **Spec Exp:** Laparoscopic Surgery; Gynecologic Cancer; **Hospital:** Mount Sinai Med Ctr (page 77), Hackensack Univ Med Ctr (page 74); **Address:** 800-A 5th Ave, Ste 405, New York, NY 10021-7215; **Phone:** 212-888-8439; **Board Cert:** Obstetrics & Gynecology 1996; Gynecologic Oncology 1996; **Med School:** Georgetown Univ 1979; **Resid:** Obstetrics & Gynecology, SUNY Downstate Med Ctr 1983; **Fellow:** Gynecologic Oncology, Mount Sinai Hosp 1985

Dunton, Charles J MD [GO] - **Spec Exp:** Ovarian Cancer; Uterine Cancer; Cervical Cancer; Pap Smear Abnormalities; **Hospital:** Lankenau Hosp; **Address:** 100 Lancaster Ave, Med Office Bldg East, Ste 661, Wynnewood, PA 19096; **Phone:** 610-649-8085; **Board Cert:** Obstetrics & Gynecology 1996; Gynecologic Oncology 1996; **Med School:** Jefferson Med Coll 1980; **Resid:** Obstetrics & Gynecology, Lankenau Hosp 1984; **Fellow:** Gynecologic Oncology, Hosp Univ Penn 1989; **Fac Appt:** Prof ObG, Jefferson Med Coll

Fishman, David A MD [GO] - **Spec Exp:** Ovarian Cancer; Ovarian Cancer-Early Detection; Gynecologic Cancer; **Hospital:** NYU Med Ctr (page 80); **Address:** NYU Clinical Cancer Ctr, 160 E 34 St Fl 4, New York, NY 10016; **Phone:** 212-731-5345; **Board Cert:** Obstetrics & Gynecology 2005; Gynecologic Oncology 2005; **Med School:** Texas Tech Univ 1988; **Resid:** Obstetrics & Gynecology, Yale-New Haven Hosp 1992; **Fellow:** Gynecologic Oncology, Yale-New Haven Hosp 1994; **Fac Appt:** Prof ObG, NYU Sch Med

Herzog, Thomas J MD [GO] - **Spec Exp:** Cervical Cancer; Gynecologic Cancer; Laparoscopic Surgery; **Hospital:** NY-Presby Hosp (page 79); **Address:** Herbert Irving Pavilion, 161 Fort Washington Ave, 8-837, New York, NY 10032; **Phone:** 212-305-3410; **Board Cert:** Obstetrics & Gynecology 2005; Gynecologic Oncology 2005; **Med School:** Univ Cincinnati 1986; **Resid:** Obstetrics & Gynecology, Good Samaritan Hosp 1990; **Fellow:** Gynecologic Oncology, Barnes Jewish Hosp 1993; **Fac Appt:** Assoc Prof ObG, Columbia P&S

Kelley III, Joseph L MD [GO] - **Spec Exp:** Breast Cancer; Gynecologic Cancer; **Hospital:** Magee-Womens Hosp - UPMC; **Address:** Magee-Womens Hosp Dept OB/GYN, 300 Halket St, Pittsburgh, PA 15213; **Phone:** 412-641-5411; **Board Cert:** Obstetrics & Gynecology 2005; Gynecologic Oncology 2005; **Med School:** St Louis Univ 1985; **Resid:** Obstetrics & Gynecology, Magee-Womens Hosp 1988; **Fellow:** Gynecologic Oncology, MD Anderson Cancer Ctr 1991; **Fac Appt:** Assoc Prof ObG, Univ Pittsburgh

Koulos, John MD [GO] - **Spec Exp:** Cervical Cancer; Uterine Cancer; Ovarian Cancer; **Hospital:** Beth Israel Med Ctr - Petrie Division (page 72); **Address:** Beth Israel Hosp Cancer Ctr, 10 Union Square F, Ste 4C, New York, NY 10003; **Phone:** 212-844-5729; **Board Cert:** Obstetrics & Gynecology 2005; Gynecologic Oncology 2005; **Med School:** Northwestern Univ 1978; **Resid:** Obstetrics & Gynecology, Northwestern Univ Med Sch 1982; **Fellow:** Gynecologic Oncology, Meml Sloan Kettering Cancer Ctr 1984; **Fac Appt:** Assoc Prof ObG, NY Med Coll

Lele, Shashikant B MD [GO] - **Spec Exp:** Gynecologic Cancer; Ovarian Cancer; **Hospital:** Roswell Park Cancer Inst; **Address:** Roswell Park Cancer Inst-Dept of Gynecology, Elm & Carlton Sts, Buffalo, NY 14263; **Phone:** 716-845-5776; **Board Cert:** Obstetrics & Gynecology 1976; Gynecologic Oncology 1979; **Med School:** India 1968; **Resid:** Obstetrics & Gynecology, JJ Hosp-Grant Med Ctr 1970; Obstetrics & Gynecology, Mt Sinai Hosp 1973; **Fellow:** Gynecologic Oncology, Roswell Park Cancer Inst 1976; **Fac Appt:** Clin Prof ObG, SUNY Buffalo

Morgan, Mark A MD [GO] - **Spec Exp:** Laparoscopic Surgery; Gynecologic Surgery-Complex; Gynecologic Cancer; **Hospital:** Fox Chase Cancer Ctr (page 73); **Address:** Fox Chase Cancer Ctr-Chief, Gyne Oncology, 333 Cottman Ave, Philadelphia, PA 19111; **Phone:** 215-214-1430; **Board Cert:** Obstetrics & Gynecology 2005; Gynecologic Oncology 2005; **Med School:** SUNY Downstate 1982; **Resid:** Obstetrics & Gynecology, Hosp Univ Penn 1986; **Fellow:** Gynecologic Oncology, Hosp Univ Penn 1988

Rosenblum, Norman G MD/PhD [GO] - **Spec Exp:** Ovarian Cancer; Uterine Cancer; Vulvar Disease/Cancer; **Hospital:** Thomas Jefferson Univ Hosp (page 82); **Address:** 834 Chesnut St, Ste 300, Philadelphia, PA 19107-5127; **Phone:** 215-955-6200; **Board Cert:** Obstetrics & Gynecology 2005; Gynecologic Oncology 2005; **Med School:** Jefferson Med Coll 1978; **Resid:** Obstetrics & Gynecology, Hosp Univ Penn 1982; **Fellow:** Gynecologic Oncology, Hosp Univ Penn 1984; **Fac Appt:** Prof ObG, Jefferson Med Coll

Rubin, Stephen C MD [GO] - **Spec Exp:** Gynecologic Cancer; Ovarian Cancer; Cervical Cancer; **Hospital:** Hosp Univ Penn - UPHS (page 84); **Address:** Hosp Univ Penn, Gynecologic Oncology, 3400 Spruce St, 1000 Courtyard Bldg, Philadelphia, PA 19104-4283; **Phone:** 215-662-3318; **Board Cert:** Obstetrics & Gynecology 2006; Gynecologic Oncology 2006; **Med School:** Univ Pennsylvania 1976; **Resid:** Obstetrics & Gynecology, Hosp Univ Penn 1980; **Fellow:** Gynecologic Oncology, Hosp Univ Penn 1982; **Fac Appt:** Prof ObG, Univ Pennsylvania

Wallach, Robert C MD [GO] - **Spec Exp:** Vulvar & Vaginal Cancer; Ovarian Cancer; Cervical Cancer; Uterine Cancer; **Hospital:** NYU Med Ctr (page 80); **Address:** NYU Clinical Cancer Ctr, 160 E 34th St, New York, NY 10016; **Phone:** 212-735-5345; **Board Cert:** Obstetrics & Gynecology 1967; Gynecologic Oncology 1974; **Med School:** Yale Univ 1960; **Resid:** Obstetrics & Gynecology, Beth Israel Med Ctr 1965; **Fellow:** Gynecologic Oncology, SUNY Downstate Med Ctr 1966; **Fac Appt:** Prof ObG, NYU Sch Med

Southeast

Alleyn, James MD [GO] - **Spec Exp:** Cervical Cancer; Ovarian Cancer; Uterine Cancer; **Hospital:** Mercy Hosp - Miami, Baptist Hosp of Miami; **Address:** 3661 S Miami Ave, Ste 308, Miami, FL 33133-4232; **Phone:** 305-854-3603; **Board Cert:** Obstetrics & Gynecology 1978; **Med School:** Indiana Univ 1972; **Resid:** Obstetrics & Gynecology, Miami-Jackson Meml Hosp 1976; **Fellow:** Gynecologic Oncology, Miami-Jackson Meml Hosp 1978; **Fac Appt:** Asst Clin Prof ObG, Univ Miami Sch Med

Alvarez, Ronald D MD [GO] - **Spec Exp:** Gynecologic Cancer; Ovarian Cancer; **Hospital:** Univ of Ala Hosp at Birmingham, Brookwood Med Ctr; **Address:** Univ Alabama, Div Gyn Oncology, 619 19th St S, OHB 538, Birmingham, AL 35249-7333; **Phone:** 205-934-4986; **Board Cert:** Obstetrics & Gynecology 2006; Gynecologic Oncology 2006; **Med School:** Louisiana State Univ 1983; **Resid:** Obstetrics & Gynecology, Univ Alabama Hosp 1987; **Fellow:** Gynecologic Oncology, Univ Alabama Hosp 1990; **Fac Appt:** Assoc Prof ObG, Univ Ala

Berchuck, Andrew MD [GO] - **Spec Exp:** Ovarian Cancer; Uterine Cancer; **Hospital:** Duke Univ Med Ctr; **Address:** Duke Univ Med Center, DUMC Box 3079, Durham, NC 27710; **Phone:** 919-684-3765; **Board Cert:** Obstetrics & Gynecology 1998; Gynecologic Oncology 1998; **Med School:** Case West Res Univ 1980; **Resid:** Obstetrics & Gynecology, Case Western Resrv 1984; **Fellow:** Gynecology, UT Southwestern 1985; Gynecologic Oncology, Meml Sloan-Kettering 1987; **Fac Appt:** Prof ObG, Duke Univ

Boronow, Richard C MD [GO] - **Spec Exp:** Gynecologic Cancer; **Hospital:** Univ Hosps & Clins - Jackson; **Address:** Jackson Gynecologic Oncology, 971 Lakeland Drive, Ste 750, Jackson, MS 39216; **Phone:** 601-987-3033; **Board Cert:** Obstetrics & Gynecology 1967; Gynecologic Oncology 1974; **Med School:** Northwestern Univ 1959; **Resid:** Obstetrics & Gynecology, Evanston Hosp 1963; Surgery, Meml Hosp Cancer 1964; **Fellow:** Gynecology, Anderson Tumor Inst 1965; **Fac Appt:** Clin Prof ObG, Univ Miss

Clarke-Pearson, Daniel L MD [GO] - **Spec Exp:** Pelvic Reconstruction; Gynecologic Surgery-Complex; Gynecologic Cancer; **Hospital:** Univ NC Hosps, Wesley Long Comm Hosp; **Address:** Univ of North Carolina, CB #7570, Chapel Hill, NC 27599; **Phone:** 919-966-5280; **Board Cert:** Obstetrics & Gynecology 2006; Gynecologic Oncology 2006; **Med School:** Case West Res Univ 1975; **Resid:** Obstetrics & Gynecology, Duke Univ Med Ctr 1979; **Fellow:** Gynecologic Oncology, Duke Univ Med Ctr 1981; **Fac Appt:** Prof ObG, Univ NC Sch Med

Creasman, William T MD [GO] - **Spec Exp:** Uterine Cancer; Ovarian Cancer; Cervical Cancer; **Hospital:** MUSC Med Ctr; **Address:** Med Univ S Carolina-Dept ObGyn, Charleston, SC 29425; **Phone:** 843-792-4509; **Board Cert:** Obstetrics & Gynecology 1991; Gynecologic Oncology 1974; **Med School:** Baylor Coll Med 1960; **Resid:** Obstetrics & Gynecology, Rochester Med Ctr 1967; **Fellow:** Gynecologic Oncology, Anderson Hosp Tumor Inst 1969; **Fac Appt:** Prof ObG, Med Univ SC

Finan, Michael A MD [GO] - **Spec Exp:** Ovarian Cancer; Cervical Cancer; Uterine Cancer; **Hospital:** Mobile Infirmary Med Ctr, USA Children & Women's Hospital; **Address:** 1700 Springhill Ave, Ste 100, Mobile, AL 36604; **Phone:** 251-435-1200; **Board Cert:** Obstetrics & Gynecology 2005; Gynecologic Oncology 2005; **Med School:** Louisiana State Univ 1986; **Resid:** Obstetrics & Gynecology, Univ South Fla Affil Hosps 1990; **Fellow:** Gynecologic Oncology, H Lee Moffitt Cancer Ctr 1992; **Fac Appt:** Prof ObG, Univ S Ala Coll Med

Fiorica, James V MD [GO] - **Spec Exp:** Gynecologic Cancer; Breast Cancer; Cervical Cancer; **Hospital:** Sarasota Meml Hosp; **Address:** 118 Hillview St, Sarasota, FL 34239; **Phone:** 941-917-8383; **Board Cert:** Obstetrics & Gynecology 2005; Gynecologic Oncology 2005; **Med School:** Tufts Univ 1982; **Resid:** Obstetrics & Gynecology, Univ South Fla Affil Hosp 1986; **Fellow:** Gynecologic Oncology, Univ South Fla Affil Hosp 1989; Breast Disease, Tufts Univ 1990; **Fac Appt:** Clin Prof ObG, Univ S Fla Coll Med

Fowler Jr, Wesley C MD [GO] - **Spec Exp:** Vulvar Disease/Cancer; DES-Exposed Females; **Hospital:** Univ NC Hosps; **Address:** U NC Chapel Hill, Div of Ob/Gyn, Campus Box 7570, Chapel Hill, NC 27599-7570; **Phone:** 919-966-1196; **Board Cert:** Obstetrics & Gynecology 1991; Gynecologic Oncology 1979; **Med School:** Univ NC Sch Med 1966; **Resid:** Obstetrics & Gynecology, NC Memorial Hosp 1971; **Fac Appt:** Prof ObG, Univ NC Sch Med

Gynecologic Oncology

Horowitz, Ira R MD [GO] - **Spec Exp:** Laparoscopic Surgery; Ovarian Cancer; Cervical Cancer; **Hospital:** Emory Univ Hosp, Crawford Long Hosp of Emory Univ; **Address:** Emory Clinic, 1365 Clifton Rd NE A Bldg Fl 4, Atlanta, GA 30322; **Phone:** 404-778-4416; **Board Cert:** Obstetrics & Gynecology 1997; Gynecologic Oncology 1997; **Med School:** Baylor Coll Med 1980; **Resid:** Obstetrics & Gynecology, Baylor Coll Med 1984; **Fellow:** Gynecologic Oncology, Johns Hopkins Hosp 1987; **Fac Appt:** Prof ObG, Emory Univ

Jones III, Howard Wilbur MD [GO] - **Spec Exp:** Pap Smear Abnormalities; Cervical Cancer; Uterine Cancer; **Hospital:** Vanderbilt Univ Med Ctr; **Address:** Vanderbilt Univ Med Ctr, Medical Center North, rm B1100, Nashville, TN 37232-2519; **Phone:** 615-322-2114; **Board Cert:** Obstetrics & Gynecology 1999; Gynecologic Oncology 1999; **Med School:** Duke Univ 1968; **Resid:** Obstetrics & Gynecology, Univ Colo Med Ctr 1972; **Fellow:** Gynecologic Oncology, Univ Tex-MD Anderson Hosp 1974; **Fac Appt:** Prof ObG, Vanderbilt Univ

Kohler, Matthew MD [GO] - **Spec Exp:** Pelvic Reconstruction; **Hospital:** MUSC Med Ctr; **Address:** MUSC Med Ctr-Women's Hlth Ob/Gyn, 96 Jonathan Lucas St, Box 250619, Charleston, SC 29425; **Phone:** 843-792-9300; **Board Cert:** Obstetrics & Gynecology 1995; Gynecologic Oncology 1997; **Med School:** Duke Univ 1987; **Resid:** Obstetrics & Gynecology, Duke University Med Ctr 1991; **Fellow:** Gynecologic Oncology, Duke University Med Ctr 1993; **Fac Appt:** Assoc Prof ObG, Med Univ SC

Lancaster, Johnathan M MD/PhD [GO] - **Spec Exp:** Ovarian Cancer; Cancer Genetics; Genetic Therapy; **Hospital:** H Lee Moffitt Cancer Ctr & Research Inst; **Address:** H Lee Moffitt Cancer Ctr - Gyn Oncology, 12902 Magnolia Drive, Tampa, FL 33612; **Phone:** 813-745-7272; **Board Cert:** Obstetrics & Gynecology 2005; **Med School:** Wales 1992; **Resid:** Obstetrics & Gynecology, Duke Univ Med Ctr 2000; **Fellow:** Gynecologic Oncology, Duke Univ Med Ctr 2003; **Fac Appt:** Asst Prof ObG, Univ S Fla Coll Med

Lentz, Samuel S MD [GO] - **Spec Exp:** Gynecologic Cancer; Pelvic Reconstruction; **Hospital:** Wake Forest Univ Baptist Med Ctr (page 85), Forsyth Med Ctr; **Address:** Wake Forest Univ Sch Med, Div Gyn Oncology, Medical Center Blvd, Winston-Salem, NC 27157; **Phone:** 336-716-6673; **Board Cert:** Obstetrics & Gynecology 2006; Gynecologic Oncology 2006; **Med School:** Wake Forest Univ 1978; **Resid:** Obstetrics & Gynecology, NC Baptist Hosp 1982; **Fellow:** Gynecologic Oncology, Mayo Clinic 1989; **Fac Appt:** Prof ObG, Wake Forest Univ

Partridge, Edward E MD [GO] - **Spec Exp:** Ovarian Cancer; **Hospital:** Univ of Ala Hosp at Birmingham; **Address:** Univ Alabama, Div Gyn Oncology, 619 19th St S, OHB 538, Birmingham, AL 35249-7333; **Phone:** 205-934-4986; **Board Cert:** Obstetrics & Gynecology 1993; Gynecologic Oncology 1981; **Med School:** Univ Ala 1973; **Resid:** Obstetrics & Gynecology, Univ Alabama Hosp 1977; **Fellow:** Gynecologic Oncology, Univ Alabama Hosp 1979; **Fac Appt:** Prof ObG, Univ Ala

Penalver, Manuel A MD [GO] - **Spec Exp:** Gynecologic Cancer; Cervical Cancer; Pelvic Tumors; **Hospital:** Doctors' Hosp, Baptist Hosp of Miami; **Address:** South Florida Gyn Oncology, 5000 University Drive, Ste 3300, Coral Gables, FL 33146; **Phone:** 305-663-7001; **Board Cert:** Obstetrics & Gynecology 1997; Gynecologic Oncology 1997; **Med School:** Univ Miami Sch Med 1977; **Resid:** Obstetrics & Gynecology, Univ Miami/Jackson Meml Hosp 1982; **Fellow:** Gynecologic Oncology, Univ Miami/Jackson Meml Hosp 1984

Poliakoff, Steven MD [GO] - **Spec Exp:** Ovarian Cancer; Minimally Invasive Surgery; Cancer Genetics; **Hospital:** Mount Sinai Med Ctr - Miami, South Miami Hosp; **Address:** 6280 Sunset Dr, Ste 502, South Miami, FL 33143-4870; **Phone:** 305-596-0870; **Board Cert:** Obstetrics & Gynecology 1983; **Med School:** Univ NC Sch Med 1975; **Resid:** Obstetrics & Gynecology, Johns Hopkins Hosp 1979; **Fellow:** Gynecologic Oncology, Jackson Meml Hosp/Univ Miami 1981

Rice, Laurel W MD [GO] - **Spec Exp:** Ovarian Cancer; Uterine Cancer; Cervical Cancer; **Hospital:** Univ Virginia Med Ctr; **Address:** UVA Health System, Dept OB/GYN, PO Box 800712, Charlottesville, VA 22908; **Phone:** 434-924-5100; **Board Cert:** Obstetrics & Gynecology 2003; Gynecologic Oncology 2003; **Med School:** Univ Colorado 1983; **Resid:** Obstetrics & Gynecology, Brigham-Womens Hosp 1987; **Fellow:** Obstetrics & Gynecology, Brigham-Womens Hosp 1989; **Fac Appt:** Assoc Prof ObG, Univ VA Sch Med

Sevin, Bernd-Uwe MD [GO] - **Spec Exp:** Ovarian Cancer; Pelvic Reconstruction; Pelvic Tumors; **Hospital:** St Luke's Hosp - Jacksonville; **Address:** Mayo Clinic-Dept Gynecology, 4500 San Pablo Rd, Jacksonville, FL 32224; **Phone:** 904-953-0612; **Board Cert:** Obstetrics & Gynecology 1980; Gynecologic Oncology 1981; **Med School:** Germany 1968; **Resid:** Obstetrics & Gynecology, Stanford U Med Ctr 1977; **Fellow:** Gynecologic Oncology, Jackson Meml Hosp 1979; **Fac Appt:** Prof ObG, Mayo Med Sch

Soper, John T MD [GO] - **Spec Exp:** Gynecologic Cancer; **Hospital:** Univ NC Hosps; **Address:** Univ North Carolina, Dept OB/GYN, 5017 Old Clinic Bldg, Chapel Hill, NC 27599; **Phone:** 919-966-1194; **Board Cert:** Obstetrics & Gynecology 1996; Gynecologic Oncology 1996; **Med School:** Univ Iowa Coll Med 1978; **Resid:** Obstetrics & Gynecology, Univ Utah Med Ctr 1982; **Fellow:** Gynecologic Oncology, Duke Univ Med Ctr 1985; **Fac Appt:** Prof ObG, Univ NC Sch Med

Spann Jr, Cyril O MD [GO] - **Spec Exp:** Gynecologic Cancer; Ovarian Cancer; **Hospital:** Emory Univ Hosp; **Address:** Emory Clinic Crawford Long, 550 Peachtree St, Ste 900, Atlanta, GA 30308; **Phone:** 404-616-3540; **Board Cert:** Obstetrics & Gynecology 2005; Gynecologic Oncology 2005; **Med School:** Meharry Med Coll 1981; **Resid:** Obstetrics & Gynecology, Emory Univ Med Ctr 1985; **Fellow:** Gynecologic Oncology, Univ NC Meml Hosp 1989; **Fac Appt:** Prof ObG, Emory Univ

Taylor Jr, Peyton T MD [GO] - **Spec Exp:** Gynecologic Surgery-Complex; Gynecologic Cancer; **Hospital:** Univ Virginia Med Ctr; **Address:** Univ VA Hlth Sys, Dept Ob/Gyn, PO Box 800712, Charlottesville, VA 22908; **Phone:** 434-924-9933; **Board Cert:** Obstetrics & Gynecology 1994; Gynecologic Oncology 1981; **Med School:** Univ Ala 1968; **Resid:** Obstetrics & Gynecology, Univ VA Hosp 1970; Obstetrics & Gynecology, Univ VA Hosp 1975; **Fellow:** Surgical Oncology, Natl Cancer Inst 1972; Gynecologic Oncology, Univ Va Hosp 1977; **Fac Appt:** Prof ObG, Univ VA Sch Med

Van Nagell Jr, John R MD [GO] - **Spec Exp:** Ovarian Cancer; Cervical Cancer; **Hospital:** Univ of Kentucky Chandler Hosp; **Address:** UKMC, Dept Ob/Gyn, 800 Rose St, Lexington, KY 40536-0001; **Phone:** 859-323-5553; **Board Cert:** Obstetrics & Gynecology 1973; Gynecologic Oncology 1976, **Med School:** Univ Pennsylvania 1967; **Resid:** Obstetrics & Gynecology, Kentucky Med Ctr 1971; **Fac Appt:** Prof ObG, Univ KY Coll Med

Gynecologic Oncology

Belinson, Jerome L MD [GO] - **Spec Exp:** Ovarian Cancer; Cervical Cancer; **Hospital:** Cleveland Clin Fdn (page 71); **Address:** 9500 Euclid Ave, Desk A81, Cleveland, OH 44195; **Phone:** 216-444-7933; **Board Cert:** Obstetrics & Gynecology 1998; Gynecologic Oncology 1980; **Med School:** Univ MO-Columbia Sch Med 1968; **Resid:** Obstetrics & Gynecology, Columbia Presby Med Ctr 1973; **Fellow:** Gynecologic Oncology, Jackson Meml Hosp 1977; **Fac Appt:** Prof ObG, Ohio State Univ

Copeland, Larry J MD [GO] - **Spec Exp:** Ovarian Cancer; Uterine Cancer; Gynecologic Cancer; **Hospital:** Arthur G James Cancer Hosp & Research Inst, Ohio St Univ Med Ctr; **Address:** 1654 Upham Drive, Ste 505, Columbus, OH 43210-1250; **Phone:** 614-293-8697; **Board Cert:** Obstetrics & Gynecology 1991; Gynecologic Oncology 1981; **Med School:** Univ Western Ontario 1973; **Resid:** Obstetrics & Gynecology, McMaster Univ Affil Hosps 1977; **Fellow:** Gynecologic Oncology, MD Anderson Cancer Ctr-Univ Tex 1979; **Fac Appt:** Prof ObG, Ohio State Univ

De Geest, Koen MD [GO] - **Spec Exp:** Ovarian Cancer; Cervical Cancer; Clinical Trials; **Hospital:** Univ Iowa Hosp & Clinics; **Address:** Univ Iowa, Div Gynecological Oncology, 200 Hawkins Drive, rm 4630 JCP, Iowa City, IA 52242; **Phone:** 319-356-2015; **Board Cert:** Obstetrics & Gynecology 1997; Gynecologic Oncology 1997; **Med School:** Belgium 1977; **Resid:** Obstetrics & Gynecology, Univ Ghent 1982; **Fellow:** Gynecologic Oncology, Penn State/Hershey Med Ctr 1990; **Fac Appt:** Prof ObG, Univ Iowa Coll Med

Fowler, Jeffrey M MD [GO] - **Spec Exp:** Laparoscopic Surgery; Gynecologic Cancer; Robotic Surgery; Pelvic Reconstruction; **Hospital:** Ohio St Univ Med Ctr; **Address:** Ohio State Univ, Div Gynecologic Oncology, 320 W Tenth Ave, M-210 SLH, Columbus, OH 43210; **Phone:** 614-293-8737; **Board Cert:** Obstetrics & Gynecology 2005; Gynecologic Oncology 2005; **Med School:** Northwestern Univ 1985; **Resid:** Obstetrics & Gynecology, Ohio State Univ Hosp 1989; **Fellow:** Gynecologic Oncology, UCLA 1991; **Fac Appt:** Prof ObG, Ohio State Univ

Johnston, Carolyn Marie MD [GO] - **Spec Exp:** Gynecologic Surgery-Complex; **Hospital:** Univ Michigan Hlth Sys; **Address:** Womens Hosp-Div Gyn Onc, 1500 E Med Ctr Drive, rm L4510, Ann Arbor, MI 48109-0276; **Phone:** 734-647-8906; **Board Cert:** Obstetrics & Gynecology 2000; Gynecologic Oncology 2000; **Med School:** Yale Univ 1984; **Resid:** Obstetrics & Gynecology, Univ Chicago Hosp 1988; **Fellow:** Gynecologic Oncology, Mt Sinai Hosp 1990; **Fac Appt:** Assoc Clin Prof ObG, Univ Mich Med Sch

Kim, Woo Shin MD [GO] - **Spec Exp:** Ovarian Cancer; Uterine Cancer; Gestational Trophoblastic Disease; **Hospital:** Henry Ford Hosp; **Address:** 3031 W Grand Blvd, Ste 800, Detroit, MI 48202-2608; **Phone:** 313-916-2465; **Board Cert:** Obstetrics & Gynecology 1977; Gynecologic Oncology 1979; **Med School:** South Korea 1966; **Resid:** Obstetrics & Gynecology, Boston City Hosp 1973; **Fellow:** Gynecologic Oncology, Meml Sloan-Kettering Cancer Ctr 1976; **Fac Appt:** Assoc Clin Prof ObG, Wayne State Univ

Look, Katherine MD [GO] - **Spec Exp:** Ovarian Cancer; Uterine Cancer; **Hospital:** Indiana Univ Hosp (page 70), Methodist Hosp - Indianapolis (page 70); **Address:** 535 Barnhill Drive, Ste 434, Indianapolis, IN 46202; **Phone:** 317-274-2130; **Board Cert:** Obstetrics & Gynecology 1996; Gynecologic Oncology 1996; **Med School:** Univ Mich Med Sch 1979; **Resid:** Obstetrics & Gynecology, Univ Illinois 1983; **Fellow:** Gynecologic Oncology, Meml Sloan Kettering Cancer Ctr 1986; **Fac Appt:** Prof ObG, Indiana Univ

Lurain, John R MD [GO] - **Spec Exp:** Gestational Trophoblastic Disease; Uterine Cancer; Ovarian Cancer; **Hospital:** Northwestern Meml Hosp; **Address:** Northwestern Univ Feinberg Sch Med, 333 E Superior St, Chicago, IL 60611-3056; **Phone:** 312-926-7365; **Board Cert:** Obstetrics & Gynecology 1977; Gynecologic Oncology 1981; **Med School:** Univ NC Sch Med 1972; **Resid:** Obstetrics & Gynecology, Univ Pittsburgh Med Ctr 1975; **Fellow:** Gynecologic Oncology, Roswell Park Cancer Inst 1979; **Fac Appt:** Prof ObG, Northwestern Univ

Moore, David H MD [GO] - **Spec Exp:** Cervical Cancer; Ovarian Cancer; **Hospital:** St Francis Hosp; **Address:** Gynecologic Oncology of Indianapolis, 5255 E Stop 11 Rd, Ste 310, Indianapolis, IN 46237; **Phone:** 317-851-2555; **Board Cert:** Obstetrics & Gynecology 2005; Gynecologic Oncology 2005; **Med School:** Indiana Univ 1982; **Resid:** Obstetrics & Gynecology, Indiana Univ Hosp 1986; **Fellow:** Gynecologic Oncology, Univ North Carolina 1988

Mutch, David MD [GO] - **Spec Exp:** Gynecologic Cancer; Pelvic Reconstruction; **Hospital:** Barnes-Jewish Hosp; **Address:** 4911 Barnes Jewish Hospital Plaza, St. Louis, MO 63110; **Phone:** 314-362-3181; **Board Cert:** Obstetrics & Gynecology 2003; Gynecologic Oncology 2003; **Med School:** Washington Univ, St Louis 1980; **Resid:** Obstetrics & Gynecology, Barnes Hosp-Wash Univ 1984; **Fellow:** Gynecologic Oncology, Duke Univ Med Ctr 1987; **Fac Appt:** Prof ObG, Washington Univ, St Louis

Podratz, Karl C MD/PhD [GO] - **Spec Exp:** Pelvic Tumors; **Hospital:** Mayo Med Ctr & Clin - Rochester; **Address:** Mayo Clinic SW, 200 1st St SW, Rochester, MN 55905-0001; **Phone:** 507-266-7712; **Board Cert:** Obstetrics & Gynecology 1993; Gynecologic Oncology 1993; **Med School:** St Louis Univ 1974; **Resid:** Obstetrics & Gynecology, Univ Chicago Hosps 1977; **Fellow:** Gynecologic Oncology, Mayo Clinic 1979; **Fac Appt:** Prof ObG, Mayo Med Sch

Potkul, Ronald MD [GO] - **Spec Exp:** Ovarian Cancer; Cervical Cancer; **Hospital:** Loyola Univ Med Ctr, Elmhurst Meml Hosp; **Address:** Loyola Univ Med Ctr, 2160 S 1st Ave Bldg 112 - rm 267, Maywood, IL 60153; **Phone:** 708-327-3500; **Board Cert:** Obstetrics & Gynecology 1997; Gynecologic Oncology 1997; **Med School:** Univ Chicago-Pritzker Sch Med 1981; **Resid:** Obstetrics & Gynecology, Univ Chicago Hosps 1985; **Fellow:** Gynecologic Oncology, Georgetown Univ 1988; **Fac Appt:** Prof ObG, Loyola Univ-Stritch Sch Med

Reynolds, R Kevin MD [GO] - **Hospital:** Univ Michigan Hlth Sys; **Address:** Women's Hosp, Div Gyn Onc, 1500 E Med Ctr Drive, rm L4510, Ann Arbor, MI 48109-0276; **Phone:** 734-764-9106; **Board Cert:** Obstetrics & Gynecology 1998; Gynecologic Oncology 1994; **Med School:** Univ New Mexico 1982; **Resid:** Obstetrics & Gynecology, Univ Vt Hosp 1986; **Fellow:** Gynecologic Oncology, Univ Mich Med Ctr 1991; **Fac Appt:** Asst Prof ObG, Univ Mich Med Sch

Rose, Peter G MD [GO] - **Spec Exp:** Cervical Cancer; Ovarian Cancer; **Hospital:** Cleveland Clin Fdn (page 71), MetroHealth Med Ctr; **Address:** Cleveland Clinic Fdn, 9500 Euclid Ave A-81, Cleveland, OH 44195; **Phone:** 216-444-1712; **Board Cert:** Obstetrics & Gynecology 1999; Gynecologic Oncology 1990; **Med School:** Boston Univ 1981; **Resid:** Surgery, Vanderbilt Med Ctr 1983; Obstetrics & Gynecology, Ohio State Univ Med Ctr 1986; **Fellow:** Gynecologic Oncology, Roswell Park Med Ctr 1988; **Fac Appt:** Prof ObG, Case West Res Univ

Rotmensch, Jacob MD [GO] - **Spec Exp:** Gynecologic Cancer; Ovarian Cancer; Cervical Cancer; **Hospital:** Rush Univ Med Ctr; **Address:** Gyn Oncology Assocs, 1725 W Harrison St, Ste 842, Chicago, IL 60612; **Phone:** 312-942-6300; **Board Cert:** Obstetrics & Gynecology 1986; Gynecologic Oncology 1990; **Med School:** Meharry Med Coll 1977; **Resid:** Obstetrics & Gynecology, Johns Hopkins Hosp 1981; **Fellow:** Gynecologic Oncology, Johns Hopkins Hosp 1984; **Fac Appt:** Prof ObG, Rush Med Coll

Savage, John MD [GO] - **Spec Exp:** Uterine Cancer; **Hospital:** Abbott - Northwestern Hosp; **Address:** 310 Smith Ave N, Ste 430, St Paul, MN 55102; **Phone:** 651-602-5333; **Board Cert:** Obstetrics & Gynecology 1981; Gynecologic Oncology 1983; **Med School:** Univ Iowa Coll Med 1974; **Resid:** Obstetrics & Gynecology, Univ Iowa 1978; **Fellow:** Gynecologic Oncology, Univ Iowa 1981

Schink, Julian C MD [GO] - **Spec Exp:** Ovarian Cancer; **Hospital:** Northwestern Meml Hosp; **Address:** 675 N St Clair St, Fl 21 - Ste 100, Chicago, IL 60611; **Phone:** 312-695-0990; **Board Cert:** Obstetrics & Gynecology 2000; Gynecologic Oncology 2000; **Med School:** Univ Tex, San Antonio 1982; **Resid:** Obstetrics & Gynecology, Northwestern Univ Med Sch 1986; **Fellow:** Gynecologic Oncology, UCLA Med Ctr 1988; **Fac Appt:** Prof ObG, Northwestern Univ

Smith, Donna Marie MD [GO] - **Spec Exp:** Cervical Cancer; Ovarian Cancer; **Hospital:** Loyola Univ Med Ctr; **Address:** Cardinal Bernardin Cancer Ctr, Clinic A, 2160 S 1st Ave Bldg 112 - rm 267, Maywood, IL 60153; **Phone:** 708-327-3500; **Board Cert:** Obstetrics & Gynecology 1997; Gynecologic Oncology 1997; **Med School:** Univ MO-Kansas City 1980; **Resid:** Obstetrics & Gynecology, Emory Univ Hosp 1984; **Fellow:** Gynecologic Oncology, Georgetown Univ Med Ctr 1987; **Fac Appt:** Assoc Prof ObG, Loyola Univ-Stritch Sch Med

Stehman, Frederick B MD [GO] - **Spec Exp:** Clinical Trials; Gynecologic Cancer; **Hospital:** Indiana Univ Hosp (page 70), Wishard Hlth Srvs; **Address:** Indiana Univ Hosp, Dept ObGyn, 550 N University Blvd, rm 2440, Indianapolis, IN 46202; **Phone:** 317-274-8609; **Board Cert:** Obstetrics & Gynecology 2004; Gynecologic Oncology 2004; **Med School:** Univ Mich Med Sch 1972; **Resid:** Obstetrics & Gynecology, Univ Kansas Medical Ctr 1975; Surgery, Univ Kansas Medical Ctr 1977; **Fellow:** Gynecologic Oncology, UCLA Medical Ctr 1979; **Fac Appt:** Prof ObG, Indiana Univ

Waggoner, Steven MD [GO] - **Spec Exp:** Ovarian Cancer; Cervical Cancer; Uterine Cancer; **Hospital:** Univ Hosps Case Med Ctr; **Address:** Dept Ob/Gyn, Div Gyn Oncology, 11100 Euclid Ave, MC 5034, Cleveland, OH 44106; **Phone:** 216-844-3954; **Board Cert:** Obstetrics & Gynecology 2002; Gynecologic Oncology 2002; **Med School:** Univ Wash 1984; **Resid:** Obstetrics & Gynecology, Univ Chicago Hosps 1988; **Fellow:** Gynecologic Oncology, Georgetown Univ 1991; **Fac Appt:** Prof ObG, Case West Res Univ

Great Plains and Mountains

Davidson, Susan MD [GO] - **Spec Exp:** Gynecologic Cancer; **Hospital:** Univ Colorado Hosp; **Address:** Univ Colorado Hosp, Dept OB/GYN, 4200 E Ninth Ave, Box B198, Denver, CO 80262; **Phone:** 303-315-7897; **Board Cert:** Obstetrics & Gynecology 2005; Gynecologic Oncology 2005; **Med School:** Univ Tex, San Antonio 1984; **Resid:** Obstetrics & Gynecology, Univ Texas Med Ctr 1988; **Fellow:** Gynecologic Oncology, Meml Sloan Kettering Cancer Ctr 1990; **Fac Appt:** Assoc Prof ObG, Univ Colorado

Soisson, Andrew MD [GO] - **Spec Exp:** Cervical Cancer; **Hospital:** LDS Hosp, Univ Utah Hosps and Clins; **Address:** Univ Utah, Div Gyn Oncology, 1950 Circle of Hope, Salt Lake City, UT 84112; **Phone:** 801-585-0100; **Board Cert:** Obstetrics & Gynecology 2002; Gynecologic Oncology 2002; **Med School:** Georgetown Univ 1981; **Resid:** Obstetrics & Gynecology, Madigan AMC 1985; **Fellow:** Gynecologic Oncology, Duke Univ Med Ctr 1990; **Fac Appt:** Assoc Prof ObG, Univ Utah

Southwest

Chambers, Setsuko K MD [GO] - **Spec Exp:** Gynecologic Cancer; Breast Cancer; Ovarian Cancer; **Hospital:** Univ Med Ctr - Tucson; **Address:** 1515 N Campbell Ave, rm 1968, Tucson, AZ 85724; **Phone:** 520-626-9285; **Board Cert:** Obstetrics & Gynecology 1997; Gynecologic Oncology 1997; **Med School:** Brown Univ 1980; **Resid:** Obstetrics & Gynecology, Yale-New Haven Hosp 1984; **Fellow:** Gynecologic Oncology, Yale-New Haven Hosp 1986; **Fac Appt:** Prof ObG, Univ Ariz Coll Med

Follen-Mitchell, Michele MD/PhD [GO] - **Spec Exp:** Gynecologic Cancer; Clinical Trials; **Hospital:** UT MD Anderson Cancer Ctr (page 81); **Address:** MD Anderson Cancer Ctr, 1515 Holcombe Blvd, Unit 193, Houston, TX 77030; **Phone:** 713-745-2564; **Board Cert:** Obstetrics & Gynecology 1999; Gynecologic Oncology 1999; **Med School:** Univ Mich Med Sch 1980; **Resid:** Obstetrics & Gynecology, Columbia-Presby Med Ctr 1983; **Fellow:** Gynecologic Oncology, MD Anderson Cancer Ctr 1986; **Fac Appt:** Prof ObG, Univ Tex, Houston

Gershenson, David M MD [GO] - **Spec Exp:** Ovarian Cancer & Borderline Tumors; Peritoneal Carcinomatosis; Fertility Preservation in Cancer; Uterine Cancer; **Hospital:** UT MD Anderson Cancer Ctr (page 81), St Luke's Episcopal Hosp - Houston; **Address:** Univ Tex MD Anderson Cancer Ctr, PO Box 301439, Houston, TX 77030-1439; **Phone:** 713-745-2565; **Board Cert:** Obstetrics & Gynecology 1991; Gynecologic Oncology 1981; **Med School:** Vanderbilt Univ 1971; **Resid:** Obstetrics & Gynecology, Yale-New Haven Hosp 1975; **Fellow:** Gynecologic Oncology, MD Anderson Cancer Ctr 1979

Hatch, Kenneth MD [GO] - **Spec Exp:** Cervical Cancer; **Hospital:** Univ Med Ctr - Tucson, NW Med Ctr; **Address:** Univ Arizona College of Medicine, 1515 N Campbell Ave, rm 1968, Tucson, AZ 85724; **Phone:** 520-626-9285; **Board Cert:** Obstetrics & Gynecology 1993; Gynecologic Oncology 1981; **Med School:** Univ Nebr Coll Med 1971; **Resid:** Obstetrics & Gynecology, Univ AL Med Ctr Birmingham 1976; **Fellow:** Gynecologic Oncology, Univ AL Med Ctr Birmingham 1978; **Fac Appt:** Prof ObG, Univ Ariz Coll Med

Levenback, Charles MD [GO] - **Spec Exp:** Vulvar Disease/Cancer; Cervical Cancer; Gynecologic Cancer; **Hospital:** UT MD Anderson Cancer Ctr (page 81); **Address:** PO Box 301439 - Unit 1362, Houston, TX 77230; **Phone:** 713-745-2563; **Board Cert:** Obstetrics & Gynecology 2005; Gynecologic Oncology 2005; **Med School:** Mount Sinai Sch Med 1983; **Resid:** Obstetrics & Gynecology, Albert Einstein Coll Med 1987; **Fellow:** Gynecologic Oncology, Meml Sloan Kettering Cancer Ctr 1989; **Fac Appt:** Prof ObG, Univ Tex, Houston

Magrina, Javier MD [GO] - **Spec Exp:** Gynecologic Cancer; Robotic Surgery; Minimally Invasive Surgery; **Hospital:** Mayo Clin Hosp - Scottsdale; **Address:** Mayo Clinic, 13400 E Shea Blvd, Scottsdale, AZ 85259-5404; **Phone:** 480-342-2668; **Board Cert:** Obstetrics & Gynecology 1994; Gynecologic Oncology 1982; **Med School:** Spain 1972; **Resid:** Obstetrics & Gynecology, Mayo Clinic 1977; **Fellow:** Gynecologic Oncology, Kansas Med Ctr 1980; **Fac Appt:** Prof ObG, Mayo Med Sch

Gynecologic Oncology

Roman-Lopez, Juan J MD [GO] - **Spec Exp:** Vulvar Disease/Cancer; Gynecologic Cancer; **Hospital:** UAMS Med Ctr; **Address:** 4301 W Markham St, Slot 793, Little Rock, AR 72205-7199; **Phone:** 501-296-1099; **Board Cert:** Obstetrics & Gynecology 1971; **Med School:** Univ Puerto Rico 1963; **Resid:** Obstetrics & Gynecology, San Juan City Hosp 1967; Obstetrics & Gynecology, Tulane-Charity Hosp 1969; **Fellow:** Gynecologic Oncology, Tulane-LSU Med Ctr 1970; **Fac Appt:** Assoc Clin Prof ObG, Univ Ark

Smith, Harriet O MD [GO] - **Spec Exp:** Uterine Cancer; Pelvic Reconstruction; Ovarian Cancer; **Hospital:** Univ NM Hlth & Sci Ctr; **Address:** 1 University of New Mexico NE, MS 105580, Albuquerque, NM 87131; **Phone:** 505-272-3392; **Board Cert:** Obstetrics & Gynecology 1995; Gynecologic Oncology 2005; **Med School:** Med Coll GA 1981; **Resid:** Obstetrics & Gynecology, Med Coll Georgia 1985; Gynecologic Oncology, MD Anderson 1988; **Fellow:** Reconstructive Pelvic Surgery, Emory Univ Hosp 1989; Gynecologic Oncology, Albert Einstein Coll Med 1990; **Fac Appt:** Prof ObG, Univ New Mexico

Walker, Joan L MD [GO] - **Spec Exp:** Ovarian Cancer; Cervical Cancer; Uterine Cancer; **Hospital:** OU Med Ctr; **Address:** OU Health Science Ctr, PO Box 26901, Oklahoma City, OK 73190; **Phone:** 405-271-8707; **Board Cert:** Obstetrics & Gynecology 2004; Gynecologic Oncology 2004; **Med School:** UCLA 1982; **Resid:** Obstetrics & Gynecology, Hosp U Penn 1986; **Fellow:** Gynecologic Oncology, UC-Irvine Med Ctr 1990; **Fac Appt:** Assoc Prof ObG, Univ Okla Coll Med

West Coast and Pacific

Berek, Jonathan S MD [GO] - **Spec Exp:** Ovarian Cancer; Uterine Cancer; Cervical Cancer; **Hospital:** Stanford Univ Med Ctr; **Address:** Stanford Univ School of Medicine, 300 Pasteur Dr, HH333, Stanford, CA 94305-5317; **Phone:** 650-498-5618; **Board Cert:** Obstetrics & Gynecology 2005; Gynecologic Oncology 2005; **Med School:** Johns Hopkins Univ 1975; **Resid:** Obstetrics & Gynecology, Brigham & Womans Hosp 1979; **Fellow:** Gynecologic Oncology, UCLA Sch Med 1981; **Fac Appt:** Prof ObG, Stanford Univ

Berman, Michael L MD [GO] - **Spec Exp:** Gynecologic Cancer; **Hospital:** UC Irvine Med Ctr, Long Beach Meml Med Ctr; **Address:** Cho Family Comprehensive Cancer Ctr, 101 The City Drive Bldg 56 - Ste 260, Orange, CA 92868-3201; **Phone:** 714-456-8020; **Board Cert:** Obstetrics & Gynecology 2005; Gynecologic Oncology 2005; **Med School:** Geo Wash Univ 1967; **Resid:** Obstetrics & Gynecology, GW Univ Hosp 1969; Obstetrics & Gynecology, Los Angeles Co-Harbor 1974; **Fellow:** Gynecologic Oncology, UCLA Med Ctr 1976; **Fac Appt:** Prof ObG, UC Irvine

Cain, Joanna MD [GO] - **Spec Exp:** Ovarian Cancer; Breast Cancer Risk Assessment; Uterine Cancer; Ovarian Cancer-Early Detection; **Hospital:** OR Hlth & Sci Univ; **Address:** 3181 SW Sam Jackson Park Rd, MC L-466, Portland, OR 97239; **Phone:** 503-494-2999; **Board Cert:** Obstetrics & Gynecology 2005; Gynecologic Oncology 2005; **Med School:** Creighton Univ 1978; **Resid:** Obstetrics & Gynecology, Univ Washington Med Ctr 1981; **Fellow:** Gynecologic Oncology, Meml Sloan Kettering Cancer Ctr 1983; **Fac Appt:** Prof ObG, Oregon Hlth Sci Univ

Di Saia, Philip J MD [GO] - **Spec Exp:** Ovarian Cancer; Gynecologic Cancer; Cervical Cancer; **Hospital:** UC Irvine Med Ctr; **Address:** Cho Family Comprehensive Cancer Ctr, 200 S Manchester, Orange, CA 92668; **Phone:** 714-456-8000; **Board Cert:** Obstetrics & Gynecology 1983; Gynecologic Oncology 1974; **Med School:** Tufts Univ 1963; **Resid:** Obstetrics & Gynecology, Yale-New Haven Hosp 1967; **Fellow:** Gynecologic Oncology, MD Anderson Hosp 1971; **Fac Appt:** Prof ObG, UC Irvine

Goff, Barbara MD [GO] - **Spec Exp:** Ovarian Cancer; Uterine Cancer; Cervical Cancer; **Hospital:** Univ Wash Med Ctr; **Address:** Univ Washington, Dept ObGyn, Box 356460, Seattle, WA 98195; **Phone:** 206-543-3669; **Board Cert:** Obstetrics & Gynecology 2004; Gynecologic Oncology 2004; **Med School:** Univ Pennsylvania 1986; **Resid:** Obstetrics & Gynecology, Mass Genl Hosp/Brigham & Womens Hosp 1990; **Fellow:** Gynecologic Oncology, Mass Genl Hosp 1993; **Fac Appt:** Assoc Prof ObG, Univ Wash

Greer, Benjamin MD [GO] - **Spec Exp:** Gynecologic Cancer; **Hospital:** Univ Wash Med Ctr; **Address:** Univ Wash, Dept OB/GYN, Box 356460, Seattle, WA 98195; **Phone:** 206-543-3669; **Board Cert:** Obstetrics & Gynecology 2002; Gynecologic Oncology 2002; **Med School:** Univ Pennsylvania 1966; **Resid:** Obstetrics & Gynecology, Univ Colorado Med Ctr 1970; **Fac Appt:** Prof ObG, Univ Wash

Karlan, Beth Young MD [GO] - **Spec Exp:** Ovarian Cancer; Gynecologic Cancer; **Hospital:** Cedars-Sinai Med Ctr, UCLA Med Ctr (page 83); **Address:** 8700 Beverly Blvd, Ste 290W, Los Angeles, CA 90048; **Phone:** 310-423-3302; **Board Cert:** Obstetrics & Gynecology 1998; Gynecologic Oncology 1998; **Med School:** Harvard Med Sch 1982; **Resid:** Obstetrics & Gynecology, Yale-New Haven Hosp 1986; **Fellow:** Gynecologic Oncology, UCLA Med Sch 1989; **Fac Appt:** Prof ObG, UCLA

Muntz, Howard G MD [GO] - **Spec Exp:** Gynecologic Cancer; Ovarian Cancer; Clinical Trials; Gynecologic Surgery-Complex; **Hospital:** Virginia Mason Med Ctr; **Address:** Virginia Mason Medical Ctr, 1100 9th Ave, MS X8-GYO, Seattle, WA 98111-0900; **Phone:** 206-223-6191; **Board Cert:** Obstetrics & Gynecology 2005; Gynecologic Oncology 2005; **Med School:** Harvard Med Sch 1984; **Resid:** Obstetrics & Gynecology, Brigham & Women's Hosp 1988; **Fellow:** Gynecologic Oncology, Mass General Hosp 1991; **Fac Appt:** Assoc Clin Prof ObG, Univ Wash

Powell, Catherine Bethan MD [GO] - **Spec Exp:** Gynecologic Cancer; Cancer Genetics; Complementary Medicine; **Hospital:** UCSF - Mt Zion Med Ctr; **Address:** UCSF Comp Cancer Ctr, 1600 Divisadero St Fl 4, San Francisco, CA 94143; **Phone:** 415-353-9838; **Board Cert:** Obstetrics & Gynecology 2005; Gynecologic Oncology 2005; **Med School:** Univ Pennsylvania 1982; **Resid:** Obstetrics & Gynecology, Pennsylvania Hosp 1987; **Fellow:** Gynecologic Oncology, Wash Univ 1990; **Fac Appt:** Asst Clin Prof ObG, UCSF

Smith, Lloyd H MD [GO] - **Spec Exp:** Ovarian Cancer; Uterine Cancer; Vulvar Disease/Cancer; Vaginal Cancer; **Hospital:** UC Davis Med Ctr, Sutter Mem Hospital - Sacramento; **Address:** UC Davis Med Ctr, Dept Ob/Gyn, 4860 Y St, Ste 2500, Sacramento, CA 95817; **Phone:** 916-734-6946; **Board Cert:** Obstetrics & Gynecology 1998; Gynecologic Oncology 1998; **Med School:** UC Davis 1981; **Resid:** Obstetrics & Gynecology, UC Davis Med Ctr 1985; **Fellow:** Gynecologic Oncology, Stanford Univ Hosp 1988; **Fac Appt:** Prof ObG, UC Davis

Spirtos, Nicola Michael MD [GO] - **Spec Exp:** Gynecologic Cancer; Ovarian Cancer; **Hospital:** Univ Med Ctr Las Vegas; **Address:** 3131 La Canada St, Ste 110, Las Vegas, NV 89109; **Phone:** 650-988-8421; **Board Cert:** Obstetrics & Gynecology 1998; Gynecologic Oncology 1998; **Med School:** Northwestern Univ 1980; **Resid:** Obstetrics & Gynecology, Women's Hosp LAC-USC Med Ctr 1984; **Fellow:** Gynecologic Oncology, Stanford Univ 1987

Stern, Jeffrey L MD [GO] - **Spec Exp:** Laparoscopic Surgery; Vulvar Disease/Cancer; **Hospital:** Alta Bates Summit Med Ctr; **Address:** Womens Cancer Ctr Northern Calif, 2500 Malvia St, Ste 224, Berkley, CA 94704; **Phone:** 510-540-8235; **Board Cert:** Obstetrics & Gynecology 1983; Gynecologic Oncology 1984; **Med School:** SUNY Upstate Med Univ 1976; **Resid:** Obstetrics & Gynecology, Johns Hopkins Hosp 1980; **Fellow:** Gynecologic Oncology, USC Med Ctr 1982

Teng, Nelson NH MD/PhD [GO] - **Spec Exp:** Ovarian Cancer; Clinical Trials; **Hospital:** Stanford Univ Med Ctr; **Address:** Stanford Univ Sch Med, Dept Gyn Oncology, 300 Pasteur Drive, Ste HH333, Stanford, CA 94305-5317; **Phone:** 650-498-8080; **Board Cert:** Obstetrics & Gynecology 1985; Gynecologic Oncology 1987; **Med School:** Univ Miami Sch Med 1977; **Resid:** Obstetrics & Gynecology, UCLA Med Ctr 1981; **Fellow:** Gynecologic Oncology, Stanford Univ Sch Med 1984; **Fac Appt:** Assoc Prof ObG, Stanford Univ

Obstetrics & Gynecology

New England

Cramer, Daniel W MD [ObG] - **Spec Exp:** Ovarian Cancer; Ovarian Cancer-High Risk; **Hospital:** Brigham & Women's Hosp, Dana-Farber Cancer Inst; **Address:** Brigham-Womens Hosp Ob/Gyn Epidemiology Ctr, 221 Longwood Ave, Boston, MA 02115; **Phone:** 617-732-4895; **Board Cert:** Obstetrics & Gynecology 1979; **Med School:** Univ Colorado 1970; **Resid:** Obstetrics & Gynecology, Boston Womens Hosp 1976; **Fellow:** Public Health, Harvard Med Sch 1982; **Fac Appt:** Prof ObG, Harvard Med Sch

Harper, Diane M MD [ObG] - **Spec Exp:** Cervical Cancer Screening; Vaccine Therapy; **Address:** 127 Mascoma St Fl 1, Lebanon, NH 03766; **Phone:** 603-448-5886; **Board Cert:** Family Medicine 2002; **Med School:** Univ Kans 1986; **Resid:** Obstetrics & Gynecology, Univ Kansas Med Ctr 1987; Family Medicine, Univ Kansas Med Ctr 1990; **Fellow:** Inter-Insts Genetics Clin-NIH 1994; Stanford Univ 1994; **Fac Appt:** Prof ObG, Dartmouth Med Sch

Noller, Kenneth L MD [ObG] - **Spec Exp:** DES-Exposed Females; Cervical Cancer; **Hospital:** Tufts-New England Med Ctr; **Address:** Tufts New England Med Ctr, Box 324, 750 Washington St, Boston, MA 02111; **Phone:** 617-636-2382; **Board Cert:** Obstetrics & Gynecology 1991; **Med School:** Creighton Univ 1970; **Resid:** Obstetrics & Gynecology, Mayo Clinic 1974; **Fac Appt:** Prof ObG, Univ Mass Sch Med

Southeast

Lipscomb, Gary H MD [ObG] - **Spec Exp:** Cervical Cancer; **Hospital:** Regional Med Ctr - Memphis, Baptist Memorial Hospital - Memphis; **Address:** Memphis Medical Ctr, 880 Madison Ave, Ste 3E01, Memphis, TN 38103-3409; **Phone:** 901-448-6632; **Board Cert:** Obstetrics & Gynecology 1997; **Med School:** Univ Tenn Coll Med, Memphis 1981; **Resid:** Obstetrics & Gynecology, Univ Tenn Affil Hosps 1985; **Fac Appt:** Prof ObG, Univ Tenn Coll Med, Memphis

Morgan, Linda S MD [ObG] - **Spec Exp:** Gynecologic Cancer; **Hospital:** Shands Hlthcre at Univ of FL; **Address:** Univ of Florida, PO Box 100294, Dept Ob/Gyn, Gainesville, FL 32610; **Phone:** 352-392-4161; **Board Cert:** Obstetrics & Gynecology 2004; Gynecologic Oncology 2004; **Med School:** Med Coll PA Hahnemann 1975; **Resid:** Obstetrics & Gynecology, Shands Hosp 1979; **Fellow:** Gynecologic Oncology, Mass Genl Hosp 1981; **Fac Appt:** Prof ObG, Univ Fla Coll Med

Midwest

Shulman, Lee MD [ObG] - **Spec Exp:** Breast Cancer Genetics; Ovarian Cancer Genetics; **Hospital:** Northwestern Meml Hosp, Rush Univ Med Ctr; **Address:** Northwestern Univ, Dept Ob/Gyn, 333 E Superior St, Ste 484, Chicago, IL 60611; **Phone:** 312-926-6627; **Board Cert:** Obstetrics & Gynecology 1999; Clinical Genetics 1990; **Med School:** Cornell Univ-Weill Med Coll 1983; **Resid:** Obstetrics & Gynecology, North Shore Univ Hosp 1987; **Fellow:** Reproductive Genetics, Univ Tenn Med Ctr 1989; **Fac Appt:** Prof ObG, Northwestern Univ

Reproductive Endocrinology

New England

Crowley, William F MD [RE] - **Spec Exp:** Fertility Preservation in Cancer; **Hospital:** Mass Genl Hosp; **Address:** Mass Genl Hosp, Reproductive Science Ctr, 55 Fruit St, Bartlett Hall-Extension 5, Boston, MA 02114; **Phone:** 617-726-5390; **Board Cert:** Internal Medicine 1974; Endocrinology 1977; **Med School:** Tufts Univ 1969; **Resid:** Internal Medicine, Mass Genl Hosp 1971; Internal Medicine, Mass Genl Hosp 1974; **Fellow:** Endocrinology, Mass Genl Hosp 1976; **Fac Appt:** Prof Med, Harvard Med Sch

Ginsburg, Elizabeth MD [RE] - **Spec Exp:** Fertility Preservation in Cancer; **Hospital:** Brigham & Women's Hosp, Dana-Farber Cancer Inst; **Address:** Brigham & Womens Hosp - Ctr Reproductive Med, 75 Francis St, Boston, MA 02115; **Phone:** 617-732-4222; **Board Cert:** Obstetrics & Gynecology 2005; Reproductive Endocrinology 2005; **Med School:** Mount Sinai Sch Med 1985; **Resid:** Obstetrics & Gynecology, Brigham & Womens Hosp 1989; **Fellow:** Reproductive Endocrinology, Brigham & Womens Hosp 1991

Patrizio, Pasquale MD [RE] - **Spec Exp:** Fertility Preservation in Cancer; **Hospital:** Yale - New Haven Hosp; **Address:** Yale Fertility Ctr, Dept OB/GYN, 150 Sargent Drive, New Haven, CT 06511; **Phone:** 203-785-4708; **Board Cert:** Obstetrics & Gynecology 1997; Reproductive Endocrinology 1999; **Med School:** Italy 1983; **Resid:** Obstetrics & Gynecology, Univ Naples 1987; Reproductive Endocrinology, Univ Pisa 1990; **Fellow:** Infertility, UC Irvine 1995; **Fac Appt:** Prof ObG, Yale Univ

Mid Atlantic

Coutifaris, Christos MD/PhD [RE] - **Spec Exp:** Fertility Preservation in Cancer; **Hospital:** Hosp Univ Penn - UPHS (page 84); **Address:** 3701 Market St Fl 8 - Ste 800, Philadelphia, PA 19104; **Phone:** 215-662-6100; **Board Cert:** Obstetrics & Gynecology 1998; Reproductive Endocrinology 1998; **Med School:** Univ Pennsylvania 1982; **Resid:** Obstetrics & Gynecology, Hosp Univ Penn 1986; **Fellow:** Reproductive Endocrinology, Univ Penn 1987; **Fac Appt:** Prof ObG, Univ Pennsylvania

Licciardi, Frederick L MD [RE] - **Spec Exp:** Fertility Preservation in Cancer; **Hospital:** NYU Med Ctr (page 80); **Address:** NYU Medical Ctr, 660 First Ave, 5th Fl, New York, NY 10016; **Phone:** 212-263-7754; **Board Cert:** Obstetrics & Gynecology 2005; Reproductive Endocrinology 2005; **Med School:** UMDNJ-Rutgers Med Sch 1986; **Resid:** Obstetrics & Gynecology, St Barnabas Med Ctr 1990; **Fellow:** Reproductive Endocrinology, New York Hosp-Cornell Med Ctr 1992; **Fac Appt:** Assoc Prof ObG, NYU Sch Med

Reproductive Endocrinology

Noyes, Nicole MD [RE] - **Spec Exp:** Fertility Preservation in Cancer; **Hospital:** NYU Med Ctr (page 80); **Address:** NYU Medical Ctr, 660 First Ave, 5th FL, New York, NY 10016; **Phone:** 212-263-7981; **Board Cert:** Obstetrics & Gynecology 2005; Reproductive Endocrinology 2005; **Med School:** Univ VT Coll Med 1986; **Resid:** Obstetrics & Gynecology, NY Hosp-Cornell Med Ctr 1990; **Fellow:** Reproductive Endocrinology, NY Hosp-Cornell Med Ctr 1992; **Fac Appt:** Assoc Prof ObG, NYU Sch Med

Rosenwaks, Zev MD [RE] - **Spec Exp:** Fertility Preservation in Cancer; **Hospital:** NY-Presby Hosp (page 79); **Address:** Ctr For Reproductive Medicine & Infertility, 505 E 70th St, Ste 340, New York, NY 10021-4872; **Phone:** 212-746-1743; **Board Cert:** Obstetrics & Gynecology 1978; Reproductive Endocrinology 1981; **Med School:** SUNY Downstate 1972; **Resid:** Obstetrics & Gynecology, LI Jewish Med Ctr 1976; **Fellow:** Reproductive Endocrinology, Johns Hopkins Hosp 1978; **Fac Appt:** Prof ObG, Cornell Univ-Weill Med Coll

Midwest

Wood Molo, Mary MD [RE] - **Spec Exp:** Fertility Preservation in Cancer; **Hospital:** Rush Univ Med Ctr; **Address:** 1725 W Harrison St, 408E, Chicago, IL 60612; **Phone:** 312-997-2229; **Board Cert:** Obstetrics & Gynecology 2004; Reproductive Endocrinology 2004; **Med School:** Southern IL Univ 1982; **Resid:** Obstetrics & Gynecology, Southern Illinois Affil Hosps 1984; Obstetrics & Gynecology, Rush Presby St Lukes Hosp 1987; **Fellow:** Reproductive Endocrinology, Rush Presby St Lukes Hosp 1989; **Fac Appt:** Asst Prof ObG, Rush Med Coll

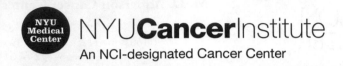

Looking for information on our expert physicians?
1-212-731-5000

NYU Clinical Cancer Center
160 East 34th Street
New York, New York 10016
www.nyuci.org/atcd

NYU Medical Center
550 First Avenue
(at 31st Street)
New York, New York 10016
www.nyumc.org/atcd

Stephen D. Hassenfeld Children's Center for Cancer and Blood Disorders
160 East 32nd Street
New York, New York 10016
www.nyumc.org/hassenfeld

A Collaborative Approach
The NYU Cancer Institute, an NCI designated center, is a "matrix cancer center" without walls operating within the larger NYU Medical Center. With over 200 members and a research funding base of over $81 million, this structure strengthens our capabilities to forge collaborations across medical and scientific disciplines, which translates to comprehensive care for our patients and discoveries that will influence the future of this disease.

Renowned Expertise
Our highly skilled Magnet™ nursing team not only plays a pivotal role in coordinating direct patient care, but is also a source of invaluable patient education. Team members' compassion and expertise help patients better manage the symptoms of their disease as well as their special needs.

A Patient-Focused Setting
The NYU Clinical Cancer Center, with over 70 faculty members from various disciplines at the New York University School of Medicine, is the principal outpatient facility of the Cancer Institute and serves as home for our patients and their caregivers. The center and its multidisciplinary team of experts provide access to the latest treatment options and clinical trials along with a variety of programs in cancer prevention, screening, diagnostics, genetic counseling, and supportive services. When it comes to kids and cancer, the Stephen D. Hassenfeld Children's Center for Cancer and Blood Disorders offers not just innovation but insight. As a leading member of the NCI-sponsored Children's Oncology Group, our physicians are known for developing new ways to treat childhood cancer. Our affiliation with Bellevue Hospital, the oldest public hospital in the country, affords clinically distinctive opportunities to learn and care for patients with cancer by observing its presentation and behavior in a variety of patient groups.

GYNECOLOGIC ONCOLOGY

Over 1,200 new patients come from around the world each year to M. D. Anderson's Gynecologic Oncology Center which specializes in diagnosis, early detection, prevention and treatment of cancers of the vagina, cervix, uterus, ovaries, vulva and fallopian tubes.

ROBOTIC AND MINIMALLY INVASIVE SURGERY

Advanced technology in the hands of cancer experts gives patients the best opportunity for a positive outcome. The DaVinci Robot is one of the latest additions to our surgical artillery against cancer. Our surgeons use laparoscopic, harmonic scalpel, and endoscopic surgical techniques to maximize outcomes. As a result, patients experience less bleeding, less scarring and pain, and enjoy faster recovery and return to normal activities.
M. D. Anderson cancer surgeons use minimally invasive surgery to treat gynecologic cancers as well as prostate, lung, and head and neck cancers.

MORE INFORMATION
For more information or to make an appointment, call 877-MDA-6789, or visit us online at http://www.mdanderson.org.

838

Ophthalmology

An ophthalmologist has the knowledge and professional skills needed to provide eye and vision care. Ophthalmologists are medically trained to diagnose, monitor and medically or surgically treat all ocular and visual disorders. This includes problems affecting the eye and its component structures, the eyelids, the orbit and the visual pathways. In so doing, an ophthalmologist prescribes vision services, including glasses and contact lenses.

Training Required: Four years

Ophthalmology

New England

Rubin, Peter A D MD [Oph] - **Spec Exp:** Oculoplastic Surgery; Orbital & Eyelid Tumors/Cancer; Eyelid Cancer & Reconstruction; **Hospital:** Mass Eye & Ear Infirmary; **Address:** Boston Eye Physicians, 44 Washington St, Brookline, MA 02245; **Phone:** 617-232-9600; **Board Cert:** Ophthalmology 1991; **Med School:** Yale Univ 1985; **Resid:** Ophthalmology, Manhattan EET Hosp 1989; **Fellow:** Oculoplastic Surgery, Mass EE Infirm 1990; **Fac Appt:** Assoc Prof Oph, Harvard Med Sch

Mid Atlantic

Abramson, David H MD [Oph] - **Spec Exp:** Eye Tumors/Cancer; Orbital Tumors/Cancer; Retinoblastoma; Melanoma-Choroidal (eye); **Hospital:** Meml Sloan Kettering Cancer Ctr (page 76); **Address:** 70 E 66th St, New York, NY 10021; **Phone:** 212-744-1700; **Board Cert:** Ophthalmology 1975; **Med School:** Albert Einstein Coll Med 1969; **Resid:** Ophthalmology, Harkness Eye Inst 1974; **Fellow:** Ocular Oncology, Columbia-Presby Med Ctr 1975; **Fac Appt:** Clin Prof Oph, Cornell Univ-Weill Med Coll

Della Rocca, Robert MD [Oph] - **Spec Exp:** Orbital Tumors/Cancer; Eyelid Tumors/Cancer; Oculoplastic Surgery; Eyelid Cancer & Reconstruction; **Hospital:** New York Eye & Ear Infirm (page 78), Sound Shore Med Ctr - Westchester; **Address:** 310 E 14th St, South Bldg, rm 319, New York, NY 10003; **Phone:** 212-979-4575; **Board Cert:** Ophthalmology 1975; **Med School:** Creighton Univ 1967; **Resid:** Ophthalmology, NY Eye & Ear Infirm 1973; **Fellow:** Oculoplastic Surgery, Albany Med Ctr

Finger, Paul T MD [Oph] - **Spec Exp:** Eye Tumors/Cancer; **Hospital:** New York Eye & Ear Infirm (page 78), NYU Med Ctr (page 80); **Address:** The New York Eye Cancer Ctr, 115 E 61st St, New York, NY 10021-8183; **Phone:** 212-832-8170; **Board Cert:** Ophthalmology 1990; **Med School:** Tulane Univ 1982; **Resid:** Ophthalmology, Manhattan EET Hosp 1986; **Fellow:** Ocular Oncology, N Shore Univ Hosp-Cornell 1987; **Fac Appt:** Clin Prof Oph, NYU Sch Med

Handa, James T MD [Oph] - **Spec Exp:** Melanoma-Choroidal (eye); Retinoblastoma; **Hospital:** Johns Hopkins Hosp - Baltimore; **Address:** Johns Hopkins-Wilmer Eye Inst, 1550 Orleans St, rm CRB-144, Baltimore, MD 21287; **Phone:** 410-614-4211; **Board Cert:** Ophthalmology 1991; **Med School:** Univ Pennsylvania 1986; **Resid:** Ophthalmology, Wills Eye Hosp 1990; **Fellow:** Retina/Vitreous, Duke Eye Ctr 1992; Ophthalmic Oncololgy, USC Sch Med 1993; **Fac Appt:** Assoc Prof Oph, Johns Hopkins Univ

Iliff, Nicholas Taylor MD [Oph] - **Spec Exp:** Oculoplastic Surgery; Orbital & Eyelid Tumors/Cancer; **Hospital:** Johns Hopkins Hosp - Baltimore; **Address:** Johns Hopkins Hosp-Wilmer Inst, Maumenee 505, 600 N Wolfe St, Baltimore, MD 21287-9218; **Phone:** 410-955-1112; **Board Cert:** Ophthalmology 1978; **Med School:** Johns Hopkins Univ 1972; **Resid:** Ophthalmology, Johns Hopkins-Wilmer Inst 1977; **Fellow:** Retinal Surgery, Johns Hopkins-Wilmer Inst 1978; Oculoplastic & Reconstructive Surgery, Johns Hopkins-Wilmer Inst 1980; **Fac Appt:** Prof Oph, Johns Hopkins Univ

Shields, Carol L MD [Oph] - Spec Exp: Orbital Tumors/Cancer; Melanoma; Retinoblastoma; **Hospital:** Wills Eye Hosp, Jefferson Hosp - Pittsburgh; **Address:** Wills Eye Hosp, Ocular Oncology Service, 840 Walnut St, Ste 1440, Phildelphia, PA 19107; **Phone:** 215-928-3105; **Board Cert:** Ophthalmology 1989; **Med School:** Univ Pittsburgh 1983; **Resid:** Ophthalmology, Willis Eye Hosp 1988; **Fellow:** Ophthalmic Pathology, Willis Eye Hosp 1988; Ophthalmic Oncololgy, Willis Eye Hosp 1989; **Fac Appt:** Prof Oph, Jefferson Med Coll

Shields, Jerry MD [Oph] - Spec Exp: Eye Tumors/Cancer; Pediatric Ophthalmology; Retinoblastoma; **Hospital:** Wills Eye Hosp; **Address:** Wills Eye Hosp, Ocular Oncology Service, 840 Walnut St, Ste 1440, Philadelphia, PA 19107; **Phone:** 215-928-3105; **Board Cert:** Ophthalmology 1972; **Med School:** Univ Mich Med Sch 1964; **Resid:** Ophthalmology, Wills Eye Hosp 1970; **Fellow:** Ophthalmology, Wills Eye Hosp 1972; **Fac Appt:** Prof Oph, Thomas Jefferson Univ

Southeast

Dutton, Jonathan J MD/PhD [Oph] - Spec Exp: Oculoplastic Surgery; Eye Tumors/Cancer; Melanoma-Choroidal (eye); **Hospital:** Univ NC Hosps; **Address:** Univ North Carolina - Dept Ophthalmology, 130 Mason Farm Rd, 5110 Bioinformatics, CB 7040, Chapel Hill, NC 27599; **Phone:** 919-966-5296; **Board Cert:** Ophthalmology 1983; **Med School:** Washington Univ, St Louis 1977; **Resid:** Ophthalmology, Washington Univ Med Ctr 1982; **Fellow:** Oculoplastic Surgery, Univ Iowa Med Ctr 1983; **Fac Appt:** Prof Oph, Univ NC Sch Med

Grossniklaus, Hans E MD [Oph] - Spec Exp: Ophthalmic Pathology; Melanoma-Choroidal (eye); **Hospital:** Emory Univ Hosp; **Address:** Emory Clinic - LF Montgomery Lab, 1365-B Clifton Rd NE, rm BT428, Atlanta, GA 30322; **Phone:** 404-778-4611; **Board Cert:** Ophthalmology 1985; Anatomic Pathology 1987; **Med School:** Ohio State Univ 1980; **Resid:** Ophthalmology, Case West Res Univ Hosp 1984; Pathology, Case West Res Univ Hosp 1987; **Fellow:** Ophthalmological Pathology, Johns Hopkins Hosp 1985; **Fac Appt:** Prof Oph, Emory Univ

Haik, Barrett MD [Oph] - Spec Exp: Eye Tumors/Cancer; **Hospital:** St Jude Children's Research Hosp; **Address:** Univ Tenn Med Group, Ophthamology, 930 Madison Ave, Ste 200, Memphis, TN 38103-3452; **Phone:** 901-448-6650; **Board Cert:** Ophthalmology 1981; **Med School:** Louisiana State Univ 1976; **Resid:** Ophthalmology, Columbia-Presby/Harkness Eye Inst 1980; **Fac Appt:** Prof Oph, Univ Tenn Coll Med, Memphis

Murray, Timothy MD [Oph] - Spec Exp: Eye Tumors/Cancer; **Hospital:** Bascom Palmer Eye Inst.; **Address:** Bascom Palmer Eye Inst, 900 NW 17th St, rm 254, Miami, FL 33136-1119; **Phone:** 305-326-6166; **Board Cert:** Ophthalmology 1990; **Med School:** Johns Hopkins Univ 1985; **Resid:** Ophthalmology, UCSF Med Ctr 1989; **Fellow:** Ophthalmology, UCSF 1999; Ophthalmology, Med Coll Wisconsin 1991; **Fac Appt:** Prof Oph, Univ Miami Sch Med

Sternberg Jr, Paul MD [Oph] - Spec Exp: Eye Tumors/Cancer; **Hospital:** Vanderbilt Univ Med Ctr, Vanderbilt Children's Hosp; **Address:** Vanderbilt Eye Institute, 8000 Medical Center E, Nashville, TN 37232-8808; **Phone:** 615-936-1453; **Board Cert:** Ophthalmology 1985; **Med School:** Univ Chicago-Pritzker Sch Med 1979; **Resid:** Ophthalmology, Johns Hopkins Hosp 1983; **Fellow:** Vitreoretinal Surgery, Duke Univ Med Ctr 1984; **Fac Appt:** Prof Oph, Vanderbilt Univ

Ophthalmology

Tse, David MD [Oph] - **Spec Exp:** Oculoplastic Surgery; Orbital Tumors/Cancer; Eyelid Tumors/Cancer; **Hospital:** Bascom Palmer Eye Inst., Jackson Meml Hosp; **Address:** Bascom Palmer Eye Inst, 900 NW 17th St, Miami, FL 33136-1119; **Phone:** 305-326-6086; **Board Cert:** Ophthalmology 2002; **Med School:** Univ Miami Sch Med 1976; **Resid:** Ophthalmology, LAC/USC Med Ctr 1981; **Fellow:** Oculoplastic Surgery, Univ Iowa Hosps 1982; **Fac Appt:** Prof Oph, Univ Miami Sch Med

Wilson, Matthew MD [Oph] - **Spec Exp:** Eye Tumors/Cancer; Retinoblastoma; Melanoma-Choroidal (eye); **Hospital:** St Jude Children's Research Hosp, Methodist Univ Hosp - Memphis; **Address:** Univ Tenn Med Grp, Ophthalmology, 930 Madison Ave, Ste 200, Memphis, TN 38103; **Phone:** 901-448-6650; **Board Cert:** Ophthalmology 1996; **Med School:** Emory Univ 1990; **Resid:** Ophthalmology, Emory Univ 1994; **Fellow:** Ophthalmological Pathology, Emory Univ 1995; Ocular Oncology, Moorfields Eye Hosp 1996; **Fac Appt:** Assoc Prof Oph, Univ Tenn Coll Med, Memphis

Midwest

Albert, Daniel M MD [Oph] - **Spec Exp:** Eye Tumors/Cancer; Ophthalmic Pathology; **Hospital:** Univ WI Hosp & Clins; **Address:** Dept Ophthalmology/VisualSci, K61412 CSC, 600 Highland Ave, Madison, WI 53792-4673; **Phone:** 608-263-9092; **Board Cert:** Ophthalmology 1969; **Med School:** Univ Pennsylvania 1962; **Resid:** Ophthalmology, Hosp Univ Penn 1966; Neurological Ophthalmology, Natl Inst Hlth 1968; **Fellow:** Pathology, Armed Forces Inst Path 1969; **Fac Appt:** Prof Oph, Univ Wisc

Augsburger, James MD [Oph] - **Spec Exp:** Eye Tumors/Cancer; Melanoma-Choroidal (eye); Retinoblastoma; **Hospital:** Univ Hosp - Cincinnati, Cincinnati Chldns Hosp Med Ctr; **Address:** Medical Arts Bldg, Ste 1500, 222 Piedmont Ave, rm ML 665-E, Cincinnati, OH 45267-0665; **Phone:** 513-475-7300; **Board Cert:** Ophthalmology 1979; **Med School:** Univ Cincinnati 1974; **Resid:** Ophthalmology, Univ Hosp-Cincinnati 1978; **Fellow:** Ocular Oncology, Wills Eye Hosp 1980; **Fac Appt:** Prof Oph, Univ Cincinnati

Blair, Norman P MD [Oph] - **Spec Exp:** Eye Tumors/Cancer; Melanoma-Choroidal (eye); **Hospital:** Univ of IL Med Ctr at Chicago; **Address:** University of Illinois Eye Ctr, 1855 W Taylor St, Chicago, IL 60612; **Phone:** 312-996-6660; **Board Cert:** Ophthalmology 1978; **Med School:** Indiana Univ 1970; **Resid:** Ophthalmology, Mass Eye Ear Infirmary 1977; **Fellow:** Retina/Vitreous, Mass Eye Ear Infirmary 1979; Ophthalmic Pathology, Univ IL Eye Ear Infirmary 1981; **Fac Appt:** Prof Oph, Univ IL Coll Med

Harbour, J William MD [Oph] - **Spec Exp:** Eye Tumors/Cancer; Melanoma-Choroidal (eye); Retinoblastoma; **Hospital:** Barnes-Jewish Hosp, St Louis Chldns Hosp; **Address:** Washington Univ Sch Med, Dept Ophthalmology, 660 S Euclid Ave, Box 8096, St Louis, MO 63110; **Phone:** 314-362-3315; **Board Cert:** Ophthalmology 1996; **Med School:** Johns Hopkins Univ 1990; **Resid:** Ophthalmology, Wills Eye Hosp 1994; **Fellow:** Retina/Vitreous, Bascom Palmer Eye Inst 1995; Ocular Oncology, UCSF Med Ctr 1996; **Fac Appt:** Prof Oph, Washington Univ, St Louis

Lee, Andrew G MD [Oph] - **Spec Exp:** Neuro-Ophthalmology; Optic Nerve Tumors; **Hospital:** Univ Iowa Hosp & Clinics; **Address:** Univ Iowa, Dept Ophthalmology, 200 Hawkins Dr, PFP 11290-E, Iowa City, IA 52242; **Phone:** 319-356-2548; **Board Cert:** Ophthalmology 1995; **Med School:** Univ VA Sch Med 1989; **Resid:** Ophthalmology, Cullen Eye Inst-Baylor 1993; **Fellow:** Neurological Ophthalmology, Wilmer Eye Inst-Johns Hopkins 1994; **Fac Appt:** Prof Oph, Univ Iowa Coll Med

Lueder, Gregg T MD [Oph] - **Spec Exp:** Retinoblastoma; Eye Tumors-Pediatric; Pediatric Ophthalmology; **Hospital:** St Louis Chldns Hosp; **Address:** St Louis Children's Hospital, One Children's Pl, rm 2S89, St Louis, MO 63110; **Phone:** 314-454-6026; **Board Cert:** Pediatrics 1989; Ophthalmology 2003; **Med School:** Univ Iowa Coll Med 1985; **Resid:** Pediatrics, St Louis Children's Hosp 1988; Ophthalmology, Univ Iowa Med Ctr 1991; **Fellow:** Pediatric Ophthalmology, Hosp for Sick Children 1993; **Fac Appt:** Assoc Prof Oph, Washington Univ, St Louis

Mieler, William F MD [Oph] - **Spec Exp:** Eye Tumors/Cancer; Retinoblastoma; **Hospital:** Univ of Chicago Hosps; **Address:** Univ Chicago, Dept Opth & Vis Sci, 5841 S Maryland, rm S-209, MC 211, Chicago, IL 60637; **Phone:** 773-702-3838; **Board Cert:** Ophthalmology 1984; **Med School:** Univ Wisc 1979; **Resid:** Ophthalmology, Bascom-Palmer Eye Inst 1983; **Fellow:** Vitreoretinal Surgery & Disease, Med Ctr Wisconsin Eye Inst 1984; Oculoplastic Surgery, Wills Eye Hosp 1986; **Fac Appt:** Prof Oph, Univ Chicago-Pritzker Sch Med

Nerad, Jeffrey MD [Oph] - **Spec Exp:** Orbital Tumors/Cancer; Eyelid Cancer & Reconstruction; Oculoplastic Surgery; **Hospital:** Univ Iowa Hosp & Clinics; **Address:** Univ Iowa, Dept Ophthalmology, 200 Hawkins Drive, Iowa City, IA 52242; **Phone:** 319-356-2864; **Board Cert:** Ophthalmology 1984; **Med School:** St Louis Univ 1979; **Resid:** Ophthalmology, St Louis Univ Med Ctr 1983; **Fellow:** Oculoplastic & Reconstructive Surgery, Univ Iowa 1984; **Fac Appt:** Prof Oph, Univ Iowa Coll Med

Vine, Andrew K MD [Oph] - **Spec Exp:** Melanoma-Choroidal (eye); **Hospital:** Univ Michigan Hlth Sys; **Address:** Univ Michigan-Kellogg Eye Ctr, 1000 Wall St, Ann Arbor, MI 48105; **Phone:** 734-763-5906; **Board Cert:** Ophthalmology 1979; **Med School:** McGill Univ 1972; **Resid:** Ophthalmology, Royal Victoria Hosp 1978; **Fellow:** Pathology, McGill Univ 1975; Retina, UCSF Med Ctr 1980; **Fac Appt:** Prof Oph, Univ Mich Med Sch

Weingeist, Thomas A MD/PhD [Oph] - **Spec Exp:** Eye Tumors/Cancer; **Hospital:** Univ Iowa Hosp & Clinics; **Address:** Univ Iowa, Dept Ophthalmology, 200 Hawkins Drive, Iowa City, IA 52242; **Phone:** 319-356-2864; **Board Cert:** Ophthalmology 1976; **Med School:** Univ Iowa Coll Med 1972; **Resid:** Ophthalmology, Univ Iowa Hosp 1975; **Fellow:** Vitreoretinal Surgery, Univ Iowa 1976; **Fac Appt:** Prof Oph, Univ Iowa Coll Med

Great Plains and Mountains

Anderson, Richard L MD [Oph] - **Spec Exp:** Orbital & Eyelid Tumors/Cancer; **Hospital:** Salt Lake Regional Med Ctr, Intermountain Shriners Hosp; **Address:** 1002 E South Temple, Ste 308, Salt Lake City, UT 84102-1525; **Phone:** 801-363-3355; **Board Cert:** Ophthalmology 1976; **Med School:** Univ Iowa Coll Med 1971; **Resid:** Ophthalmology, Univ Iowa Hosps-Clins 1975; **Fellow:** Oculoplastic & Reconstructive Surgery, Albany Med Ctr 1975; Oculoplastic & Reconstructive Surgery, UCSF Med Ctr 1976; **Fac Appt:** Prof PlS, Univ Utah

Southwest

Gigantelli, James W MD [Oph] - **Spec Exp:** Orbital Tumors/Cancer; Eyelid Cancer & Reconstruction; Lymphoma-Ocular (eye); **Hospital:** OU Med Ctr; **Address:** McGee Eye Institute, 608 Stanton L Young Blvd, Oklahoma City, OK 73104; **Phone:** 405-271-6060; **Board Cert:** Ophthalmology 1991; **Med School:** Vanderbilt Univ 1985; **Resid:** Ophthalmology, Baylor Coll Med 1989; **Fellow:** Oculoplastic Surgery, Duke Unv Med Ctr 1990; **Fac Appt:** Assoc Prof Oph, Univ Okla Coll Med

Ophthalmology

Piest, Kenneth L MD [Oph] - **Spec Exp:** Eyelid Cancer & Reconstruction; Pediatric Eye Reconstructive Surgery; Orbital Tumors/Cancer; Oculoplastic Surgery; **Hospital:** Metro Methodist Hosp, Baptist Med Ctr - San Antonio; **Address:** Texas Ophthalmic Plastic Surgery, 225 E Sonterra Blvd, Ste 201, San Antonio, TX 78258; **Phone:** 210-494-8859; **Board Cert:** Ophthalmology 1991; **Med School:** Univ IL Coll Med 1984; **Resid:** Ophthalmology, Univ Tex Hlth Scis Ctr 1989; **Fellow:** Ophthalmic Plastic Surgery, Chldns Hosp/Sheie Eye Inst/Univ Penn 1990; Craniofacial Ophthalmic Plastic Surgery, Chldns Hosp/Univ Penn 1991; **Fac Appt:** Assoc Clin Prof Oph, Univ Tex, San Antonio

Soparkar, Charles MD [Oph] - **Spec Exp:** Eye Tumors/Cancer; Orbital & Eyelid Tumors/Cancer; Oculoplastic Surgery; **Hospital:** Methodist Hosp - Houston, Texas Chldns Hosp - Houston; **Address:** Plastic Eye Surg Assocs, 3730 Kirby Drive, Ste 900, Houston, TX 77098; **Phone:** 713-795-0705; **Board Cert:** Ophthalmology 1996; **Med School:** Univ Mass Sch Med 1990; **Resid:** Ophthalmology, Baylor Affil Hosps 1994; **Fellow:** Ophthalmic Oncololgy, Texas Med Ctr 1995

West Coast and Pacific

Boxrud, Cynthia Ann MD [Oph] - **Spec Exp:** Oculoplastic Surgery; Eye Tumors/Cancer; **Hospital:** UCLA Med Ctr (page 83), St John's Hlth Ctr, Santa Monica; **Address:** 2021 Santa Monica Blvd, Ste 700E, Santa Monica, CA 90404-2208; **Phone:** 310-829-9060; **Board Cert:** Ophthalmology 1997; **Med School:** Case West Res Univ 1986; **Resid:** Ophthalmology, NYU-Bellevue Hosp Ctr 1990; **Fellow:** Ophthalmic Oncololgy, New York Hosp-Cornell Med Ctr 1992; Ophthalmic Plastic Surgery, UCLA - Jules Stein Eye Inst 1993; **Fac Appt:** Asst Prof Oph, UCLA

Char, Devron H MD [Oph] - **Spec Exp:** Eye Tumors/Cancer; Oculoplastic Surgery; **Hospital:** CA Pacific Med Ctr - Pacific Campus, UCSF Med Ctr; **Address:** 45 Castro St, Ste 309, San Francisco, CA 94114; **Phone:** 415-522-0700; **Board Cert:** Ophthalmology 1978; **Med School:** Univ Minn 1970; **Resid:** Internal Medicine, Mass Genl Hosp 1972; Ophthalmology, UCSF Med Ctr 1977; **Fellow:** Medical Oncology, Natl Cancer Inst 1974; Ophthalmology, UCSF Med Ctr 1978; **Fac Appt:** Prof Oph, Stanford Univ

Cockerham, Kimberly P MD [Oph] - **Spec Exp:** Meningioma-Orbital (eye); Orbital Tumors/Cancer; Eyelid Cancer & Reconstruction; Neuro-Ophthalmology; **Hospital:** Stanford Univ Med Ctr; **Address:** Stanford Eye Center, 900 Blake Wilbur Dr, #3002, Palo Alto, CA 94304; **Phone:** 650-723-6695; **Board Cert:** Ophthalmology 2004; **Med School:** Geo Wash Univ 1987; **Resid:** Ophthalmology, Walter Reed Army Med Ctr 1992; **Fellow:** Neurological Ophthalmology, Walter Reed Army Med Ctr 1993; Neurological Ophthalmology, Allegheny General Hosp 1995

Murphree, A Linn MD [Oph] - **Spec Exp:** Pediatric Ophthalmology; Retinoblastoma; Orbital Tumors/Cancer; **Hospital:** Chldns Hosp - Los Angeles, USC Univ Hosp - R K Eamer Med Plz; **Address:** Chldns Hosp, Div Oph, 4650 Sunset Blvd, MS 88, Los Angeles, CA 90027-6016; **Phone:** 323-669-2299; **Board Cert:** Ophthalmology 1978; **Med School:** Baylor Coll Med 1972; **Resid:** Clinical Genetics, Baylor Heed 1973; Ophthalmology, Baylor Coll Med 1976; **Fellow:** Ophthalmology, Wilmer Inst/Johns Hopkins 1977; **Fac Appt:** Prof Oph, USC Sch Med

O'Brien, Joan M MD [Oph] - **Spec Exp:** Eye Tumors/Cancer; Retinoblastoma; **Hospital:** UCSF Med Ctr; **Address:** UCSF, Dept Ophthalmology, 533 Parnassus Ave Fl 5, San Francisco, CA 94143; **Phone:** 415-476-3705; **Board Cert:** Ophthalmology 1996; **Med School:** Dartmouth Med Sch 1986; **Resid:** Ophthalmology, Mass Eye & Ear Infirm 1992; **Fellow:** Ophthalmic Pathology, Mass Eye & Ear Infirm 1989; UCSF Med Ctr 1993; **Fac Appt:** Prof Oph, UCSF

Seiff, Stuart R MD [Oph] - **Spec Exp:** Oculoplastic Surgery; Orbital Tumors/Cancer; **Hospital:** UCSF Med Ctr, CA Pacific Med Ctr; **Address:** 2100 Webster St, Ste 214, San Francisco, CA 94115; **Phone:** 415-923-3007; **Board Cert:** Ophthalmology 1986; **Med School:** UCSF 1980; **Resid:** Ophthalmology, UCSF Med Ctr 1984; **Fellow:** Ophthalmic Plastic & Reconstructive Surgery, UCLA Med Ctr 1985; Oculoplastic Surgery, Moorfield's Eye Hosp 1986; **Fac Appt:** Prof Oph, UCSF

Stout, John Timothy MD/PhD [Oph] - **Spec Exp:** Retinoblastoma; **Hospital:** OR Hlth & Sci Univ, Providence St Vincent Med Ctr; **Address:** 3375 SW Terwilliger Blvd, Portland, OR 97239; **Phone:** 503-494-2435; **Board Cert:** Ophthalmology 1999; **Med School:** Baylor Coll Med 1989; **Resid:** Ophthalmology, Doheny Eye Inst 1993; **Fellow:** Ophthalmology, Moorfields Eye Hosp 1994; Retinal Surgery, Doheny Eye Inst 1995; **Fac Appt:** Assoc Prof Oph, Oregon Hlth Sci Univ

Wilson, David Jean MD [Oph] - **Spec Exp:** Eye Tumors/Cancer; Ophthalmic Pathology; **Hospital:** OR Hlth & Sci Univ; **Address:** 3375 SW Terwilliger Blvd, Portland, OR 97239; **Phone:** 503-494-7891; **Board Cert:** Ophthalmology 1986; **Med School:** Baylor Coll Med 1981; **Resid:** Ophthalmology, Univ Oregon 1985; **Fellow:** Ophthalmic Pathology, John Hopkins Hosp 1987; Retina/Vitreous, Mass Eye & Ear Infirm 1988; **Fac Appt:** Prof Oph, Oregon Hlth Sci Univ

THE NEW YORK EYE AND EAR INFIRMARY

310 East 14th Street
New York, New York 10003
Tel. 212.979.4000   Fax. 212.228.0664
www.nyee.edu

OCULAR TUMOR SERVICE

The Infirmary is a national referral center within the Collaborative Ocular Melanoma Study of the National Eye Institute/National Institutes of Health. New and innovative treatments for patients with eye cancer include radioactive plaques to treat intraocular tumors and chemotherapy for conjunctival neoplasia. Tumors of the eyelids, iris, retina, choroid and optic nerve are also treated by specialists in this service. A multidisciplinary Ocular Tumor Board meets monthly to discuss the most difficult cases and formulate therapeutic options.

OTOLARYNGOLOGY/ HEAD & NECK SURGERY

Head & Neck Oncology: A team comprised of board-certified surgeons, medical & radiation oncologists, nutritionists and rehabilitation specialists ensure rapid recovery from complex, life saving surgical procedures and return to daily activities.

Thyroid Center: A unique center concentrates on streamlining the diagnosis and treatment of thyroid diseases and cancers with a highly skilled team of surgeons, endocrinologists and radiologists to manage the patient's care. An area of expertise is cancer resulting from radiation exposure such as Chernobyl.

Facial Plastics and Reconstructive Surgery: Treatment of facial tumors, both benign and cancerous, frequently requires expert reconstruction. Designed to restore the function and appearance of the face, these procedures may be required after appropriate treatment of skin cancers or deep tumors.

Otology–Neuro-otology: These rare cancers can be treated by our highly skilled team of surgeons which includes a neuro-otologist and a neurosurgeon.

Center for the Voice and Swallowing: The Center is cooperatively staffed by a team of specialists able to diagnose cancer of the vocal cords early and rehabilitate the voice after surgical and radiation treatment.

PATHOLOGY & LABORATORY MEDICINE

The Ocular Pathology Service is the leading laboratory in the Northeast and utilized by ophthalmologists throughout the region. The Infirmary is the site of some of the most promising studies into diseases and cancers of the eye, ear, nose and throat. Among them: cellular markers of oral cancer risk, non-invasive detection of thyroid cancer, basic cell biology of the growth of ocular melanoma cells, and persistence of biomaterials for repair in plastic and reconstructive surgery.

About The New York Eye and Ear Infirmary

Established in 1820, the Infirmary is the oldest continuously operating specialty hospital in the nation and one of the most experienced in terms of the number of patients it treats and complexity of cases. Each year the Ophthalmology Department performs more than 16,000 surgeries and sees more than 80,000 visits from outpatients. The Otolaryngology Department performs more than 6,000 surgeries and has some 60,000 outpatient visits. A third clinical department, the Department of Plastic & Reconstructive Surgery, is a natural complement to the Infirmary's other services and annually treats more than 1,000 patients who seek reconstructive surgery as a result of accident, birth defect or cancer, and those who elect cosmetic surgery.

NYEEI is a teaching affiliate of New York Medical College and a member of Continuum Health Partners, Inc.

**Physician Referral
1.800.449.HOPE (4673)**

Orthopaedic Surgery

An orthopaedic surgeon is trained in the preservation, investigation and restoration of the form and function of the extremities, spine and associated structures by medical, surgical and physical means.

An orthopaedic surgeon is involved with the care of patients whose musculoskeletal problems include congenital deformities, trauma, infections, tumors, metabolic disturbances of the musculoskeletal system, deformities, injuries and degenerative diseases of the spine, hands, feet, knee, hip, shoulder and elbow in children and adults. An orthopaedic surgeon is also concerned with primary and secondary muscular problems and the effects of central or peripheral nervous system lesions of the musculoskeletal system.

Training Required: Five years (including general surgery training) plus two years in clinical practice before final certification is achieved.

Note: There are many Orthopaedic Surgeons who are trained in Sports Medicine and prefer to be listed under that heading; some trained in Sports Medicine prefer to be listed under Orthopaedics.

Hand Surgery: A specialist trained in the investigation, preservation and restoration by medical, surgical and rehabilitative means of all structures of the upper extremity directly affecting the form and function of the hand and wrist.

Training Required: Training required for Orthopaedic Surgery certification plus an additional year in hand surgery.

Orthopaedic Surgery

New England

Friedlaender, Gary E MD [OrS] - **Spec Exp:** Bone & Soft Tissue Tumors; Bone Tumors-Metastatic; **Hospital:** Yale - New Haven Hosp; **Address:** Yale Univ Sch Med, Dept Orthopedic Surg, 800 Howard Ave YPB Bldg - rm 133, Box 208071, New Haven, CT 06520-8071; **Phone:** 203-737-5656; **Board Cert:** Orthopaedic Surgery 1975; **Med School:** Univ Mich Med Sch 1969; **Resid:** Surgery, Michigan Med Ctr 1971; Orthopaedic Surgery, Yale-New Haven Hosp 1974; **Fellow:** Musculoskeletal Oncology, Mass Genl Hosp 1983; **Fac Appt:** Prof OrS, Yale Univ

Gebhardt, Mark MD [OrS] - **Spec Exp:** Musculoskeletal Tumors; Bone Tumors; **Hospital:** Beth Israel Deaconess Med Ctr - Boston, Children's Hospital - Boston; **Address:** 330 Brookline Ave, Shapiro 2, Boston, MA 02215; **Phone:** 617-667-3940; **Board Cert:** Orthopaedic Surgery 1992; **Med School:** Univ Cincinnati 1975; **Resid:** Surgery, Univ Pittsburg Med Ctr 1977; Orthopaedic Surgery, Harvard 1982; **Fellow:** Pediatric Orthopaedic Surgery, Boston Chldns Hosp 1983; Orthopaedic Oncology, Mass Genl Hosp 1983; **Fac Appt:** Prof OrS, Harvard Med Sch

Ready, John E MD [OrS] - **Spec Exp:** Bone Cancer; Sarcoma-Soft Tissue; Hip & Knee Replacement in Bone Tumors; **Hospital:** Brigham & Women's Hosp, Dana-Farber Cancer Inst; **Address:** Brigham & Women's Hospital, Dept Orthopaedics, 75 Francis St, Boston, MA 02115; **Phone:** 617-732-5368; **Board Cert:** Orthopaedic Surgery 2002; **Med School:** Dalhousie Univ 1982; **Resid:** Orthopaedic Surgery, Dalhousie Univ Hosp 1987; **Fellow:** Orthopaedic Oncology, St Michael's Hosp 1988; Orthopaedic Oncology, Mass Genl Hosp/Childns Hosp 1989

Springfield, Dempsey MD [OrS] - **Spec Exp:** Bone Tumors; Soft Tissue Tumors; **Hospital:** Mass Genl Hosp; **Address:** 55 Fruit St, YAW 3700, Boston, MA 02114-2621; **Phone:** 617-724-3700; **Board Cert:** Orthopaedic Surgery 1992; **Med School:** Univ Fla Coll Med 1971; **Resid:** Orthopaedic Surgery, Univ Florida/Shands 1976; **Fellow:** Orthopaedic Surgery, Univ Florida/Shands 1979

Weinstein, James DO [OrS] - **Spec Exp:** Pain-Back; Spinal Tumors; **Hospital:** Dartmouth - Hitchcock Med Ctr; **Address:** DHMC, Dept Orthopaedic Surgery, One Medical Ctr Drive, Lebanon, NH 03756; **Phone:** 603-653-3580; **Board Cert:** Orthopaedic Surgery 2002; **Med School:** Chicago Coll Osteo Med 1973; **Resid:** Orthopaedic Surgery, Rush Presby-St Lukes Med Ctr 1983; **Fac Appt:** Prof OrS, Dartmouth Med Sch

Mid Atlantic

Benevenia, Joseph MD [OrS] - **Spec Exp:** Limb Sparing Surgery; Bone Cancer; Sarcoma-Soft Tissue; **Hospital:** UMDNJ-Univ Hosp-Newark; **Address:** 140 Bergen St, Ste D-1610, Newark, NJ 07103; **Phone:** 973-972-2153; **Board Cert:** Orthopaedic Surgery 2003; **Med School:** UMDNJ-NJ Med Sch, Newark 1984; **Resid:** Orthopaedic Surgery, UMDNJ-NJ Med Sch Hosp 1988; **Fellow:** Orthopaedic Oncology, Case Western Reserve Univ 1991; **Fac Appt:** Prof OrS, UMDNJ-NJ Med Sch, Newark

Dormans, John P MD [OrS] - **Spec Exp:** Tumor Surgery-Pediatric; Pediatric Orthopedic Surgery; **Hospital:** Chldns Hosp of Philadelphia, The; **Address:** Childrens Hosp Philadelphia, 34 St & Civic Center Blvd, Wood Bldg Fl 2-rm 2315, Philadelphia, PA 19104; **Phone:** 215-590-1527; **Board Cert:** Orthopaedic Surgery 2002; **Med School:** Indiana Univ 1983; **Resid:** Orthopaedic Surgery, Michigan State Univ Hosps 1988; **Fellow:** Pediatric Orthopaedic Surgery, Hosp Sick Children 1989; **Fac Appt:** Prof OrS, Univ Pennsylvania

Frassica, Frank J MD [OrS] - **Spec Exp:** Bone Cancer; **Hospital:** Johns Hopkins Hosp - Baltimore; **Address:** 601 N Caroline St, Ste 5215, Baltimore, MD 21287-0882; **Phone:** 410-955-9300; **Board Cert:** Orthopaedic Surgery 2001; **Med School:** Univ SC Sch Med 1982; **Resid:** Orthopaedic Surgery, Mayo Clinic 1987; **Fellow:** Orthopaedic Oncology, Mayo Clinic 1988; **Fac Appt:** Prof OrS, Johns Hopkins Univ

Healey, John H MD [OrS] - **Spec Exp:** Bone Tumors; Hip & Knee Replacement in Bone Tumors; Prosthetic Reconstruction; Sarcoma-Soft Tissue; **Hospital:** Meml Sloan Kettering Cancer Ctr (page 76), Hosp For Special Surgery; **Address:** 1275 York Ave, Ste A-342, New York, NY 10021-6007; **Phone:** 212-639-7610; **Board Cert:** Orthopaedic Surgery 2005; **Med School:** Univ VT Coll Med 1978; **Resid:** Orthopaedic Surgery, Hosp Special Surg 1983; **Fellow:** Orthopaedic Oncology, Meml Sloan Kettering Cancer Ctr 1984; Orthopaedic Surgery, Hosp Special Surgery 1984; **Fac Appt:** Prof OrS, Cornell Univ-Weill Med Coll

Kenan, Samuel MD [OrS] - **Spec Exp:** Bone Tumors; **Hospital:** Hosp For Joint Diseases, NYU Med Ctr (page 80); **Address:** 317 E 34th St, Ste 903, New York, NY 10016; **Phone:** 212-684-5511; **Med School:** Israel 1976; **Resid:** Orthopaedic Surgery, Hadassah Univ Hosp 1984; **Fellow:** Orthopaedic Pathology, Hosp for Joint Diseases 1987; **Fac Appt:** Prof OrS, NYU Sch Med

Lackman, Richard D MD [OrS] - **Spec Exp:** Bone Cancer; Sarcoma; Limb Sparing Surgery; **Hospital:** Hosp Univ Penn - UPHS (page 84), Pennsylvania Hosp (page 84); **Address:** Hosp Univ Penn - Dept Orthopaedic Surg, 3400 Spruce St, 2 Silverstein, Philadelphia, PA 19104; **Phone:** 215-662-3340; **Board Cert:** Orthopaedic Surgery 1985; **Med School:** Univ Pennsylvania 1977; **Resid:** Orthopaedic Surgery, Hosp Univ Penn 1982; **Fellow:** Orthopaedic Oncology, Mayo Clinic 1983; **Fac Appt:** Assoc Prof OrS, Univ Pennsylvania

Lane, Joseph MD [OrS] - **Spec Exp:** Bone Cancer; **Hospital:** Hosp For Special Surgery, NY-Presby Hosp (page 79); **Address:** Hosp for Special Surgery, 535 E 70th St, New York, NY 10021; **Phone:** 212-606-1172; **Board Cert:** Orthopaedic Surgery 1998; **Med School:** Harvard Med Sch 1965; **Resid:** Surgery, Hosp Univ Penn 1967; Orthopaedic Surgery, Hosp Univ Penn 1973; **Fac Appt:** Prof OrS, Cornell Univ-Weill Med Coll

Malawer, Martin M MD [OrS] - **Spec Exp:** Bone Tumors; Limb Sparing Surgery; Pediatric Orthopaedic Surgery; Sarcoma; **Hospital:** Washington Hosp Ctr, G Washington Univ Hosp; **Address:** Washington Cancer Institute, 110 Irving St NW, Ste C2173, Washington, DC 20010; **Phone:** 202-877-3970; **Board Cert:** Orthopaedic Surgery 1993; **Med School:** NYU Sch Med 1969; **Resid:** Surgery, Bronx Muni Hosp 1972; Orthopaedic Surgery, Bellevue Hosp Ctr 1975; **Fellow:** Orthopaedic Oncology, Shands Hosp-Univ Florida 1978; **Fac Appt:** Prof OrS, Geo Wash Univ

O'Keefe, Regis J MD/PhD [OrS] - **Spec Exp:** Bone & Soft Tissue Tumors; Reconstructive Surgery; **Hospital:** Univ of Rochester Strong Meml Hosp, Highland Hosp - Rochester; **Address:** Univ Rochester, Dept Orthopaedic Surgery, 601 Elmwood Ave, Box 665, Rochester, NY 14642; **Phone:** 585-275-3100; **Board Cert:** Orthopaedic Surgery 1996; **Med School:** Harvard Med Sch 1985; **Resid:** Surgery, New Eng Deaconess Hosp/Harvard 1986; Orthopaedic Surgery, Univ Rochester 1992; **Fellow:** Orthopaedic Oncology, Mass Genl Hosp 1993; **Fac Appt:** Prof S, Univ Rochester

Orthopaedic Surgery

Southeast

Berrey, B Hudson MD [OrS] - **Spec Exp:** Musculoskeletal Tumors; **Hospital:** Shands Jacksonville; **Address:** Univ of FL Col of Med Dept of Orth Surg, 655 W Eighth St, Jacksonville, FL 32209; **Phone:** 904-244-5942; **Board Cert:** Orthopaedic Surgery 1982; **Med School:** Univ Tex Med Br, Galveston 1977; **Resid:** Orthopaedic Surgery, Tripler Army Med Ctr 1981; **Fellow:** Medical Oncology, Mass Genl Hosp Harvard 1985; **Fac Appt:** Prof OrS, Univ Fla Coll Med

Kneisl, Jeffrey S MD [OrS] - **Spec Exp:** Bone Cancer; Musculoskeletal Tumors; **Hospital:** Carolinas Med Ctr; **Address:** Carolinas Med Ctr, 1001 Blythe Blvd, Ste 602, Charlotte, NC 28203; **Phone:** 704-355-5982; **Board Cert:** Orthopaedic Surgery 2000; **Med School:** Northwestern Univ 1980; **Resid:** Orthopaedic Surgery, Northwestern Univ 1987; **Fellow:** Orthopaedic Oncology, Univ Chicago 1990

Scarborough, Mark MD [OrS] - **Spec Exp:** Bone Tumors; Sarcoma; **Hospital:** Shands Hlthcre at Univ of FL; **Address:** Shands Healthcare Univ FL, 3450 Hull Rd, Gainesville, FL 32611; **Phone:** 352-273-7000; **Board Cert:** Orthopaedic Surgery 2003; **Med School:** Univ Fla Coll Med 1985; **Resid:** Orthopaedic Surgery, Univ Texas Med Ctr 1990; **Fellow:** Orthopaedic Surgery, Mass Genl Hosp 1991; **Fac Appt:** Prof OrS, Univ Fla Coll Med

Schwartz, Herbert S MD [OrS] - **Spec Exp:** Bone Tumors-Metastatic; Bone Tumors; **Hospital:** Vanderbilt Univ Med Ctr, Baptist Hosp - Nashville; **Address:** Vanderbilt Med Ctr Ortho Institute, South Tower, rm 4200, Medical Ctr East, Nashville, TN 37232-8774; **Phone:** 615-343-8612; **Board Cert:** Orthopaedic Surgery 1992; **Med School:** Univ Chicago-Pritzker Sch Med 1981; **Resid:** Orthopaedic Surgery, Univ Chicago Hosps 1986; **Fellow:** Orthopaedic Oncology, Mayo Clinic 1987; **Fac Appt:** Prof OrS, Vanderbilt Univ

Scully, Sean P MD [OrS] - **Spec Exp:** Bone Cancer; Sarcoma; Musculoskeletal Tumors; **Hospital:** Cedars Med Ctr - Miami; **Address:** Cedars Medical Ctr, East Bldg, 1400 NW 12th Ave Fl 4, Miami, FL 33136; **Phone:** 305-325-4683; **Board Cert:** Orthopaedic Surgery 1995; **Med School:** Univ Rochester 1980; **Resid:** Orthopaedic Surgery, Duke Univ Med Ctr 1985; **Fellow:** Orthopaedic Oncology, Mass General Hosp 1987; Research, Natl Inst Health 1988; **Fac Appt:** Prof OrS, Univ Miami Sch Med

Siegel, Herrick J MD [OrS] - **Spec Exp:** Bone Cancer; Sarcoma; Metastic Bone Disease; **Hospital:** Univ of Ala Hosp at Birmingham; **Address:** UAB Kirklin Clinic, 2000 6th Ave S, Birmingham, AL 35294; **Phone:** 205-975-0415; **Board Cert:** Orthopaedic Surgery 2005; **Med School:** NYU Sch Med 1995; **Resid:** Orthopaedic Surgery, USC 2000; **Fellow:** Orthopaedic Oncology, Mayo Clinic 2002; **Fac Appt:** Asst Prof OrS, Univ Ala

Walling, Arthur MD [OrS] - **Spec Exp:** Bone Tumors; Soft Tissue Tumors; **Hospital:** H Lee Moffitt Cancer Ctr & Research Inst, Tampa Genl Hosp; **Address:** Florida Orthopedic Inst, 13020 Telecom Pkwy N, Temple Terrace, FL 33637; **Phone:** 813-978-9700; **Board Cert:** Orthopaedic Surgery 1982; **Med School:** Creighton Univ 1976; **Resid:** Orthopaedic Surgery, Univ South Florida Affil Hosps 1980; **Fellow:** Surgical Oncology, Univ Florida 1981; **Fac Appt:** Assoc Clin Prof OrS, Univ S Fla Coll Med

Ward, William G MD [OrS] - **Spec Exp:** Bone Tumors; Soft Tissue Tumors; Reconstructive Surgery; **Hospital:** Wake Forest Univ Baptist Med Ctr (page 85), Forsyth Med Ctr; **Address:** Wake Forest Med Ctr, Comprehensive Rehab, 131 Miller St, Winston Salem, NC 77103; **Phone:** 336-716-8200; **Board Cert:** Orthopaedic Surgery 2004; **Med School:** Duke Univ 1975; **Resid:** Surgery, Duke Univ Med Ctr 1985; Orthopaedic Surgery, Duke Univ Med Ctr 1989; **Fellow:** Sports Medicine, Cleveland Clinic 1990; Orthopaedic Oncology, UCLA Med Ctr 1991; **Fac Appt:** Prof OrS, Wake Forest Univ

Midwest

Biermann, J Sybil MD [OrS] - **Spec Exp:** Sarcoma; Bone Cancer; Multiple Myeloma; Limb Sparing Surgery; **Hospital:** Univ Michigan Hlth Sys; **Address:** Univ Michigan Cancer Ctr, 1500 E Medical Ctr Drive, 7304 CCGC, Ann Arbor, MI 48109-0948; **Phone:** 734-647-8902; **Board Cert:** Orthopaedic Surgery 2004; **Med School:** Stanford Univ 1987; **Resid:** Orthopaedic Surgery, Univ Iowa Hosp 1992; **Fellow:** Orthopaedic Oncology, Univ Chicago Hosps 1993; **Fac Appt:** Assoc Prof OrS, Univ Mich Med Sch

Buckwalter, Joseph MD [OrS] - **Spec Exp:** Bone Cancer; Bone Tumors-Metastatic; **Hospital:** Univ Iowa Hosp & Clinics; **Address:** Univ Iowa Hosps, Orthopaedics, 200 Hawkins Drive, Iowa City, IA 52242; **Phone:** 319-356-2595; **Board Cert:** Orthopaedic Surgery 1991; **Med School:** Univ Iowa Coll Med 1974; **Resid:** Orthopaedic Surgery, Iowa Hosp 1979; **Fac Appt:** Prof OrS, Univ Iowa Coll Med

Cheng, Edward MD [OrS] - **Spec Exp:** Bone & Soft Tissue Tumors; **Hospital:** Univ Minn Med Ctr, Fairview - Univ Campus; **Address:** Dept Orthopedic Surgery, Univ Minnesota, 2450 Riverside Ave S, Ste R-200, Minneapolis, MN 55455; **Phone:** 612-273-1177; **Board Cert:** Orthopaedic Surgery 2003; **Med School:** Northwestern Univ 1983; **Resid:** Surgery, Northwestern Univ 1985; Orthopaedic Surgery, Beth Israel Hosp 1989; **Fellow:** Surgical Oncology, Mass Genl Hosp 1990; **Fac Appt:** Prof OrS, Univ Minn

Clohisy, Denis MD [OrS] - **Spec Exp:** Bone Cancer; **Hospital:** Univ Minn Med Ctr, Fairview - Univ Campus; **Address:** Oncology Clin @ Masonic Cancer Ctr, 420 Deleware St. SE, MMC 806, Minneapolis, MN 55455; **Phone:** 612-273-1177; **Board Cert:** Orthopaedic Surgery 2004; **Med School:** Northwestern Univ 1983; **Resid:** Orthopaedic Surgery, Univ Minn 1990; **Fellow:** Pathology, Wash Univ Med Ctr 1987; Musculoskeletal Oncology, Mass Genl Hosp/Harvard 1991; **Fac Appt:** Prof OrS, Univ Minn

Irwin, Ronald B MD [OrS] - **Spec Exp:** Bone Cancer; Limb Sparing Surgery; Sarcoma-Soft Tissue; **Hospital:** William Beaumont Hosp; **Address:** Rose Cancer Treatment Ctr, 3577 W 13 Mile Rd, Ste 402, Royal Oak, MI 48073-6769; **Phone:** 248-551-9910; **Board Cert:** Orthopaedic Surgery 1979; **Med School:** Univ Mich Med Sch 1971; **Resid:** Orthopaedic Surgery, William Beaumont Hosp 1978; **Fellow:** Orthopaedic Oncology, Mayo Clinic 1978

Joyce, Michael J MD [OrS] - **Spec Exp:** Bone & Soft Tissue Tumors; **Hospital:** Cleveland Clin Fdn (page 71); **Address:** Cleveland Clinic, Dept Orthopaedic Surgery, 9500 Euclid Ave, Desk A41, Cleveland, OH 44195; **Phone:** 216-444-4282; **Board Cert:** Orthopaedic Surgery 1985; **Med School:** Univ Louisville Sch Med 1976; **Resid:** Surgery, Johns Hopkins Hosp 1978; Orthopaedic Surgery, Harvard Combined Program 1981; **Fellow:** Orthopaedic Oncology, Mass General Hosp 1982; Trauma, Univ Toronto-Sunnybrook Hosp 1983; **Fac Appt:** Assoc Clin Prof OrS, Case West Res Univ

McDonald, Douglas J MD [OrS] - **Spec Exp:** Bone Tumors; Ewing's Sarcoma; Reconstructive Surgery; **Hospital:** Barnes-Jewish Hosp; **Address:** Ctr Advanced Med, Orthopaedic Surg Ctr, 4921 Parkview Pl Fl 6 - Ste A, Box 8605, St Louis, MO 63110; **Phone:** 314-747-2500; **Board Cert:** Orthopaedic Surgery 2001; **Med School:** Univ Minn 1982; **Resid:** Orthopaedic Surgery, Mayo Clinic 1987; **Fellow:** Orthopaedic Oncology, Mayo Clinic 1988; **Fac Appt:** Prof OrS, Washington Univ, St Louis

Orthopaedic Surgery

Peabody, Terrance MD [OrS] - **Spec Exp:** Soft Tissue Tumors; Bone Tumors; Pediatric Orthopaedic Cancers; **Hospital:** Univ of Chicago Hosps; **Address:** Univ of Chicago Hospital, 5841 S Maryland Ave, MC 3079, Chicago, IL 60637-1463; **Phone:** 773-702-3442; **Board Cert:** Orthopaedic Surgery 2004; **Med School:** UC Irvine 1985; **Resid:** Orthopaedic Surgery, UC Irvine Med Ctr 1990; **Fellow:** Orthopaedic Oncology, Univ Chicago 1991; **Fac Appt:** Prof S, Univ Chicago-Pritzker Sch Med

Sim, Franklin MD [OrS] - **Spec Exp:** Sarcoma; Bone Cancer; **Hospital:** Mayo Med Ctr & Clin - Rochester; **Address:** Mayo Clin W-14A, 200 1st St SW, Rochester, MN 55905; **Phone:** 507-284-2511; **Board Cert:** Orthopaedic Surgery 1971; **Med School:** Dalhousie Univ 1965; **Resid:** Orthopaedic Surgery, Mayo Clinic 1970; **Fac Appt:** Prof OrS, Mayo Med Sch

Simon, Michael MD [OrS] - **Spec Exp:** Bone Tumors; Soft Tissue Tumors; Pediatric Orthopaedic Cancers; **Hospital:** Univ of Chicago Hosps; **Address:** 5841 S Maryland Ave, MC 3079, Univ of Chicago, Chicago, IL 60637; **Phone:** 773-702-6144; **Board Cert:** Orthopaedic Surgery 1992; **Med School:** Univ Mich Med Sch 1967; **Resid:** Surgery, Univ Mich Med Ctr 1969; Orthopaedic Surgery, Univ Mich Med Ctr 1974; **Fellow:** Orthopaedic Oncology, Univ Fla 1975; **Fac Appt:** Prof S, Univ Chicago-Pritzker Sch Med

Yasko, Alan MD [OrS] - **Spec Exp:** Sarcoma; **Hospital:** Children's Mem Hosp; **Address:** Children's Memorial Hosp, 645 N Michigan Ave, Ste 910, Chicago, IL 60611; **Phone:** 312-503-7987; **Board Cert:** Orthopaedic Surgery 2004; **Med School:** Northwestern Univ 1984; **Resid:** Orthopaedic Surgery, Case Western 1989; **Fellow:** Orthopaedic Oncology, Meml Sloan Kettering 1991; Metabolic Diseases, Hosp for Special Surgery 1991; **Fac Appt:** Prof S, Northwestern Univ-Feinberg Sch Med

Great Plains and Mountains

Randall, R Lor MD [OrS] - **Spec Exp:** Bone Tumors; Sarcoma-Soft Tissue; Pediatric Orthopaedic Surgery; **Hospital:** Univ Utah Hosps and Clins, Primary Children's Med Ctr; **Address:** Ped Ortho Surg, Primary Chlds Med Ctr, 100 N Medical Drive, Ste 4550, SLC, UT 84113, Salt Lake City, UT 84113; **Phone:** 801-662-5600; **Board Cert:** Orthopaedic Surgery 2001; **Med School:** Yale Univ 1992; **Resid:** Orthopaedic Surgery, UCSF Med Ctr 1997; **Fellow:** Musculoskeletal Oncology, Univ WA Med Ctr 1998; **Fac Appt:** Assoc Prof OrS, Univ Utah

Wilkins, Ross M MD [OrS] - **Spec Exp:** Bone Cancer; **Hospital:** Presby - St Luke's Med Ctr, Porter Adventist Hosp; **Address:** 1601 E 19th Ave, Ste 3300, Denver, CO 80218; **Phone:** 303-837-0072; **Board Cert:** Orthopaedic Surgery 2006; **Med School:** Wayne State Univ 1978; **Resid:** Orthopaedic Surgery, Univ Colorado Med Ctr 1983; **Fellow:** Orthopaedic Oncology, Mayo Clinic 1984

Southwest

Williams, Ronald Paul MD [OrS] - **Spec Exp:** Bone Tumors; **Hospital:** Univ Hlth Sys - Univ Hosp; **Address:** Dept of Orthopaedics, 7703 Floyd Curl Drive, MC 7774, San Antonio, TX 78229-3900; **Phone:** 210-567-6446; **Board Cert:** Orthopaedic Surgery 2003; **Med School:** Univ Tex, San Antonio 1984; **Resid:** Orthopaedic Surgery, U Kans Sch Med. 1989; **Fellow:** Orthopaedic Surgery, Case West Res. U. 1990; **Fac Appt:** Prof OrS, Univ Tex, San Antonio

West Coast and Pacific

Bos, Gary D MD [OrS] - **Spec Exp:** Musculoskeletal Tumors; Sarcoma; Reconstructive Surgery; **Hospital:** Yakima Valley Mem Hosp; **Address:** 16th Avenue Station, 1470 16th Ave, Yakima, WA 98902; **Phone:** 509-574-3300; **Board Cert:** Orthopaedic Surgery 1998; **Med School:** Univ Chicago-Pritzker Sch Med 1978; **Resid:** Orthopaedic Surgery, Case West Reserve 1984; **Fellow:** Orthopaedic Surgery, Case West Reserve 1980; Orthopaedic Oncology, Mayo Clinic 1985

Conrad, Ernest U MD [OrS] - **Spec Exp:** Pediatric Orthopaedic Surgery; Bone Tumors; Sarcoma; **Hospital:** Chldns Hosp and Regl Med Ctr - Seattle, Univ Wash Med Ctr; **Address:** Children's Hosp & Regional Med Ctr, 4800 Sand Point Way, MS B6553, Seattle, WA 98105; **Phone:** 206-987-5096; **Board Cert:** Orthopaedic Surgery 1999; **Med School:** Univ VA Sch Med 1979; **Resid:** Orthopaedic Surgery, Hosp for Special Surgery 1984; **Fellow:** Orthopaedic Oncology, Univ Fla Coll Med 1985; Pediatric Orthopaedic Surgery, Hosp for Sick Chldn 1986; **Fac Appt:** Prof OrS, Univ Wash

Eckardt, Jeffrey J MD [OrS] - **Spec Exp:** Bone Tumors; Soft Tissue Tumors; Limb Sparing Surgery; **Hospital:** Santa Monica - UCLA Med Ctr, UCLA Med Ctr (page 83); **Address:** UCLA Med Ctr, Dept Ortho Surg/Oncology, 1250 16th St Tower # 745, Santa Monica, CA 90404; **Phone:** 310-319-3816; **Board Cert:** Orthopaedic Surgery 1981; **Med School:** Cornell Univ-Weill Med Coll 1971; **Resid:** Orthopaedic Surgery, UCLA Med Ctr 1979; **Fellow:** Orthopaedic Oncology, Mayo Clinic 1980; **Fac Appt:** Prof OrS, UCLA

Luck Jr, James V MD [OrS] - **Spec Exp:** Musculoskeletal Tumors; **Hospital:** Santa Monica - UCLA Med Ctr; **Address:** 2400 S Flower St, Fl 3, Los Angeles, CA 90007-2660; **Phone:** 213-749-8255; **Board Cert:** Orthopaedic Surgery 2000; **Med School:** USC Sch Med 1967; **Resid:** Orthopaedic Surgery, Orthopaedic Hosp 1973; **Fellow:** Orthopaedic Oncology, Orthopaedic Hosp 1974; Reconstructive Surgery, Rancho Los Amigos 1974; **Fac Appt:** Prof OrS, UCLA

O'Donnell, Richard John MD [OrS] - **Spec Exp:** Bone Cancer; Sarcoma-Soft Tissue; Pediatric Orthopaedic Cancers; **Hospital:** UCSF Med Ctr; **Address:** 1600 Divisadero St Fl 4th, San Francisco, CA 94115; **Phone:** 415-885-3800; **Board Cert:** Orthopaedic Surgery 1999; **Med School:** Harvard Med Sch 1989; **Resid:** Orthopaedic Surgery, Mass Genl Hosp 1995; **Fellow:** Musculoskeletal Oncology, Univ WA Med Ctr 1996; **Fac Appt:** Assoc Prof OrS, UCSF

Singer, Daniel I MD [OrS] - **Spec Exp:** Bone Cancer; Hand & Upper Extremity Tumors; **Hospital:** Queen's Med Ctr - Honolulu, Kapiolani Med Ctr @ Pali Momi; **Address:** Queen's Physicians' Office Blg 1, 1380 Lusitana St, Ste 615, Honolulu, HI 96813-2442; **Phone:** 808-521-8109; **Board Cert:** Orthopaedic Surgery 2000; Hand Surgery 2000; **Med School:** Boston Univ 1979; **Resid:** Surgery, Univ Conn Hlth Ctr 1981; Orthopaedic Surgery, Univ Hawaii 1984; **Fellow:** Hand Surgery, Thomas Jefferson Univ Med Ctr 1985; Microvascular Surgery, St Vincent's Hosp 1985; **Fac Appt:** Assoc Prof OrS, Univ Hawaii JA Burns Sch Med

Hand Surgery

Athanasian, Edward MD [HS] - **Spec Exp:** Bone & Soft Tissue Tumors; Hand & Upper Extremity Tumors; **Hospital:** Hosp For Special Surgery, Meml Sloan Kettering Cancer Ctr (page 76); **Address:** Hospital for Special Surgery, 535 E 72th St, New York, NY 10021; **Phone:** 212-606-1962; **Board Cert:** Orthopaedic Surgery 1997; Hand Surgery 1999; **Med School:** Columbia P&S 1988; **Resid:** Surgery, Beth Israel Hosp 1989; Orthopaedic Surgery, Hosp Special Surgery 1993; **Fellow:** Hand Surgery, Mayo Clinic 1994; Orthopaedic Oncology, Meml Sloan Kettering Cancer Ctr 1995; **Fac Appt:** Asst Prof OrS, Cornell Univ-Weill Med Coll

West Coast and Pacific

Szabo, Robert M MD [HS] - **Spec Exp:** Hand & Upper Extremity Tumors; **Hospital:** UC Davis Med Ctr, Mercy General Hosp - Sacramento; **Address:** UC Davis, Dept Orthopaedics, 4860 Y St, Ste 3800, Sacramento, CA 95817-2307; **Phone:** 916-734-3678; **Board Cert:** Orthopaedic Surgery 1998; Hand Surgery 1998; **Med School:** SUNY Buffalo 1977; **Resid:** Surgery, Mt Sinai Hosp 1979; Orthopaedic Surgery, Mt Sinai Hosp 1982; **Fellow:** Hand Surgery, UCSD Med Ctr 1983; Epidemiology, UC Berkeley 1995; **Fac Appt:** Prof OrS, UC Davis

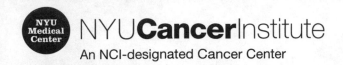

NYU**Cancer**Institute
An NCI-designated Cancer Center

NYU Clinical Cancer Center
160 East 34th Street
New York, New York 10016
www.nyuci.org/atcd

NYU Medical Center
550 First Avenue
(at 31st Street)
New York, New York 10016
www.nyumc.org/atcd

Stephen D. Hassenfeld
Children's Center
for Cancer and Blood
Disorders
160 East 32nd Street
New York, New York 10016
www.nyumc.org/hassenfeld

A Collaborative Approach

The NYU Cancer Institute, an NCI designated center, is a "matrix cancer center" without walls operating within the larger NYU Medical Center. With over 200 members and a research funding base of over $81 million, this structure strengthens our capabilities to forge collaborations across medical and scientific disciplines, which translates to comprehensive care for our patients and discoveries that will influence the future of this disease.

Renowned Expertise

Our highly skilled Magnet™ nursing team not only plays a pivotal role in coordinating direct patient care, but is also a source of invaluable patient education. Team members' compassion and expertise help patients better manage the symptoms of their disease as well as their special needs.

A Patient-Focused Setting

The NYU Clinical Cancer Center, with over 70 faculty members from various disciplines at the New York University School of Medicine, is the principal outpatient facility of the Cancer Institute and serves as home for our patients and their caregivers. The center and its multidisciplinary team of experts provide access to the latest treatment options and clinical trials along with a variety of programs in cancer prevention, screening, diagnostics, genetic counseling, and supportive services. When it comes to kids and cancer, the Stephen D. Hassenfeld Children's Center for Cancer and Blood Disorders offers not just innovation but insight. As a leading member of the NCI-sponsored Children's Oncology Group, our physicians are known for developing new ways to treat childhood cancer. Our affiliation with Bellevue Hospital, the oldest public hospital in the country, affords clinically distinctive opportunities to learn and care for patients with cancer by observing its presentation and behavior in a variety of patient groups.

Otolaryngology

An otolaryngologist diagnoses and provides medical and/or surgical therapy prevention of diseases, allergies, neoplasms, deformities, disorders and/or injuries of the ears, nose, sinuses, throat, respiratory and upper alimentary systems, face, jaws and the other head and neck systems. Head and neck oncology, facial plastic and reconstructive surgery and the treatment of disorders of hearing and voice are fundamental areas of expertise.

An otolarayngologist-head and neck surgeon provides comprehensive medical and surgical care for patients with diseases and disorders that affect the ears, nose, throat, the respiratory and upper alimentary systems and related structures of the head and neck.

Training Required: Five years

Certification in the following subspecialty requires additional training and examination.

Plastic Surgery within the Head and Neck: An otolaryngologist with additional training in plastic and reconstructive procedures within the head, face, neck and associated structures, including cutaneous head and neck oncology and reconstructioin, management of maxillofacial trauma, soft tissue repair and neural surgery.

This field is diverse and involves a wide range of patients, from the newborn to the aged. While both cosmetic and reconstructive surgeries are practiced, there are many additional procedures which interface with them.

Otolaryngology

New England

Deschler, Daniel G MD [Oto] - **Spec Exp:** Head & Neck Cancer; Head & Neck Reconstruction; Salivary Gland Tumors & Surgery; **Hospital:** Mass Eye & Ear Infirmary; **Address:** Mass Eye & Ear Infirmary, Head & Neck Surgery, 243 Charles St, Boston, MA 02114; **Phone:** 617-573-4100; **Board Cert:** Otolaryngology 1996; **Med School:** Harvard Med Sch 1990; **Resid:** Otolaryngology, UCSF Med Ctr 1995; **Fellow:** Facial Plastic & Reconstructive Surgery, Hahneman U Med Ctr 1996; **Fac Appt:** Assoc Prof Oto, Harvard Med Sch

Sasaki, Clarence T MD [Oto] - **Spec Exp:** Head & Neck Cancer; Skull Base Surgery; Voice Disorders; Swallowing Disorders; **Hospital:** Yale - New Haven Hosp, Hosp of St Raphael; **Address:** Yale Sch Med, Dept Otolaryngology, 333 Cedar St, Box 208041, New Haven, CT 06520-8041; **Phone:** 203-785-2592; **Board Cert:** Otolaryngology 1973; **Med School:** Yale Univ 1966; **Resid:** Surgery, Mary Hitchcock Hosp 1968; Otolaryngology, Yale-New Haven Hosp 1973; **Fellow:** Head and Neck Surgery, Univ of Milan 1978; Skull Base Surgery, Univ Zurich 1982; **Fac Appt:** Prof Oto, Yale Univ

Mid Atlantic

Abramson, Allan MD [Oto] - **Spec Exp:** Head & Neck Cancer & Surgery; Laryngeal Cancer; **Hospital:** Long Island Jewish Med Ctr; **Address:** LIJ Med Ctr, Dept Otolaryngology, 270-05 76th Ave, Ste 1120, New Hyde Park, NY 11040; **Phone:** 516-470-7555; **Board Cert:** Otolaryngology 1972; **Med School:** SUNY Downstate 1967; **Resid:** Surgery, LI Jewish-Hillside Med Ctr 1969; Otolaryngology, Mount Sinai Med Ctr 1972; **Fac Appt:** Prof Oto, Albert Einstein Coll Med

Carrau, Ricardo L MD [Oto] - **Spec Exp:** Skull Base Tumors & Surgery; Nasal & Sinus Cancer & Surgery; Swallowing Disorders; **Hospital:** UPMC Presby, Pittsburgh; **Address:** Eye & Ear Institute, 200 Lothrop St, Ste 500, Pittsburgh, PA 15213; **Phone:** 412-647-2100; **Board Cert:** Otolaryngology 1987; **Med School:** Univ Puerto Rico 1981; **Resid:** Surgery, University Hosp 1984; Head and Neck Surgery, University Hosp 1987; **Fellow:** Head and Neck Oncology, Univ Pittsburgh Med Ctr 1990; **Fac Appt:** Assoc Prof Oto, Univ Pittsburgh

Chalian, Ara A MD [Oto] - **Spec Exp:** Head & Neck Cancer; Head & Neck Reconstruction; Thyroid Cancer; **Hospital:** Hosp Univ Penn - UPHS (page 84); **Address:** Hosp U Penn, Dept Otolaryngology, 3400 Spruce St, Silverstein Bldg, Philadelphia, PA 19104; **Phone:** 215-349-5559; **Board Cert:** Otolaryngology 1994; **Med School:** Indiana Univ 1988; **Resid:** Surgery, Indiana Univ Hosp 1990; Otolaryngology, Indiana Univ Hosp 1993; **Fellow:** Molecular Biology, Hosp U Penn 1994; Head and Neck Surgery, Hosp U Penn 1995; **Fac Appt:** Assoc Prof Oto, Univ Pennsylvania

Close, Lanny G MD [Oto] - **Spec Exp:** Skull Base Surgery; Head & Neck Cancer; **Hospital:** NY-Presby Hosp (page 79); **Address:** 16 E 60th St, Ste 470, New York, NY 10022; **Phone:** 212-326-8475; **Board Cert:** Otolaryngology 1977; **Med School:** Baylor Coll Med 1972; **Resid:** Surgery, Johns Hopkins Hosp 1974; Otolaryngology, Baylor Affil Hosps 1977; **Fellow:** Head and Neck Surgery, MD Anderson Cancer Ctr 1979; **Fac Appt:** Prof Oto, Columbia P&S

Costantino, Peter D MD [Oto] - **Spec Exp:** Skull Base Tumors; Head & Neck Cancer; Craniofacial Surgery/Reconstruction; **Hospital:** St Luke's - Roosevelt Hosp Ctr - Roosevelt Div (page 72), NY-Presby Hosp (page 79); **Address:** 1000 W 10th Ave, Ste 5G-80, New York, NY 10019-1104; **Phone:** 212-523-6756; **Board Cert:** Otolaryngology 1990; Facial Plastic & Reconstructive Surgery 2000; **Med School:** Northwestern Univ 1984; **Resid:** Surgery, Northwestern Meml Hosp 1986; Otolaryngology, Northwestern Meml Hosp 1989; **Fellow:** Head and Neck Surgery, Northwestern Meml Hosp 1990; Skull Base Surgery, Univ Pittsburgh 1991; **Fac Appt:** Prof Oto, Columbia P&S

Cummings, Charles MD [Oto] - **Spec Exp:** Head & Neck Cancer & Surgery; Laryngeal Cancer; **Hospital:** Johns Hopkins Hosp - Baltimore; **Address:** Johns Hopkins Outpt Ctr, Otolaryngology, 601 N Caroline St Fl 6, Baltimore, MD 21287; **Phone:** 410-955-7400; **Board Cert:** Otolaryngology 1968; **Med School:** Univ VA Sch Med 1961; **Resid:** Surgery, Univ Virginia Hosp 1965; Otolaryngology, Mass Genl Hosp 1968; **Fac Appt:** Prof Oto, Johns Hopkins Univ

Davidson, Bruce J MD [Oto] - **Spec Exp:** Head & Neck Cancer; Thyroid Disorders; **Hospital:** Georgetown Univ Hosp; **Address:** Georgetown Univ Med Ctr, Dept Oto, 3800 Reservoir Rd NW, 1st fl Gorman, Washington, DC 20007; **Phone:** 202-444-8186; **Board Cert:** Otolaryngology 1993; **Med School:** W VA Univ 1987; **Resid:** Otolaryngology, Georgetown Univ Med Ctr 1992; **Fellow:** Otolaryngology, Memorial Sloan-Kettering Cancer Ctr 1994; **Fac Appt:** Asst Prof Oto, Georgetown Univ

Genden, Eric M MD [Oto] - **Spec Exp:** Head & Neck Cancer & Surgery; Head & Neck Reconstruction; Airway Reconstruction; Thyroid & Parathyroid Cancer & Surgery; **Hospital:** Mount Sinai Med Ctr (page 77); **Address:** Mt Sinai Sch Med Dept Otolar, 1 Gustave L. Levy Pl, Box 1191, New York, NY 10029; **Phone:** 212-241-9410; **Board Cert:** Otolaryngology 1999; Facial Plastic & Reconstructive Surgery 2000; **Med School:** Mount Sinai Sch Med 1992; **Resid:** Otolaryngology, Barnes Jewish Hosp 1998; **Fellow:** Head and Neck Surgery, Mount Sinai Med Ctr 1999; **Fac Appt:** Assoc Prof Oto, Mount Sinai Sch Med

Grandis, Jennifer MD [Oto] - **Spec Exp:** Head & Neck Cancer; **Hospital:** UPMC Presby, Pittsburgh, Magee-Womens Hosp - UPMC; **Address:** Univ Pittsburgh Med Ctr EELB, 200 Lothrop St, Ste 500, Pittsburgh, PA 15213; **Phone:** 412-647-5280; **Board Cert:** Otolaryngology 1994; **Med School:** Univ Pittsburgh 1987; **Resid:** Otolaryngology, Univ Pittsburgh Med Ctr 1993; **Fac Appt:** Prof Oto, Univ Pittsburgh

Har-El, Gady MD [Oto] - **Spec Exp:** Head & Neck Cancer; Thyroid & Parathyroid Surgery; Skull Base Surgery; **Hospital:** Lenox Hill Hosp, Long Island Coll Hosp (page 72); **Address:** 110 E 59th St, New York, NY 10022; **Phone:** 212-223-1333; **Board Cert:** Otolaryngology 1992; **Med School:** Israel 1982; **Resid:** Otolaryngology, SUNY Downstate Med Ctr 1991; **Fac Appt:** Prof Oto, SUNY Hlth Sci Ctr

Hicks Jr, Wesley L MD/DDS [Oto] - **Spec Exp:** Head & Neck Cancer & Surgery; Reconstructive Surgery; **Hospital:** Roswell Park Cancer Inst; **Address:** Roswell Park Cancer Inst, Head & Neck Surg, Elm & Carlton Sts, Buffalo, NY 14263; **Phone:** 716-845-3158; **Board Cert:** Otolaryngology 1993; **Med School:** SUNY Buffalo 1984; **Resid:** Otolaryngology, Manhattan Eye Ear & Throat Hosp 1988; Otolaryngology, New York Hosp/Meml Sloan Kettering Cancer Ctr 1989; **Fellow:** Head and Neck Surgery, Stanford Univ Med Ctr 1990; **Fac Appt:** Assoc Prof Oto, SUNY Buffalo

Otolaryngology

Hirsch, Barry MD [Oto] - **Spec Exp:** Ear Tumors; Skull Base Tumors; **Hospital:** UPMC Presby, Pittsburgh; **Address:** 200 Lothrop St, Ste 500, Ear Nose Throat Inst, Dept Otolaryngology, Pittsburgh, PA 15213; **Phone:** 412-647-2100; **Board Cert:** Otolaryngology 1982; Neurotology 2005; **Med School:** Univ Pennsylvania 1977; **Resid:** Otolaryngology, Univ Pittsburgh Med Ctr 1982; **Fellow:** Neurotology, Univ Pittsburgh 1985; Neurotology, Univ Zurich 1986; **Fac Appt:** Prof Oto, Univ Pittsburgh

Holliday, Michael J MD [Oto] - **Spec Exp:** Head & Neck Cancer; Skull Base Surgery; Neuro-Otology; **Hospital:** Johns Hopkins Hosp - Baltimore; **Address:** Johns Hopkins Hosp-Otology Division, 601 N Caroline St Fl 6, Baltimore, MD 21287; **Phone:** 410-955-3492; **Board Cert:** Otolaryngology 1976; **Med School:** Marquette Sch Med 1969; **Resid:** Otolaryngology, Johns Hopkins Hosp 1976; **Fellow:** Neurotology, Univ Zurich; **Fac Appt:** Assoc Prof Oto, Johns Hopkins Univ

Johnson, Jonas T MD [Oto] - **Spec Exp:** Head & Neck Surgery; Head & Neck Cancer; **Hospital:** UPMC Presby, Pittsburgh, Magee-Womens Hosp - UPMC; **Address:** Univ Physicians UPMC, Eye & Ear Inst, 200 Lothrop St, Ste 300, Pittsburgh, PA 15213; **Phone:** 412-647-2100; **Board Cert:** Otolaryngology 1977; **Med School:** SUNY Upstate Med Univ 1972; **Resid:** Surgery, Med Coll Virginia Hosps 1974; Otolaryngology, SUNY-Univ Hosp 1977; **Fac Appt:** Prof Oto, Univ Pittsburgh

Keane, William M MD [Oto] - **Spec Exp:** Head & Neck Cancer & Surgery; Thyroid Cancer; Sinus Disorders/Surgery; **Hospital:** Thomas Jefferson Univ Hosp (page 82); **Address:** Thomas Jefferson Hosp, 925 Chestnut St Fl 6, Philadelphia, PA 19107; **Phone:** 215-955-6760; **Board Cert:** Otolaryngology 1978; **Med School:** Harvard Med Sch 1970; **Resid:** Surgery, Strong Meml Hosp 1972; Otolaryngology, Univ Penn Hosp 1977; **Fac Appt:** Prof Oto, Thomas Jefferson Univ

Kennedy, David W MD [Oto] - **Spec Exp:** Sinus Disorders/Surgery; Skull Base Tumors & Surgery; **Hospital:** Hosp Univ Penn - UPHS (page 84), Pennsylvania Hosp (page 84); **Address:** Hosp Univ Penn, Dept Oto/Head & Neck Surg, 3400 Spruce St Ravdin Bldg Fl 5, Philadelphia, PA 19104; **Phone:** 215-662-6971; **Board Cert:** Otolaryngology 1978; **Med School:** Ireland 1972; **Resid:** Surgery, Johns Hopkins Hosp 1974; Otolaryngology, Johns Hopkins Hosp 1978; **Fac Appt:** Prof Oto, Univ Pennsylvania

Koch, Wayne Martin MD [Oto] - **Spec Exp:** Head & Neck Cancer; Sinus Tumors; **Hospital:** Johns Hopkins Hosp - Baltimore; **Address:** Johns Hopkins Hosp, Dept Otolaryngology, 601 N Caroline St, rm 6221, Baltimore, MD 21287; **Phone:** 410-955-4906; **Board Cert:** Otolaryngology 1987; **Med School:** Univ Pittsburgh 1982; **Resid:** Otolaryngology, Tufts-Boston Univ Hosps 1987; **Fellow:** Surgical Oncology, Johns Hopkins Hosp 1989; **Fac Appt:** Assoc Prof Oto, Johns Hopkins Univ

Kraus, Dennis MD [Oto] - **Spec Exp:** Head & Neck Cancer; Skull Base Tumors; Thyroid & Parathyroid Surgery; **Hospital:** Meml Sloan Kettering Cancer Ctr (page 76); **Address:** Memorial Sloan Kettering Cancer Ctr, 1275 York Ave, Box 285, New York, NY 10021-6007; **Phone:** 212-639-5621; **Board Cert:** Otolaryngology 1990; **Med School:** Univ Rochester 1985; **Resid:** Surgery, Cleveland Clinic Hosp 1987; Otolaryngology, Cleveland Clinic Hosp 1990; **Fellow:** Head and Neck Surgery, Meml Sloan Kettering Cancer Ctr 1991; **Fac Appt:** Prof Oto, Cornell Univ-Weill Med Coll

Krespi, Yosef MD [Oto] - **Spec Exp:** Nasal & Sinus Cancer & Surgery; Head & Neck Cancer & Surgery; **Hospital:** St Luke's - Roosevelt Hosp Ctr - Roosevelt Div (page 72); **Address:** 425 W 59th St Fl 10, New York, NY 10019-1128; **Phone:** 212-262-4444; **Board Cert:** Otolaryngology 1981; **Med School:** Israel 1973; **Resid:** Surgery, Mount Sinai Hosp 1976; Otolaryngology, Mount Sinai Hosp 1980; **Fellow:** Surgery, Northwestern Meml Hosp 1981; **Fac Appt:** Clin Prof Oto, Columbia P&S

Lawson, William MD [Oto] - **Spec Exp:** Sinus Disorders/Surgery; Head & Neck Cancer; Skull Base Surgery; **Hospital:** Mount Sinai Med Ctr (page 77); **Address:** 5 E 98th St Fl 8, Box 1191, New York, NY 10029-6501; **Phone:** 212-241-9410; **Board Cert:** Otolaryngology 1974; **Med School:** NYU Sch Med 1965; **Resid:** Surgery, Bronx VA Hosp 1967; Otolaryngology, Mount Sinai Hosp 1973; **Fellow:** Otolaryngology, Mount Sinai Hosp 1970; **Fac Appt:** Prof Oto, Mount Sinai Sch Med

Myers, Eugene MD [Oto] - **Spec Exp:** Head & Neck Surgery; Parotid Gland Tumors; **Hospital:** UPMC Montefiore, Western Penn Hosp; **Address:** UPMC Health System, Dept Otolaryngology, 200 Lothrop St, EEI Inst Fl 3 - Ste 300, Pittsburgh, PA 15213-2546; **Phone:** 412-647-2111; **Board Cert:** Otolaryngology 1966; **Med School:** Temple Univ 1960; **Resid:** Surgery, VA Hosp 1962; Otolaryngology, Mass EE Infirm 1965; **Fellow:** Otolaryngology, Harvard Med Sch 1965; Head and Neck Surgery, St Vincent's Hosp 1968; **Fac Appt:** Prof Oto, Univ Pittsburgh

O'Malley Jr, Bert W MD [Oto] - **Spec Exp:** Head & Neck Cancer; Sinus Tumors; Skull Base Tumors; **Hospital:** Hosp Univ Penn - UPHS (page 84); **Address:** Hosp Univ Penn, Dept Oto, 3400 Spruce St, 5 Ravdin, Philadelphia, PA 19104; **Phone:** 215-615-4325; **Board Cert:** Otolaryngology 1995; **Med School:** Univ Tex SW, Dallas 1988; **Resid:** Surgery, UTSW Med Ctr/Parkland Meml Hosp 1989; Otolaryngology, Baylor Coll Med 1993; **Fellow:** Head and Neck Oncology, Univ Pittsburgh 1994; Skull Base Surgery, Univ Pittsburgh 1995; **Fac Appt:** Prof Oto, Univ Pennsylvania

Papel, Ira D MD [Oto] - **Spec Exp:** Reconstructive Surgery-Face; Skin Cancer/Facial Reconstruction; **Hospital:** Greater Baltimore Med Ctr, Johns Hopkins Hosp - Baltimore; **Address:** 1838 Greene Tree Rd, Ste 370, Baltimore, MD 21208; **Phone:** 410-486-3400; **Board Cert:** Otolaryngology 1986; Facial Plastic & Reconstructive Surgery 1991; **Med School:** Boston Univ 1981; **Resid:** Otolaryngology, Johns Hopkins Hosp 1986; **Fellow:** Facial Plastic Surgery, UCSF Med Ctr 1987; **Fac Appt:** Assoc Prof Oto, Johns Hopkins Univ

Persky, Mark S MD [Oto] - **Spec Exp:** Head & Neck Cancer; Skull Base Tumors; Thyroid Cancer; **Hospital:** Beth Israel Med Ctr - Petrie Division (page 72); **Address:** 10 Union Square East, Ste 4J, New York, NY 10003; **Phone:** 212-844-8648; **Board Cert:** Otolaryngology 1976; **Med School:** SUNY Upstate Med Univ 1972; **Resid:** Otolaryngology, Bellevue Hosp 1976; **Fellow:** Head and Neck Surgery, Beth Israel Med Ctr 1977; **Fac Appt:** Clin Prof Oto, Albert Einstein Coll Med

Rassekh, Christopher MD [Oto] - **Spec Exp:** Laryngeal Cancer-Organ Preservation; Skull Base Tumors; Salivary Gland Tumors & Surgery; **Hospital:** WV Univ Hosp - Ruby Memorial, Monongalia Genl Hosp; **Address:** West Virginia Univ Dept Otolaryngology, PO Box 9200, Morgantown, WV 26506; **Phone:** 800-982-8242; **Board Cert:** Otolaryngology 1993; **Med School:** Univ Iowa Coll Med 1986; **Resid:** Otolaryngology, U Iowa Med Ctr 1992; **Fellow:** Head and Neck Surgery, U Pittsburgh Med Ctr 1993; **Fac Appt:** Assoc Prof Oto, W VA Univ

Otolaryngology

Schantz, Stimson P MD [Oto] - **Spec Exp:** Head & Neck Surgery; Head & Neck Cancer; Thyroid Cancer & Surgery; **Hospital:** New York Eye & Ear Infirm (page 78), Beth Israel Med Ctr - Petrie Division (page 72); **Address:** 310 E 14th St Fl 6N, New York, NY 10003; **Phone:** 212-979-4535; **Board Cert:** Surgery 2005; **Med School:** Univ Cincinnati 1975; **Resid:** Surgery, Georgetown Univ Med Ctr 1982; Otolaryngology, Univ Illinois Eye & Ear Infirm 1980; **Fellow:** Surgical Oncology, MD Anderson Cancer Ctr 1984; **Fac Appt:** Prof Oto, NY Med Coll

Shapshay, Stanley M MD [Oto] - **Spec Exp:** Laryngeal Cancer; **Hospital:** Albany Med Ctr; **Address:** University Ear, Nose & Throat Ctr, 35 Hackett Blvd, Albany, NY 12208; **Phone:** 518-262-5575; **Board Cert:** Otolaryngology 1975; **Med School:** Med Coll VA 1968; **Resid:** Surgery, New England Med Ctr 1971; Otolaryngology, Boston Med Ctr 1975; **Fellow:** Surgery, Serafimer Hosp/Karolinska Med Sch 1972

Shindo, Maisie L MD [Oto] - **Spec Exp:** Head & Neck Cancer & Surgery; Thyroid Cancer; Laryngeal Cancer; Parathyroid Cancer; **Hospital:** Stony Brook Univ Med Ctr; **Address:** Stony Brook Univ Hosp, HSC T19-064, Stony Brook, NY 11794-8191; **Phone:** 631-444-8242; **Board Cert:** Otolaryngology 1989; **Med School:** Univ Saskatchewan 1984; **Resid:** Otolaryngology, LAC& USC Med Ctr 1989; **Fellow:** Head and Neck Surgery, Northwestern Univ 1991; **Fac Appt:** Assoc Prof Oto, SUNY Stony Brook

Snyderman, Carl H MD [Oto] - **Spec Exp:** Skull Base Tumors & Surgery; Sinus Tumors; Head & Neck Cancer; Endoscopic Surgery; **Hospital:** UPMC Presby, Pittsburgh; **Address:** Eye Ear Inst, Dept of Otolaryngology, 200 Lothrop St, Ste 500, Pittsburgh, PA 15213; **Phone:** 412-647-2100; **Board Cert:** Otolaryngology 1987; **Med School:** Univ Chicago-Pritzker Sch Med 1982; **Resid:** Otolaryngology, Eye-Ear Hosp/Univ Pittsburgh 1987; **Fellow:** Skull Base Surgery, Eye-Ear Hosp/Univ Pittsburgh 1988; **Fac Appt:** Prof Oto, Univ Pittsburgh

Urken, Mark MD [Oto] - **Spec Exp:** Head & Neck Cancer & Surgery; Head & Neck Cancer Reconstruction; Thyroid & Parathyroid Cancer & Surgery; Salivary Gland Tumors & Surgery; **Hospital:** Beth Israel Med Ctr - Petrie Division (page 72); **Address:** Inst for Head, Neck & Thyroid Cancer, 10 Union Square E, Ste 5B, New York, NY 10003-3314; **Phone:** 212-844-8775; **Board Cert:** Otolaryngology 1986; **Med School:** Univ VA Sch Med 1981; **Resid:** Otolaryngology, Mount Sinai Hosp 1986; **Fellow:** Microvascular Surgery, Mercy Hosp 1987; **Fac Appt:** Prof Oto, Albert Einstein Coll Med

Weinstein, Gregory MD [Oto] - **Spec Exp:** Head & Neck Cancer; Laryngeal Cancer; **Hospital:** Hosp Univ Penn - UPHS (page 84); **Address:** Hosp Univ Penn, Dept Otolaryngology, 3400 Spruce St, 5 Ravdin, Philadelphia, PA 19104; **Phone:** 215-349-5390; **Board Cert:** Otolaryngology 1990; **Med School:** NY Med Coll 1985; **Resid:** Otolaryngology, Univ Iowa Hosp 1990; **Fellow:** Head and Neck Oncology, UC Davis Med Ctr 1991; **Fac Appt:** Assoc Prof Oto, Univ Pennsylvania

Woo, Peak MD [Oto] - **Spec Exp:** Voice Disorders; Laryngeal Cancer; **Hospital:** Mount Sinai Med Ctr (page 77); **Address:** 5 E 98th St Fl 1, Box 1653, New York, NY 10029-6501; **Phone:** 212-241-9425; **Board Cert:** Otolaryngology 1983; **Med School:** Boston Univ 1978; **Resid:** Otolaryngology, Boston Univ Med Ctr 1983; **Fac Appt:** Prof Oto, Mount Sinai Sch Med

Southeast

Bumpous, Jeffrey MD [Oto] - **Spec Exp:** Head & Neck Cancer; Head & Neck Reconstruction; Thyroid & Parathyroid Cancer & Surgery; **Hospital:** Univ of Louisville Hosp, Norton Hosp; **Address:** 601 S Floyd St, Ste 700, Louisville, KY 40202-1845; **Phone:** 502-583-8303; **Board Cert:** Otolaryngology 1994; **Med School:** Univ Louisville Sch Med 1989; **Resid:** Otolaryngology, Univ Louisville Hosp 1993; **Fellow:** Head and Neck Surgery, Univ Pittsburgh 1994; **Fac Appt:** Prof Oto, Univ Louisville Sch Med

Burkey, Brian MD [Oto] - **Spec Exp:** Parotid Gland Tumors; Head & Neck Cancer; Reconstructive Microvascular Surgery; **Hospital:** Vanderbilt Univ Med Ctr, Saint Thomas Hosp - Nashville; **Address:** Vanderbilt Univ, Dept Otolaryngology, 1215 21st Ave South, 7209 MCE-South Tower, Nashville, TN 37232-0014; **Phone:** 615-322-6180; **Board Cert:** Otolaryngology 1992; **Med School:** Univ VA Sch Med 1986; **Resid:** Otolaryngology, Univ Mich Med Ctr 1991; **Fellow:** Microsurgery, Ohio State Univ 1991; **Fac Appt:** Assoc Prof Oto, Vanderbilt Univ

Cassisi, Nicholas J MD [Oto] - **Spec Exp:** Head & Neck Cancer; **Hospital:** Shands Hlthcre at Univ of FL; **Address:** Shands Healthcare at Univ FL, 1600 SW Archer Rd, Box 100383, Gainesville, FL 32610; **Phone:** 352-265-8989; **Board Cert:** Otolaryngology 1971; **Med School:** Univ Miami Sch Med 1965; **Resid:** Surgery, Jackson Memorial Hosp 1967; Otolaryngology, Barnes Hosp - Washington U 1971; **Fac Appt:** Prof Oto, Univ Fla Coll Med

Couch, Marion E MD [Oto] - **Spec Exp:** Head & Neck Cancer; Thyroid Cancer; **Hospital:** Univ NC Hosps; **Address:** Univ N Carolina Sch Med, Dept Otolaryngology, CB 7070, Chapel Hill, NC 27599-7070; **Phone:** 919-966-3342; **Board Cert:** Otolaryngology 1997; **Med School:** Rush Med Coll 1990; **Resid:** Surgery, Johns Hopkins Hosp 1991; Otolaryngology, Johns Hopkins Hosp 1995; **Fac Appt:** Asst Prof Oto, Univ NC Sch Med

Day, Terrence A MD [Oto] - **Spec Exp:** Head & Neck Cancer; Reconstructive Microvascular Surgery; Skull Base Surgery; Facial Plastic & Reconstructive Surgery; **Hospital:** MUSC Med Ctr; **Address:** MUSC, Dept Otolaryngology, 135 Rutledge Ave, Ste 1130, Box 250550, Charleston, SC 29425; **Phone:** 843-792-0719; **Board Cert:** Otolaryngology 1996; **Med School:** Univ Okla Coll Med 1989; **Resid:** Otolaryngology, LSU Med Ctr 1995; **Fellow:** Head & Neck Surgical Oncology, UC Davis Med Ctr 1996; Maxillofacial Surgery, Univ Hosp; **Fac Appt:** Assoc Prof Oto, Med Univ SC

Goodwin, W Jarrard Jarrard MD [Oto] - **Spec Exp:** Head & Neck Cancer; **Hospital:** Univ of Miami Hosp & Clins/Sylvester Comp Canc Ctr, Jackson Meml Hosp; **Address:** Dept Otolaryngology, 1475 NW 12th Ave, Ste 4037, Miami, FL 33136-1015; **Phone:** 305-243-4387; **Board Cert:** Otolaryngology 1978; **Med School:** Albany Med Coll 1972; **Resid:** Surgery, Univ Miami/Jackson Hosp Meml Hosp 1973; Otolaryngology, Univ Miami/Jackson Hosp 1977; **Fellow:** Head & Neck Surgical Oncology, MD Anderson Hosp 1980; **Fac Appt:** Prof Oto, Univ Miami Sch Med

Lanza, Donald MD [Oto] - **Spec Exp:** Skull Base Tumors; Sinus Disorders/Surgery; **Hospital:** St Anthony's Hosp - St Petersburg, All Children's Hosp; **Address:** 900 Carillon Pkwy, Ste 200, St. Petersburg, FL 33716-1108; **Phone:** 727-573-0074; **Board Cert:** Otolaryngology 1990; **Med School:** SUNY Hlth Sci Ctr 1985; **Resid:** Surgery, Albany Med Ctr 1987; Otolaryngology, Albany Med Ctr 1990; **Fellow:** Rhinology, Johns Hopkins Univ 1990; Rhinology, Univ Penn 1991

Otolaryngology

Levine, Paul A MD [Oto] - **Spec Exp:** Head & Neck Cancer; Head & Neck Reconstruction; Skull Base Tumors; **Hospital:** Univ Virginia Med Ctr; **Address:** UVA Hlth Systems, Dept Otolaryngology, PO Box 800713, Charlottesville, VA 22908; **Phone:** 434-924-5593; **Board Cert:** Otolaryngology 1978; **Med School:** Albany Med Coll 1973; **Resid:** Otolaryngology, Yale-New Haven Hosp 1977; **Fellow:** Head and Neck Surgery, Stanford Med Ctr 1978; **Fac Appt:** Prof Oto, Univ VA Sch Med

Mattox, Douglas MD [Oto] - **Spec Exp:** Neuro-Otology; Ear Tumors; Skull Base Surgery; **Hospital:** Emory Univ Hosp, Chldns Hlthcare Atlanta - Scottish Rite; **Address:** Emory Univ Hospital, Dept Otolaryngology, 1365-A Clifton Rd NE, Atlanta, GA 30322; **Phone:** 404-778-3381; **Board Cert:** Otolaryngology 1977; Neurotology 2004; **Med School:** Yale Univ 1973; **Resid:** Otolaryngology, Stanford Univ Hosp 1977; **Fellow:** Neurotology, Ugo Fisch, MD 1985; **Fac Appt:** Prof Oto, Emory Univ

McCaffrey, Thomas MD [Oto] - **Spec Exp:** Head & Neck Cancer; Thyroid Cancer; Tracheal Surgery; **Hospital:** H Lee Moffitt Cancer Ctr & Research Inst, Tampa Genl Hosp; **Address:** H Lee Moffitt Cancer Ctr-Dept Otolaryngology-HNS, 12902 Magnolia Drive, Tampa, FL 33612; **Phone:** 813-745-8463; **Board Cert:** Otolaryngology 1980; **Med School:** Loyola Univ-Stritch Sch Med 1974; **Resid:** Surgery, Mayo Grad Sch Med 1976; Otolaryngology, Mayo Grad Med 1980; **Fac Appt:** Prof Oto, Univ S Fla Coll Med

Netterville, James MD [Oto] - **Spec Exp:** Head & Neck Surgery; Head & Neck Cancer; Skull Base Tumors; **Hospital:** Vanderbilt Univ Med Ctr, Vanderbilt Children's Hosp; **Address:** Vanderbilt Univ Med Ctr, Dept Oto, 7209 Med Ctr East, South Twr, 1215 21st Ave S, Nashville, TN 37232-8605; **Phone:** 615-343-8840; **Board Cert:** Otolaryngology 1985; **Med School:** Univ Tenn Coll Med, Memphis 1980; **Resid:** Surgery, Methodist Hosp 1982; Otolaryngology, Univ Tenn 1985; **Fellow:** Surgical Oncology, Univ Iowa 1986; **Fac Appt:** Prof Oto, Vanderbilt Univ

Osguthorpe, John D MD [Oto] - **Spec Exp:** Head & Neck Cancer; Thyroid & Parathyroid Cancer & Surgery; Salivary Gland Tumors & Surgery; Laryngeal Cancer; **Hospital:** MUSC Med Ctr; **Address:** MUSC Med Ctr-Dept Otolaryngology, 135 Rutledge Ave, Ste 1130, Box 250550, Charleston, SC 29425; **Phone:** 843-792-3533; **Board Cert:** Otolaryngology 1978; **Med School:** Univ Utah 1973; **Resid:** Surgery, UCLA 1975; Otolaryngology, UCLA 1978; **Fellow:** Skull Base Surgery, Univ Zurich 1989; **Fac Appt:** Prof Oto, Med Univ SC

Peters, Glenn E MD [Oto] - **Spec Exp:** Head & Neck Cancer & Surgery; Skull Base Surgery; Thyroid & Parathyroid Cancer & Surgery; **Hospital:** Univ of Ala Hosp at Birmingham; **Address:** UAB Med Ctr, Div of Head & Neck Surgery, 1530 3rd Ave S, BDB 563 Ave S, Birmingham, AL 35294-0012; **Phone:** 205-934-9777; **Board Cert:** Otolaryngology 1985; **Med School:** Louisiana State Univ 1980; **Resid:** Surgery, Bapt Med Ctr 1982; Otolaryngology, Univ Alabama Hosp 1984; **Fellow:** Head & Neck Surgical Oncology, Johns Hopkins Hosp 1987; **Fac Appt:** Prof S, Univ Ala

Pitman, Karen MD [Oto] - **Spec Exp:** Head & Neck Cancer & Surgery; Swallowing Disorders; Thyroid & Parathyroid Cancer & Surgery; Sentinel Node Surgery; **Hospital:** Univ Hosps & Clins - Jackson; **Address:** Univ Mississippi Med Ctr, 2500 N State St, Jackson, MS 39216; **Phone:** 601-984-5160; **Board Cert:** Otolaryngology 1995; **Med School:** Uniformed Srvs Univ, Bethesda 1987; **Resid:** Otolaryngology, Naval Med Ctr 1994; **Fellow:** Head and Neck Oncology, Univ Pittsburgh 1996; **Fac Appt:** Assoc Prof Oto, Univ Miss

Stringer, Scott P MD [Oto] - Spec Exp: Head & Neck Cancer; Thyroid & Parathyroid Cancer & Surgery; **Hospital:** Univ Hosps & Clins - Jackson; **Address:** Univ Mississippi Med Ctr, Dept Otolaryngology, 2500 N State St, Jackson, MS 39216-4505; **Phone:** 601-984-5160; **Board Cert:** Otolaryngology 1987; **Med School:** Univ Tex SW, Dallas 1982; **Resid:** Surgery, Univ Tex SW Med Ctr 1984; Otolaryngology, Univ Tex SW Med Ctr 1988; **Fac Appt:** Prof Oto, Univ Miss

Terris, David J MD [Oto] - Spec Exp: Head & Neck Cancer; **Hospital:** Med Coll of GA Hosp and Clin; **Address:** MCG Health System-Dept of Otolaryngology, 1120 15th St, rm BP4134, Augusta, GA 30912; **Phone:** 706-721-4400; **Board Cert:** Otolaryngology 1994; **Med School:** Duke Univ 1988; **Resid:** Surgery, Stanford Univ Med Ctr 1989; Otolaryngology, Stanford Univ Med Ctr 1993; **Fellow:** Head and Neck Surgery, Stanford Univ Med Ctr 1994; **Fac Appt:** Prof Oto, Med Coll GA

Valentino, Joseph MD [Oto] - Spec Exp: Head & Neck Cancer; Reconstructive Microvascular Surgery; Thyroid Cancer; **Hospital:** Univ of Kentucky Chandler Hosp; **Address:** 740 S Limestone St, rm B-317, Lexington, KY 40536-0284; **Phone:** 859-257-5405; **Board Cert:** Otolaryngology 1993; **Med School:** UMDNJ-RW Johnson Med Sch 1987; **Resid:** Otolaryngology, Univ Minn 1992; **Fellow:** Otolaryngology, Univ Iowa Coll Med 1993; **Fac Appt:** Assoc Prof Oto, Univ KY Coll Med

Wazen, Jack J MD [Oto] - Spec Exp: Skull Base Surgery; **Hospital:** Sarasota Meml Hosp; **Address:** 1901 Floyd St, Silverstein Inst, Sarasota, FL 34239; **Phone:** 941-366-9222; **Board Cert:** Otolaryngology 1983; **Med School:** Lebanon 1978; **Resid:** Surgery, St Lukes Hosp 1980; Otolaryngology, Columbia Presby Hosp 1983; **Fellow:** Neurotology, Ear Rsch Fdn 1984; **Fac Appt:** Assoc Clin Prof Oto, Columbia P&S

Weissler, Mark Christian MD [Oto] - Spec Exp: Head & Neck Cancer; **Hospital:** Univ NC Hosps; **Address:** G0412 Neurosciences Hosp UNC, CB 7070, Chapel Hill, NC 27599-7070; **Phone:** 919-843-3796; **Board Cert:** Otolaryngology 1985; **Med School:** Boston Univ 1980; **Resid:** Surgery, Mass Genl Hosp 1982; Otolaryngology, Mass Eye & Ear Infirm 1985; **Fellow:** Head and Neck Oncology, Univ Cincinnati 1986; **Fac Appt:** Prof Oto, Univ NC Sch Med

Yarbrough, Wendell G MD [Oto] - Spec Exp: Head & Neck Cancer; **Hospital:** Vanderbilt Univ Med Ctr; **Address:** Vanderbilt Otolaryngology, 7209 Med Ctr East, South Tower Ave, 1215 21st Ave S, Nashville, TN 37232-8605; **Phone:** 615-348-8840; **Board Cert:** Otolaryngology 1995; **Med School:** Univ NC Sch Med 1989; **Resid:** Otolaryngology, Univ NC Hosps 1994; **Fellow:** Surgical Oncology, Univ NC Hosps 1996; **Fac Appt:** Assoc Prof Oto, Vanderbilt Univ

Midwest

Arts, H Alexander MD [Oto] - Spec Exp: Skull Base Tumors & Surgery; Neuro-Otology; **Hospital:** Univ Michigan Hlth Sys; **Address:** Univ Michigan Health Systems, Dept Otolaryngology, 1500 E Medical Ctr Dr, 1904 Taubman Ctr, Ann Arbor, MI 48109; **Phone:** 734-936-8006; **Board Cert:** Otolaryngology 1992; Neurotology 2004; **Med School:** Baylor Coll Med 1983; **Resid:** Surgery, Univ Washington Med Ctr 1985; Otolaryngology, Univ Washington Med Ctr 1990; **Fellow:** Neurotology, Univ Virginia 1991; **Fac Appt:** Prof Oto, Univ Mich Med Sch

Otolaryngology

Bojrab, Dennis I MD [Oto] - **Spec Exp:** Skull Base Tumors; **Hospital:** Providence Hosp - Southfield, William Beaumont Hosp; **Address:** Michigan Ear Inst, 30055 Northwestern Hwy, Ste 101, Farmington Hills, MI 48334; **Phone:** 248-865-4444; **Board Cert:** Otolaryngology 1985; **Med School:** Indiana Univ 1979; **Resid:** Surgery, Butterworth Hosp 1981; Otolaryngology, Univ Indiana Sch Med 1984; **Fellow:** Skull Base Surgery, Vanderbilt Univ Med Ctr 1985; **Fac Appt:** Prof Oto, Wayne State Univ

Bradford, Carol MD [Oto] - **Spec Exp:** Head & Neck Cancer; Melanoma-Head & Neck; Skin Cancer-Head & Neck; **Hospital:** Univ Michigan Hlth Sys; **Address:** A A Taubman Health Care Ctr, 1500 E Medical Center Drive, rm 1904-TC, Ann Arbor, MI 48109-0312; **Phone:** 734-936-8050; **Board Cert:** Otolaryngology 1993; **Med School:** Univ Mich Med Sch 1986; **Resid:** Otolaryngology, Univ Michigan Med Ctr 1992; **Fellow:** Head and Neck Surgery, Univ Michigan Med Ctr 1988; **Fac Appt:** Prof Oto, Univ Mich Med Sch

Campbell, Bruce H MD [Oto] - **Spec Exp:** Head & Neck Surgery; Head & Neck Cancer; **Hospital:** Froedtert Meml Lutheran Hosp, Chldns Hosp - Wisconsin; **Address:** Med Coll Wisc-Dept Oto, 9200 W Wisconsin Ave, Milwaukee, WI 53226; **Phone:** 414-805-5583; **Board Cert:** Otolaryngology 1986; **Med School:** Rush Med Coll 1980; **Resid:** Otolaryngology, Med Coll Wisconsin 1985; **Fellow:** Head and Neck Surgery, MD Anderson Cancer Ctr 1987; **Fac Appt:** Prof Oto, Med Coll Wisc

Funk, Gerry F MD [Oto] - **Spec Exp:** Head & Neck Cancer; Head & Neck Reconstruction; **Hospital:** Univ Iowa Hosp & Clinics; **Address:** UIHC, Dept Otolaryngology, 200 Hawkins Drive, Iowa City, IA 52242-1009; **Phone:** 319-356-2165; **Board Cert:** Otolaryngology 1992; **Med School:** Univ Chicago-Pritzker Sch Med 1986; **Resid:** Surgery, LAC-USC Med Ctr 1987; Otolaryngology, LAC-USC Med Ctr 1991; **Fellow:** Head and Neck Surgery, Univ Iowa Hosp 1992; **Fac Appt:** Prof Oto, Univ Iowa Coll Med

Gluckman, Jack L MD [Oto] - **Spec Exp:** Head & Neck Cancer; Head & Neck Surgery; **Hospital:** Univ Hosp - Cincinnati, Good Samaritan Hosp - Cincinnati; **Address:** Univ Cincinnati Medical Center, Head & Neck Surgery MSB 6505, 231 Albert B Sabin Way, Box 670528, Cincinnati, OH 45267-0528; **Phone:** 513-558-0017; **Board Cert:** Otolaryngology 1990; **Med School:** South Africa 1967; **Resid:** Surgery, St James Hosp 1971; Otolaryngology, Groote Schuur Hosp 1974; **Fellow:** Otolaryngology, Univ Cincinnati Med Ctr 1979; **Fac Appt:** Prof Oto, Univ Cincinnati

Haughey, Bruce MD [Oto] - **Spec Exp:** Reconstructive Surgery-Face; Head & Neck Cancer; Head & Neck Reconstruction; **Hospital:** Barnes-Jewish Hosp; **Address:** Barnes Jewish Hosp South, 660 S Euclid Ave, Box 8115, St Louis, MO 63110; **Phone:** 314-362-7509; **Board Cert:** Otolaryngology 1984; **Med School:** New Zealand 1976; **Resid:** Surgery, Univ Auckland 1980; Otolaryngology, Univ Iowa Med Ctr 1984; **Fac Appt:** Prof Oto, Washington Univ, St Louis

Hoffman, Henry T MD [Oto] - **Spec Exp:** Head & Neck Cancer; Head & Neck Surgery; Voice Disorders; **Hospital:** Univ Iowa Hosp & Clinics; **Address:** Univ Iowa Hosp & Clins-Dept Oto, 200 Hawkins Drive, Iowa City, IA 52242; **Phone:** 319-356-2166; **Board Cert:** Otolaryngology 1985; **Med School:** UCSD 1980; **Resid:** Otolaryngology, Univ Iowa Hosp & Clinics 1985; **Fellow:** Head and Neck Oncology, Univ Michigan Hosp 1989; **Fac Appt:** Clin Prof Oto, Univ Iowa Coll Med

Kern, Robert MD [Oto] - **Spec Exp:** Head & Neck Cancer; **Hospital:** Northwestern Meml Hosp, Stroger Hosp of Cook Co; **Address:** 675 N St Clair St, Ste 15-200, Chicago, IL 60611; **Phone:** 312-695-8182; **Board Cert:** Otolaryngology 1990; **Med School:** Jefferson Med Coll 1985; **Resid:** Otolaryngology, Wayne State Affil Hosp 1990; **Fellow:** Research, Natl Inst Hlth 1991; **Fac Appt:** Prof Oto, Northwestern Univ

Lavertu, Pierre MD [Oto] - **Spec Exp:** Thyroid Cancer; Head & Neck Cancer; Skull Base Tumors; **Hospital:** Univ Hosps Case Med Ctr; **Address:** Univ Hosps, Dept Oto-Head & Neck Surg, 11100 Euclid Ave, Cleveland, OH 44106-5045; **Phone:** 216-844-4773; **Board Cert:** Otolaryngology 1981; **Med School:** Univ Montreal 1976; **Resid:** Otolaryngology, Univ Montreal Med Ctr 1981; **Fellow:** Head and Neck Surgery, Univ Montreal Med Ctr 1982; Head and Neck Surgery, Cleveland Clinic 1983; **Fac Appt:** Prof Oto, Case West Res Univ

Leonetti, John P MD [Oto] - **Spec Exp:** Skull Base Tumors & Surgery; Neuro-Otology; **Hospital:** Loyola Univ Med Ctr; **Address:** Loyola University Medical Ctr, Dept Otolaryngology, 2160 S First Ave Bldg 105 - rm 1870, Maywood, IL 60153; **Phone:** 708-216-4804; **Board Cert:** Otolaryngology 1987; **Med School:** Loyola Univ-Stritch Sch Med 1982; **Resid:** Otolaryngology, Loyola Univ Med Ctr 1987; Research, House Ear Inst; **Fellow:** Neurotology, Barnes Hosp 1988; **Fac Appt:** Prof Oto, Loyola Univ-Stritch Sch Med

Marentette, Lawrence MD [Oto] - **Spec Exp:** Skull Base Tumors & Surgery; Facial Plastic & Reconstructive Surgery; **Hospital:** Univ Michigan Hlth Sys; **Address:** Univ Michigan Health Systems, Dept Oto, 1500 E Med Ctr Drive, 1904 Taubman Ctr, Ann Arbor, MI 48109; **Phone:** 734-936-8051; **Board Cert:** Otolaryngology 1981; Facial Plastic & Reconstructive Surgery 1995; **Med School:** Wayne State Univ 1976; **Resid:** Otolaryngology, Wayne State Univ 1980; **Fellow:** Maxillofacial Surgery, Univ of Zurich 1985; **Fac Appt:** Prof Oto, Univ Mich Med Sch

Olsen, Kerry D MD [Oto] - **Spec Exp:** Head & Neck Cancer & Surgery; Esthesioneuroblastoma; Salivary Gland Tumors & Surgery; Skull Base Tumors; **Hospital:** Mayo Med Ctr & Clin - Rochester; **Address:** Mayo Clinic, Dept Otolaryngology, 200 1st St SW, Rochester, MN 55905-0001; **Phone:** 507-284-3542; **Board Cert:** Otolaryngology 1981; **Med School:** Mayo Med Sch 1976; **Resid:** Otolaryngology, Mayo Clinic 1981; **Fac Appt:** Prof Oto, Mayo Med Sch

Pelzer, Harold J MD/DDS [Oto] - **Spec Exp:** Head & Neck Cancer; **Hospital:** Northwestern Meml Hosp; **Address:** 675 N St Clair, Ste 15-200, Chicago, IL 60611; **Phone:** 312-695-8182; **Board Cert:** Otolaryngology 1985; **Med School:** Northwestern Univ 1979; **Resid:** Surgery, Northwestern Meml Hosp 1983; **Fellow:** Head and Neck Surgery, Northwestern Meml Hosp 1985; **Fac Appt:** Assoc Prof Oto, Northwestern Univ

Pensak, Myles MD [Oto] - **Spec Exp:** Skull Base Tumors; **Hospital:** Univ Hosp - Cincinnati, Good Samaritan Hosp - Cincinnati; **Address:** Univ Medical Arts Building, 222 Piedmont Ave, Ste 5200, Cincinnati, OH 45219; **Phone:** 513-475-8400; **Board Cert:** Otolaryngology 1983; Neurotology 2004; **Med School:** NY Med Coll 1978; **Resid:** Surgery, Upstate Med Ctr 1980; Otolaryngology, Yale Univ 1983; **Fellow:** Otology & Neurotology, The Otology Group 1984; **Fac Appt:** Prof Oto, Univ Cincinnati

Petruzzelli, Guy MD/PhD [Oto] - **Spec Exp:** Head & Neck Cancer & Surgery; Skull Base Tumors; Thyroid Cancer; **Hospital:** Loyola Univ Med Ctr; **Address:** Loyola Univ Med Ctr, 2160 S 1st Ave, Bldg 105 - rm 1870, Maywood, IL 60153; **Phone:** 708-216-9183; **Board Cert:** Otolaryngology 1993; **Med School:** Rush Med Coll 1987; **Resid:** Otolaryngology, Univ Pittsburgh Med Ctr 1992; **Fellow:** Head and Neck Oncology, Univ Pittsburgh Med Ctr 1993; Skull Base Surgery, Univ Pittsburgh Ctr Cranial Base Surg; **Fac Appt:** Prof Oto, Loyola Univ-Stritch Sch Med

Otolaryngology

Schuller, David MD [Oto] - **Spec Exp:** Head & Neck Cancer; Head & Neck Surgery; **Hospital:** Arthur G James Cancer Hosp & Research Inst, Ohio St Univ Med Ctr; **Address:** 300 W 10th Ave, rm 518, Columbus, OH 43210; **Phone:** 614-293-8074; **Board Cert:** Otolaryngology 1975; **Med School:** Ohio State Univ 1970; **Resid:** Otolaryngology, Ohio State Univ Affil Hosps 1975; Surgery, Univ Hosps 1973; **Fellow:** Head and Neck Surgery, Pack Med Fdn 1973; Head and Neck Oncology, Univ Iowa 1976; **Fac Appt:** Prof Oto, Ohio State Univ

Siegel, Gordon J MD [Oto] - **Spec Exp:** Head & Neck Cancer; **Hospital:** Northwestern Meml Hosp; **Address:** 3 E Huron St Fl 1, Chicago, IL 60611-2705; **Phone:** 312-988-7777; **Board Cert:** Otolaryngology 1984; **Med School:** Ros Franklin Univ/Chicago Med Sch 1978; **Resid:** Otolaryngology, Northwestern Univ 1982; **Fac Appt:** Asst Clin Prof Oto, Northwestern Univ

Strome, Marshall MD [Oto] - **Spec Exp:** Voice Disorders; Head & Neck Cancer; **Hospital:** Cleveland Clin Fdn (page 71); **Address:** Cleveland Clinic Fdn, 9500 Euclid Ave, Ste A71, Cleveland, OH 44195; **Phone:** 216-444-6686; **Board Cert:** Otolaryngology 1970; **Med School:** Univ Mich Med Sch 1964; **Resid:** Surgery, Harper Hosp 1966; Otolaryngology, Univ Michigan Hosp 1970; **Fac Appt:** Prof Oto, Cleveland Cl Coll Med/Case West Res

Teknos, Theodoros N MD [Oto] - **Spec Exp:** Head & Neck Cancer; Thyroid Cancer; Facial Plastic & Reconstructive Surgery; Skull Base Surgery; **Hospital:** Univ Michigan Hlth Sys; **Address:** Univ Mich Med Ctr, TC 1904, 1500 E Med Ctr Drive, Ann Arbor, MI 48109; **Phone:** 734-936-3172; **Board Cert:** Otolaryngology 1997; **Med School:** Harvard Med Sch 1991; **Resid:** Otolaryngology, Mass Eye & Ear Hosp 1996; **Fellow:** Head and Neck Surgery, Vanderbilt Univ Med Ctr 1997; **Fac Appt:** Assoc Prof Oto, Univ Mich Med Sch

Wilson, Keith M MD [Oto] - **Spec Exp:** Head & Neck Cancer & Surgery; Voice Disorders; **Hospital:** Univ Hosp - Cincinnati; **Address:** Univ Cincinnati Medical Ctr, 222 Piedmont Ave, Ste 5200, Cincinnati, OH 45219; **Phone:** 513-475-8351; **Board Cert:** Otolaryngology 1992; **Med School:** Cornell Univ-Weill Med Coll 1986; **Resid:** Otolaryngology, St Louis Univ Med Ctr 1991; **Fellow:** Head & Neck Surgical Oncology, Ohio State Med Ctr 1992; **Fac Appt:** Assoc Prof Oto, Univ Cincinnati

Wolf, Gregory T MD [Oto] - **Spec Exp:** Head & Neck Cancer; Laryngeal Cancer; **Hospital:** Univ Michigan Hlth Sys; **Address:** Univ Mich Med Ctr, Dept Oto-HNS, 1500 E Med Ctr, Taubman Ctr, rm 1904, Ann Arbor, MI 48109-0312; **Phone:** 734-936-8029; **Board Cert:** Otolaryngology 1978; **Med School:** Univ Mich Med Sch 1973; **Resid:** Surgery, Georgetown Univ Hosp 1975; Otolaryngology, SUNY Upstate Med Ctr 1978; **Fac Appt:** Prof Oto, Univ Mich Med Sch

Great Plains and Mountains

Bentz, Brandon G MD [Oto] - **Spec Exp:** Head & Neck Cancer & Surgery; Skull Base Tumors; **Hospital:** Univ Utah Hosps and Clins; **Address:** Univ Utah Hospitals, Dept Otolaryngology, 50 N Medical Drive, rm 3C120, Salt Lake City, UT 84132; **Phone:** 801-581-7515; **Board Cert:** Otolaryngology 2001; **Med School:** Northwestern Univ 1993; **Resid:** Otolaryngology, Northwestern Univ Med Ctr 1997; **Fellow:** Head & Neck Surgical Oncology, Meml Sloan Kettering Cancer Ctr 1999; **Fac Appt:** Asst Prof Oto, Univ Utah

Chowdhury, Khalid MD [Oto] - **Spec Exp:** Skull Base Tumors & Surgery; Craniofacial Surgery; **Hospital:** Presby - St Luke's Med Ctr, Chldn's Hosp - Denver, The; **Address:** Center for Craniofacial Surgery, 1601 E 19th Ave, Ste 3000, Denver, CO 80218; **Phone:** 303-839-5155; **Board Cert:** Otolaryngology 1990; Facial Plastic & Reconstructive Surgery 1995; **Med School:** Univ Saskatchewan 1982; **Resid:** Surgery, Univ Saskatchewan Hosp 1985; Otolaryngology, McGill Univ Hosps 1989; **Fellow:** Craniofacial Surgery, Univ Bern Hosp 1990; Facial Plastic & Reconstructive Surgery, Univ Bern Hosp 1990; **Fac Appt:** Assoc Prof Oto, Univ Colorado

Lydiatt, Daniel D MD/DDS [Oto] - **Spec Exp:** Head & Neck Cancer; **Hospital:** Nebraska Med Ctr; **Address:** 981225 Nebraska Medical Ctr, Omaha, NE 68198-1225; **Phone:** 402-559-5268; **Board Cert:** Otolaryngology 1992; **Med School:** Univ Nebr Coll Med 1983; **Resid:** Otolaryngology, Univ Nebraska Med Ctr 1990; **Fellow:** Head and Neck Surgery, MD Anderson Med Ctr 1991; **Fac Appt:** Assoc Prof Oto, Univ Nebr Coll Med

Lydiatt, William M MD [Oto] - **Spec Exp:** Head & Neck Cancer; Thyroid Cancer; Salivary Gland Tumors & Surgery; **Hospital:** Nebraska Med Ctr, Nebraska Meth Hosp; **Address:** 981225 Nebraska Medical Ctr, Omaha, NE 68198-1225; **Phone:** 402-559-8007; **Board Cert:** Otolaryngology 1994; **Med School:** Univ Nebr Coll Med 1988; **Resid:** Otolaryngology, Univ Nebraska Med Ctr 1993; **Fellow:** Head and Neck Surgery, Meml Sloan Kettering Cancer Ctr 1995; **Fac Appt:** Assoc Prof Oto, Univ Nebr Coll Med

Southwest

Clayman, Gary Lee MD/DMD [Oto] - **Spec Exp:** Thyroid Cancer & Surgery; Salivary Gland Tumors & Surgery; Head & Neck Cancer; **Hospital:** UT MD Anderson Cancer Ctr (page 81); **Address:** Univ TX/MD Anderson Cancer Center, 1515 Holcombe Blvd, Box 441, Houston, TX 77030-4009; **Phone:** 713-792-8837; **Board Cert:** Otolaryngology 1992; **Med School:** NE Ohio Univ 1986; **Resid:** Surgery, Hennepin Co Med Ctr 1987; Otolaryngology, Univ Minn 1991; **Fellow:** Head and Neck Surgery, MD Anderson Cancer Ctr 1993; **Fac Appt:** Prof Oto, Univ Tex, Houston

Coker, Newton J MD [Oto] - **Spec Exp:** Skull Base Tumors; **Hospital:** Methodist Hosp - Houston, Texas Chldns Hosp - Houston; **Address:** Baylor Coll Medicine, One Baylor Plaza, MS NA-102, Houston, TX 77030; **Phone:** 713-798-3200; **Board Cert:** Otolaryngology 1981; Neurotology 2004; **Med School:** Med Coll GA 1976; **Resid:** Surgery, Med Coll Georgia 1978; Otolaryngology, Med Coll Georgia 1981; **Fellow:** Otology & Neurotology, University Hosp 1982; **Fac Appt:** Prof Oto, Baylor Coll Med

Daspit, C Phillip MD [Oto] - **Spec Exp:** Skull Base Tumors & Surgery; **Hospital:** St Joseph's Hosp & Med Ctr - Phoenix; **Address:** 222 W Thomas Rd, Ste 114, Phoenix, AZ 85013; **Phone:** 602-279-5444; **Board Cert:** Otolaryngology 1977; **Med School:** Louisiana State Univ 1968; **Resid:** Surgery, UCSF Med Ctr 1973; Otolaryngology, Ft Miley VA Hosp 1977; **Fellow:** Otology & Neurotology, House Ear Inst 1978; Skull Base Surgery, House Ear Inst 1978; **Fac Appt:** Clin Prof S, Univ Ariz Coll Med

Donovan, Donald T MD [Oto] - **Spec Exp:** Head & Neck Cancer; Voice Disorders; Thyroid Disorders; **Hospital:** Methodist Hosp - Houston, St Luke's Episcopal Hosp - Houston; **Address:** 6550 Fannin St, Ste 1727, Houston, TX 77030; **Phone:** 713-798-3380; **Board Cert:** Otolaryngology 1981; **Med School:** Baylor Coll Med 1976; **Resid:** Surgery, Baylor Affil Hosps 1978; Otolaryngology, Baylor Affil Hosps 1981; **Fellow:** Head and Neck Surgery, Columbia-Presby Med Ctr 1982; **Fac Appt:** Prof Oto, Baylor Coll Med

Hanna, Ehab YN MD [Oto] - **Spec Exp:** Skull Base Tumors & Surgery; Head & Neck Cancer & Surgery; **Hospital:** UT MD Anderson Cancer Ctr (page 81); **Address:** Univ Tex MD Anderson Cancer Ctr, 1515 Holcolmbe Blvd, Unit 441, Houston, TX 77030; **Phone:** 713-745-1815; **Board Cert:** Otolaryngology 1994; **Med School:** Egypt 1982; **Resid:** Otolaryngology, Cleveland Clinic 1989; Otolaryngology, Cleveland Clinic 1993; **Fellow:** Otolaryngology, Univ Pittsburgh Med Ctr 1994; **Fac Appt:** Asst Prof Oto, Univ Tex, Houston

Medina, Jesus MD [Oto] - **Spec Exp:** Head & Neck Cancer; **Hospital:** OU Med Ctr; **Address:** Univ OK Hlth Sci Ctr, Dept Oto-WP 1290, PO Box 26901, Oklahoma City, OK 73190; **Phone:** 405-271-8047; **Board Cert:** Otolaryngology 1980; **Med School:** Peru 1974; **Resid:** Surgery, Wayne St Univ Affil Hosp 1977; Otolaryngology, Wayne St Univ Affil Hosp 1980; **Fellow:** Head and Neck Surgery, Univ Tex Sys Cancer Ctrs 1981; **Fac Appt:** Prof Oto, Univ Okla Coll Med

Myers, Jeffrey N MD/PhD [Oto] - **Spec Exp:** Head & Neck Cancer; Melanoma-Head & Neck; Tongue Cancer; **Hospital:** UT MD Anderson Cancer Ctr (page 81); **Address:** Univ Texas MD Anderson Cancer Ctr, 1515 Holcombe Blvd, Box 441, Houston, TX 77030; **Phone:** 713-745-2667; **Board Cert:** Otolaryngology 1997; **Med School:** Univ Pennsylvania 1991; **Resid:** Otolaryngology, Univ Pittsburgh Med Ctr 1996; **Fellow:** Head & Neck Surgical Oncology, MD Anderson Cancer Ctr 1997; **Fac Appt:** Assoc Prof Oto, Univ Tex, Houston

Nuss, Daniel W MD [Oto] - **Spec Exp:** Head & Neck Cancer; Skull Base Tumors & Surgery; **Hospital:** Our Lady of the Lake Regl Med Ctr; **Address:** LSU Sch Med, Dept Otolaryngology, 533 Bolivar St Fl 5, New Orleans, LA 70112; **Phone:** 225-765-1475; **Board Cert:** Otolaryngology 1987; **Med School:** Louisiana State Univ 1981; **Resid:** Surgery, Charity Hosp 1983; Otolaryngology, LSU Med Ctr 1987; **Fellow:** Surgical Oncology, MD Anderson Hosp & Tumor Inst 1984; Head and Neck Surgery, Ctr Cranial Base Surg-Univ Pittsbur 1991; **Fac Appt:** Prof Oto, Louisiana State Univ

Otto, Randal A MD [Oto] - **Spec Exp:** Head & Neck Cancer; Thyroid & Parathyroid Cancer & Surgery; **Hospital:** Univ Hlth Sys - Univ Hosp, Audie L Murphy Meml Vets Hosp; **Address:** 7703 Floyd Curl Drive, MS 7777, San Antonio, TX 78229-3900; **Phone:** 210-358-0490; **Board Cert:** Otolaryngology 1987; **Med School:** Univ MO-Columbia Sch Med 1981; **Resid:** Pathology, Queens Med Ctr 1982; Otolaryngology, Univ Missouri 1987; **Fac Appt:** Prof Oto, Univ Tex, San Antonio

Suen, James Y MD [Oto] - **Spec Exp:** Head & Neck Cancer; **Hospital:** UAMS Med Ctr, Arkansas Chldns Hosp; **Address:** Univ Hosp Arkansas Med Scis, 4301 W Markham St, Slot 543, Little Rock, AR 72205; **Phone:** 501-686-8224; **Board Cert:** Otolaryngology 1973; **Med School:** Univ Ark 1966; **Resid:** Surgery, Univ Arkansas Med Ctr 1970; Otolaryngology, Univ Arkansas Med Ctr 1973; **Fellow:** Head and Neck Surgery, MD Anderson Cancer Ctr-Tumor Inst 1974; **Fac Appt:** Prof Oto, Univ Ark

Weber, Randal S MD [Oto] - **Spec Exp:** Skin Cancer; Thyroid & Parathyroid Cancer & Surgery; Salivary Gland Tumors & Surgery; Head & Neck Cancer; **Hospital:** UT MD Anderson Cancer Ctr (page 81); **Address:** 1515 Holcombe Blvd, Unit 441, Houston, TX 77030-4009; **Phone:** 713-745-0497; **Board Cert:** Otolaryngology 1985; **Med School:** Univ Tenn Coll Med, Memphis 1976; **Resid:** Surgery, Baylor Coll Med 1982; Otolaryngology, Baylor Coll Med 1985; **Fellow:** Head and Neck Surgery, MD Anderson Cancer Ctr 1986; **Fac Appt:** Prof Oto, Univ Tex, Houston

Weber, Samuel C MD [Oto] - **Spec Exp:** Thyroid Cancer; Parathyroid Cancer; Nasal & Sinus Cancer & Surgery; Head & Neck Surgery; **Hospital:** St Luke's Episcopal Hosp - Houston, Texas Chldns Hosp - Houston; **Address:** 6624 Fannin St, Ste 1480, Houston, TX 77030-2385; **Phone:** 713-795-5343; **Board Cert:** Otolaryngology 1972; **Med School:** Univ Tenn Coll Med, Memphis 1965; **Resid:** Surgery, Baylor Coll Med 1971; Otolaryngology, Baylor Coll Med 1972; **Fac Appt:** Clin Prof Oto, Baylor Coll Med

West Coast and Pacific

Berke, Gerald S MD [Oto] - **Spec Exp:** Head & Neck Surgery; Head & Neck Cancer; Voice Disorders; **Hospital:** UCLA Med Ctr (page 83); **Address:** 200 UCLA Med Plaza, Ste 550, Los Angeles, CA 90095; **Phone:** 310-825-5179; **Board Cert:** Otolaryngology 1984; **Med School:** USC Sch Med 1978; **Resid:** Otolaryngology, LAC-USC Med Ctr 1979; **Fellow:** Head and Neck Surgery, UCLA Med Ctr 1984; **Fac Appt:** Prof Oto, UCLA

Cohen, James I MD [Oto] - **Spec Exp:** Thyroid & Parathyroid Cancer & Surgery; **Hospital:** OR Hlth & Sci Univ, Providence St Vincent Med Ctr; **Address:** Oregon Hlth Scis U-PV-01, 3181 SW Sam Jackson Park Rd, Portland, OR 97239; **Phone:** 503-494-5355; **Board Cert:** Otolaryngology 1984; **Med School:** Canada 1978; **Resid:** Surgery, Univ Minn Med Ctr 1980; Otolaryngology, Univ Minn Med Ctr 1984; **Fellow:** Head & Neck Surgical Oncology, MD Anderson Hosp 1985; **Fac Appt:** Prof Oto, Oregon Hlth Sci Univ

Courey, Mark S MD [Oto] - **Spec Exp:** Swallowing Disorders; Laryngeal Cancer; **Hospital:** UCSF - Mt Zion Med Ctr, UCSF Med Ctr; **Address:** UCSF Voice & Swallowing Ctr, 2330 Post St Fl 5, San Francisco, CA 94115; **Phone:** 415-885-7700; **Board Cert:** Otolaryngology 1993; **Med School:** SUNY Buffalo 1987; **Resid:** Otolaryngology, SUNY-Buffalo Med Ctr 1992; **Fellow:** Laryngology, Vanderbilt Univ 1993; **Fac Appt:** Prof Oto, UCSF

Donald, Paul MD [Oto] - **Spec Exp:** Skull Base Tumors & Surgery; Head & Neck Cancer; **Hospital:** UC Davis Med Ctr; **Address:** 2521 Stockton Blvd, rm 7200, Sacramento, CA 95817; **Phone:** 916-734-2832; **Board Cert:** Otolaryngology 1973; **Med School:** Univ British Columbia Fac Med 1964; **Resid:** Surgery, St Pauls Hosp 1969; Otolaryngology, Univ Iowa Hosp 1973; **Fac Appt:** Prof Oto, UC Davis

Eisele, David W MD [Oto] - **Spec Exp:** Salivary Gland Tumors & Surgery; Head & Neck Cancer; Thyroid Cancer; **Hospital:** UCSF Med Ctr; **Address:** UCSF, Dept Head & Neck Surgery, 400 Parnassus Ave, Ste A 730, San Francisco, CA 94143-0342; **Phone:** 415-502-0498; **Board Cert:** Otolaryngology 1988; **Med School:** Cornell Univ-Weill Med Coll 1982; **Resid:** Surgery, Univ Wash Med Ctr 1984; Otolaryngology, Univ Wash Med Ctr 1988; **Fac Appt:** Prof Oto, UCSF

Fee Jr, Willard E MD [Oto] - **Spec Exp:** Head & Neck Cancer; Parotid Gland Tumors; Thyroid Cancer; **Hospital:** Stanford Univ Med Ctr; **Address:** Stanford Cancer Ctr, 875 Lake Wilber Dr, CC-2227, Stanford, CA 94305-5826; **Phone:** 650-725-6500; **Board Cert:** Otolaryngology 1974; **Med School:** Univ Colorado 1969; **Resid:** Surgery, Wadsworth VA Hosp 1971; Otolaryngology, UCLA Med Ctr 1974; **Fac Appt:** Prof Oto, Stanford Univ

Otolaryngology

Futran, Neal D MD/DMD [Oto] - **Spec Exp:** Head & Neck Cancer & Surgery; Head & Neck Cancer Reconstruction; Skull Base Surgery; **Hospital:** Univ Wash Med Ctr, Harborview Med Ctr; **Address:** U Wash Med Ctr, Oto Office, 1959 NE Pacific St, Box 356515, Seattle, WA 98195-6515; **Phone:** 206-543-3060; **Board Cert:** Otolaryngology 1993; **Med School:** SUNY Downstate 1987; **Resid:** Surgery, Kings Co-SUNY Downstate 1985; Otolaryngology, U Rochester Med Ctr 1992; **Fellow:** Microvascular Surgery, Mt Sinai Hosp 1993; **Fac Appt:** Prof Oto, Univ Wash

Jackler, Robert K MD [Oto] - **Spec Exp:** Neuro-Otology; Skull Base Surgery; Ear Tumors; **Hospital:** Stanford Univ Med Ctr; **Address:** Stanford Univ Med Ctr, Dept Head & Neck Surg, 801 Welch Rd, Stanford, CA 94305-5739; **Phone:** 650-725-6500; **Board Cert:** Otolaryngology 1984; Neurotology 2004; **Med School:** Boston Univ 1979; **Resid:** Otolaryngology, UCSF Med Ctr 1984; **Fellow:** Otolaryngology, Oto Med Grp 1985; **Fac Appt:** Prof Oto, Stanford Univ

Kaplan, Michael J MD [Oto] - **Spec Exp:** Head & Neck Surgery; Skull Base Surgery; Head & Neck Cancer; **Hospital:** Stanford Univ Med Ctr; **Address:** Stanford Cancer Ctr, Dept Otolaryngology, 801 Welch Rd, Stanford, CA 94305-5739; **Phone:** 650-723-5416; **Board Cert:** Otolaryngology 1982; **Med School:** Harvard Med Sch 1977; **Resid:** Surgery, Beth Israel-Chldns Hosps 1979; Otolaryngology, Mass EE Infirm 1982; **Fellow:** Head and Neck Surgery, Univ Virginia 1984; **Fac Appt:** Prof Oto, Stanford Univ

McMenomey, Sean O MD [Oto] - **Spec Exp:** Skull Base Tumors & Surgery; Head & Neck Surgery; Gamma Knife Surgery; **Hospital:** OR Hlth & Sci Univ, Providence St Vincent Med Ctr; **Address:** Oregon Hlth & Sci Univ, Dept Otolaryngology, 3181 SW Sam Jackson Park Rd, MC PV-01, Portland, OR 97239; **Phone:** 503-494-8135; **Board Cert:** Otolaryngology 1993; **Med School:** St Louis Univ 1987; **Resid:** Otolaryngology, Oregon Health Sci Ctr 1992; **Fellow:** Otology & Neurotology, Baptist Hosp 1993; **Fac Appt:** Assoc Prof Oto, Oregon Hlth Sci Univ

Rice, Dale MD [Oto] - **Spec Exp:** Head & Neck Cancer; Sinus Disorders/Surgery; **Hospital:** USC Univ Hosp - R K Eamer Med Plz; **Address:** USC Keck Sch Med, 1200 N State St, Box 795, Los Angeles, CA 90033-1029; **Phone:** 323-442-5790; **Board Cert:** Otolaryngology 1976; **Med School:** Univ Mich Med Sch 1968; **Resid:** Surgery, Univ Mich Med Ctr 1976; Otolaryngology, Univ Mich Med Ctr 1976; **Fac Appt:** Prof Oto, USC Sch Med

Singer, Mark I MD [Oto] - **Spec Exp:** Head & Neck Surgery; Head & Neck Cancer; Melanoma; **Hospital:** UCSF - Mt Zion Med Ctr; **Address:** 3801 Sacramento St, Ste 230, San Francisco, CA 94118; **Phone:** 415-600-2450; **Board Cert:** Otolaryngology 1976; **Med School:** Columbia P&S 1970; **Resid:** Surgery, Northwestern Meml Hosp 1973; Otolaryngology, Northwestern Meml Hosp 1976; **Fellow:** Oncology, Northwestern Meml Hosp 1976; **Fac Appt:** Prof Oto, UCSF

Sinha, Uttam K MD [Oto] - **Spec Exp:** Head & Neck Cancer; Voice Disorders; **Hospital:** USC Univ Hosp - R K Eamer Med Plz, House Ear Inst; **Address:** 1200 N State St, rm 4136, Los Angeles, CA 90033; **Phone:** 323-226-7315; **Board Cert:** Otolaryngology 1998; **Med School:** India 1985; **Resid:** Otolaryngology, LAC-USC Med Ctr 1995; **Fellow:** Mount Sinai Med Sch 1988; LAC-USC Med Ctr 1990; **Fac Appt:** Asst Prof Oto, USC Sch Med

Wax, Mark K MD [Oto] - **Spec Exp:** Skull Base Tumors & Surgery; Facial Plastic & Reconstructive Surgery; **Hospital:** OR Hlth & Sci Univ; **Address:** Oregon Hlth Scis Univ-Dept Otolaryngology, 3181 SW Sam Jackson Park Rd, Ste PV-01, Portland, OR 97201; **Phone:** 503-494-5355; **Board Cert:** Otolaryngology 1985; Facial Plastic & Reconstructive Surgery 1987; **Med School:** Univ Toronto 1980; **Resid:** Otolaryngology, Univ Toronto 1985; Surgery, Cedars-Sinai Med Ctr 1983; **Fellow:** Head and Neck Surgery, St Michaels Hosp 1991; **Fac Appt:** Prof Oto, Oregon Hlth Sci Univ

Weisman, Robert A MD [Oto] - **Spec Exp:** Head & Neck Cancer; Clinical Trials; Thyroid & Parathyroid Cancer & Surgery; Head & Neck Cancer Reconstruction; **Hospital:** UCSD Med Ctr; **Address:** Moores-UCSD Cancer Center, 3855 Health Sciences Drive, MC 0987, La Jolla, CA 92093-0987; **Phone:** 858-822-6197; **Board Cert:** Otolaryngology 1978; **Med School:** Washington Univ, St Louis 1973; **Resid:** Head and Neck Surgery, UCLA Med Ctr 1978; **Fac Appt:** Prof S, UCSD

Weymuller, Ernest MD [Oto] - **Spec Exp:** Head & Neck Cancer; Sinus Disorders/Surgery; **Hospital:** Univ Wash Med Ctr; **Address:** 1959 NE Pacific St, Box 356161, Seattle, WA 98195-6161; **Phone:** 206-598-4022; **Board Cert:** Otolaryngology 1973; **Med School:** Harvard Med Sch 1966; **Resid:** Surgery, Vanderbilt Univ Hosp 1968; Otolaryngology, Mass Eye and Ear Infirm 1973; **Fac Appt:** Prof Oto, Univ Wash

Yueh, Bevan MD [Oto] - **Spec Exp:** Head & Neck Cancer; **Hospital:** Univ Wash Med Ctr, VA Puget Sound Hlth Care Sys; **Address:** Surgery Section, VA Puget Sound, 1660 S Columbian Way, MS 98108-112-OTO, Seattle, WA 98108; **Phone:** 206-764-2424; **Board Cert:** Otolaryngology 1995; **Med School:** Stanford Univ 1989; **Resid:** Otolaryngology, Johns Hopkins Hosp 1994; **Fellow:** Otolaryngology, Johns Hopkins Hosp 1995; **Fac Appt:** Assoc Prof Oto, Univ Wash

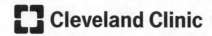

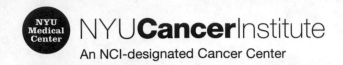

NYU**Cancer**Institute

An NCI-designated Cancer Center

A Collaborative Approach
The NYU Cancer Institute, an NCI designated center, is a "matrix cancer center" without walls operating within the larger NYU Medical Center. With over 200 members and a research funding base of over $81 million, this structure strengthens our capabilities to forge collaborations across medical and scientific disciplines, which translates to comprehensive care for our patients and discoveries that will influence the future of this disease.

Renowned Expertise
Our highly skilled Magnet™ nursing team not only plays a pivotal role in coordinating direct patient care, but is also a source of invaluable patient education. Team members' compassion and expertise help patients better manage the symptoms of their disease as well as their special needs.

A Patient-Focused Setting
The NYU Clinical Cancer Center, with over 70 faculty members from various disciplines at the New York University School of Medicine, is the principal outpatient facility of the Cancer Institute and serves as home for our patients and their caregivers. The center and its multidisciplinary team of experts provide access to the latest treatment options and clinical trials along with a variety of programs in cancer prevention, screening, diagnostics, genetic counseling, and supportive services. When it comes to kids and cancer, the Stephen D. Hassenfeld Children's Center for Cancer and Blood Disorders offers not just innovation but insight. As a leading member of the NCI-sponsored Children's Oncology Group, our physicians are known for developing new ways to treat childhood cancer. Our affiliation with Bellevue Hospital, the oldest public hospital in the country, affords clinically distinctive opportunities to learn and care for patients with cancer by observing its presentation and behavior in a variety of patient groups.

Pain Medicine

a subspecialty of Anesthesiology, Neurology, Physical Medicine & Rehabilitation or Psychiatry

Some physicians who have their primary board certification in anesthesiology, neurology, physical medicine and rehabilitation, or psychiatry have completed additional training and passed an examination in the subspecialty called pain management. These doctors provide a high level of care, either as a primary physcian or consultant, for patients experiencing problems with acute, chronic and/or cancer pain in both hospital and ambulatory settings.

For more information about the main specialties of these physicians, see Anesthesiology, Neurology, Physical Medicine and Rehabilitation or Psychiatry.

Training Required: Number of years required for primary specialty plus additional training and examination.

Pain Medicine

New England

Abrahm, Janet L MD [PM] - **Spec Exp:** Palliative Care; Pain-Cancer; **Hospital:** Dana-Farber Cancer Inst; **Address:** Dana-Farber Cancer Institute, 44 Binney St, Shields-Warren 420, Boston, MA 02115; **Phone:** 617-632-6464; **Board Cert:** Internal Medicine 1976; Medical Oncology 1981; Hematology 1978; **Med School:** UCSF 1973; **Resid:** Internal Medicine, Mass Genl Hosp 1975; Internal Medicine, Moffitt Hosp-UCSF 1977; **Fellow:** Hematology, Mass Genl Hosp 1976; Hematology & Oncology, Hosp Univ Penn 1980; **Fac Appt:** Assoc Prof Med, Harvard Med Sch

Mid Atlantic

De Leon-Casasola, Oscar MD [PM] - **Spec Exp:** Pain-Acute; Pain-Chronic; Pain-Cancer; **Hospital:** Roswell Park Cancer Inst; **Address:** Roswell Park Cancer Inst, Anesthesia/Pain Med, Elm & Carlton Sts, Buffalo, NY 14263; **Phone:** 716-845-4595; **Board Cert:** Anesthesiology 1991; Critical Care Medicine 1993; Pain Medicine 2005; **Med School:** Guatemala 1982; **Resid:** Surgery, SUNY-Downstate Med Ctr 1986; Anesthesiology, Univ Buffalo 1989; **Fac Appt:** Prof Anes, SUNY Buffalo

Foley, Kathleen M MD [PM] - **Spec Exp:** Palliative Care; Pain-Cancer; **Hospital:** Meml Sloan Kettering Cancer Ctr (page 76); **Address:** Meml Sloan Kettering Cancer Ctr, Pain Care, 1275 York Ave, Box 52, New York, NY 10021-6007; **Phone:** 212-639-7050; **Board Cert:** Neurology 1977; **Med School:** Cornell Univ-Weill Med Coll 1969; **Resid:** Neurology, New York Hosp 1974; **Fellow:** Clinical Genetics, New York Hosp 1971; **Fac Appt:** Prof N, Cornell Univ-Weill Med Coll

Jain, Subhash MD [PM] - **Spec Exp:** Pain-Cancer; Pain-Neuropathic; **Hospital:** NY-Presby Hosp (page 79), Beth Israel Med Ctr - Petrie Division (page 72); **Address:** 360 S 72nd St, Ste C, New York, NY 10021; **Phone:** 212-439-6100; **Board Cert:** Anesthesiology 1994; Pain Medicine 1998; **Med School:** India 1968; **Resid:** Surgery, St Vincent Med Ctr 1977; Anesthesiology, New York Hosp 1979; **Fellow:** Pain Medicine, New York Hosp/Meml Sloan Kettering Cancer Ctr 1980; **Fac Appt:** Assoc Prof Anes, Cornell Univ-Weill Med Coll

Kreitzer, Joel MD [PM] - **Spec Exp:** Pain-Back; Pain-Cancer; Pain-Neuropathic; **Hospital:** Mount Sinai Med Ctr (page 77), Mount Sinai Hosp of Queens (page 77); **Address:** Upper East Side Pain Medicine, 1540 York Ave, New York, NY 10028; **Phone:** 212-288-2180; **Board Cert:** Anesthesiology 1990; Pain Medicine 2003; **Med School:** Albert Einstein Coll Med 1985; **Resid:** Anesthesiology, Mount Sinai Hosp 1989; **Fellow:** Pain Medicine, Mount Sinai Hosp 1989; **Fac Appt:** Assoc Clin Prof Anes, Mount Sinai Sch Med

Lema, Mark J MD/PhD [PM] - **Spec Exp:** Pain-Cancer; Pain-Acute; Pain-Neuropathic; **Hospital:** Roswell Park Cancer Inst; **Address:** Roswell Park Cancer Inst, Dept Pain Medicine, Elm & Carlton St, Buffalo, NY 14263-0001; **Phone:** 716-845-3240; **Board Cert:** Anesthesiology 1987; Pain Medicine 2004; **Med School:** SUNY Downstate 1982; **Resid:** Anesthesiology, Brigham & Women's Hosp 1984; **Fellow:** Physiology, SUNY Buffalo Genl Hosp 1978; **Fac Appt:** Prof Anes, SUNY Buffalo

Portenoy, Russell MD [PM] - **Spec Exp:** Pain-Cancer; Palliative Care; **Hospital:** Beth Israel Med Ctr - Petrie Division (page 72); **Address:** Beth Israel Med Ctr, Dept Pain Medicine/Palliative Care, First Ave at 16th St, New York, NY 10003; **Phone:** 212-844-1403; **Board Cert:** Neurology 1985; **Med School:** Univ MD Sch Med 1980; **Resid:** Neurology, Albert Einstein 1984; **Fellow:** Pain Medicine, Meml Sloan-Kettering Cancer Ctr 1985; **Fac Appt:** Prof N, Albert Einstein Coll Med

Staats, Peter MD [PM] - **Spec Exp:** Pain-Cancer; **Hospital:** Riverview Med Ctr, CentraState Med Ctr; **Address:** Metzger Staats Pain Mgmt, LLC, 160 Avenue at the Commons, Ste 1, Shrewsbury, NJ 07702; **Phone:** 732-380-0200; **Board Cert:** Anesthesiology 1994; Pain Medicine 2005; **Med School:** Univ Mich Med Sch 1989; **Resid:** Anesthesiology, Johns Hopkins Hosp 1993; **Fellow:** Pain Medicine, Johns Hopkins Hosp 1994

Weinberger, Michael L MD [PM] - **Spec Exp:** Pain-Cancer; Pain-Back; **Hospital:** NY-Presby Hosp (page 79); **Address:** 630 W 168th St, PH5, rm 500, New York, NY 10032-3720; **Phone:** 212-305-7114; **Board Cert:** Internal Medicine 1986; Anesthesiology 1990; Pain Medicine 2004; Hospice & Palliative Medicine 2006; **Med School:** Columbia P&S 1983; **Resid:** Internal Medicine, St Vincent's Hosp 1986; Anesthesiology, Columbia-Presby Med Ctr 1989; **Fellow:** Pain Medicine, Meml Sloan Kettering Cancer Ctr 1990; **Fac Appt:** Assoc Prof Anes, Columbia P&S

Southeast

Anghelescu, Doralina L MD [PM] - **Spec Exp:** Pain Management-Pediatric; Pain-Cancer; **Hospital:** St Jude Children's Research Hosp; **Address:** St Jude Chldn's Rsch Hosp, Anesthesiology, 332 N Lauderdale, rm B3035, MS 130, Memphis, TN 38105; **Phone:** 901-495-4034; **Board Cert:** Anesthesiology 1998; Pain Medicine 2001; **Med School:** Romania 1985; **Resid:** Anesthesiology, Univ NMex Hosp 1997; **Fellow:** Pain Medicine, Chldns Natl Med Ctr 1998; Pain Medicine, Univ NMex Hosp 1999

Payne, Richard MD [PM] - **Spec Exp:** Palliative Care; Pain-Neuropathic; **Hospital:** Duke Univ Med Ctr; **Address:** Duke Inst on Care at the End of Life, Box 90968, Durham, NC 27705; **Phone:** 919-660-3553; **Board Cert:** Neurology 1984; **Med School:** Harvard Med Sch 1977; **Resid:** Internal Medicine, Peter Bent Brigham Hosp 1979; Neurology, New York Hosp 1982; **Fellow:** Neuro-Oncology, Meml Sloan Kettering Cancer Ctr 1984

Rauck, Richard L MD [PM] - **Spec Exp:** Pain-Cancer; **Hospital:** Forsyth Med Ctr, Wake Forest Univ Baptist Med Ctr (page 85); **Address:** Carolinas Pain Institute, 145 Kimel Park Drive, Ste 330, Winston Salem, NC 27103; **Phone:** 336-765-6181; **Board Cert:** Anesthesiology 1987; Pain Medicine 2005; **Med School:** Bowman Gray 1982; **Resid:** Anesthesiology, Univ Cincinnati Hosp 1985; **Fellow:** Pain Medicine, Univ Cincinnati Hosp 1986; **Fac Appt:** Assoc Prof Anes, Wake Forest Univ

Midwest

Benedetti, Costantino MD [PM] - **Spec Exp:** Pain-Cancer; Palliative Care; **Hospital:** Ohio St Univ Med Ctr, Arthur G James Cancer Hosp & Research Inst; **Address:** Ohio State Univ Med Ctr, 300 W 10th Ave, Ste 519, Columbus, OH 43210; **Phone:** 614-293-6599; **Med School:** Italy 1972; **Resid:** Anesthesiology, Univ Colorado Hosp 1976; Anesthesiology, Univ Wash Med Ctr 1976; **Fellow:** Pain Medicine, Univ Wash Med Ctr 1978; **Fac Appt:** Clin Prof Anes, Ohio State Univ

Pain Medicine

Huntoon, Marc MD [PM] - **Spec Exp:** Pain-Cancer; Pain-after Spinal Intervention; Palliative Care; **Hospital:** Mayo Med Ctr & Clin - Rochester; **Address:** Mayo Clinic - Pain Medicine, 200 First St SW, Rochester, MN 55905; **Phone:** 507-266-9240; **Board Cert:** Anesthesiology 2003; Pain Medicine 2004; **Med School:** Wayne State Univ 1985; **Resid:** Anesthesiology, Naval Hosp Med Ctr 1991; **Fellow:** Pain Medicine, Naval Hosp Med Ctr 1992

Swarm, Robert A MD [PM] - **Spec Exp:** Pain-Acute; Pain-Chronic; Pain-Cancer; **Hospital:** Barnes-Jewish Hosp; **Address:** Ctr for Advanced Med-Pain Mngmt Ctr, 4921 Parkview Pl, Ste 10A, MS 90-35-706, St Louis, MO 63110; **Phone:** 314-362-8820; **Board Cert:** Anesthesiology 1990; Pain Medicine 2004; **Med School:** Washington Univ, St Louis 1983; **Resid:** Surgery, Barnes Hosp 1986; Anesthesiology, Barnes Hosp 1989; **Fellow:** Pain Medicine, Univ Sydney; **Fac Appt:** Assoc Prof Anes, Washington Univ, St Louis

Great Plains and Mountains

Weinstein, Sharon MD [PM] - **Spec Exp:** Pain-Cancer; **Hospital:** Univ Utah Hosps and Clins; **Address:** Huntsman Cancer Institute, 2000 Circle of Hope, Salt Lake City, UT 84112; **Phone:** 801-585-0262; **Board Cert:** Neurology 1993; Pain Medicine 2000; **Med School:** Albert Einstein Coll Med 1986; **Resid:** Neurology, Albert Einstein Coll Med 1990; **Fellow:** Pain Medicine, Meml Sloan Kettering Cancer Ctr; **Fac Appt:** Assoc Prof Anes, Univ Utah

Southwest

Burton, Allen W MD [PM] - **Spec Exp:** Pain-Cancer; Palliative Care; **Hospital:** UT MD Anderson Cancer Ctr (page 81); **Address:** MD Anderson Cancer Ctr, Dept Anesth, 1400 Holcombe Blvd, Unit 409, Houston, TX 77030; **Phone:** 713-745-7246; **Board Cert:** Anesthesiology 1996; Pain Medicine 1998; **Med School:** Baylor Coll Med 1991; **Resid:** Anesthesiology, Brigham & Women's Hosp 1995; **Fellow:** Pain Medicine, U Texas Med Branch Hosp 1998; **Fac Appt:** Assoc Prof Anes, Univ Tex Med Br, Galveston

Driver, Larry C MD [PM] - **Spec Exp:** Pain-Cancer; Palliative Care; **Hospital:** UT MD Anderson Cancer Ctr (page 81); **Address:** MD Andeson Cancer Ctr, Dept Pain Medicine, 1400 Holcombe Blvd, Unit 409, Houston, TX 77030; **Phone:** 713-745-7246; **Board Cert:** Anesthesiology 1992; Pain Medicine 2002; **Med School:** Univ Tex, San Antonio 1980; **Resid:** Anesthesiology, Univ Colorado Hlth Sci Ctr 1984; **Fellow:** Pain Medicine, MD Anderson Cancer Ctr 1999; Pain Medicine, The Mayday Fund 2006; **Fac Appt:** Assoc Prof Anes, Univ Tex, Houston

West Coast and Pacific

Du Pen, Stuart L MD [PM] - **Spec Exp:** Pain-Cancer; Pain-Chronic; **Hospital:** Overlake Hosp Med Ctr, Harrison Meml Hosp; **Address:** 1135 116th Ave NE, Ste 110, Bellevue, WA 98004; **Phone:** 425-289-3140; **Board Cert:** Anesthesiology 1972; Pain Medicine 1993; **Med School:** St Louis Univ 1967; **Resid:** Anesthesiology, Virginia Mason Med Ctr 1971; **Fac Appt:** Assoc Clin Prof Anes, Univ Wash

Fishman, Scott M MD [PM] - **Spec Exp:** Pain-Cancer; Pain-Chronic; Psychiatry in Pain Management; **Hospital:** UC Davis Med Ctr; **Address:** UC Davis Med Ctr, Pain Management Clinic, 4860 Y St, Ste 2700, Sacramento, CA 95817; **Phone:** 916-734-7246; **Board Cert:** Internal Medicine 1994; Psychiatry 1998; **Med School:** Univ Mass Sch Med 1990; **Resid:** Internal Medicine, Greenwich Hosp 1993; Psychiatry, Mass Genl Hosp 1996; **Fellow:** Pain Medicine, Mass Genl Hosp 1995; **Fac Appt:** Assoc Prof Anes, UC Davis

Fitzgibbon, Dermot R MD [PM] - **Spec Exp:** Pain-Cancer; **Hospital:** Univ Wash Med Ctr; **Address:** Univ Wash Med Ctr, Dept Anesthesiology, 1959 NE Pacific St, Box 356540, Seattle, WA 98195; **Phone:** 206-598-4260; **Board Cert:** Anesthesiology 1996; Pain Medicine 1998; **Med School:** Ireland 1983; **Resid:** Anesthesiology, St Vincent's Hosp 1992; Anesthesiology, Univ Washington Med Ctr 1995; **Fellow:** Pain Medicine, Univ Wash-Pain Mngmt Clinic 1994; **Fac Appt:** Assoc Prof Anes, Univ Wash

Ready, L Brian MD [PM] - **Spec Exp:** Pain-Cancer; **Hospital:** Tacoma Genl Hosp; **Address:** 1901 S Union Ave, Ste A244, Tacoma, WA 98405; **Phone:** 253-459-6509; **Med School:** Canada 1967; **Resid:** Anesthesiology, Univ Washington Med Ctr 1975

Rosner, Howard L MD [PM] - **Spec Exp:** Pain-after Spinal Intervention; Pain-Cancer; Pain-Back; **Hospital:** Cedars-Sinai Med Ctr; **Address:** 444 S San Vincente Blvd, Ste 1101, Cedars-Sinai Med Ctr,Mark Goodson Bldg, Los Angeles, CA 90048; **Phone:** 310-423-9612; **Board Cert:** Anesthesiology 1989; Pain Medicine 2004; **Med School:** Univ Miami Sch Med 1980; **Resid:** Anesthesiology, Mass Genl Hosp 1983; **Fellow:** Pain Medicine, Columbia-Presby Med Ctr

Slatkin, Neal E MD [PM] - **Spec Exp:** Pain-Cancer; Palliative Care; **Hospital:** City of Hope Natl Med Ctr & Beckman Rsch (page 69); **Address:** City of Hope Supportive Care NW Bldg, 1500 E Duarte Rd, rm 1218, Duarte, CA 91010; **Phone:** 626-256-4673 x63991; **Board Cert:** Neurology 1982; Pain Medicine 2000; **Med School:** SUNY Stony Brook 1976; **Resid:** Neurology, Bellevue Hosp Ctr-NYU 1978; Neurology, Med Coll Va 1981; **Fellow:** Neurology, Med Coll Va 1982; Neuro-Oncology, Meml Sloan-Kettering Cancer Ctr 1984; **Fac Appt:** Asst Clin Prof Med, USC-Keck School of Medicine

Wallace, Mark S MD [PM] - **Spec Exp:** Pain-Chronic; Pain-Cancer; Palliative Care; **Hospital:** UCSD Med Ctr; **Address:** 9300 Campus Point Drive, MC 7651, La Jolla, CA 92037; **Phone:** 858-657-6035; **Board Cert:** Anesthesiology 1992; Pain Medicine 2005; **Med School:** Creighton Univ 1987; **Resid:** Anesthesiology, Univ Maryland Hosp 1991; **Fellow:** Pain Medicine, UCSD Med Ctr 1994; **Fac Appt:** Assoc Prof Anes, UCSD

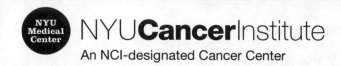

NYUCancerInstitute
An NCI-designated Cancer Center

A Collaborative Approach

The NYU Cancer Institute, an NCI designated center, is a "matrix cancer center" without walls operating within the larger NYU Medical Center. With over 200 members and a research funding base of over $81 million, this structure strengthens our capabilities to forge collaborations across medical and scientific disciplines, which translates to comprehensive care for our patients and discoveries that will influence the future of this disease.

Renowned Expertise

Our highly skilled Magnet™ nursing team not only plays a pivotal role in coordinating direct patient care, but is also a source of invaluable patient education. Team members' compassion and expertise help patients better manage the symptoms of their disease as well as their special needs.

A Patient-Focused Setting

The NYU Clinical Cancer Center, with over 70 faculty members from various disciplines at the New York University School of Medicine, is the principal outpatient facility of the Cancer Institute and serves as home for our patients and their caregivers. The center and its multidisciplinary team of experts provide access to the latest treatment options and clinical trials along with a variety of programs in cancer prevention, screening, diagnostics, genetic counseling, and supportive services. When it comes to kids and cancer, the Stephen D. Hassenfeld Children's Center for Cancer and Blood Disorders offers not just innovation but insight. As a leading member of the NCI-sponsored Children's Oncology Group, our physicians are known for developing new ways to treat childhood cancer. Our affiliation with Bellevue Hospital, the oldest public hospital in the country, affords clinically distinctive opportunities to learn and care for patients with cancer by observing its presentation and behavior in a variety of patient groups.

Pathology

A pathologist deals with the causes and nature of disease and contributes to diagnosis, prognosis and treatment through knowledge gained by the laboratory application of the biologic, chemical and physical sciences.

A pathologist uses information gathered from the microscopic examination of tissue specimens, cells and body fluids, and from clinical laboratory tests on body fluids and secretions for the diagnosis, exclusion and monitoring of the disease.

Training Required: Three to four years

Certification in the following subspecialty requires additional training and examination.

Dermatopathology: A dermatopathologist has the expertise to diagnose and monitor diseases of the skin including infectious, immunologic, degenerative and neoplastic diseases. This entails the examination and interpretation of specially prepared tissue sections, cellular scrapings and smears of skin lesions by means of routine and special (electron and fluorescent) microscopes.

Pathology

Bell, Debra A MD [Path] - **Spec Exp:** Gynecologic Pathology; Ovarian Cancer; **Hospital:** Mass Genl Hosp; **Address:** Pathology Assocs, 55 Fruit St, WRN 105, Boston, MA 02114; **Phone:** 617-726-3977; **Board Cert:** Anatomic Pathology 1980; Cytopathology 1989; **Med School:** Albany Med Coll 1976; **Resid:** Pathology, NYU Med Ctr 1981; **Fellow:** Cytopathology, Meml Sloan Kettering Cancer Ctr 1982; **Fac Appt:** Assoc Prof Path, Harvard Med Sch

Bhan, Atul Kumar MD [Path] - **Spec Exp:** Immunopathology; Liver Pathology; Liver Cancer; **Hospital:** Mass Genl Hosp; **Address:** Mass Genl Hosp, Dept Path, 55 Fruit St, Warren 501, Boston, MA 02114-2620; **Phone:** 617-726-2588; **Board Cert:** Anatomic Pathology 1976; Immunopathology 1985; **Med School:** India 1965; **Resid:** Pathology, Boston Univ Hosp 1971; Pathology, Chldns Univ Hosp 1974; **Fac Appt:** Prof Path, Harvard Med Sch

Connolly, James Leo MD [Path] - **Spec Exp:** Breast Pathology; Breast Cancer; **Hospital:** Beth Israel Deaconess Med Ctr - Boston; **Address:** BIDMC, Dept Path, 330 Brookline Ave, rm ES 112, Boston, MA 02215-5400; **Phone:** 617-667-4344; **Board Cert:** Anatomic Pathology 1980; **Med School:** Vanderbilt Univ 1974; **Resid:** Anatomic Pathology, Beth Israel Hosp 1978; **Fac Appt:** Prof Path, Harvard Med Sch

DeLellis, Ronald A MD [Path] - **Spec Exp:** Thyroid Cancer; Endocrine Pathology; **Hospital:** Rhode Island Hosp, Miriam Hosp; **Address:** Rhode Island Hospital, Dept Pathology, 593 Eddy St, Providence, RI 02903-4923; **Phone:** 401-444-5154; **Board Cert:** Anatomic Pathology 1997; **Med School:** Tufts Univ 1966; **Resid:** Anatomic Pathology, Natl Inst Hlth 1971; **Fellow:** Pathology, Univ Hosp 1973; **Fac Appt:** Prof Path, Brown Univ

Fletcher, Christopher MD [Path] - **Spec Exp:** Soft Tissue Tumors; Sarcoma; Surgical Pathology; **Hospital:** Brigham & Women's Hosp, Dana-Farber Cancer Inst; **Address:** Brigham & Women's Hospital, Dept Pathology, 75 Francis St, Boston, MA 02115-6110; **Phone:** 617-732-8558; **Med School:** England 1981; **Resid:** Pathology, St Thomas Hosp 1985; **Fellow:** Pathology, St Thomas Hosp 1986; **Fac Appt:** Prof Path, Harvard Med Sch

Harris, Nancy L MD [Path] - **Spec Exp:** Lymphoma; Hematopathology; **Hospital:** Mass Genl Hosp; **Address:** Mass Genl Hosp, Dept Path, 55 Fruit St, Warren 211, Boston, MA 02114; **Phone:** 617-726-5155; **Board Cert:** Anatomic Pathology 1978; Clinical Pathology 1978; **Med School:** Stanford Univ 1970; **Resid:** Pathology, Beth Israel Hosp 1978; **Fellow:** Immunopathology, Mass Genl Hosp 1980; **Fac Appt:** Prof Path, Harvard Med Sch

Mark, Eugene J MD [Path] - **Spec Exp:** Lung Pathology; Cardiac Pathology; **Hospital:** Mass Genl Hosp; **Address:** Mass Genl Hosp, Dept Path, 55 Fruit St, Warren 246, Boston, MA 02114; **Phone:** 617-726-8891; **Board Cert:** Anatomic & Clinical Pathology 1973; Dermatopathology 1975; **Med School:** Harvard Med Sch 1967; **Resid:** Pathology, Mass Genl Hosp 1972; **Fellow:** Pathology, Kantons Hospital 1966; **Fac Appt:** Prof Path, Harvard Med Sch

Odze, Robert D MD [Path] - **Spec Exp:** Gastrointestinal Pathology; Liver Pathology; **Hospital:** Brigham & Women's Hosp; **Address:** Brigham & Women's Hosp, Dept Pathology, 75 Francis St, Boston, MA 02115; **Phone:** 617-732-7549; **Board Cert:** Anatomic Pathology 1990; **Med School:** McGill Univ 1984; **Resid:** Surgery, McGill Univ 1987; Pathology, McGill Univ 1990; **Fellow:** Gastrointestinal Pathology, New England Deaconess Med Ctr 1991; **Fac Appt:** Assoc Prof Path, Harvard Med Sch

Schnitt, Stuart J MD [Path] - **Spec Exp:** Breast Pathology; Breast Cancer; **Hospital:** Beth Israel Deaconess Med Ctr - Boston; **Address:** Beth Israel Deaconess Med Ctr, Dept Pathology, 330 Brookline Ave, rm ES 112, Boston, MA 02215-5400; **Phone:** 617-667-4344; **Board Cert:** Anatomic & Clinical Pathology 1983; **Med School:** Albany Med Coll 1979; **Resid:** Anatomic Pathology, Beth Israel Deaconess Med Ctr; **Fellow:** Surgical Pathology, Beth Israel Deaconess Med Ctr; **Fac Appt:** Assoc Prof Path, Harvard Med Sch

Young, Robert H MD [Path] - **Spec Exp:** Ovarian Cancer; Breast Cancer; **Hospital:** Mass Genl Hosp; **Address:** Mass Genl Hosp, Dept Pathology, 55 Fruit St, Warren 215, Boston, MA 02114; **Phone:** 617-726-8892; **Board Cert:** Anatomic Pathology 1980; **Med School:** Ireland 1974; **Resid:** Pathology, Mass Genl Hosp 1979; Pathology, Dublin Univ 1977; **Fac Appt:** Prof Path, Harvard Med Sch

Mid Atlantic

Brooks, John S MD [Path] - **Spec Exp:** Tumor Diagnosis; Sarcoma; Bone & Soft Tissue Pathology; **Hospital:** Pennsylvania Hosp (page 84), Hosp Univ Penn - UPHS (page 84); **Address:** Pennsylvania Hospital, Preston 6 FL, 800 Spruce St, Philadelphia, PA 19107; **Phone:** 215-829-3541; **Board Cert:** Anatomic Pathology 1978; Immunopathology 1983; **Med School:** Thomas Jefferson Univ 1974; **Resid:** Pathology, osp U Penn 1978; **Fellow:** Immunopathology, Hosp U Penn 1978; **Fac Appt:** Prof Path, Univ Pennsylvania

Burger, Peter MD [Path] - **Spec Exp:** Brain Tumors; Neuro-Pathology; **Hospital:** Johns Hopkins Hosp - Baltimore; **Address:** Johns Hopkins Hosp-Division Pathology, 600 N Wolfe St, rm 710, Baltimore, MD 21287; **Phone:** 410-955-8378; **Board Cert:** Anatomic Pathology 1976; Neuropathology 1976; **Med School:** Northwestern Univ 1966; **Resid:** Anatomic Pathology, Duke Univ Med Ctr 1973; **Fellow:** Neuropathology, Duke Univ Med Ctr 1973

Dorfman, Howard D MD [Path] - **Spec Exp:** Bone Tumors; Soft Tissue Tumors; **Hospital:** Montefiore Med Ctr, Montefiore Med Ctr - Weiler-Einstein Div; **Address:** Montefiore-Orthopaedic Pathology Div, 111 E 210th St, Bronx, NY 10467-2401; **Phone:** 718-920-5622; **Board Cert:** Anatomic Pathology 1958; **Med School:** SUNY Downstate 1951; **Resid:** Pathology, Mt Sinai Hosp 1953; Surgical Pathology, Columbia-Presby Med Ctr 1958; **Fellow:** Pathology, Mt Sinai Med Ctr 1954; **Fac Appt:** Prof Path, Albert Einstein Coll Med

Ehya, Hormoz MD [Path] - **Spec Exp:** Cytopathology; Breast Pathology; Lung Pathology; **Hospital:** Fox Chase Cancer Ctr (page 73); **Address:** Fox Chase Cancer Center, 333 Cottman Ave, rm C427, Philadelphia, PA 19111-2497; **Phone:** 215-728-5389; **Board Cert:** Anatomic Pathology 1979; Cytopathology 1989; **Med School:** Iran 1974; **Resid:** Pathology, Univ Miss Med Ctr 1979; **Fellow:** Cytopathology, Meml Sloan-Kettering Cancer Ctr 1980

Epstein, Jonathan MD [Path] - **Spec Exp:** Bladder Cancer; Urologic Cancer; Prostate Cancer; Urologic Pathology; **Hospital:** Johns Hopkins Hosp - Baltimore; **Address:** 401 N Broadway, Weinberg 2242, Baltimore, MD 21231; **Phone:** 410-955-5043; **Board Cert:** Anatomic Pathology 1986; **Med School:** Boston Univ 1981; **Resid:** Pathology, Johns Hopkins Hosp 1985; **Fellow:** Pathology, Meml Sloan Kettering Cancer Ctr 1984; **Fac Appt:** Prof Path, Johns Hopkins Univ

Pathology

Gupta, Prabodh K MD [Path] - **Spec Exp:** Lung Pathology; Cervical Cancer; Fine Needle Aspiration Biopsy; **Hospital:** Hosp Univ Penn - UPHS (page 84); **Address:** Hosp Univ Penn - Cytopathology, 3400 Spruce St, 6 Founders, Philadelphia, PA 19104; **Phone:** 215-662-3238; **Board Cert:** Anatomic Pathology 1975; Cytopathology 1989; **Med School:** India 1965; **Resid:** Pathology, All India Inst Med Scis 1967; **Fellow:** Pathology, Mass Genl Hosp 1968; Johns Hopkins Hosp 1969; **Fac Appt:** Prof Path, Univ Pennsylvania

Hoda, Syed A MD [Path] - **Spec Exp:** Breast Cancer; Surgical Pathology; **Hospital:** NY-Presby Hosp (page 79); **Address:** 525 E 68th St, 1028 Starr, New York, NY 10021; **Phone:** 212-746-2700; **Board Cert:** Anatomic & Clinical Pathology 2001; Cytopathology 1991; **Med School:** Pakistan 1984; **Resid:** Anatomic & Clinical Pathology, Tulane Univ Affil Hosps 1990; **Fellow:** Cytopathology, Meml Sloan Kettering Cancer Ctr 1991; Pathology, Meml Sloan Kettering Cancer Ctr 1992; **Fac Appt:** Clin Prof Path, Cornell Univ-Weill Med Coll

Hruban, Ralph H MD [Path] - **Spec Exp:** Gastrointestinal Pathology; Pancreatic Cancer; **Hospital:** Johns Hopkins Hosp - Baltimore; **Address:** Johns Hopkins Hosp, Dept Pathology, 401 N Broadway Bldg Weinberg - rm 2242, Baltimore, MD 21231; **Phone:** 410-955-9132; **Board Cert:** Anatomic Pathology 1990; **Med School:** Johns Hopkins Univ 1985; **Resid:** Pathology, Johns Hopkins Hosp 1990; **Fellow:** Meml Sloan Kettering Cancer Ctr 1989; **Fac Appt:** Prof Path, Johns Hopkins Univ

Jaffe, Elaine S MD [Path] - **Spec Exp:** Lymphoma; Hematopathology; **Hospital:** Natl Inst of Hlth - Clin Ctr; **Address:** NIH/NCI - Lab Pathology, 10 Center Drive Bldg 10 - rm 2N202, Bethesda, MD 20892; **Phone:** 301-496-0183; **Board Cert:** Anatomic Pathology 1974; **Med School:** Univ Pennsylvania 1969; **Resid:** Pathology, Clinical Ctr/NIH 1972; **Fellow:** Hematopathology, Natl Cancer Inst 1974; **Fac Appt:** Clin Prof Path, Geo Wash Univ

Jones, Robert V MD [Path] - **Spec Exp:** Neuro-Pathology; Brain Tumors; **Hospital:** Georgetown Univ Hosp; **Address:** GWUMC, Dept Path, 2300 Eye St NW, Ross Hall, Ste 502, Washington, DC 20037; **Phone:** 202-994-3391; **Board Cert:** Anatomic & Clinical Pathology 1981; Neuropathology 1994; **Med School:** Univ VA Sch Med 1977; **Resid:** Anatomic & Clinical Pathology, Walter Reed AMC 1981; **Fellow:** Neurological Pathology, ARmed Forces Inst Path 1990; **Fac Appt:** Assoc Prof Path, Geo Wash Univ

Katzenstein, Anna-Luise A MD [Path] - **Spec Exp:** Lung Cancer; Pulmonary Pathology; **Hospital:** Univ. Hosp.-SUNY Upstate, Crouse Hosp; **Address:** SUNY Upstate Medical Univ, 766 Irving Ave, Weiskotten, rm 2106, Syracuse, NY 13210; **Phone:** 315-464-7125; **Board Cert:** Anatomic Pathology 1976; **Med School:** Johns Hopkins Univ 1971; **Resid:** Pathology, Univ Hospital 1975; **Fellow:** Surgical Pathology, Barnes Hosp-Wash Univ 1976; **Fac Appt:** Prof Path, SUNY Upstate Med Univ

Knowles, Daniel MD [Path] - **Spec Exp:** Lymph Node Pathology; Bone Marrow Pathology; Lymphoma; **Hospital:** NY-Presby Hosp (page 79); **Address:** Cornell-Weill Med Coll- Dept Pathology, 1300 York Ave, rm C302, New York, NY 10021; **Phone:** 212-746-6464; **Board Cert:** Anatomic Pathology 1978; Immunopathology 1984; **Med School:** Univ Chicago-Pritzker Sch Med 1973; **Resid:** Anatomic Pathology, Columbia-Presby Med Ctr 1975; **Fellow:** Immunopathology, Rockefeller Univ 1977; **Fac Appt:** Prof Path, Cornell Univ-Weill Med Coll

Kurman, Robert J MD [Path] - **Spec Exp:** Gynecologic Pathology; Ovarian Cancer; Uterine Cancer; **Hospital:** Johns Hopkins Hosp - Baltimore; **Address:** Johns Hopkins Hosp, Dept Pathology, 401 N Broadway, Weinberg-2242, Baltimore, MD 21231; **Phone:** 410-955-0471; **Board Cert:** Anatomic Pathology 1972; Obstetrics & Gynecology 1980; **Med School:** SUNY Upstate Med Univ 1968; **Resid:** Pathology, Peter Bent Brigham Hosp/Mass Genl Hosp 1977; Obstetrics & Gynecology, LAC Hosp/USC 1978; **Fellow:** Obstetrics & Gynecology, Harvard Univ 1973; **Fac Appt:** Prof Path, Johns Hopkins Univ

Li Volsi, Virginia A MD [Path] - **Spec Exp:** Endocrine Cancers; Thyroid Cancer; Gynecologic Cancer; **Hospital:** Hosp Univ Penn - UPHS (page 84); **Address:** Hosp Univ Penn - Pathology, 3400 Spruce St 6 Founders Bldg - Ste 6030, Philadelphia, PA 19104; **Phone:** 215-662-6545; **Board Cert:** Anatomic Pathology 1974; **Med School:** Columbia P&S 1969; **Resid:** Anatomic Pathology, Presbyterian Hosp 1974; **Fac Appt:** Prof Path, Univ Pennsylvania

McCormick, Steven MD [Path] - **Spec Exp:** Ophthalmic Pathology; Head & Neck Pathology; Fine Needle Aspiration Biopsy; **Hospital:** New York Eye & Ear Infirm (page 78); **Address:** 310 E 14th St, New York, NY 10003; **Phone:** 212-979-4156; **Board Cert:** Anatomic Pathology 1988; **Med School:** W VA Univ 1984; **Resid:** Anatomic Pathology, West Va Univ Hosp 1988; **Fellow:** Ophthalmic Pathology, West Va Univ Hosp 1988; **Fac Appt:** Assoc Prof Path, NY Med Coll

Melamed, Jonathan MD [Path] - **Spec Exp:** Prostate Cancer; Tumor Banking; **Hospital:** NYU Med Ctr (page 80); **Address:** NYU Medical Ctr, Dept Pathology, TH-461, 560 First Ave, New York, NY 10016; **Phone:** 212-263-8927; **Board Cert:** Anatomic & Clinical Pathology 1992; **Med School:** South Africa 1985; **Resid:** Pathology, Lenox Hill Hosp 1991; **Fellow:** Pathology, Meml Sloan Kettering Cancer Ctr 1992; Urologic Pathology, Meml Sloan Kettering Cancer Ctr 1993; **Fac Appt:** Assoc Prof Path, NYU Sch Med

Mies, Carolyn MD [Path] - **Spec Exp:** Breast Cancer; **Hospital:** Hosp Univ Penn - UPHS (page 84); **Address:** Hosp Univ Penn - Surgical Pathology, 3400 Spruce St, Founders 6, Philadelphia, PA 19104; **Phone:** 215-662-6503; **Board Cert:** Anatomic Pathology 1980; **Med School:** Rush Med Coll 1980; **Resid:** Pathology, Tufts-New England Med Ctr 1982; Pathology, New England Deaconess Hosp 1984; **Fellow:** Surgical Pathology, Meml Sloan Kettering Cancer Ctr 1986; **Fac Appt:** Assoc Prof Path, Univ Pennsylvania

Montgomery, Elizabeth A MD [Path] - **Spec Exp:** Barrett's Esophagus; Esophageal Cancer; Gastrointestinal Pathology; **Hospital:** Johns Hopkins Hosp - Baltimore; **Address:** Johns Hopkins Univ, Dept Pathology, 401 N Broadway Weinberg Bldg - rm 2242, Baltimore, MD 21231; **Phone:** 410-614-2308; **Board Cert:** Anatomic Pathology 1988; Cytopathology 1994; **Med School:** Geo Wash Univ 1984; **Resid:** Pathology, Walter Reed AMC 1988; **Fac Appt:** Assoc Prof Path, Johns Hopkins Univ

Orenstein, Jan M MD/PhD [Path] - **Spec Exp:** Prostate Cancer; Tumor Banking; AIDS/HIV; **Hospital:** G Washington Univ Hosp; **Address:** Geo Wash Univ Med Ctr Dept Path, 502 Ross Hall, 2300 Eye St NW, Washington, DC 20037; **Phone:** 202-994-2943; **Board Cert:** Anatomic Pathology 1977; **Med School:** SUNY Downstate 1971; **Resid:** Pathology, Presby Hosp 1973; Pathology, Natl Cancer Inst 1977; **Fac Appt:** Prof Path, Geo Wash Univ

Patchefsky, Arthur S MD [Path] - **Spec Exp:** Breast Cancer; Pulmonary Pathology; Sarcoma; **Hospital:** Fox Chase Cancer Ctr (page 73); **Address:** Fox Chase Cancer Center, 7701 Burholme Ave, rm C4333, Philadelphia, PA 19111; **Phone:** 215-728-5390; **Board Cert:** Anatomic Pathology 1969; **Med School:** Hahnemann Univ 1963; **Resid:** Pathology, John Hopkins Hosp 1966; Pathology, Hosp U Penn 1967; **Fellow:** Pathology, Meml Sloan Kettering Cancer Ctr 1968; **Fac Appt:** Prof Path, Thomas Jefferson Univ

Rosen, Paul P MD [Path] - **Spec Exp:** Breast Pathology; Breast Cancer; **Hospital:** NY-Presby Hosp (page 79); **Address:** New York Presbyterian, Dept Pathology, 525 E 68th St, Starr 1031, New York, NY 10021-4870; **Phone:** 212-746-6482; **Board Cert:** Anatomic & Clinical Pathology 1969; Pathology 1998; **Med School:** Columbia P&S 1964; **Resid:** Pathology, Presby Hosp 1966; Pathology, VA Hosp 1968; **Fellow:** Pathology, Meml Hosp Cancer Ctr 1970; **Fac Appt:** Prof Path, Cornell Univ-Weill Med Coll

Ross, Jeffrey S MD [Path] - Spec Exp: Urologic Cancer; Prostate Cancer; Breast Cancer; **Hospital:** Albany Med Ctr; **Address:** Albany Med Coll, Dept Path, 47 New Scotland Ave, MC 8, Albany, NY 12208; **Phone:** 518-262-5471; **Board Cert:** Anatomic & Clinical Pathology 1974; **Med School:** SUNY Buffalo 1970; **Resid:** Pathology, Mass Genl Hosp 1974; **Fellow:** Pathology, Harvard Med Sch 1974; **Fac Appt:** Prof Path, Albany Med Coll

Sanchez, Miguel A MD [Path] - Spec Exp: Breast Cancer; Thyroid Cancer; **Hospital:** Englewood Hosp & Med Ctr; **Address:** Englewood Hosp & Med Ctr, Dept Pathology, 350 Engle St, Englewood, NJ 07631-1898; **Phone:** 201-894-3423; **Board Cert:** Anatomic Pathology 1975; Clinical Pathology 1979; Cytopathology 1991; **Med School:** Spain 1969; **Resid:** Pathology, Englewood Hosp 1972; Pathology, Temple Univ 1973; **Fellow:** Pathology, Meml Sloan Kettering Cancer Ctr 1974; **Fac Appt:** Assoc Prof Path, Mount Sinai Sch Med

Schiller, Alan L MD [Path] - Spec Exp: Bone & Joint Pathology; Soft Tissue Pathology; Bone Tumors; **Hospital:** Mount Sinai Med Ctr (page 77); **Address:** Mt Sinai Sch Med, Dept Pathology, 1 Gustave Levy Pl, Box 1194, New York, NY 10029-6500; **Phone:** 212-241-8014; **Board Cert:** Anatomic Pathology 1973; **Med School:** Ros Franklin Univ/Chicago Med Sch 1967; **Resid:** Pathology, Mass Genl Hosp 1972; **Fac Appt:** Prof Path, Mount Sinai Sch Med

Silverberg, Steven G MD [Path] - Spec Exp: Gynecologic Pathology; Breast Pathology; Urologic Pathology; Endocrine Pathology; **Hospital:** Univ of MD Med Sys; **Address:** Univ Maryland Med Ctr, Dept Pathology, 22 S Greene St, Baltimore, MD 21201; **Phone:** 410-328-5072; **Board Cert:** Anatomic Pathology 1969; **Med School:** Johns Hopkins Univ 1962; **Resid:** Pathology, Yale-New Haven Hosp 1965; **Fellow:** Surgical Pathology, Meml Sloan Kettering Cancer Ctr 1966; **Fac Appt:** Prof Path, Univ MD Sch Med

Silverman, Jan F MD [Path] - Spec Exp: Breast Cancer; Lung Cancer; Gastrointestinal Pathology; Fine Needle Aspiration Biopsy; **Hospital:** Allegheny General Hosp; **Address:** Allegheny Gen Hosp-Dept Lab Medicine, 320 E North Ave, Pittsburgh, PA 15212; **Phone:** 412-359-6886; **Board Cert:** Anatomic & Clinical Pathology 1975; Cytopathology 1989; **Med School:** Med Coll VA 1970; **Resid:** Pathology, Med Coll Virginia 1975; **Fellow:** Surgical Pathology, Med Coll Virginia 1975; **Fac Appt:** Prof Path, Drexel Univ Coll Med

Swerdlow, Steven H MD [Path] - Spec Exp: Lymphoma; Hematopathology; **Hospital:** UPMC Presby, Pittsburgh; **Address:** UPMC-Presby Hosp, Div Hematopathology, 200 Lothrop St, rm C606, Pittsburgh, PA 15213-2536; **Phone:** 412-647-5191; **Board Cert:** Anatomic Pathology 2005; Clinical Pathology 2005; **Med School:** Harvard Med Sch 1975; **Resid:** Pathology, Beth Israel Hosp 1979; **Fellow:** Hematopathology, Vanderbilt Univ 1981; Hematopathology, St Bartholmew's Hosp 1983; **Fac Appt:** Prof Path, Univ Pittsburgh

Tomaszewski, John E MD [Path] - Spec Exp: Breast Cancer; Head & Neck Pathology; Ovarian Cancer; Uterine Cancer; **Hospital:** Hosp Univ Penn - UPHS (page 84); **Address:** Hosp Univ Penn, Dept Pathology & Lab Med, 3400 Spruce St, 6 Founders Bldg, Ste 6042, Philadelphia, PA 19104; **Phone:** 215-662-6852; **Board Cert:** Anatomic Pathology 1982; Immunopathology 1983; **Med School:** Univ Pennsylvania 1977; **Resid:** Pathology, Hosp Univ Penn 1982; **Fellow:** Surgical Pathology, Hosp Univ Penn 1983; **Fac Appt:** Prof Path, Univ Pennsylvania

Tornos, Carmen MD [Path] - Spec Exp: Gynecologic Cancer; Breast Cancer; Ovarian Cancer; Hospital: Stony Brook Univ Med Ctr; Address: Stony Brook Univ Hosp, Dept Pathology, Level 2, rm 766, Stony Brook, NY 11794-7025; Phone: 631-444-2222; Board Cert: Anatomic & Clinical Pathology 1997; Med School: Spain 1977; Resid: Hematology, Ciudad Sanitaria Valle de Hebron 1982; Anatomic & Clinical Pathology, Univ Texas HSC 1989; Fellow: Surgical Pathology, MD Anderson Cancer Ctr 1990; Fac Appt: Prof Path, SUNY Stony Brook

Travis, William MD [Path] - Spec Exp: Pulmonary Pathology; Lung Cancer; Hospital: Meml Sloan Kettering Cancer Ctr (page 76); Address: Meml Sloan-Kettering Canc Ctr, Dept Path, 1275 York Ave, New York, NY 10021; Phone: 212-639-5905; Board Cert: Anatomic & Clinical Pathology 1985; Med School: Univ Fla Coll Med 1981; Resid: Anatomic Pathology, New England Deaconess Hosp 1983; Clinical Pathology, Mayo Clinic 1985; Fellow: Surgical Pathology, Mayo Clinic 1986

Yousem, Samuel A MD [Path] - Spec Exp: Pulmonary Pathology; Transplant-Lung (Pathology); Lung Cancer; Hospital: UPMC Presby, Pittsburgh; Address: Dept Pathology, A-610, Presbyterian Campus, 200 Lothrop St, Pittsburgh, PA 15213; Phone: 412-647-6193; Board Cert: Anatomic Pathology 1985; Cytopathology 1997; Med School: Univ MD Sch Med 1981; Resid: Pathology, Stanford Univ Med Ctr 1983; Fellow: Surgical Pathology, Stanford Univ Med Ctr 1984; Fac Appt: Prof Path, Univ Pittsburgh

Southeast

Banks, Peter MD [Path] - Spec Exp: Hematopathology; Lymphoma; Hospital: Carolinas Med Ctr; Address: Dept Pathology, 1000 Blythe Blvd, 4th Fl Lab, Charlotte, NC 28232; Phone: 704-355-2251; Board Cert: Anatomic Pathology 1997; Med School: Harvard Med Sch 1971; Resid: Pathology, National Cancer Inst 1974; Pathology, Duke Univ Med Ctr 1975; Fellow: Surgical Pathology, Univ Minn Med Ctr 1976; Fac Appt: Prof Path, Univ NC Sch Med

Bostwick, David MD [Path] - Spec Exp: Urologic Pathology; Prostate Cancer; Bladder Cancer; Address: 4355 Innslake Drive, Glen Allen, VA 23060; Phone: 804-967-9225; Board Cert: Anatomic Pathology 1985; Med School: Univ MD Sch Med 1979; Resid: Pathology, Stanford Univ Med Ctr 1981; Fellow: Surgical Pathology, Stanford Univ Med Ctr 1984

Braylan, Raul MD [Path] - Spec Exp: Hematopathology; Leukemia; Lymphoma; Hospital: Shands Hlthcre at Univ of FL; Address: Univ Florida, Dept Hematopathology, PO Box 100275, Gainesville, Fl 32610; Phone: 352-392-3477; Board Cert: Anatomic Pathology 1972; Med School: Argentina 1960; Resid: Anatomic Pathology, Mt Sinai Hosp 1965; Anatomic Pathology, Einstein Affil Hosps 1967; Fellow: Anatomic Pathology, Meml Sloan Kettering Cancer Hosp 1968; Hematopathology, Univ Chicago Hosps 1973; Fac Appt: Prof Path, Univ Fla Coll Med

Crawford, James M MD/PhD [Path] - Spec Exp: Liver Pathology; Gastrointestinal Pathology; Gastrointestinal Cancer; Hospital: Shands Hlthcre at Univ of FL; Address: Univ Florida, Dept Pathology, 1600 SW Archer Rd, rm M649, Box 100275, Gainesville, FL 32610-0275; Phone: 352-392-3741; Board Cert: Anatomic Pathology 1987; Med School: Duke Univ 1982; Resid: Pathology, Brigham & Women's Hosp 1984; Fellow: Gastrointestinal Pathology, Brigham & Women's Hosp 1987; Fac Appt: Prof Path, Univ Fla Coll Med

Pathology

Lage, Janice MD [Path] - Spec Exp: Gynecologic Pathology; Breast Pathology; **Hospital:** MUSC Med Ctr; **Address:** MUSC Med Ctr, Dept Path, 165 Ashley Ave, Ste 309, Box 250908, Charleston, SC 29425; **Phone:** 843-792-3121; **Board Cert:** Anatomic Pathology 2001; **Med School:** Washington Univ, St Louis 1980; **Resid:** Pathology, Barnes Hosp/Wash Univ 1982; Obstetrics & Gynecology, Barnes Hosp/Wash Univ 1983; **Fellow:** Surgical Pathology, Barnes Hosp/Wash Univ 1984; **Fac Appt:** Prof Path, Med Univ SC

Masood, Shahla MD [Path] - Spec Exp: Breast Cancer; Breast Pathology; **Hospital:** Shands Jacksonville; **Address:** Univ of Florida, Dept Pathology, 655 W 8th St, Jacksonville, FL 32209-6511; **Phone:** 904-244-4387; **Board Cert:** Anatomic & Clinical Pathology 1998; Cytopathology 1990; **Med School:** Iran 1973; **Resid:** Anatomic Pathology, University Hosp 1977; **Fac Appt:** Prof Path, Univ Fla Coll Med

McCurley, Thomas L MD [Path] - Spec Exp: Hematopathology; Immunopathology; **Hospital:** Vanderbilt Univ Med Ctr, VA Med Ctr - Nashville; **Address:** Vanderbilt Univ Hosp, Dept Pathology, 21st & Garland Ave, Nashville, TN 37232; **Phone:** 615-343-9167; **Board Cert:** Anatomic & Clinical Pathology 1981; Immunopathology 1986; Hematology 1999; **Med School:** Vanderbilt Univ 1974; **Resid:** Internal Medicine, UCSF Med Ctr 1976; Pathology, Vanderbilt Univ Med Ctr 1981; **Fellow:** Hematopathology, Vanderbilt Univ Med Ctr 1984; **Fac Appt:** Assoc Prof Path, Vanderbilt Univ

Mills, Stacey E MD [Path] - Spec Exp: Breast Pathology; Ear, Nose & Throat Cancer; Surgical Pathology; **Hospital:** Univ Virginia Med Ctr; **Address:** Univ VA Hlth System, Dept Pathology, PO Box 800214, Charlottesville, VA 22908-0214; **Phone:** 434-982-4406; **Board Cert:** Anatomic Pathology 1999; **Med School:** Univ VA Sch Med 1977; **Resid:** Pathology, Univ Virginia Med Ctr 1980; **Fellow:** Pathology, Univ Virginia 1981; **Fac Appt:** Prof Path, Univ VA Sch Med

Nicosia, Santo MD [Path] - Spec Exp: Ovarian Cancer; **Hospital:** H Lee Moffitt Cancer Ctr & Research Inst; **Address:** 12901 Bruce B Downs Blvd, MDC Box 11, Tampa, FL 33612-4742; **Phone:** 813-974-3133; **Board Cert:** Anatomic Pathology 1978; Cytopathology 1990; **Med School:** Italy 1967; **Resid:** Anatomic Pathology, Michael Reese Hosp 1972; **Fellow:** Hosp Univ Penn 1973; **Fac Appt:** Prof Path, Univ S Fla Coll Med

Page, David L MD [Path] - Spec Exp: Breast Cancer; **Hospital:** Vanderbilt Univ Med Ctr; **Address:** Vanderbilt Univ, MCN, 1161 21st Ave S, rm C 3309, Nashville, TN 37232-2561; **Phone:** 615-322-3759; **Board Cert:** Anatomic Pathology 1972; Dermatopathology 1974; **Med School:** Johns Hopkins Univ 1966; **Resid:** Pathology, Mass Genl Hosp 1969; Pathology, Johns Hopkins Hosp 1972; **Fac Appt:** Prof Path, Vanderbilt Univ

Sewell, C Whitaker MD [Path] - Spec Exp: Breast Pathology; Surgical Pathology; **Hospital:** Emory Univ Hosp; **Address:** Emory Univ Hosp, Dept Pathology, 1364 Clifton Rd NE, rm H185, Atlanta, GA 30322; **Phone:** 404-712-7003; **Board Cert:** Anatomic Pathology 1974; Clinical Pathology 1974; **Med School:** Emory Univ 1969; **Resid:** Pathology, Emory Univ Hosp 1974; **Fac Appt:** Prof Path, Emory Univ

Weiss, Sharon MD [Path] - Spec Exp: Soft Tissue Pathology; Surgical Pathology; Sarcoma; **Hospital:** Emory Univ Hosp, Crawford Long Hosp of Emory Univ; **Address:** Emory Univ Hosp, Dept Path, 1364 Clifton Rd NE, rm H180, Atlanta, GA 30322; **Phone:** 404-712-0708; **Board Cert:** Anatomic Pathology 1974; **Med School:** Johns Hopkins Univ 1971; **Resid:** Pathology, Johns Hopkins Hosp 1975; **Fac Appt:** Prof Path, Emory Univ

Midwest

Allred, D Craig MD [Path] - **Spec Exp:** Breast Cancer; Breast Pathology; Breast Cancer Risk Assessment; **Hospital:** Barnes-Jewish Hosp; **Address:** Washington Univ Sch Med, Path & Immunology, 660 S Euclid Ave, Box 8118, St Louis, MO 63110; **Phone:** 314-362-6313; **Board Cert:** Anatomic Pathology 1984; **Med School:** Univ Utah 1979; **Resid:** Anatomic Pathology, Univ Conn Hlth Ctr 1983; **Fellow:** Immunopathology, Univ Conn Hlth Ctr 1982; **Fac Appt:** Prof Path, Baylor Coll Med

Balla, Andre K MD/PhD [Path] - **Spec Exp:** Prostate Cancer; Gynecologic Pathology; Tumor Banking; **Hospital:** Univ of IL Med Ctr at Chicago; **Address:** Univ IL at Chicago, Dept Path, 840 S Wood St, rm 130, MC 847, Chicago, IL 60612; **Phone:** 312-996-3879; **Board Cert:** Anatomic & Clinical Pathology 1988; **Med School:** Brazil 1972; **Resid:** Pathology, Hahnemann Univ Hosp 1988; **Fellow:** Clinical Immunology, Scripps Clin Rsch Fdn 1981; **Fac Appt:** Prof Path, Univ IL Coll Med

Behm, Frederick G MD [Path] - **Spec Exp:** Hematopathology; **Hospital:** Univ of IL Med Ctr at Chicago; **Address:** Univ Illinois Chicago, Dept Pathology, 130 CSN, MC 847, 840 S Wood St, Chicago, IL 60612-7335; **Phone:** 312-996-3150; **Board Cert:** Anatomic & Clinical Pathology 1980; Hematology 1983; **Med School:** Med Coll Wisc 1974; **Resid:** Pathology, Med Coll Va Hosps 1979; **Fac Appt:** Prof Path, Univ IL Coll Med

Cho, Kathleen R MD [Path] - **Spec Exp:** Gynecologic Pathology; Ovarian Cancer; Cervical Cancer; **Hospital:** Univ Michigan Hlth Sys; **Address:** Univ Michigan Med Sch, 109 Zina Pitcher Pl, rm 1506BSRB, Ann Arbor, MI 48109-2200; **Phone:** 734-764-1549; **Board Cert:** Anatomic Pathology 1990; **Med School:** Vanderbilt Univ 1984; **Resid:** Pathology, Johns Hopkins Hosp 1988; **Fellow:** Gynecologic Pathology, Johns Hopkins Hosp 1990; **Fac Appt:** Prof Path, Univ Mich Med Sch

Cohen, Michael B MD [Path] - **Spec Exp:** Urologic Cancer; Cytopathology; **Hospital:** Univ Iowa Hosp & Clinics, VA Med Ctr - Iowa City; **Address:** Univ Iowa - Dept Pathology, 200 Hawkins Drive, C670GH, Iowa City, IA 52242; **Phone:** 319-384-9609; **Board Cert:** Anatomic Pathology 1998; Cytopathology 1996; **Med School:** Albany Med Coll 1982; **Resid:** Pathology, UCSF Hosps & Clinics 1986; **Fellow:** Cytopathology, UCSF Hosps & Clinics 1987; **Fac Appt:** Prof Path, Univ Iowa Coll Med

Goldblum, John R MD [Path] - **Spec Exp:** Soft Tissue Pathology; Esophageal Cancer; Gastrointestinal Pathology; Sarcoma; **Hospital:** Cleveland Clin Fdn (page 71); **Address:** Cleveland Clinic, Anatomic Pathology L25, 9500 Euclid Ave, Cleveland, OH 44195; **Phone:** 216-444-8238; **Board Cert:** Anatomic Pathology 1993; **Med School:** Univ Mich Med Sch 1989; **Resid:** Anatomic Pathology, Univ Michigan Hosps 1993; **Fac Appt:** Prof Path, Cleveland Cl Coll Med/Case West Res

Greenson, Joel K MD [Path] - **Spec Exp:** Liver Cancer; Gastrointestinal Pathology; Liver Pathology; **Hospital:** Univ Michigan Hlth Sys; **Address:** Univ Michigan Hospitals, Dept Pathology, 1500 E Medical Center Drive, rm 2G332, Ann arbor, MI 48109-0054; **Phone:** 734-936-6776; **Board Cert:** Anatomic & Clinical Pathology 1988; **Med School:** Univ Mich Med Sch 1984; **Resid:** Pathology, Cedars-Sinai Med Ctr 1988; **Fellow:** Gastrointestinal Pathology, Johns Hopkins Hosp 1990; **Fac Appt:** Prof Path, Univ Mich Med Sch

Hart, William R MD [Path] - **Spec Exp:** Gynecologic Pathology; Surgical Pathology; **Hospital:** Cleveland Clin Fdn (page 71); **Address:** 9500 Euclid Ave, MS L21, Cleveland, OH 44195; **Phone:** 216-444-2840; **Board Cert:** Anatomic & Clinical Pathology 1970; **Med School:** Univ Mich Med Sch 1965; **Resid:** Anatomic & Clinical Pathology, Univ Mich Med Ctr 1970; **Fac Appt:** Prof Path, Cleveland Cl Coll Med/Case West Res

Pathology

Kurtin, Paul J MD [Path] - **Spec Exp:** Lymph Node Pathology; Bone Marrow Pathology; Lymphoma; **Hospital:** Mayo Med Ctr & Clin - Rochester; **Address:** Mayo Clinic - Dept Pathology, 200 First St SW, Hilton 1156A, Rochester, MN 55905; **Phone:** 507-284-4939; **Board Cert:** Anatomic & Clinical Pathology 1983; Hematology 1988; **Med School:** Med Coll Wisc 1979; **Resid:** Anatomic & Clinical Pathology, Vanderbilt Univ mED cTR 1983; **Fellow:** Hematopathology, Brigham & Women's Hosp 1984; Surgical Pathology, Brigham & Women's Hosp 1986; **Fac Appt:** Prof Path, Mayo Med Sch

Myers, Jeffrey L MD [Path] - **Spec Exp:** Lung Cancer; Lung Pathology; **Hospital:** Univ Michigan Hlth Sys; **Address:** Univ Michigan, 2G332 UH, 1500 E Medical Ctr Drive, Ann Arbor, MI 48109; **Phone:** 734-936-1888; **Board Cert:** Anatomic Pathology 1986; **Med School:** Washington Univ, St Louis 1981; **Resid:** Anatomic Pathology, Barnes Jewish Hosp 1984; **Fellow:** Surgical Pathology, U Alabama Med Ctr 1985; **Fac Appt:** Prof Path, Univ Mich Med Sch

Nascimento, Antonio G MD [Path] - **Spec Exp:** Bone & Soft Tissue Pathology; Head & Neck Pathology; **Hospital:** Mayo Med Ctr & Clin - Rochester; **Address:** Mayo Clinic - Dept Pathology, 200 First St SW, Hilton 1160A, Rochester, MN 55905; **Phone:** 507-284-4939; **Board Cert:** Anatomic Pathology 1979; **Med School:** Brazil ; **Resid:** Pathology, Univ Mississippi Med Ctr; **Fellow:** Anatomic Pathology, Meml Sloan-Kettering Cancer Ctr; Surgical Pathology, Mayo Clinic

Perry, Arie MD [Path] - **Spec Exp:** Neuro-Pathology; Brain Tumors; **Hospital:** Washington Univ Med Ctr; **Address:** Washington Univ Sch Med, Dept Path-Div Neuropath, 660 S Euclid Ave, St Louis, MO 63110; **Phone:** 314-362-7426; **Board Cert:** Anatomic & Clinical Pathology 1995; Neuropathology 1997; **Med School:** Univ Tex SW, Dallas 1990; **Resid:** Pathology, Univ Tex SW 1994; **Fellow:** Surgical Pathology, Mayo Clinic 1995; Neurological Pathology, Mayo Clinic 1998; **Fac Appt:** Assoc Prof Path, Washington Univ, St Louis

Rubin, Brian P MD [Path] - **Spec Exp:** Bone & Soft Tissue Tumors; Sarcoma; **Hospital:** Cleveland Clin Fdn (page 71); **Address:** Cleveland Clinic, Dept Anatomic Pathology, L25, 9500 Euclid Ave, Cleveland, OH 44195; **Phone:** 216-445-5551; **Board Cert:** Anatomic Pathology 1999; **Med School:** Cornell Univ-Weill Med Coll 1995; **Resid:** Pathology, Brigham & Women's Hosp 2000; **Fac Appt:** Asst Prof Path, Univ Wash

Scheithauer, Bernd MD [Path] - **Spec Exp:** Brain Tumors; Pituitary Tumors; Neuro-Pathology; **Hospital:** Mayo Med Ctr & Clin - Rochester, St Mary's Hosp - Rochester; **Address:** Mayo Clinic, Dept Pathology, 200 First St SW, Rochester, MN 55905; **Phone:** 507-284-8350; **Board Cert:** Anatomic Pathology 1979; Neuropathology 1979; **Med School:** Loma Linda Univ 1973; **Resid:** Anatomic Pathology, Stanford Univ Med Ctr 1976; Neuropathology, Stanford Univ Med Ctr 1978; **Fac Appt:** Prof Path, Mayo Med Sch

Suster, Saul M MD [Path] - **Spec Exp:** Lung Cancer; Mediastinal Tumors; Surgical Pathology; **Hospital:** Ohio St Univ Med Ctr; **Address:** Ohio State Univ Med Ctr, E-411 Doan Hall, 410 W 10th Ave, Columbus, OH 43210-1240; **Phone:** 614-293-7625; **Board Cert:** Anatomic & Clinical Pathology 1988; **Med School:** Ecuador 1976; **Resid:** Anatomic Pathology, Tel Aviv Univ Med Ctr 1984; Anatomic & Clinical Pathology, Mt Sinai Med Ctr 1988; **Fellow:** Surgical Pathology, Yale-New Haven Hosp 1990; **Fac Appt:** Prof Path, Ohio State Univ

Ulbright, Thomas M MD [Path] - **Spec Exp:** Testicular Cancer; Gynecologic Pathology; **Hospital:** Indiana Univ Hosp (page 70); **Address:** Clarion Pathology Laboratory, 350 W 11th St, rm 4014, Indianapolis, IN 46202; **Phone:** 317-491-6498; **Board Cert:** Anatomic Pathology 1980; **Med School:** Washington Univ, St Louis 1975; **Resid:** Pathology, Barnes Jewish Hosp 1978; Surgical Pathology, Barnes Jewish Hosp 1979; **Fellow:** Gynecologic Pathology, St Johns Mercy Med Ctr 1980; **Fac Appt:** Prof Path, Indiana Univ

Great Plains and Mountains

De Masters, Bette K MD [Path] - **Spec Exp:** Neuro-Pathology; Brain Tumors; **Hospital:** Univ Colorado Hosp, Chldn's Hosp - Denver, The; **Address:** Univ Colo Hlth Sci Ctr, Dept Path, Box 6511, MS 8104, Denver, CO 80262; **Phone:** 303-724-3704; **Board Cert:** Anatomic & Clinical Pathology 1982; Neuropathology 1985; **Med School:** Univ Wisc 1977; **Resid:** Internal Medicine, Presby Hosp 1979; Pathology, Univ Colo Med Sch 1982; **Fellow:** Neurological Pathology, Univ Colo/Univ Kansas 1984; **Fac Appt:** Prof Path, Univ Colorado

Rodgers III, George M MD/PhD [Path] - **Spec Exp:** Hematopathology; Anemia-Cancer Related; **Hospital:** Univ Utah Hosps and Clins; **Address:** Univ Utah Med Ctr - Div Hematology, 30 N 1900 E, rm 4C416, Salt Lake City, UT 84132; **Phone:** 801-585-3229; **Board Cert:** Internal Medicine 1979; Hematology 1982; **Med School:** Tulane Univ 1976; **Resid:** Internal Medicine, Baylor Affil Hosps 1979; **Fellow:** Hematology, UCSF Med Ctr 1982; **Fac Appt:** Prof Med, Univ Utah

Thor, Ann D MD [Path] - **Spec Exp:** Breast Cancer; Gynecologic Cancer; **Hospital:** Univ Colorado Hosp; **Address:** Univ Colorado Hlth Sci Ctr, Dept Pathology, Box 6511, MS 8104, Aurora, CO 80045-0508; **Phone:** 303-724-3704; **Board Cert:** Anatomic Pathology 1987; Cytopathology 1989; **Med School:** Vanderbilt Univ 1981; **Resid:** Pathology, Vanderbilt Univ 1983; **Fellow:** Immunopathology, Natl Cancer Inst 1986; Gynecologic Pathology, Mass Genl Hosp 1990; **Fac Appt:** Prof Path, Univ Colorado

Weisenburger, Dennis MD [Path] - **Spec Exp:** Hematopathology; Lymphoma; **Hospital:** Nebraska Med Ctr; **Address:** Univ Nebraska Med Ctr, Dept Pathology, 983135 Nebraska Medical Center, Omaha, NE 68198-3135; **Phone:** 402-559-7688; **Board Cert:** Anatomic & Clinical Pathology 1979; **Med School:** Univ Minn 1974; **Resid:** Anatomic Pathology, Univ Iowa Hosps 1978; **Fellow:** Hematopathology, City of Hope Natl Med Ctr 1980; **Fac Appt:** Prof Path, Univ Nebr Coll Med

Southwest

Bruner, Janet M MD [Path] - **Spec Exp:** Brain Tumors; Neuro Pathology; **Hospital:** UT MD Anderson Cancer Ctr (page 81); **Address:** MD Anderson Cancer Ctr, 1515 Holcombe Blvd, Ste 85, Houston, TX 77030; **Phone:** 713-792-6127; **Board Cert:** Anatomic Pathology 1997; Neuropathology 1984; **Med School:** Med Coll OH 1979; **Resid:** Anatomic & Clinical Pathology, Med Coll Ohio Hosp 1982; **Fellow:** Neurological Pathology, Baylor Coll Med 1984

Cagle, Philip MD [Path] - **Spec Exp:** Pulmonary Pathology; Lung Cancer; Mesothelioma; **Hospital:** Methodist Hosp - Houston; **Address:** Methodist Hospital, Dept Pathology, 6565 Fannin St, Ste 227, Houston, TX 77030; **Phone:** 713-441-6478; **Board Cert:** Anatomic & Clinical Pathology 1985; **Med School:** Univ Tenn Coll Med, Memphis 1981; **Fac Appt:** Prof Path, Baylor Coll Med

Colby, Thomas V MD [Path] - **Spec Exp:** Pulmonary Pathology; Surgical Pathology; Lung Cancer; **Hospital:** Mayo Clin Hosp - Scottsdale; **Address:** Mayo Clinic, Dept Path, 13400 E Shea Blvd, Scottsdale, AZ 85259; **Phone:** 480-301-8021; **Board Cert:** Anatomic Pathology 1978; **Med School:** Univ Mich Med Sch 1974; **Resid:** Anatomic Pathology, Stanford Univ Hosp 1978; **Fellow:** Surgical Pathology, Stanford Univ Hosp; **Fac Appt:** Prof Path, Mayo Med Sch

Pathology

Foucar, M Kathryn MD [Path] - **Spec Exp:** Leukemia; Lymph Node Pathology; Bone Marrow Pathology; **Hospital:** Univ NM Hlth & Sci Ctr; **Address:** TriCore Reference Lab, Hematopathology, 1001 Woodward Pl NE, Albuquerque, NM 87102; **Phone:** 505-938-8457; **Board Cert:** Anatomic & Clinical Pathology 1978; **Med School:** Ohio State Univ 1974; **Resid:** Anatomic Pathology, Univ NM Health & Sci Ctr 1976; Anatomic Pathology, Univ Minn Med Ctr 1978; **Fellow:** Surgical Pathology, Univ Minn Med Ctr 1979; **Fac Appt:** Prof Path, Univ New Mexico

Grogan, Thomas M MD [Path] - **Spec Exp:** Immunopathology; Lymphoma; **Hospital:** Univ Med Ctr - Tucson; **Address:** Univ Med Ctr, Dept Pathology, 1501 N Campbell Ave, rm 5212, Tucson, AZ 85724; **Phone:** 520-626-7477; **Board Cert:** Anatomic Pathology 1976; **Med School:** Geo Wash Univ 1971; **Resid:** Pathology, Letterman Army Med Ctr 1976; **Fellow:** Immunopathology, Stanford Univ Sch Med 1979; **Fac Appt:** Prof Path, Univ Ariz Coll Med

Hamilton, Stanley R MD [Path] - **Spec Exp:** Surgical Pathology; Gastrointestinal Pathology; Liver Pathology; **Hospital:** UT MD Anderson Cancer Ctr (page 81); **Address:** Univ Texas MD Anderson Cancer Ctr, 1515 Holcombe Blvd, Unit 85, Houston, TX 77030-4009; **Phone:** 713-792-2040; **Board Cert:** Anatomic & Clinical Pathology 1978; **Med School:** Indiana Univ 1973; **Resid:** Pathology, Johns Hopkins Hosp 1978; **Fellow:** St Marks Hosp 1979; **Fac Appt:** Prof Path, Univ Tex, Houston

Kinney, Marsha C MD [Path] - **Spec Exp:** Hematopathology; Lymphoma; Leukemia; **Hospital:** Univ Hlth Sys - Univ Hosp; **Address:** Univ Tex Hlth & Sci Ctr, Dept Path, 7703 Floyd Curl Drive, MC 775, San Antonio, TX 78229-3900; **Phone:** 210-567-4098; **Board Cert:** Anatomic & Clinical Pathology 1985; Hematology 1998; **Med School:** Univ Tex SW, Dallas 1981; **Resid:** Pathology, Vanderbilt Univ Med Ctr 1985; **Fellow:** Hematopathology, Vanderbilt Univ Med Ctr 1988; **Fac Appt:** Prof Path, Univ Tex, San Antonio

Leslie, Kevin O MD [Path] - **Spec Exp:** Pulmonary Pathology; Lung Cancer; Surgical Pathology; **Hospital:** Mayo Clin Hosp - Scottsdale; **Address:** Mayo Clinic, Scottsdale, 13400 E Shea Blvd, Scottsdale, AZ 85259; **Phone:** 480-301-8021; **Board Cert:** Anatomic & Clinical Pathology 1982; **Med School:** Albert Einstein Coll Med 1976; **Resid:** Anatomic & Clinical Pathology, Univ Colorado Health Sci Ctr 1982; **Fellow:** Surgical Pathology, Stanford Univ Med Ctr 1983; **Fac Appt:** Prof Path, Mayo Med Sch

Moran, Cesar A MD [Path] - **Spec Exp:** Lung Cancer; Mediastinal Tumors; Mesothelioma; **Hospital:** UT MD Anderson Cancer Ctr (page 81); **Address:** MD Anderson Cancer Ctr, Dept Pathology, 1515 Holcombe Blvd, rm G1-3738, Houston, TX 77030; **Phone:** 713-792-8134; **Board Cert:** Anatomic Pathology 1992; **Med School:** Guatemala 1981; **Resid:** Anatomic Pathology, Mt Sinai Med Ctr 1988; **Fellow:** Surgical Pathology, Yale-New Haven Med Ctr 1989; **Fac Appt:** Prof Path, Univ Tex, Houston

Prieto, Victor G MD/PhD [Path] - **Spec Exp:** Dermatopathology; Melanoma; Skin Cancer; **Hospital:** UT MD Anderson Cancer Ctr (page 81); **Address:** MD Anderson Cancer Ctr, Dept Pathology, 1515 Holcombe Blvd, Box 85, Houston, TX 77030; **Phone:** 713-792-0918; **Board Cert:** Anatomic Pathology 1995; Dermatopathology 1997; **Med School:** Spain 1986; **Resid:** Pathology, New York Hosp-Cornell Med Ctr 1993; **Fellow:** Pathology, Meml Sloan Kettering Cancer Ctr 1995; Dermatopathology, New York Hosp-Cornell Med Ctr 1996; **Fac Appt:** Prof Path, Univ Tex, Houston

Rashid, Asif MD/PhD [Path] - **Spec Exp:** Gastrointestinal Pathology; Liver Pathology; **Hospital:** UT MD Anderson Cancer Ctr (page 81); **Address:** MD Anderson Cancer Ctr, Dept Pathology, 1515 Holcombe Blvd, Box 85, Houston, TX 77030; **Phone:** 713-745-1101; **Board Cert:** Anatomic Pathology 1994; **Med School:** Pakistan 1984; **Resid:** Anatomic Pathology, Mass Gnrl Hosp 1993; **Fellow:** Anatomic Pathology, Mass Gnrl Hosp 1994; Anatomic Pathology, Johns Hopkins Med Inst 1996

Silva, Elvio G MD [Path] - **Spec Exp:** Gynecologic Pathology; Gynecologic Cancer; **Hospital:** UT MD Anderson Cancer Ctr (page 81), Cedars-Sinai Med Ctr; **Address:** MD Anderson Cancer Ctr, Dept Pathology, 1515 Holcombe Blvd, Box 85, Houston, TX 77030; **Phone:** 713-792-3154; **Board Cert:** Anatomic Pathology 1997; **Med School:** Argentina 1969; **Resid:** Pathology, National Univ Med Ctr 1975; Anatomic Pathology, Univ Toronto 1978; **Fellow:** Surgical Pathology, MD Anderson Cancer Ctr 1979; **Fac Appt:** Prof Path

Wheeler, Thomas M MD [Path] - **Spec Exp:** Thyroid Disorders; Thyroid Cancer; **Hospital:** Ben Taub General Hosp; **Address:** Baylor Coll Med, Dept Pathology, One Baylor Plaza, rm T203, Houston, TX 77030; **Phone:** 713-798-4664; **Board Cert:** Anatomic & Clinical Pathology 1999; Cytopathology 1990; **Med School:** Baylor Coll Med 1977; **Resid:** Pathology, Baylor Coll Med 1981; **Fac Appt:** Prof Path, Baylor Coll Med

West Coast and Pacific

Amin, Mahul MD [Path] - **Spec Exp:** Genitourinary Pathology; Bladder Pathology; **Hospital:** Cedars-Sinai Med Ctr; **Address:** Cedars Sinai Hosp, 8700 Beverly Blvd, Ste 8728, Los Angeles, CA 90048; **Phone:** 310-423-6631; **Board Cert:** Anatomic & Clinical Pathology 1996; **Med School:** India 1983; **Resid:** Pathology, Henry Ford Hosp 1992; **Fellow:** Surgical Pathology, MD Anderson Cancer Ctr 1993; **Fac Appt:** Prof Path, Emory Univ

Arber, Daniel A MD [Path] - **Spec Exp:** Bone Marrow Pathology; Lymph Node Pathology; Spleen Pathology; **Hospital:** Stanford Univ Med Ctr, Lucile Packard Chldns Hosp/Stanford Univ Med Ctr; **Address:** Clinic Laboratories, Stanford Univ Med Ctr, 300 Pasteur Drive, rm H1507, MC 5627, Stanford, CA 94305; **Phone:** 650-725-5604; **Board Cert:** Anatomic & Clinical Pathology 1991; Hematology 1993; **Med School:** Univ Tex, San Antonio 1986; **Resid:** Anatomic & Clinical Pathology, Scott & White Meml Hosp 1991; **Fellow:** Hematopathology, City of Hope Natl Med Ctr 1993; **Fac Appt:** Prof Path, Stanford Univ

Bastian, Boris C MD [Path] - **Spec Exp:** Melanoma; Skin Cancer; **Hospital:** UCSF Med Ctr; **Address:** UCSF Comprehensive Cancer Center, Box 0808, San Francisco, CA 94143; **Phone:** 415-476-5132; **Med School:** Germany 1988; **Resid:** Dermatology, University of Wurzburg 1994; **Fellow:** Hematology, Ludwig-Maximilian-University 1989; **Fac Appt:** Asst Prof D, UCSF

Bollen, Andrew W MD [Path] - **Spec Exp:** Neuro-Pathology; Brain Tumors; **Hospital:** UCSF Med Ctr, CA Pacific Med Ctr - Pacific Campus; **Address:** Dept Pathology/Neuropathology, 505 Parnassus Ave, M551, Box 0102, San Francisco, CA 94143-0511; **Phone:** 415-476-5236; **Board Cert:** Clinical Pathology 1993; Anatomic Pathology 1992; Neuropathology 1992; **Med School:** UCSD 1985; **Resid:** Anatomic Pathology, UCSF Med Ctr 1991; **Fellow:** Neuropathology, UCSF Med Ctr 1989; **Fac Appt:** Prof Path, UCSF

Chandrasoma, Parakrama T MD [Path] - **Spec Exp:** Gastrointestinal Pathology; Gastrointestinal Cancer; Neuro-Pathology; **Hospital:** LAC & USC Med Ctr; **Address:** LAC-USC Med Ctr, Dept Path, 1200 N State St, rm 16-905, Los Angeles, CA 90033; **Phone:** 323-226-4600; **Board Cert:** Anatomic Pathology 1982; **Med School:** Sri Lanka 1971; **Resid:** Anatomic Pathology, Univ Sri Lanka 1978; Anatomic Pathology, LAC-USC Med Ctr 1982; **Fac Appt:** Prof Path, USC Sch Med

Pathology

Cochran, Alistair J MD [Path] - **Spec Exp:** Melanoma; Dermatopathology; **Hospital:** UCLA Med Ctr (page 83); **Address:** UCLA Med Ctr, Dept Path & Med, 10833 Le Conte Ave, rm 13145CHS, MC 173216, Los Angeles, CA 90095-1713; **Phone:** 310-825-2743; **Med School:** Scotland 1966; **Resid:** Dermatopathology, Western Infirmary 1968; **Fellow:** Immunology, Karolinska Inst 1970; **Fac Appt:** Prof Path, UCLA

Cote, Richard J MD [Path] - **Spec Exp:** Lymph Node Pathology; Bladder Cancer; Breast Cancer; **Hospital:** USC Norris Comp Cancer Ctr, USC Univ Hosp - R K Eamer Med Plz; **Address:** 1441 Eastlake Ave, rm 2424, Los Angeles, CA 90033; **Phone:** 323-865-0212; **Board Cert:** Anatomic Pathology 1987; **Med School:** Univ Chicago-Pritzker Sch Med 1980; **Resid:** Pathology, New York Hosp-Cornell 1987; **Fellow:** Pathology, Meml Sloan-Kettering Cancer Ctr 1990; **Fac Appt:** Prof Path, USC-Keck School of Medicine

Dubeau, Louis MD/PhD [Path] - **Spec Exp:** Ovarian Cancer; Breast Cancer; **Hospital:** USC Norris Comp Cancer Ctr; **Address:** USC Norris Cancer Ctr, Dept Pathology, 1441 Eastlake Ave, rm 7320, Los Angeles, CA 90033-1048; **Phone:** 323-865-0720; **Board Cert:** Anatomic Pathology 1984; **Med School:** McGill Univ 1979; **Resid:** Anatomic Pathology, McGill Univ Med Ctr 1984; **Fac Appt:** Prof Path, USC Sch Med

Hammar, Samuel P MD [Path] - **Spec Exp:** Lung Cancer; Pulmonary Pathology; **Hospital:** Harrison Meml Hosp; **Address:** Diagnostic Specialties Laboratory, 700 Lebo Blvd, Bremerton, WA 98310; **Phone:** 360-479-7707; **Board Cert:** Anatomic & Clinical Pathology 1975; **Med School:** Univ Wash 1970

Hendrickson, Michael MD [Path] - **Spec Exp:** Gynecologic Cancer; Gynecologic Pathology; **Hospital:** Stanford Univ Med Ctr; **Address:** Stanford Univ Med Ctr, Surg Path Lab, 300 Pasteur Drive, rm L230, MC 5324, Stanford, CA 94305; **Phone:** 650-725-5169; **Board Cert:** Anatomic Pathology 1975; **Med School:** Stanford Univ 1971; **Resid:** Anatomic Pathology, Stanford Univ Med Sch 1974; **Fac Appt:** Prof Path, Stanford Univ

Koss, Michael N MD [Path] - **Spec Exp:** Pulmonary Pathology; Lung Cancer; Mediastinal Tumors; **Hospital:** USC Norris Comp Cancer Ctr, USC Univ Hosp - R K Eamer Med Plz; **Address:** Hoffman Medical Research Bldg, rm 209, 2011 Zonal Ave, Los Angeles, CA 90033; **Phone:** 323-226-6507; **Board Cert:** Anatomic Pathology 1979; **Med School:** Stanford Univ 1970; **Resid:** Pathology, Columbia Presby Med Ctr 1974; **Fellow:** Renal Pathology, Columbia Presby Med Ctr 1975; Pulmonary Pathology, Armed Forces Inst Path 1978; **Fac Appt:** Prof Path, USC Sch Med

Le Boit, Philip E MD [Path] - **Spec Exp:** Cutaneous Lymphoma; Skin Cancer; Dermatopathology; **Hospital:** UCSF Med Ctr; **Address:** UCSF - Dermatopathology Section, 1701 Divisadero St, Ste 350, San Francisco, CA 94115; **Phone:** 415-353-7546; **Board Cert:** Anatomic Pathology 1983; Clinical Pathology 1986; Dermatopathology 1983; **Med School:** Albany Med Coll 1979; **Resid:** Anatomic Pathology, UCSF Med Ctr 1981; Clinical Pathology, Mt Sinai Hosp 1982; **Fellow:** Dermatopathology, New York Hosp-Cornell Med Ctr 1983; **Fac Appt:** Prof Path, UCSF

Ljung, Britt-Marie E MD [Path] - **Spec Exp:** Breast Cancer; Cytopathology; Fine Needle Aspiration Biopsy; **Hospital:** UCSF - Mt Zion Med Ctr; **Address:** UCSF - Dept Pathology, Box 1785, San Francisco, CA 94143-1785; **Phone:** 415-353-7320; **Board Cert:** Anatomic Pathology 1985; Cytopathology 1989; **Med School:** Sweden 1975; **Resid:** Pathology, Karolinska Hosp 1979; Anatomic Pathology, UCLA Med Ctr 1983; **Fac Appt:** Prof Path, UCSF

Mischel, Paul MD [Path] - **Spec Exp:** Neuro-Pathology; Brain Tumors; **Hospital:** UCLA Med Ctr (page 83); **Address:** UCLA Med Ctr, Div Neuropathology, 10833 Le Conte Ave, rm 13-317 CHS, Los Angeles, CA 90095-1732; **Phone:** 310-825-0377; **Board Cert:** Anatomic Pathology 1997; Neuropathology 1997; **Med School:** Cornell Univ-Weill Med Coll 1991; **Resid:** Anatomic & Clinical Pathology, UCLA Med Sch 1996; **Fellow:** Neurological Pathology, UCLA Med Sch 1995; Research, Howard Hughes Med Inst/UCSF 1998; **Fac Appt:** Assoc Prof Path, UCLA

Nathwani, Bharat N MD [Path] - **Spec Exp:** Hematopathology; Leukemia; Lymphoma; **Hospital:** LAC & USC Med Ctr; **Address:** LAC & USC Med Ctr, Dept Pathology, 1200 N State St, rm 2422, Los Angeles, CA 90033-4526; **Phone:** 323-226-7064; **Board Cert:** Anatomic Pathology 1977; **Med School:** India 1969; **Resid:** Pathology, JJ Group-Grant Med Ctr 1972; Pathology, Rush-Presby-St Lukes Med Ctr 1974; **Fellow:** Hematopathology, City Hope Natl Med Ctr 1975; **Fac Appt:** Prof Path, USC Sch Med

Rutgers, Joanne MD [Path] - **Spec Exp:** Gynecologic Cancer; Gastrointestinal Pathology; **Hospital:** Long Beach Meml Med Ctr; **Address:** 2801 Atlantic Ave, Dept of Pathology, Long Beach, CA 90806; **Phone:** 562-933-0717; **Board Cert:** Clinical Pathology 1992; Anatomic Pathology 1985; Pathology 1997; Cytopathology 1997; **Med School:** UCSD 1981; **Resid:** Pathology, Montefiore Med Ctr 1983; Pathology, NYU 1985; **Fellow:** Gynecologic Pathology, Mass Genl Hosp 1989; **Fac Appt:** Assoc Clin Prof Path, UCLA

Sibley, Richard K MD [Path] - **Spec Exp:** Kidney Pathology; Breast Pathology; Liver Pathology; **Hospital:** Stanford Univ Med Ctr; **Address:** Stanford Univ Med Ctr, Dept Pathology, 300 Pasteur Drive, rm H2110, MC 5243, Stanford, CA 94305; **Phone:** 650-723-7211; **Board Cert:** Anatomic Pathology 1975; **Med School:** Univ Tex SW, Dallas 1971; **Resid:** Anatomic Pathology, Univ Chicago Hosps 1974; **Fellow:** Stanford Univ Med Ctr 1975; **Fac Appt:** Prof Path, Stanford Univ

Triche, Timothy J MD/PhD [Path] - **Spec Exp:** Pediatric Pathology; Pediatric Cancers; Sarcoma; **Hospital:** Chldns Hosp - Los Angeles; **Address:** Chldns Hosp of Los Angeles, Dept Path, 4650 Sunset Blvd, MS 43, Los Angeles, CA 90027; **Phone:** 323-669-4516; **Board Cert:** Anatomic Pathology 1975; **Med School:** Tulane Univ 1971; **Resid:** Anatomic Pathology, Barnes Hosp-Wash Univ 1973; Surgical Pathology, Barnes Hosp 1974; **Fellow:** Pathology, Natl Cancer Inst 1975; **Fac Appt:** Prof Path, USC Sch Med

True, Lawrence D MD [Path] - **Spec Exp:** Urologic Pathology; Prostate Cancer; Bladder Cancer; **Hospital:** Univ Wash Med Ctr; **Address:** Univ Wash Med Ctr, Dept Anatomic Path, 1959 NE Pacific St, rm BB220, Box 356100, Seattle, WA 98195-6100; **Phone:** 206-598-6400; **Board Cert:** Anatomic Pathology 1981; **Med School:** Tulane Univ 1971; **Resid:** Pathology, Univ Colo Hlth Sci Ctr 1980; **Fac Appt:** Prof Path, Univ Wash

Warnke, Roger A MD [Path] - **Spec Exp:** Lymphoma; Hematopathology; **Hospital:** Stanford Univ Med Ctr; **Address:** Stanford Univ, Dept Pathology, 300 Pasteur Drive, Ste L235, Stanford, CA 94305; **Phone:** 650-725-5167; **Board Cert:** Anatomic Pathology 1975; **Med School:** Washington Univ, St Louis 1971; **Resid:** Pathology, Stanford Univ Med Ctr 1973, **Fellow:** Surgical Pathology, Stanford Univ Med Ctr 1975; Immunology, Stanford Univ Med Ctr 1976; **Fac Appt:** Prof Path, Stanford Univ

Weiss, Lawrence M MD [Path] - **Spec Exp:** Lymphoma; Hematopathology; Adrenal Pathology; **Hospital:** City of Hope Natl Med Ctr & Beckman Rsch (page 69); **Address:** City of Hope Natl Med Ctr, Div Pathology, 1500 E Duarte Rd, Duarte, CA 91010-0269; **Phone:** 626-359-8111 x62456; **Board Cert:** Anatomic Pathology 1985; **Med School:** Univ MD Sch Med 1981; **Resid:** Pathology, Brigham & Women's Hosp 1983; **Fellow:** Pathology, Stanford Univ Hosp 1984

Pathology

Wilczynski, Sharon P MD/PhD [Path] - **Spec Exp:** Gynecologic Cancer; Breast Cancer; Ovarian Cancer; Clinical Trials; **Hospital:** City of Hope Natl Med Ctr & Beckman Rsch (page 69); **Address:** City Hope Natl Med Ctr-Dept of Pathology, 1500 E Duarte Blvd, Duarte, CA 91010; **Phone:** 626-256-4673 x62456; **Board Cert:** Anatomic & Clinical Pathology 1985; Cytopathology 1991; **Med School:** Med Coll PA Hahnemann 1981; **Resid:** Pathology, Hosp Univ Penn 1983; Anatomic & Clinical Pathology, Long Beach Meml Hosp 1985; **Fac Appt:** Prof Path, USC-Keck School of Medicine

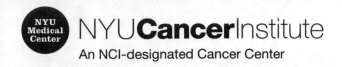

NYUCancerInstitute
An NCI-designated Cancer Center

A Collaborative Approach

The NYU Cancer Institute, an NCI designated center, is a "matrix cancer center" without walls operating within the larger NYU Medical Center. With over 200 members and a research funding base of over $81 million, this structure strengthens our capabilities to forge collaborations across medical and scientific disciplines, which translates to comprehensive care for our patients and discoveries that will influence the future of this disease.

Renowned Expertise

Our highly skilled Magnet™ nursing team not only plays a pivotal role in coordinating direct patient care, but is also a source of invaluable patient education. Team members' compassion and expertise help patients better manage the symptoms of their disease as well as their special needs.

A Patient-Focused Setting

The NYU Clinical Cancer Center, with over 70 faculty members from various disciplines at the New York University School of Medicine, is the principal outpatient facility of the Cancer Institute and serves as home for our patients and their caregivers. The center and its multidisciplinary team of experts provide access to the latest treatment options and clinical trials along with a variety of programs in cancer prevention, screening, diagnostics, genetic counseling, and supportive services. When it comes to kids and cancer, the Stephen D. Hassenfeld Children's Center for Cancer and Blood Disorders offers not just innovation but insight. As a leading member of the NCI-sponsored Children's Oncology Group, our physicians are known for developing new ways to treat childhood cancer. Our affiliation with Bellevue Hospital, the oldest public hospital in the country, affords clinically distinctive opportunities to learn and care for patients with cancer by observing its presentation and behavior in a variety of patient groups.

Pediatrics

A pediatrician is concerned with the physical, emotional and social health of children from birth to young adulthood. Care encompasses a broad spectrum of health services ranging from preventive healthcare to the diagnosis and treatment of acute and chronic diseases.

A pediatrician deals with biological, social and environmental influences on the developing child, and with the impact of disease and dysfunction on development.

Training Required: Three years

Certification in one or more of the following specialties additional training is required

Pediatric Hematology/Oncology: A pediatrician trained in the combination of pediatrics, hematology and oncology to recognize and manage pediatric blood disorders and cancerous diseases.

Pediatric Allergy and Immunology: An allergist-immunologist is trained in evaluation, physical and laboratory diagnosis and management of disorders involving the immune system. Selected examples of such conditions include asthma, anaphylaxis, rhinitis, eczema and adverse reactions to drugs, foods and insect stings as well as immune deficiency diseases (both acquired and congenital), defects in host defense and problems related to autoimmune disease, organ transplantation or malignancies of the immune system. As our understanding of the immune system develops, the scope of this specialty is widening.

Training programs are available at some medical centers to provide individuals with expertise in both allergy/immunology and pediatric pulmonology. Such individuals are candidates for dual certification.

Pediatric Endocrinology: A pediatrician who provides expert care to infants, children and adolescents who have diseases that result from an abnormality in the endocrine glands (glands which secrete hormones) These diseases include diabetes mellitus, growth failure, unusual size for age, early or late pubertal development, birth defects, the genital region and disorders of the thyroid, the adrenal and pituitary glands.

Pediatric Otolaryngology: A pediatric otolaryngologist has special expertise in the management of infants and children with disorders that include congenital and acquired conditions involving the aerodigestive tract, nose and paranasal sinuses, the ear and other areas of the head and neck. The pediatric otolaryngologist has special skills in the diagnosis, treatment and management of childhood disorders of voice, speech, language and hearing.

Pediatric Surgery: A surgeon with expertise in the management of surgical conditions in premature and newborn infants, children and adolescents.

Pediatric Hematology-Oncology

New England

Albritton, Karen H MD [PHO] - **Spec Exp:** Sarcoma; Adolescent/Young Adult Cancers; **Hospital:** Dana-Farber Cancer Inst; **Address:** Dana Farber Cancer Inst, 44 Binney St, Boston, MA 02115; **Phone:** 617-582-7976; **Board Cert:** Internal Medicine 1996; Pediatrics 1996; Medical Oncology 2001; Pediatric Hematology-Oncology 2002; **Med School:** Univ Tex, San Antonio 1992; **Resid:** Internal Medicine & Pediatrics, Univ NC Hosps 1996; **Fellow:** Hematology & Oncology, Univ NC Hosps 2000

Altman, Arnold MD [PHO] - **Spec Exp:** Leukemia; **Hospital:** CT Chldns Med Ctr; **Address:** CT Childrens Med Ctr, Hematology/Oncology, 282 Washington St, Ste 2J, Hartford, CT 06106; **Phone:** 860-545-9630; **Board Cert:** Pediatrics 1971; Pediatric Hematology-Oncology 1974; **Med School:** Johns Hopkins Univ 1965; **Resid:** Pediatrics, Chldns Hosp Med Ctr 1970; **Fellow:** Pediatric Hematology-Oncology, Chldns Hosp Med Ctr 1972; **Fac Appt:** Prof Ped, Univ Conn

Diller, Lisa R MD [PHO] - **Spec Exp:** Brain Tumors; Neuroblastoma; Cancer Survivors-Late Effects of Therapy; **Hospital:** Dana-Farber Cancer Inst; **Address:** Dana-Farber Cancer Inst, 44 Binney St, Dana 1646, Boston, MA 02115; **Phone:** 617-632-5642; **Board Cert:** Pediatric Hematology-Oncology 2000; **Med School:** UCSD 1985; **Resid:** Pediatrics, Chldns Hosp 1988; **Fellow:** Pediatric Hematology-Oncology, Chldns Hosp-Dana Farber Cancer Inst 1991; **Fac Appt:** Assoc Prof Ped, Harvard Med Sch

Fisher, David E MD/PhD [PHO] - **Spec Exp:** Melanoma; **Hospital:** Dana-Farber Cancer Inst; **Address:** Dana-Faber Cancer Inst, Dana 630, 44 Binney St, Boston, MA 02115; **Phone:** 617-632-4916; **Board Cert:** Internal Medicine 1989; Medical Oncology 1991; **Med School:** Cornell Univ-Weill Med Coll 1985; **Resid:** Internal Medicine, Mass Genl Hosp 1988; **Fellow:** Pediatric Hematology-Oncology, Dana-Faber CAncer Inst 1992; **Fac Appt:** Prof Ped, Harvard Med Sch

Grier, Holcombe E MD [PHO] - **Spec Exp:** Bone Cancer; Ewing's Sarcoma; **Hospital:** Dana-Farber Cancer Inst, Children's Hospital - Boston; **Address:** Dana Farber Cancer Inst, 44 Binney St, G350, Boston, MA 02115; **Phone:** 617-632-3971; **Board Cert:** Pediatrics 1983; Internal Medicine 1980; Pediatric Hematology-Oncology 1998; **Med School:** Univ Pennsylvania 1976; **Resid:** Pediatrics, NC Meml Hosp 1980; Internal Medicine, NC Meml Hosp 1980; **Fellow:** Pediatric Oncology, Dana Farber Children's Hosp 1984; **Fac Appt:** Assoc Prof Ped, Harvard Med Sch

Homans, Alan C MD [PHO] - **Spec Exp:** Leukemia; **Hospital:** FAHC - Med Ctr Campus; **Address:** Vermont Childrens Hosp, 111 Colchester Ave, Smith 5-rm 559, Burlington, VT 05401; **Phone:** 802-847-2850; **Board Cert:** Pediatrics 1985; Pediatric Hematology-Oncology 1987; **Med School:** Ohio State Univ 1979; **Resid:** Pediatrics, Med Ctr Hosp 1981; Pediatrics, Univ Massachusetts Med Ctr 1981; **Fellow:** Pediatric Hematology Oncology, Rhode Island Hosp 1985; **Fac Appt:** Prof Ped, Univ VT Coll Med

Hurwitz, Craig A MD [PHO] - **Spec Exp:** Leukemia; Brain Tumors; **Hospital:** Maine Med Ctr; **Address:** Maine Childrens Cancer Program, 100 Campus Drive, Unit 107, Scarborough, ME 04074; **Phone:** 207-885-7565; **Board Cert:** Pediatrics 1986; Pediatric Hematology-Oncology 2000; **Med School:** Univ Tex SW, Dallas 1982; **Resid:** Pediatrics, Duke Univ Med Ctr 1985; **Fellow:** Pediatric Hematology-Oncology, Duke Univ Med Ctr 1988; **Fac Appt:** Assoc Clin Prof Ped, Univ VT Coll Med

Pediatric Hematology-Oncology

Israel, Mark A MD [PHO] - **Spec Exp:** Neuro-Oncology; Brain Tumors; Neuroblastoma; **Hospital:** Dartmouth - Hitchcock Med Ctr; **Address:** Norris Cotton Cancer Ctr, One Medical Center Drive, Lebanon, NH 03756; **Phone:** 603-653-3611; **Board Cert:** Pediatrics 1982; **Med School:** Albert Einstein Coll Med 1973; **Resid:** Pediatrics, Chldns Hosp Med Ctr 1975; **Fellow:** Pediatric Hematology-Oncology, Natl Cancer Inst 1981; **Fac Appt:** Prof Ped, Dartmouth Med Sch

Kieran, Mark MD/PhD [PHO] - **Spec Exp:** Brain Tumors; **Hospital:** Children's Hospital - Boston, Dana-Farber Cancer Inst; **Address:** Dana Farber Cancer Inst, 44 Binney St, Shields Warren Ste 331, Boston, MA 02115; **Phone:** 617-632-2680; **Board Cert:** Pediatrics 2000; Pediatric Hematology-Oncology 1996; **Med School:** Canada 1986; **Resid:** Pediatrics, Montreal Chldns Hosp 1992; **Fellow:** Pediatric Hematology-Oncology, Chldns Hosp 1995; **Fac Appt:** Asst Prof Ped, Harvard Med Sch

Kretschmar, Cynthia S MD [PHO] - **Spec Exp:** Brain Tumors; Neuroblastoma; Drug Discovery & Development; **Hospital:** Tufts-New England Med Ctr; **Address:** Floating Hosp, Div Pediatric Hem/Onc, 750 Washington St, NEMC 14, Boston, MA 02111; **Phone:** 617-636-5535; **Board Cert:** Pediatrics 1984; Pediatric Hematology-Oncology 1987; **Med School:** Yale Univ 1978; **Resid:** Pediatrics, Yale-New Haven Hosp 1981; **Fellow:** Pediatric Hematology-Oncology, Dana Farber Cancer Inst 1984; **Fac Appt:** Prof Ped, Tufts Univ

Schwartz, Cindy Lee MD [PHO] - **Spec Exp:** Hodgkin's Disease; Bone Cancer; Cancer Survivors-Late Effects of Therapy; **Hospital:** Rhode Island Hosp; **Address:** RI Hospital, Dept Ped-Div Ped Hem/Onc, 593 Eddy St, MPS, rm 117, Providence, RI 02903-4923; **Phone:** 401-444-5171; **Board Cert:** Pediatrics 1985; Pediatric Hematology-Oncology 2002; **Med School:** Brown Univ 1979; **Resid:** Pediatrics, Johns Hopkins Hosp 1982; **Fellow:** Pediatric Hematology-Oncology, Johns Hopkins Hosp 1985; **Fac Appt:** Prof Med, Brown Univ

Weinstein, Howard J MD [PHO] - **Spec Exp:** Bone Marrow Transplant; Leukemia; Lymphoma; **Hospital:** Mass Genl Hosp; **Address:** 55 Fruit St, Yawkey 8B-8893, Boston, MA 02114-2622; **Phone:** 617-724-3315; **Board Cert:** Pediatrics 1977; **Med School:** Univ MD Sch Med 1972; **Resid:** Pediatrics, Mass Genl Hosp 1974; **Fellow:** Pediatric Hematology-Oncology, Dana Farber Cancer Inst/Chldns Hosp 1977; **Fac Appt:** Prof Ped, Harvard Med Sch

Wolfe, Lawrence C MD [PHO] - **Spec Exp:** Leukemia; Neuro-Oncology; Cancer Survivors-Late Effects of Therapy; Transfusion Medicine; **Hospital:** Tufts-New England Med Ctr, St Anne's Hosp; **Address:** Floating Hosp, Div Pediatric Hem/Onc, 750 Washington St, NEMC 014, Boston, MA 02111; **Phone:** 617-636-5535; **Board Cert:** Pediatrics 1981; Pediatric Hematology-Oncology 1987; **Med School:** Harvard Med Sch 1976; **Resid:** Pediatrics, Chldns Hosp 1978; **Fellow:** Pediatric Hematology-Oncology, Chldns Hosp 1991; **Fac Appt:** Assoc Prof Ped, Tulane Univ

Mid Atlantic

Adamson, Peter C MD [PHO] - **Spec Exp:** Drug Development; Clinical Trials; Rhabdomyosarcoma; **Hospital:** Chldns Hosp of Philadelphia, The; **Address:** Chldns Hosp of Philadelphia, 34th St & Civic Ctr Blvd Abramson Bldg, Philadelphia, PA 19104; **Phone:** 215-590-2299; **Board Cert:** Pediatrics 1988; Pediatric Hematology-Oncology 2005; **Med School:** Cornell Univ-Weill Med Coll 1984; **Resid:** Pediatrics, Children's Hosp 1987; **Fellow:** Pediatric Hematology-Oncology, Natl Cancer Inst 1990; **Fac Appt:** Assoc Prof Pharm, Univ Pennsylvania

Arceci, Robert J MD/PhD [PHO] - **Spec Exp:** Leukemia; Histiocytoma; Bone Marrow Transplant; **Hospital:** Johns Hopkins Hosp - Baltimore; **Address:** Kimmel Cancer Ctr, Bunting-Blaustein Bldg, 1650 Orleans St, CRB 2M51, Baltimore, MD 21231-1000; **Phone:** 410-502-7519; **Board Cert:** Pediatrics 1987; Pediatric Hematology-Oncology 2005; **Med School:** Univ Rochester 1981; **Resid:** Pediatrics, Chldns Hosp 1983; **Fellow:** Pediatric Hematology-Oncology, Chldns Hosp/Dana Farber Cancer Ctr 1986; **Fac Appt:** Prof Ped, Johns Hopkins Univ

Brecher, Martin L MD [PHO] - **Spec Exp:** Brain Tumors; Lymphoma; Hodgkin's Disease; Leukemia; **Hospital:** Roswell Park Cancer Inst, Women's & Chldn's Hosp of Buffalo, The; **Address:** Roswell Park Cancer Inst, Dept Pediatrics, Elm & Carlton Sts, Buffalo, NY 14263; **Phone:** 716-845-2333; **Board Cert:** Pediatrics 1977; Pediatric Hematology-Oncology 1978; **Med School:** SUNY Buffalo 1972; **Resid:** Pediatrics, Buffalo Chldns Hosp 1975; **Fellow:** Hematology & Oncology, Buffalo Chldns Hosp/Roswell Park Cancer Inst 1977; **Fac Appt:** Prof Ped, SUNY Buffalo

Brodeur, Garrett MD [PHO] - **Spec Exp:** Neuroblastoma; **Hospital:** Chldns Hosp of Philadelphia, The; **Address:** Chldns Hosp Philadelphia, 34th St & Civic Ctr Blvd Abramson Bldg, Philadelphia, PA 19104; **Phone:** 215-590-2817; **Board Cert:** Pediatrics 1980; Pediatric Hematology-Oncology 1980; **Med School:** Washington Univ, St Louis 1975; **Resid:** Pediatrics, St Louis Childrens Hosp 1977; **Fellow:** Pediatric Hematology-Oncology, St Jude Childrens Rsch Hosp 1979; **Fac Appt:** Prof Ped, Univ Pennsylvania

Bussel, James MD [PHO] - **Spec Exp:** Autoimmune Disease; Bleeding/Coagulation Disorders; **Hospital:** NY-Presby Hosp (page 79), Lenox Hill Hosp; **Address:** 525 E 68th St, rm P-695, New York, NY 10021; **Phone:** 212-746-3474; **Board Cert:** Pediatrics 1979; Pediatric Hematology-Oncology 1981; **Med School:** Columbia P&S 1975; **Resid:** Pediatrics, Chldns Hosp 1978; **Fellow:** Pediatric Hematology-Oncology, NY Hosp 1981; **Fac Appt:** Prof Ped, Cornell Univ-Weill Med Coll

Cairo, Mitchell S MD [PHO] - **Spec Exp:** Bone Marrow Transplant; Leukemia; Lymphoma; **Hospital:** NY-Presby Hosp (page 79); **Address:** Babies/Chldns Hosp-Presby Med Ctr, 3959 Broadway, CHONY-11, Central-1114, New York, NY 10032; **Phone:** 212-305-8316; **Board Cert:** Pediatrics 1980; Pediatric Hematology-Oncology 1982; **Med School:** UCSF 1976; **Resid:** Pediatrics, UCLA Med Ctr 1978; **Fellow:** Pediatric Hematology-Oncology, Indiana Univ Med Ctr 1981; **Fac Appt:** Prof Ped, Columbia P&S

Carroll, William L MD [PHO] - **Spec Exp:** Pediatric Cancers; Leukemia; **Hospital:** NYU Med Ctr (page 80); **Address:** NYU Med Ctr, Div Ped Hem/Onc, 160 E 32nd St Fl 2, New York, NY 10016; **Phone:** 212-263-9947; **Board Cert:** Pediatrics 1984; Pediatric Hematology-Oncology 1987; **Med School:** UC Irvine 1978; **Resid:** Pediatrics, Chldns Hosp Med Ctr 1981; **Fellow:** Pediatric Hematology-Oncology, Stanford Univ 1987; **Fac Appt:** Prof Ped, NYU Sch Med

Chen, Allen R MD/PhD [PHO] - **Spec Exp:** Bone Marrow Transplant; Hodgkin's Disease; Immunotherapy; Graft vs Host Disease; **Hospital:** Johns Hopkins Hosp - Baltimore; **Address:** Johns Hopkins Hosp, Div Peds Oncology, 1650 Orleans St, CRB 2M53, Baltimore, MD 21231; **Phone:** 410-955-7385; **Board Cert:** Pediatrics 2002; **Med School:** Duke Univ 1986; **Resid:** Pediatrics, Chldns Hosp Med Ctr 1989; **Fellow:** Pediatric Hematology-Oncology, Fred Hutchinson Canc Ctr 1993; Bone Marrow Transplant, Fred Hutchinson Canc Ctr 1994; **Fac Appt:** Assoc Prof Ped, Johns Hopkins Univ

Pediatric Hematology-Oncology

Civin, Curt Ingraham MD [PHO] - **Spec Exp:** Pediatric Cancers; Leukemia; Bone Marrow Transplant; **Hospital:** Johns Hopkins Hosp - Baltimore; **Address:** 1650 Orleans St, rm CRB-2M44, Baltimore, MD 21231-1000; **Phone:** 410-955-8816; **Board Cert:** Pediatrics 1979; Pediatric Hematology-Oncology 1980; **Med School:** Harvard Med Sch 1974; **Resid:** Pediatrics, Chldns Hosp 1976; **Fellow:** Pediatric Hematology-Oncology, Natl Cancer Inst 1979; **Fac Appt:** Prof Ped, Johns Hopkins Univ

Drachtman, Richard MD [PHO] - **Spec Exp:** Pediatric Cancers; **Hospital:** Robert Wood Johnson Univ Hosp - New Brunswick, Jersey Shore Univ Med Ctr; **Address:** Cancer Inst of New Jersey, 195 Little Albany St, New Brunswick, NJ 08903-2681; **Phone:** 732-235-5437; **Board Cert:** Pediatrics 2000; Pediatric Hematology-Oncology 2000; **Med School:** Ros Franklin Univ/Chicago Med Sch 1984; **Resid:** Pediatrics, N Shore Univ Hosp 1988; **Fellow:** Pediatric Hematology-Oncology, Mount Sinai Hosp 1991; **Fac Appt:** Assoc Prof Ped, UMDNJ-RW Johnson Med Sch

Dunkel, Ira J MD [PHO] - **Spec Exp:** Retinoblastoma; Brain & Spinal Cord Tumors; Brain Tumors; Pediatric Cancers; **Hospital:** Meml Sloan Kettering Cancer Ctr (page 76); **Address:** Meml Sloan-Kettering Cancer Ctr, Dept Peds, 1275 York Ave, rm H-1102, New York, NY 10021; **Phone:** 212-639-2153; **Board Cert:** Pediatric Hematology-Oncology 2000; **Med School:** Duke Univ 1985; **Resid:** Pediatrics, Duke Univ Med Ctr 1988; **Fellow:** Pediatric Hematology-Oncology, Memorial-Sloan Kettering 1992; **Fac Appt:** Asst Prof Ped, Cornell Univ-Weill Med Coll

Felix, Carolyn A MD [PHO] - **Spec Exp:** Leukemia; Leukemia in Infants; **Hospital:** Chldns Hosp of Philadelphia, The; **Address:** Chldns Hosp of Philadelphia, 34th St & Civic Ctr Blvd Abramson Bldg, Philadelphia, PA 19104; **Phone:** 215-590-2831; **Board Cert:** Pediatrics 1987; Pediatric Hematology-Oncology 1987; **Med School:** Boston Univ 1981; **Resid:** Pediatrics, Chldns Hosp 1984; **Fellow:** Pediatric Hematology-Oncology, Natl Cancer Inst-Pediatric Br 1987; **Fac Appt:** Assoc Prof Ped, Univ Pennsylvania

Frantz, Christopher N MD [PHO] - **Spec Exp:** Solid Tumors; Neuroblastoma; Leukemia; **Hospital:** Alfred I duPont Hosp for Children, Christiana Care Hlth Svs; **Address:** Alfred I duPont Hosp for Chldn, 1600 Rockland Rd, Box 269, Wilmington, DE 19899; **Phone:** 302-651-5500; **Board Cert:** Pediatrics 1977; Pediatric Hematology-Oncology 2005; **Med School:** Albert Einstein Coll Med 1971; **Resid:** Pediatrics, Chldns Hosp 1976; **Fellow:** Pediatric Hematology-Oncology, Chldns Hosp/Dana Farber Cancer Inst 1979

Garvin, James MD/PhD [PHO] - **Spec Exp:** Bone Marrow Transplant; Brain Tumors; Pediatric Cancers; **Hospital:** NY-Presby Hosp (page 79), St Joseph's Regl Med Ctr - Paterson; **Address:** 161 Fort Washington Ave Fl 7 - rm 708, New York, NY 10032; **Phone:** 212-305-8685; **Board Cert:** Pediatrics 1982; Pediatric Hematology-Oncology 1984; **Med School:** Jefferson Med Coll 1976; **Resid:** Pediatrics, Chldns Hosp 1978; Pediatrics, Middlesex Hosp 1979; **Fellow:** Pediatric Hematology-Oncology, Dana Farber Cancer Inst/Childrens Hosp 1982; **Fac Appt:** Clin Prof Ped, Columbia P&S

Green, Daniel M MD [PHO] - **Spec Exp:** Wilms' Tumor; Fertility in Cancer Survivors; Cancer Survivors-Late Effects of Therapy; **Hospital:** Roswell Park Cancer Inst, Women's & Chldn's Hosp of Buffalo, The; **Address:** Roswell Park Cancer Inst, Dept Pediatrics, Elm & Carlton Sts, Buffalo, NY 14263; **Phone:** 716-845-2334; **Board Cert:** Pediatrics 1986; Pediatric Hematology-Oncology 1997; **Med School:** St Louis Univ 1973; **Resid:** Pediatrics, Boston City Hosp 1975; **Fellow:** Pediatric Hematology-Oncology, Chldn's Hosp Med Ctr 1978; **Fac Appt:** Prof Ped, SUNY Buffalo

Grupp, Stephan A MD [PHO] - **Spec Exp:** Stem Cell Transplant; Neuroblastoma; Bone Marrow Transplant; **Hospital:** Chldns Hosp of Philadelphia, The; **Address:** Childrens Hosp - Oncology, 34th St & Civic Ctr Blvd Abramson Bldg, Philadelphia, PA 19104; **Phone:** 215-590-2821; **Board Cert:** Pediatric Hematology-Oncology 2002; **Med School:** Univ Cincinnati 1987; **Resid:** Pediatrics, Chldns Hosp 1990; **Fellow:** Pediatric Hematology-Oncology, Dana Farber Cancer Inst/Chldns Hosp 1992; **Fac Appt:** Asst Prof Ped, Univ Pennsylvania

Halpern, Steven MD [PHO] - **Spec Exp:** Leukemia; Brain Tumors; **Hospital:** Hackensack Univ Med Ctr (page 74), Overlook Hosp; **Address:** 30 Prospect Ave, Ste TCI, Hackensack, NJ 07601; **Phone:** 201-996-5437; **Board Cert:** Pediatrics 1981; Pediatric Hematology-Oncology 1982; **Med School:** Ros Franklin Univ/Chicago Med Sch 1976; **Resid:** Pediatrics, St Christopher's Hosp for Children 1979; **Fellow:** Pediatric Hematology-Oncology, Childrens Hosp 1982; **Fac Appt:** Asst Prof Ped, UMDNJ-NJ Med Sch, Newark

Harris, Michael B MD [PHO] - **Spec Exp:** Leukemia & Lymphoma; Bone Tumors; Cancer Survivors-Late Effects of Therapy; **Hospital:** Hackensack Univ Med Ctr (page 74); **Address:** Tomorrows Chldns Inst, JM Sanzari Chldns Hosp, 30 Prospect Ave, Imus 1-TCI, rm PC116, Hackensack, NJ 07601; **Phone:** 201-996-5437; **Board Cert:** Pediatrics 1974; Pediatric Hematology-Oncology 1974; **Med School:** Albert Einstein Coll Med 1969; **Resid:** Pediatrics, Chldns Hosp 1971; **Fellow:** Pediatric Hematology-Oncology, Chldns Hosp 1974; **Fac Appt:** Prof Ped, UMDNJ-NJ Med Sch, Newark

Helman, Lee Jay MD [PHO] - **Spec Exp:** Solid Tumors; **Hospital:** Natl Inst of Hlth - Clin Ctr; **Address:** National Cancer Inst, NIH, 31 Center Drive, rm 3A11, Bethesda, MD 20892-2440; **Phone:** 301-496-4257; **Board Cert:** Internal Medicine 1983; Medical Oncology 1985; **Med School:** Univ MD Sch Med 1980; **Resid:** Internal Medicine, Barnes Hosp 1983; **Fellow:** Oncology, Natl Inst Hlth 1986

Hinkle, Andrea S MD [PHO] - **Spec Exp:** Cancer Survivors-Late Effects of Therapy; **Hospital:** Univ of Rochester Strong Meml Hosp; **Address:** Golisano Childrens Hosp at Strong, 601 Elmwood Ave, Box 667, Rochester, NY 14642; **Phone:** 585-275-8138; **Board Cert:** Pediatrics 1999; Pediatric Hematology-Oncology 2000; **Med School:** Brown Univ 1987; **Resid:** Pediatrics, Boston City Hosp 1991; **Fellow:** Pediatric Hematology-Oncology, Chldns Natl Med Ctr 1994; **Fac Appt:** Asst Prof Ped, Univ Rochester

Jakacki, Regina MD [PHO] - **Spec Exp:** Neuro-Oncology; Clinical Trials; Palliative Care; **Hospital:** Chldns Hosp of Pittsburgh - UPMC; **Address:** Children's Hospital Pittsburgh, 3705 Fifth Ave, rm 4B 220, Pittsburgh, PA 15213; **Phone:** 412-692-7056; **Board Cert:** Pediatric Hematology-Oncology 2000; **Med School:** Univ Pennsylvania 1985; **Resid:** Pediatrics, Childrens Hosp 1988; **Fellow:** Pediatric Hematology-Oncology, Childrens Hosp 1991; **Fac Appt:** Assoc Prof Ped, Univ Pittsburgh

Kamen, Barton A MD/PhD [PHO] - **Spec Exp:** Drug Development; Leukemia; **Hospital:** Robert Wood Johnson Univ Hosp - New Brunswick; **Address:** Cancer Inst of New Jersey, 195 Little Albany St, rm 3507, New Brunswick, NJ 08903; **Phone:** 732-235-8864; **Board Cert:** Pediatrics 1981; Pediatric Hematology-Oncology 1987; **Med School:** Case West Res Univ 1976; **Resid:** Pediatrics, Yale-New Haven Hosp 1978; **Fellow:** Pediatric Hematology-Oncology, Yale-New Haven Hosp 1980; **Fac Appt:** Prof Ped, UMDNJ-RW Johnson Med Sch

Pediatric Hematology-Oncology

Korones, David MD [PHO] - **Spec Exp:** Brain Tumors; Palliative Care; Pediatric Cancers; **Hospital:** Univ of Rochester Strong Meml Hosp; **Address:** Golisano Childrens Hosp at Strong, 601 Elmwood Ave, Box 777, Rochester, NY 14642-8777; **Phone:** 585-275-2981; **Board Cert:** Pediatrics 1987; Pediatric Hematology-Oncology 1998; **Med School:** Vanderbilt Univ 1983; **Resid:** Pediatrics, Strong Meml Hosp 1986; **Fellow:** Pediatrics, Yale Univ 1988; Pediatric Hematology-Oncology, Strong Meml Hosp 1991; **Fac Appt:** Assoc Prof Ped, Univ Rochester

Kushner, Brian H MD [PHO] - **Spec Exp:** Neuroblastoma; Bone Marrow Transplant; Immunotherapy; **Hospital:** Meml Sloan Kettering Cancer Ctr (page 76); **Address:** 1275 York Ave, rm H1113, New York, NY 10021-6007; **Phone:** 212-639-6793; **Board Cert:** Pediatrics 1983; Pediatric Hematology-Oncology 1987; **Med School:** Johns Hopkins Univ 1976; **Resid:** Pediatrics, Columbia-Presby Med Ctr 1978; Pediatrics, New York Hosp 1979; **Fellow:** Pediatric Hematology-Oncology, Boston Chldns Hosp 1980; Pediatric Hematology-Oncology, Meml Sloan Kettering Cancer Ctr 1986; **Fac Appt:** Prof Ped, Cornell Univ-Weill Med Coll

Lange, Beverly MD [PHO] - **Spec Exp:** Leukemia; Brain & Spinal Cord Tumors; **Hospital:** Chldns Hosp of Philadelphia, The; **Address:** Chldns Hosp Philadelphia, Div of Oncol, 34th St & Civic Ctr Blvd Abramson Bldg, Philadelphia, PA 19104; **Phone:** 215-590-2249; **Board Cert:** Pediatrics 1976; Pediatric Hematology-Oncology 1997; **Med School:** Temple Univ 1971; **Resid:** Pediatrics, Philadelphia Genl Hosp 1973; **Fellow:** Pediatric Oncology, Chldns Hosp; **Fac Appt:** Prof Ped, Univ Pennsylvania

Lanzkowsky, Philip MD [PHO] - **Spec Exp:** Solid Tumors; Leukemia; **Hospital:** Schneider Chldn's Hosp, N Shore Univ Hosp at Manhasset; **Address:** 269-01 76th Ave, Ste CH102, New Hyde Park, NY 11040-1434; **Phone:** 718-470-3460; **Board Cert:** Pediatrics 1966; Pediatric Hematology-Oncology 1974; **Med School:** South Africa 1954; **Resid:** Pediatrics, Red Cross War Meml Chldns Hosp 1960; Pediatrics, St Mary's Hosp 1961; **Fellow:** Pediatric Hematology-Oncology, Duke Univ Med Ctr 1962; Pediatric Hematology-Oncology, Univ UT Hosp 1963; **Fac Appt:** Prof Ped, Albert Einstein Coll Med

Lipton, Jeffrey M MD/PhD [PHO] - **Spec Exp:** Bone Marrow Failure Disorders; Stem Cell Transplant; Bone Marrow Transplant; **Hospital:** Schneider Chldn's Hosp; **Address:** Div Hem-Onc & Stem Cell Transplant, 269-01 76th Ave, rm 255, MC-07670, New Hyde Park, NY 11040-1433; **Phone:** 718-470-3460; **Board Cert:** Pediatrics 1981; **Med School:** St Louis Univ 1975; **Resid:** Pediatrics, Boston Chldns Hosp 1977; **Fellow:** Pediatric Hematology-Oncology, Boston Chldns Hosp/Dana Farber Cancer Inst 1979; **Fac Appt:** Prof Ped, Albert Einstein Coll Med

Maris, John M MD [PHO] - **Spec Exp:** Neuroblastoma; Clinical Trials; **Hospital:** Chldns Hosp of Philadelphia, The; **Address:** Chldns Hosp Philadelphia - Oncology, 34th St & Civic Ctr Blvd Abramson Bldg, Philadelphia, PA 19104-4318; **Phone:** 215-590-2821; **Board Cert:** Pediatric Hematology-Oncology 2004; **Med School:** Univ Pennsylvania 1989; **Resid:** Pediatrics, Chldns Hosp 1992; **Fellow:** Pediatric Hematology-Oncology, Chldns Hosp 1996

Meadows, Anna T MD [PHO] - **Spec Exp:** Cancer Survivors-Late Effects of Therapy; Clinical Trials; Retinoblastoma; **Hospital:** Chldns Hosp of Philadelphia, The; **Address:** Childrens Hospital, Div Oncology, 34th St & Civic Center Blvd, Philadelphia, PA 19104; **Phone:** 215-590-2279; **Board Cert:** Pediatrics 1974; Pediatric Hematology-Oncology 1974; **Med School:** Med Coll PA 1969; **Resid:** Pediatrics, St Christophers Hosp 1971; **Fellow:** Pediatric Hematology-Oncology, St Christophers Hosp 1972; **Fac Appt:** Prof Ped, Univ Pennsylvania

Meek, Rita S MD [PHO] - **Hospital:** Alfred I duPont Hosp for Children, Christiana Care Hlth Svs; **Address:** Dupont Hosp for Children, Div Hem-Onc, 1600 Rockland Rd, Wilmington, DE 19899; **Phone:** 302-651-5500; **Board Cert:** Pediatrics 1979; Pediatric Hematology-Oncology 1980; **Med School:** Geo Wash Univ 1974; **Resid:** Pediatrics, Childns Hosp Natl Med Ctr 1977; **Fellow:** Pediatric Hematology-Oncology, Chldns Hosp Natl Med Ctr 1979; **Fac Appt:** Assoc Clin Prof Ped, Jefferson Med Coll

Meyers, Paul MD [PHO] - **Spec Exp:** Pediatric Cancers; Bone Tumors; Sarcoma; **Hospital:** Meml Sloan Kettering Cancer Ctr (page 76), NY-Presby Hosp (page 79); **Address:** 1275 York Ave, Box 471, New York, NY 10021-6007; **Phone:** 212-639-5952; **Board Cert:** Pediatrics 1978; Pediatric Hematology-Oncology 1978; **Med School:** Mount Sinai Sch Med 1973; **Resid:** Pediatrics, Mt Sinai Hosp 1976; **Fellow:** Pediatric Hematology-Oncology, New York Hosp-Cornell 1979; **Fac Appt:** Prof Ped, Cornell Univ-Weill Med Coll

O'Reilly, Richard MD [PHO] - **Spec Exp:** Bone Marrow Transplant; **Hospital:** Meml Sloan Kettering Cancer Ctr (page 76), NY-Presby Hosp (page 79); **Address:** 1275 York Ave, rm H1409, New York, NY 10021; **Phone:** 212-639-5957; **Board Cert:** Pediatrics 1974; **Med School:** Univ Rochester 1968; **Resid:** Pediatrics, Chldrns Hosp 1972; **Fellow:** Infectious Disease, Chldrns Hosp 1973; **Fac Appt:** Prof Ped, Cornell Univ-Weill Med Coll

Parker, Robert MD [PHO] - **Spec Exp:** Pediatric Cancers; Bleeding/Coagulation Disorders; Lymphoma; **Hospital:** Stony Brook Univ Med Ctr; **Address:** Stony Brook Univ Hosp, Dept Peds, HSC T-11, Rm 029, Stony Brook, NY 11794-8111; **Phone:** 631-444-7720; **Board Cert:** Pediatrics 1983; Pediatric Hematology-Oncology 1984; **Med School:** Brown Univ 1976; **Resid:** Internal Medicine, Roger Williams Med Ctr 1977; Pediatrics, Rhode Island Hosp 1979; **Fellow:** Pediatric Hematology-Oncology, Natl Cancer Inst 1981; Hematology, Natl Cancer Inst 1984; **Fac Appt:** Prof Ped, SUNY Stony Brook

Rausen, Aaron R MD [PHO] - **Spec Exp:** Leukemia & Lymphoma; Bone Tumors; Retinoblastoma; **Hospital:** NYU Med Ctr (page 80), Lenox Hill Hosp; **Address:** NYU Medical Ctr, 160 E 32nd St Fl 2, New York, NY 10016; **Phone:** 212-263-7144; **Board Cert:** Pediatrics 1960; Pediatric Hematology-Oncology 1974; **Med School:** SUNY Downstate 1954; **Resid:** Pediatrics, Bellevue Hosp 1956; Pediatrics, Mount Sinai 1959; **Fellow:** Hematology, Chldns Hosp 1961; **Fac Appt:** Prof Ped, NYU Sch Med

Reaman, Gregory MD [PHO] - **Spec Exp:** Leukemia; Lymphoma; Cancer Survivors-Late Effects of Therapy; **Hospital:** Chldns Natl Med Ctr; **Address:** Childrens National Med Ctr, 111 Michigan Ave NW, Washington, DC 20010-2916; **Phone:** 202-884-2800; **Board Cert:** Pediatrics 1978; Pediatric Hematology-Oncology 1978; **Med School:** Loyola Univ-Stritch Sch Med 1973; **Resid:** Hematology, Montreal Chldns Hosp 1975; Pediatrics, Montreal Chldns Hosp 1976; **Fellow:** Pediatric Oncology, Natl Cancer Inst 1979; **Fac Appt:** Prof Ped, Geo Wash Univ

Rheingold, Susan R MD [PHO] - **Spec Exp:** Leukemia; Clinical Trials; Complementary Medicine; **Hospital:** Chldns Hosp of Philadelphia, The; **Address:** Chldns Hosp Phila - Div Oncology, 34th & Civic Ctr Blvd, Philadelphia, PA 19104; **Phone:** 215-590-3025; **Board Cert:** Pediatrics 2003; Pediatric Hematology-Oncology 2000; **Med School:** Univ Pennsylvania 1992; **Resid:** Pediatrics, Johns Hopkins Hosp 1995; **Fellow:** Pediatric Hematology-Oncology, Chldns Hosp 1999; **Fac Appt:** Asst Prof Ped, Univ Pennsylvania

Pediatric Hematology-Oncology

Ritchey, Arthur MD [PHO] - **Spec Exp:** Leukemia; **Hospital:** Chldns Hosp of Pittsburgh - UPMC; **Address:** Chldns Hosp, Div Hematology/Oncology, 3705 Fifth Ave, Desoto Wing 4B, Ste 385, Pittsburgh, PA 15213; **Phone:** 412-692-5055; **Board Cert:** Pediatrics 1977; Pediatric Hematology-Oncology 2000; **Med School:** Univ Cincinnati 1972; **Resid:** Pediatrics, Johns Hopkins Hosp 1975; **Fellow:** Pediatric Hematology-Oncology, Yale-New Haven Hosp 1980; **Fac Appt:** Prof Ped, Univ Pittsburgh

Steinherz, Peter G MD [PHO] - **Spec Exp:** Leukemia & Lymphoma; Pediatric Cancers; Wilms' Tumor; **Hospital:** Meml Sloan Kettering Cancer Ctr (page 76), NY-Presby Hosp (page 79); **Address:** Memorial Sloan Kettering Cancer Ctr, 1275 York Ave, Box 411, New York, NY 10021; **Phone:** 212-639-7951; **Board Cert:** Pediatrics 1973; Pediatric Hematology-Oncology 1978; **Med School:** Albert Einstein Coll Med 1968; **Resid:** Pediatrics, New York Hosp-Cornell 1971; **Fellow:** Pediatric Hematology-Oncology, New York Hosp-Cornell 1975; **Fac Appt:** Prof Ped, Cornell Univ-Weill Med Coll

Weinblatt, Mark E MD [PHO] - **Spec Exp:** Leukemia; Lymphoma; Bleeding/Coagulation Disorders; **Hospital:** Winthrop - Univ Hosp; **Address:** Winthrop Univ Hosp, 200 Old Country Rd, Mineola, NY 11501; **Phone:** 516-663-9400; **Board Cert:** Pediatrics 1980; Pediatric Hematology-Oncology 1982; **Med School:** Albert Einstein Coll Med 1976; **Resid:** Pediatrics, Jacobi Med Ctr 1979; **Fellow:** Pediatric Hematology-Oncology, Children's Hosp 1981; **Fac Appt:** Prof Ped, SUNY Stony Brook

Weiner, Michael MD [PHO] - **Spec Exp:** Hodgkin's Disease; Lymphoma; Leukemia; **Hospital:** NY-Presby Hosp (page 79), St Joseph's Regl Med Ctr - Paterson; **Address:** 161 Fort Washington Ave, Irving Pavilion-FL 7, New York, NY 10032-3710; **Phone:** 212-305-9770; **Board Cert:** Pediatrics 1980; Pediatric Hematology-Oncology 1980; **Med School:** SUNY Hlth Sci Ctr 1972; **Resid:** Pediatrics, Montefiore Med Ctr 1974; **Fellow:** Pediatric Hematology-Oncology, NYU Med Ctr 1976; Pediatric Hematology-Oncology, Johns Hopkins Hosp 1977; **Fac Appt:** Prof Ped, Columbia P&S

Wexler, Leonard MD [PHO] - **Spec Exp:** Rhabdomyosarcoma; Bone Cancer; Gastrointestinal Stromal Tumors; Sarcoma-Soft Tissue; **Hospital:** Meml Sloan Kettering Cancer Ctr (page 76); **Address:** 1275 York Ave, Box 210, New York, NY 10021; **Phone:** 212-639-7990; **Board Cert:** Pediatrics 2000; Pediatric Hematology-Oncology 2000; **Med School:** Boston Univ 1985; **Resid:** Pediatrics, Montefiore Med Ctr 1988; **Fellow:** Pediatric Hematology-Oncology, National Cancer Inst 1991; **Fac Appt:** Assoc Prof Ped, Columbia P&S

Southeast

Barredo, Julio C MD [PHO] - **Spec Exp:** Cancer Survivors-Late Effects of Therapy; Clinical Trials; **Hospital:** Univ of Miami Hosp & Clins/Sylvester Comp Canc Ctr; **Address:** Univ Miami Hosp, Dept Pediatrics, R131 PO Box 016960, Miami, FL; **Phone:** 305-585-5635; **Board Cert:** Pediatrics 2000; Pediatric Hematology-Oncology 2000; **Med School:** Peru 1982; **Resid:** Pediatrics, Kings Co Hosp 1987; **Fellow:** Pediatric Hematology-Oncology, Chldns Hosp/USC; **Fac Appt:** Prof Ped, Med Univ SC

Bertolone, Salvatore MD [PHO] - **Spec Exp:** Bone Marrow Transplant; Kasabach-Merritt Syndrome (KMS); **Hospital:** Kosair Chldn's Hosp, Norton Hosp; **Address:** Kosair Childrens Hosp, Ped Hem/Onc, 571 S Floyd, rm 445, Louisville, KY 40202-3820; **Phone:** 502-852-8450; **Board Cert:** Pediatrics 1975; Pediatric Hematology-Oncology 1976; **Med School:** Univ Louisville Sch Med 1970; **Resid:** Pediatrics, Univ Louisville 1972; **Fellow:** Pediatric Hematology-Oncology, Univ Colorado 1974; **Fac Appt:** Prof Ped, Univ Louisville Sch Med

Blatt, Julie MD [PHO] - **Spec Exp:** Neuroblastoma; Cancer Survivors-Late Effects of Therapy; **Hospital:** Univ NC Hosps; **Address:** UNC, Dept Ped Hematology Oncology, CB 7220, Chapel Hill, NC 27599-7220; **Phone:** 919-966-1178; **Board Cert:** Pediatrics 1981; Pediatric Hematology-Oncology 1982; **Med School:** Johns Hopkins Univ 1976; **Resid:** Pediatrics, Columbia-Presby Hosp 1978; **Fellow:** Pediatric Oncology, Natl Cancer Inst 1982; **Fac Appt:** Prof Ped, Univ NC Sch Med

Castleberry Jr, Robert P MD [PHO] - **Spec Exp:** Neuroblastoma; Leukemia; **Hospital:** Children's Hospital - Birmingham, Univ of Ala Hosp at Birmingham; **Address:** Univ of Ala Hosp at Birmingham-Dept Ped, 1600 7th Ave S, Ste ACC 512, Birmingham, AL 35233; **Phone:** 205-939-9285; **Board Cert:** Pediatrics 1977; Pediatric Hematology-Oncology 1998; **Med School:** Med Coll GA 1971; **Resid:** Pediatrics, Chldns Hosp-Univ Ala 1973; **Fellow:** Pediatric Hematology-Oncology, Univ of Ala Hosp 1975; **Fac Appt:** Prof Ped, Univ Ala

Falletta, John MD [PHO] - **Spec Exp:** Hematologic Malignancies; **Hospital:** Duke Univ Med Ctr; **Address:** Duke Univ Med Ctr, 2424 Erwin Rd, Durham, NC 27710; **Phone:** 919-668-5111; **Board Cert:** Pediatrics 1972; Pediatric Hematology-Oncology 1974; **Med School:** Univ Kans 1966; **Resid:** Pediatrics, Texas Childrens Hosp 1971; **Fellow:** Pediatric Hematology-Oncology, Baylor Coll Med 1973; **Fac Appt:** Prof Ped, Duke Univ

Frangoul, Haydar MD [PHO] - **Spec Exp:** Stem Cell Transplant; **Hospital:** Vanderbilt Univ Med Ctr; **Address:** Ped Hem/Onc Clinic, 1215 21st Ave S, 397 PRB, Nashville, TN 37232-6310; **Phone:** 615-936-1762; **Board Cert:** Pediatrics 2001; Pediatric Hematology-Oncology 2000; **Med School:** Amer Univ Beirut 1990; **Resid:** Pediatrics, Duke Univ Med Ctr 1993; **Fellow:** Pediatric Hematology-Oncology, Duke Univ Med Ctr 1994; **Fac Appt:** Assoc Prof Ped, Vanderbilt Univ

Friedman, Henry S MD [PHO] - **Spec Exp:** Neuro-Oncology; Brain & Spinal Cord Tumors; **Hospital:** Duke Univ Med Ctr; **Address:** Brain Tumor Ctr-Duke Univ, Baker House, DUMC, rm 047, Box 3624, Durham, NC 27710; **Phone:** 919-684-5301; **Board Cert:** Pediatrics 1982; Pediatric Hematology-Oncology 1982; **Med School:** SUNY Upstate Med Univ 1977; **Resid:** Pediatrics, SUNY Upstate Med Ctr 1980; **Fellow:** Pediatric Hematology-Oncology, Duke Univ Med Ctr 1983; **Fac Appt:** Prof Ped, Duke Univ

Furman, Wayne L MD [PHO] - **Spec Exp:** Neuroblastoma; Liver Cancer; Drug Development; **Hospital:** St Jude Children's Research Hosp; **Address:** St Jude Children's Research Hospital, 332 N Lauderdale St, MS 260, Memphis, TN 38105; **Phone:** 901-495-2800; **Board Cert:** Pediatrics 1985; Pediatric Hematology-Oncology 1987; **Med School:** Ohio State Univ 1979; **Resid:** Pediatrics, Children's Hosp 1983; **Fellow:** Pediatric Hematology-Oncology, St Jude Children's Rsch Hosp 1985; **Fac Appt:** Prof Ped, Univ Tenn Coll Med, Memphis

Gajjar, Amar MD [PHO] - **Spec Exp:** Brain Tumors; Medulloblastoma; Neuro-Oncology; Drug Development; **Hospital:** St Jude Children's Research Hosp; **Address:** St Judes Children's Hosp, Dept Oncology, 332 N Lauderdale, rm C6024, MS 260, Memphis, TN 38105-2794; **Phone:** 901-495-4599; **Board Cert:** Pediatrics 1989; Pediatric Hematology-Oncology 2000; **Med School:** India 1984; **Resid:** Pediatrics, All Children's Hosp 1989; **Fellow:** Hematology & Oncology, St Jude Children's Hosp 1990; **Fac Appt:** Prof Ped, Univ Tenn Coll Med, Memphis

Godder, Kamar MD/PhD [PHO] - **Spec Exp:** Stem Cell Transplant; Leukemia; Palliative Care; **Hospital:** Med Coll of VA Hosp; **Address:** Va Commonwealth Univ, Sanger Hall-12th Fl, 1101 E Marshall St, Box 980121, Richmond, VA 23219; **Phone:** 804-828-9605; **Board Cert:** Pediatrics 1989; Pediatric Hematology-Oncology 1998; **Med School:** Israel 1980; **Resid:** Pediatrics, Hadassah-Mt Scopus 1984; **Fellow:** Pediatric Hematology-Oncology, Meml Sloan Kettering Cancer Ctr 1988; **Fac Appt:** Prof Ped, Va Commonwealth Univ

Gold, Stuart H MD [PHO] - **Spec Exp:** Leukemia; Brain Tumors; Cancer Survivors-Late Effects of Therapy; **Hospital:** Univ NC Hosps; **Address:** UNC, Dept Ped Hematology Oncology, CB 7220, Chapel Hill, NC 27599-7220; **Phone:** 919-966-1178; **Board Cert:** Pediatrics 1986; Pediatric Hematology-Oncology 1987; **Med School:** Vanderbilt Univ 1981; **Resid:** Pediatrics, Univ Colorado Hlth Sci Ctr 1984; **Fellow:** Pediatric Hematology-Oncology, Univ Colorado Hlth Sci Ctr 1989; **Fac Appt:** Prof Ped, Univ NC Sch Med

Graham-Pole, John R MD [PHO] - **Spec Exp:** Bone Marrow Transplant; Palliative Care; Arts in the Healing Process; **Hospital:** Shands Hlthcre at Univ of FL; **Address:** Shands Hosp, Dept Ped Hem-Onc, 1600 SW Archer Rd, rm M401, Gainesville, FL 32610-0296; **Phone:** 352-392-5633; **Board Cert:** Pediatrics 1983; Pediatric Hematology-Oncology 1987; **Med School:** England 1966; **Resid:** Pediatrics, Hosp Sick Chldn 1968; Pediatrics, Royal Hosp Sick Chldn 1970; **Fellow:** Pediatric Hematology-Oncology, Royal Hosp Sick Chldn 1971; **Fac Appt:** Prof Ped, Univ Fla Coll Med

Hudson, Melissa MD [PHO] - **Spec Exp:** Cancer Survivors-Late Effects of Therapy; Hodgkin's Disease; **Hospital:** St Jude Children's Research Hosp; **Address:** St Jude Children's Research Hosp, 332 N Lauderdale St, MS 73, Memphis, TN 38103; **Phone:** 901-495-3384; **Board Cert:** Pediatrics 1988; Pediatric Hematology-Oncology 1998; **Med School:** Univ Tex SW, Dallas 1983; **Resid:** Pediatrics, Univ Texas Affil Hosps 1986; **Fellow:** Pediatric Hematology-Oncology, MD Anderson Cancer Ctr 1989

Kane, Javier R MD [PHO] - **Spec Exp:** Palliative Care; **Hospital:** St Jude Children's Research Hosp; **Address:** St Jude Chldns Rsch Hosp, Dept Oncology, 332 N Lauderdale St, rm C6040, MS 260, Memphis, TN 38105-2794; **Phone:** 901-495-4152; **Board Cert:** Pediatrics 2000; **Med School:** Mexico 1986; **Resid:** Pediatrics, Austin Med Ed Prog; **Fellow:** Pediatric Hematology-Oncology, Univ Tennessee

Keller Jr, Frank G MD [PHO] - **Spec Exp:** Leukemia; Hodgkin's Disease; **Hospital:** Emory Univ Hosp; **Address:** Emory Healthcare Pediatrics Dept, 2105 Uppergate Drive NE Fl 4, Atlanta, GA 30322; **Phone:** 404-727-5740; **Board Cert:** Pediatric Hematology-Oncology 2002; **Med School:** Univ NC Sch Med 1986; **Resid:** Pediatrics, Vanderbilt Univ Med Ctr 1990; **Fellow:** Pediatric Hematology-Oncology, Duke Univ Med Ctr 1993; **Fac Appt:** Assoc Prof Ped, Emory Univ

Kreissman, Susan G MD [PHO] - **Spec Exp:** Neuroblastoma; Clinical Trials; **Hospital:** Duke Univ Med Ctr; **Address:** Duke Univ Med Ctr, Box 2916, Durham, NC 27710; **Phone:** 919-684-3401; **Board Cert:** Pediatrics 1998; Pediatric Hematology-Oncology 2004; **Med School:** Mount Sinai Sch Med 1985; **Resid:** Pediatrics, Chldns Hosp 1988; **Fellow:** Pediatric Hematology-Oncology, Chldns Hosp/Dana Farber Cancer Inst 1991; **Fac Appt:** Assoc Prof Ped, Duke Univ

Kurtzberg, Joanne MD [PHO] - **Spec Exp:** Stem Cell Transplant; Bone Marrow Transplant; **Hospital:** Duke Univ Med Ctr; **Address:** Duke Univ Med Ctr, 2400 Pratt St, Ste 1400, Durham, NC 27705; **Phone:** 919-668-1100; **Board Cert:** Pediatrics 1982; Pediatric Hematology-Oncology 1982; **Med School:** NY Med Coll 1976; **Resid:** Pediatrics, Dartmouth Med Ctr 1977; Pediatrics, Upstate Med Ctr 1979; **Fellow:** Pediatric Hematology-Oncology, Upstate Med Ctr 1980; Pediatric Hematology-Oncology, Duke Med Ctr 1983; **Fac Appt:** Prof Ped, Duke Univ

Kuttesch, John F MD [PHO] - **Spec Exp:** Brain Tumors; Brain Tumors-Recurrent; **Hospital:** Vanderbilt Children's Hosp; **Address:** Vanderbilt Univ Med Ctr, 2220 Pierce Ave, Rm 397 PRB, Nashville, TN 37232-6310; **Phone:** 615-936-1762; **Board Cert:** Pediatrics 2000; Pediatric Hematology-Oncology 2000; **Med School:** Univ Tex, Houston 1985; **Resid:** Pediatrics, Vanderbilt Univ Med Ctr 1988; **Fellow:** Pediatric Hematology-Oncology, St Judes Chldns Hosp 1992; **Fac Appt:** Assoc Prof Ped, Vanderbilt Univ

Moscow, Jeffrey A MD [PHO] - **Spec Exp:** Pediatric Cancers; **Hospital:** Univ of Kentucky Chandler Hosp; **Address:** Univ Kentucky - Kentucky Clinic, 740 S Limestone, rm J457, Lexington, KY 40536; **Phone:** 859-257-4554; **Board Cert:** Pediatrics 1988; Pediatric Hematology-Oncology 2000; **Med School:** Dartmouth Med Sch 1982; **Resid:** Pediatrics, Univ Texas SW Med Ctr 1985; **Fellow:** Pediatric Hematology-Oncology, Natl Cancer Inst 1986; **Fac Appt:** Prof Ped, Univ KY Coll Med

Neuberg, Ronnie W MD [PHO] - **Spec Exp:** Pediatric Cancers; Gene Therapy; Clinical Trials; Brain Tumors; **Hospital:** Palmetto Richland Mem Hosp; **Address:** Palmetto Health Richland, 7 Richland Medical Park Drive, Ste 203, Columbia, SC 29203; **Phone:** 803-434-3533; **Board Cert:** Pediatrics 1982; Pediatric Hematology-Oncology 1982; **Med School:** SUNY Buffalo 1977; **Resid:** Pediatrics, Childrens Hosp 1980; **Fellow:** Pediatric Hematology-Oncology, SUNY Upstate Med Ctr 1982; **Fac Appt:** Assoc Prof Ped, Univ SC Sch Med

Nieder, Michael L MD [PHO] - **Spec Exp:** Bone Marrow Transplant; **Hospital:** All Children's Hosp; **Address:** 801 6th St S, Dept 7865, St Petersburg, FL 33701; **Phone:** 727-767-6856; **Board Cert:** Pediatrics 1986; Pediatric Hematology-Oncology 1987; **Med School:** Univ IL Coll Med 1982; **Resid:** Pediatrics, Children's Meml Hosp 1985; **Fellow:** Pediatric Hematology-Oncology, Children's Meml Hosp 1988; **Fac Appt:** Prof Ped, Univ Fla Coll Med

Olson, Thomas A MD [PHO] - **Spec Exp:** Sarcoma; Brain Tumors; **Hospital:** Emory Univ Hosp; **Address:** 3 W AFLAC Outpatient Ctr, 1405 Clifton Rd NE, Atlanta, GA 30322; **Phone:** 404-785-1200; **Board Cert:** Pediatrics 1982; Pediatric Hematology-Oncology 1984; **Med School:** Loyola Univ-Stritch Sch Med 1978; **Resid:** Pediatrics, Walter Reed AMC 1981; **Fellow:** Pediatric Hematology-Oncology, Walter Reed AMC 1983; **Fac Appt:** Assoc Prof Ped, Emory Univ

Pui, Ching Hon MD [PHO] - **Spec Exp:** Leukemia; Lymphoma; **Hospital:** St Jude Children's Research Hosp; **Address:** St Jude Chldns Rsch Hosp, 332 N Lauderdale St, Memphis, TN 38105; **Phone:** 901-495-3335; **Board Cert:** Pediatrics 1980; Pediatric Hematology-Oncology 1982; **Med School:** Taiwan 1976; **Resid:** Pediatrics, St Jude Chldns Rsch Hosp 1979; **Fellow:** Hematology & Oncology, St Jude Chldns Rsch Hosp 1981; **Fac Appt:** Prof Ped, Univ Tenn Coll Med, Memphis

Pediatric Hematology-Oncology

Rosoff, Phillip M MD [PHO] - **Spec Exp:** Cancer Survivors-Late Effects of Therapy; Leukemia; **Hospital:** Duke Univ Med Ctr; **Address:** Duke Univ Med Ctr, Box 2916, Durham, NC 27710-0001; **Phone:** 919-684-3401; **Board Cert:** Pediatrics 1984; Pediatric Hematology-Oncology 2002; **Med School:** Case West Res Univ 1978; **Resid:** Pediatrics, Chldns Hosp 1980; **Fellow:** Pediatric Hematology-Oncology, Chldns Hosp/Dana Farber Cancer Inst 1984; **Fac Appt:** Assoc Prof Ped, Duke Univ

Sandler, Eric MD [PHO] - **Spec Exp:** Bone Marrow Transplant; Leukemia; Clinical Trials; **Hospital:** Wolfson Chldns Hosp; **Address:** 807 Childrens Way, Jacksonville, FL 32207; **Phone:** 904-390-3793; **Board Cert:** Pediatrics 2000; Pediatric Hematology-Oncology 2000; **Med School:** Univ VT Coll Med 1985; **Resid:** Pediatrics, UCSF Med Ctr 1988; **Fellow:** Pediatric Hematology-Oncology, Univ Fla Med Sch 1991; **Fac Appt:** Assoc Prof Ped, Mayo Med Sch

Sandlund Jr, John T MD [PHO] - **Spec Exp:** Lymphoma, Non-Hodgkin's; Leukemia & Lymphoma; **Hospital:** St Jude Children's Research Hosp; **Address:** St Jude Children's Research Hosp, 332 N Lauderdale St, MS 260, Memphis, TN 38105; **Phone:** 901-495-3300; **Board Cert:** Pediatrics 1986; Pediatric Hematology-Oncology 1987; **Med School:** Ohio State Univ 1980; **Resid:** Pediatrics, Columbus Chldns Hosp 1983; **Fellow:** Hematology, Natl Cancer Inst 1986; Research, Natl Cancer Inst 1987

Santana, Victor M MD [PHO] - **Spec Exp:** Solid Tumors; **Hospital:** St Jude Children's Research Hosp; **Address:** St Jude Chldn's Rsch Hosp, Dept Oncology, 332 N Lauderdale, rm C6017, MS 260, Memphis, TN 38105-2794; **Phone:** 901-495-2424; **Board Cert:** Pediatrics 1982; Pediatric Hematology-Oncology 1984; **Med School:** Puerto Rico 1978; **Resid:** Pediatrics, Johns Hopkins Hosp 1981; **Fellow:** Pediatric Hematology-Oncology, Johns Hopkins Hosp 1984

Shearer, Patricia C MD [PHO] - **Spec Exp:** Wilms' Tumor; **Hospital:** Shands Hlthcre at Univ of FL; **Address:** Univ Florida HSC, Div Ped Hem/Oncology, PO Box 100296, Gainesville, FL 32610; **Phone:** 352-273-5625; **Board Cert:** Pediatric Hematology-Oncology 2000; **Med School:** Louisiana State Univ 1986; **Resid:** Pediatrics, Johns Hopkins Hosp 1989; **Fellow:** Hematology & Oncology, St Jude Chldns Rsch Hosp 1992

Tebbi, Cameron MD [PHO] - **Spec Exp:** Adolescent/Young Adult Cancers; Hodgkin's Disease; **Hospital:** St Josephs Chldns Hosp, Tampa Genl Hosp; **Address:** 3001 W Martin Luther King Jr Blvd, Tampa, FL 33607; **Phone:** 813-870-4824; **Board Cert:** Pediatrics 1974; Pediatric Hematology-Oncology 1980; **Med School:** Iran 1968; **Resid:** Pediatrics, Cincinnati Chldns Hosp 1972; Pediatric Hematology-Oncology, MD Anderson Cancer Inst 1972; **Fellow:** Pediatric Hematology-Oncology, St Louis Chldns Hosp 1973; Medical Oncology, Ontario Cancer Inst 1974

Toledano, Stuart R MD [PHO] - **Spec Exp:** Leukemia; Solid Tumors; Retinoblastoma; **Hospital:** Jackson Meml Hosp; **Address:** Univ Miami, Dept Peds-Div Ped Hem/Onc, (R-131) P.O. Box 016960, Miami, FL 33101; **Phone:** 305-585-5635; **Board Cert:** Pediatrics 1986; Pediatric Hematology-Oncology 1986; **Med School:** SUNY Buffalo 1972; **Resid:** Pediatrics, Montefiore Med Ctr 1975; **Fellow:** Pediatric Hematology-Oncology, Montefiore Med Ctr 1975; Pediatric Oncology, Childrens Hosp 1979; **Fac Appt:** Prof Ped, Univ Miami Sch Med

Whitlock, James A MD [PHO] - **Spec Exp:** Leukemia; Drug Development; **Hospital:** Vanderbilt Children's Hosp, Vanderbilt Univ Med Ctr; **Address:** Vanderbilt Univ Med Ctr, Dept Peds, 2220 Pierce Ave, rm 397 PRB, Nashville, TN 37232-6310; **Phone:** 615-936-1762; **Board Cert:** Pediatric Hematology-Oncology 2000; **Med School:** Vanderbilt Univ 1984; **Resid:** Pediatrics, Vanderbilt Univ Med Ctr 1987; **Fellow:** Pediatric Hematology-Oncology, Vanderbilt Univ Med Ctr 1990; **Fac Appt:** Assoc Prof Ped, Vanderbilt Univ

Woods, William G MD [PHO] - **Spec Exp:** Leukemia; Neuroblastoma; **Hospital:** Chldns Hlthcare Atlanta - Egleston, Chldns Hlthcare Atlanta - Scottish Rite; **Address:** AFLAC Cancer Ctr, 2015 Uppergate Drive, rm 404, Atlanta, GA 30322; **Phone:** 404-785-6170; **Board Cert:** Pediatrics 1976; Pediatric Hematology-Oncology 1978; **Med School:** Univ Pennsylvania 1972; **Resid:** Pediatrics, Univ Minnesota Hosps 1975; **Fellow:** Hematology, Univ Minnesota Hosps 1977; **Fac Appt:** Prof Ped, Emory Univ

Midwest

Arndt, Carola A MD [PHO] - **Spec Exp:** Sarcoma; Brain Tumors; Stem Cell Transplant; **Hospital:** Mayo Med Ctr & Clin - Rochester; **Address:** Mayo Clinic, Dept Pediatrics, 200 1st St SW, Rochester, MN 55905; **Phone:** 507-284-2652; **Board Cert:** Pediatrics 1982; Pediatric Hematology-Oncology 1987; **Med School:** Boston Univ 1978; **Resid:** Pediatrics, Naval Reg Med Ctr 1981; **Fellow:** Pediatric Hematology-Oncology, Natl Inst Hlth 1984

Camitta, Bruce M MD [PHO] - **Spec Exp:** Anemia-Aplastic; Leukemia; Bone Marrow Transplant; **Hospital:** Chldns Hosp - Wisconsin; **Address:** Midwest Childrens Cancer Ctr, 8701 Watertown Plank Rd, Ste 3018, Milwaukee, WI 53226; **Phone:** 414-456-4170; **Board Cert:** Pediatrics 1971; Pediatric Hematology-Oncology 1976; **Med School:** Johns Hopkins Univ 1966; **Resid:** Pediatrics, Children's Hosp 1968; Pediatrics, Johns Hopkins Hosp 1969; **Fellow:** Pediatric Hematology-Oncology, Children's Hosp 1973; **Fac Appt:** Prof Ped, Med Coll Wisc

Castle, Valerie MD [PHO] - **Spec Exp:** Neuroblastoma; Cancer Survivors-Late Effects of Therapy; **Hospital:** Univ Michigan Hlth Sys; **Address:** Univ Mich Comp Cancer Ctr & Geriatric Ctr, 1500 E Med Ctr Drive, Desk B1-358, Ann Arbor, MI 48109-0911; **Phone:** 734-936-9814; **Board Cert:** Pediatrics 2000; Pediatric Hematology-Oncology 1998; **Med School:** McMaster Univ 1983; **Resid:** Pediatrics, McMaster Univ Med Ctr 1986; **Fellow:** Pediatric Hematology-Oncology, Univ Mich Hosps 1989; **Fac Appt:** Prof Ped, Univ Mich Med Sch

Cohn, Susan L MD [PHO] - **Spec Exp:** Neuroblastoma; **Hospital:** Children's Mem Hosp, Evanston Hosp; **Address:** Children's Memorial Hosp, 2300 Children's Plaza, Box 30, Chicago, IL 60614; **Phone:** 773-880-4562; **Board Cert:** Pediatrics 1985; Pediatric Hematology-Oncology 1987; **Med School:** Univ IL Coll Med 1980; **Resid:** Pediatrics, Michael Reese Hosp 1984; **Fellow:** Hematology & Oncology, Children's Memorial Hosp 1985; **Fac Appt:** Prof Ped, Northwestern Univ

Davies, Stella M MD/PhD [PHO] - **Spec Exp:** Leukemia; Bone Marrow Transplant; Stem Cell Transplant; **Hospital:** Cincinnati Chldns Hosp Med Ctr; **Address:** Cincinnati Chldns Hosp Med Ctr, 3333 Burnet Ave, MLC 7015, Cincinnati, OH 45229-3039; **Phone:** 513-636-2469; **Med School:** England 1981; **Resid:** Pediatrics, Univ Newcastle Med Ctr 1985; **Fellow:** Pediatric Hematology-Oncology, Univ Minn Med Ctr 1993; **Fac Appt:** Prof Ped, Univ Cincinnati

Fallon, Robert J MD/PhD [PHO] - **Spec Exp:** Lymphoma; Hodgkin's Disease; Stem Cell Transplant; **Hospital:** Riley Hosp for Children (page 70); **Address:** Riley Childrens Hospital, 702 Barnhill Drive, rm Riley 4340, Indianapolis, IN 46202; **Phone:** 317-274-8784; **Board Cert:** Internal Medicine 1983; Medical Oncology 1985; **Med School:** NYU Sch Med 1980; **Resid:** Internal Medicine, Brigham & Womens Hosp 1983; **Fellow:** Hematology & Oncology, Brigham & Womens Hosp/Dana Farber Cancer Inst 1985; **Fac Appt:** Prof Ped, Indiana Univ

Ferrara, James MD [PHO] - **Spec Exp:** Bone Marrow Transplant; Graft vs Host Disease; **Hospital:** Univ Michigan Hlth Sys; **Address:** Univ Michigan Comprehensive Cancer Ctr, 1500 E Medical Center Drive, Ste 6308, Ann Arbor, MI 48109-0942; **Phone:** 734-615-1340; **Board Cert:** Pediatrics 2004; **Med School:** Georgetown Univ 1980; **Resid:** Pediatrics, Children's Hosp 1982; **Fellow:** Pediatric Hematology-Oncology, Children's Hosp 1985; **Fac Appt:** Prof Ped, Univ Mich Med Sch

Friebert, Sarah E MD [PHO] - **Spec Exp:** Palliative Care; Cancer Survivors-Late Effects of Therapy; **Hospital:** Children's Hosp & Med Ctr- Akron; **Address:** Children's Hospital Medical Ctr of Akron, One Perkins Sq Fl 5, Akron, OH 44308; **Phone:** 330-543-8730; **Board Cert:** Pediatrics 2004; Pediatric Hematology-Oncology 2000; **Med School:** Case West Res Univ 1993; **Resid:** Pediatrics, Chldns Hosp 1996; **Fellow:** Pediatric Hematology-Oncology, Rainbow Babies-Chldns Hosp 1999; **Fac Appt:** Asst Prof Ped, NE Ohio Univ

Goldman, Stewart MD [PHO] - **Spec Exp:** Neuro-Oncology; Brain Tumors; Clinical Trials; **Hospital:** Children's Mem Hosp; **Address:** Childrens Meml Hosp, Div Hem/Onc, 2300 Childrens Plaza, Box 30, Chicago, IL 60614; **Phone:** 773-880-4562; **Board Cert:** Pediatrics 1997; Pediatric Hematology-Oncology 2004; **Med School:** Loyola Univ-Stritch Sch Med 1985; **Resid:** Pediatrics, Univ Chicago Hosps 1988; **Fellow:** Pediatric Hematology-Oncology, Univ Chicago 1991

Hayani, Ammar MD [PHO] - **Spec Exp:** Leukemia; Solid Tumors; **Hospital:** Adv Christ Med Ctr, Central DuPage Hosp; **Address:** Hope Children's Hospital, 4440 W 95th St, Oak Lawn, IL 60453-2600; **Phone:** 708-684-4094; **Board Cert:** Pediatrics 1989; Pediatric Hematology-Oncology 2005; **Med School:** Syria 1982; **Resid:** Pediatrics, Louisiana State Univ 1987; **Fellow:** Pediatric Hematology-Oncology, Baylor Coll Med 1991

Hayashi, Robert J MD [PHO] - **Spec Exp:** Bone Marrow Transplant; Cancer Survivors-Late Effects of Therapy; Leukemia; **Hospital:** St Louis Chldns Hosp; **Address:** St Louis Chldns Hosp, Div Ped Hem Onc, One Children's Pl Fl 9S, Box 8116, St Louis, MO 63110; **Phone:** 314-454-6018; **Board Cert:** Pediatrics 2000; Pediatric Hematology-Oncology 2000; **Med School:** Washington Univ, St Louis 1986; **Resid:** Pediatrics, St Louis Children's Hosp 1989; **Fellow:** Pediatric Hematology-Oncology, Johns Hopkins Hosp 1992; **Fac Appt:** Asst Prof Ped, Washington Univ, St Louis

Hetherington, Maxine MD [PHO] - **Spec Exp:** Brain Tumors; **Hospital:** Chldns Mercy Hosps & Clinics; **Address:** Childrens Mercy Hosptial, 2401 Gillham Rd, Kansas City, MO 64108; **Phone:** 816-234-3265; **Board Cert:** Pediatrics 1983; Pediatric Hematology-Oncology 1987; **Med School:** Univ Tenn Coll Med, Memphis 1978; **Resid:** Pediatrics, Childrens Med Ctr 1981; **Fellow:** Pediatric Hematology-Oncology, Univ Texas Hlth Sci Ctr 1987; **Fac Appt:** Assoc Prof Ped, Univ MO-Kansas City

Hilden, Joanne M MD [PHO] - **Spec Exp:** Brain Tumors; Leukemia & Lymphoma; Bone Tumors; Soft Tissue Tumors; **Hospital:** Cleveland Clin Fdn (page 71); **Address:** Cleveland Clinic Children's Hospital, Dept of Pediatric Hematology/Oncology, 9500 9500 Euclid Ave, Desk S20, Cleveland, OH 44195; **Phone:** 216-444-8407; **Board Cert:** Pediatrics 1999; Pediatric Hematology-Oncology 2002; **Med School:** Univ Minn 1988; **Resid:** Pediatrics, Univ Minn Med Ctr 1991; **Fellow:** Pediatric Hematology-Oncology, Univ Minn Med Ctr 1994; **Fac Appt:** Assoc Prof Ped, Cleveland Cl Coll Med/Case West Res

Hord, Jeffrey D MD [PHO] - **Spec Exp:** Hematologic Malignancies; Bone Marrow Failure Disorders; **Hospital:** Children's Hosp & Med Ctr- Akron; **Address:** Akron Childrens Hosp, Hematology/Oncology, One Perkins Square, Akron, OH 44308; **Phone:** 330-543-8580; **Board Cert:** Pediatrics 2000; Pediatric Hematology-Oncology 2004; **Med School:** Univ KY Coll Med 1989; **Resid:** Pediatrics, Childrens Hosp 1992; **Fellow:** Pediatric Hematology-Oncology, Vanderbilt Univ Med Ctr 1995; **Fac Appt:** Assoc Prof Ped, NE Ohio Univ

Hutchinson, Raymond MD [PHO] - **Spec Exp:** Leukemia; Hodgkin's Disease; **Hospital:** Univ Michigan Hlth Sys; **Address:** Univ Michigan, Cancer Ctr, 1500 E Med Ctr Drive, rm L2110, Box 0238, Ann Arbor, MI 48109-0238; **Phone:** 734-764-7126; **Board Cert:** Pediatrics 1979; Pediatric Hematology-Oncology 1980; **Med School:** Harvard Med Sch 1973; **Resid:** Pediatrics, New England Med Ctr 1975; **Fellow:** Pediatric Hematology-Oncology, Childrens Hosp 1978; **Fac Appt:** Prof Ped, Univ Mich Med Sch

Luchtman-Jones, Lori MD [PHO] - **Spec Exp:** Leukemia; Bleeding/Coagulation Disorders; Brain Tumors; **Hospital:** St Louis Chldns Hosp; **Address:** Pediatric Hematology-Oncology, 1 Childrens Place, Ste 9 South, Box 8116, Saint Louis, MO 63110; **Phone:** 314-454-6018; **Board Cert:** Pediatrics 1999; Pediatric Hematology-Oncology 2004; **Med School:** UCSD 1987; **Resid:** Pediatrics, UCSD School Med 1990; **Fellow:** Pediatric Hematology-Oncology, Washington Univ 1995; **Fac Appt:** Asst Prof Ped, Washington Univ, St Louis

Lusher, Jeanne M MD [PHO] - **Hospital:** Chldns Hosp of Michigan; **Address:** Children's Hospital Michigan, Div Hem/Onc, 3901 Beaubien Blvd, Detroit, MI 48201; **Phone:** 313-745-5515; **Board Cert:** Pediatrics 1986; Pediatric Hematology-Oncology 1986; **Med School:** Univ Cincinnati 1960; **Resid:** Pediatrics, Charity Hosp/Tulane Univ 1963; **Fellow:** Hematology & Oncology, Charity Hosp/Tulane Univ 1965; Hematology & Oncology, Saint Louis Children's Hosp 1966; **Fac Appt:** Prof Ped, Wayne State Univ

Manera, Ricarchito MD [PHO] - **Spec Exp:** Leukemia; Brain Tumors; Lymphoma; **Hospital:** Loyola Univ Med Ctr; **Address:** Loyola University Med Ctr, 2160 S First Ave, Maywood, IL 60611; **Phone:** 708 327 9136; **Board Cert:** Pediatrics 2003; Pediatric Hematology-Oncology 2004; **Med School:** Philippines 1984; **Resid:** Pediatrics, Bronx-Lebanon Hosp Ctr 1995; **Fellow:** Pediatric Hematology-Oncology, MD Anderson Cancer Ctr 1994; Pediatric Hematology-Oncology, Columbia-Presbyterian Med Ctr 1996; **Fac Appt:** Assoc Prof Ped, Loyola Univ-Stritch Sch Med

Morgan, Elaine MD [PHO] - **Spec Exp:** Leukemia; Palliative Care; Ethics; **Hospital:** Children's Mem Hosp; **Address:** Children's Meml Hosp, Div Hem/Onc, 2300 Children's Plaza, Box 30, Chicago, IL 60614; **Phone:** 773-880-4562; **Board Cert:** Pediatrics 1976; Pediatric Hematology-Oncology 1978; Hospice & Palliative Medicine 2005; **Med School:** Univ Pennsylvania 1971; **Resid:** Pediatrics, Chldns Hosp 1974; **Fellow:** Pediatric Hematology-Oncology, Chldns Hosp Med Ctr 1975; Pediatric Hematology-Oncology, Chldns Meml Med Ctr 1976; **Fac Appt:** Prof Ped, Northwestern Univ-Feinberg Sch Med

Pediatric Hematology-Oncology

Nachman, James MD [PHO] - **Spec Exp:** Leukemia & Lymphoma; Bone Tumors; Hodgkin's Disease; **Hospital:** Univ of Chicago Hosps; **Address:** Univ Chicago Hosps, 5841 S Maryland Ave, rm C-429, MC 406, Chicago, IL 60637; **Phone:** 773-702-6808; **Board Cert:** Pediatrics 1979; Pediatric Hematology-Oncology 1980; **Med School:** Johns Hopkins Univ 1974; **Resid:** Pediatrics, Chldns Meml Hosp 1977; Pediatrics, Fell-Wylers Chldns Hosp 1980; **Fellow:** Pediatric Hematology-Oncology, Chldns Meml Hosp 1979; **Fac Appt:** Prof Ped, Univ Chicago-Pritzker Sch Med

Neglia, Joseph MD [PHO] - **Spec Exp:** Cancer Survivors-Late Effects of Therapy; **Hospital:** Univ Minn Med Ctr, Fairview - Univ Campus; **Address:** Univ Minnesota-Div Ped Hem/Oncology, 420 Delaware St SE, MMC 484, Minneapolis, MN 55455; **Phone:** 612-626-2778; **Board Cert:** Pediatrics 1986; Pediatric Hematology-Oncology 1987; **Med School:** Loma Linda Univ 1981; **Resid:** Pediatrics, Baylor Coll Med 1984; **Fellow:** Pediatric Hematology-Oncology, Univ Minn Hosp 1987; **Fac Appt:** Prof Ped, Univ Minn

Puccetti, Diane MD [PHO] - **Spec Exp:** Brain Tumors; Neuro-Oncology; Cancer Survivors-Late Effects of Therapy; **Hospital:** Univ WI Hosp & Clins; **Address:** Univ Wisconsin Childrens Hosp, 600 Highland Ave, MC 4116, Madison, WI 53792; **Phone:** 608-263-6420; **Board Cert:** Pediatrics 1989; Pediatric Hematology-Oncology 1998; **Med School:** Med Coll OH 1985; **Resid:** Pediatrics, UC-Irvine Med Ctr 1986; Pediatrics, Med Coll Ohio 1988; **Fellow:** Pediatric Hematology-Oncology, Riley Hosp Chldn 1991; **Fac Appt:** Assoc Clin Prof Ped, Univ Wisc

Salvi, Sharad MD [PHO] - **Spec Exp:** Leukemia; **Hospital:** Adv Christ Med Ctr, Central DuPage Hosp; **Address:** Hope Chldns Hosp, 4440 W 95th St, Oak Lawn, IL 60453; **Phone:** 708-684-4094; **Board Cert:** Pediatrics 1982; Pediatric Hematology-Oncology 1982; **Med School:** India 1974; **Resid:** Pediatrics, Lincoln Meml Hosp 1979; **Fellow:** Pediatric Hematology-Oncology, Chldns Hosp/Roswell Park Meml Cancer Inst 1981

Sencer, Susan F MD [PHO] - **Spec Exp:** Pediatric Cancers; Complementary Medicine; **Hospital:** Chldns Hosp and Clinics - Minneapolis; **Address:** Chldns Specialty Clin, Hem/Onc, 2525 Chicago Ave S, Ste 4150, Minneapolis, MN 55404; **Phone:** 612-813-5940; **Board Cert:** Pediatrics 1989; Pediatric Hematology-Oncology 2000; **Med School:** Univ Minn 1984; **Resid:** Pediatrics, Univ Minn 1988; **Fellow:** Pediatric Hematology-Oncology, Univ Minn 1991

Sondel, Paul M MD [PHO] - **Spec Exp:** Immunotherapy; Stem Cell Transplant; Pediatric Cancers; **Hospital:** Univ WI Hosp & Clins; **Address:** Univ Wisconsin Childrens Hosp, 600 Highland Ave, K4-448 Clin Sci Ctr, Madison, WI 53792-4672; **Phone:** 608-263-6200; **Board Cert:** Pediatrics 1981; **Med School:** Harvard Med Sch 1977; **Resid:** Pediatrics, Univ Wisconsin Hosp 1980; **Fellow:** Research, Sidney Farber Cancer Inst/Harvard 1975; **Fac Appt:** Prof Ped, Univ Wisc

Tannous, Raymond MD [PHO] - **Spec Exp:** Wilms' Tumor; Leukemia & Lymphoma; Pain-Cancer; **Hospital:** Univ Iowa Hosp & Clinics; **Address:** Univ Iowa Hosps & Clinics, Dept Peds, 200 Hawkins Drive, rm 2528 JCP, Iowa City, IA 52242; **Phone:** 319-356-1905; **Board Cert:** Pediatrics 1976; Pediatric Hematology-Oncology 1978; **Med School:** France 1972; **Resid:** Pediatrics, St Jude Chldns Rsch Hosp 1976; **Fellow:** Pediatric Hematology-Oncology, St Jude Chldns Rsch Hosp 1977; **Fac Appt:** Assoc Prof Ped, Univ Iowa Coll Med

Vik, Terry A MD [PHO] - **Spec Exp:** Neuroblastoma; Clinical Trials; Cancer Survivors-Late Effects of Therapy; Leukemia; **Hospital:** Riley Hosp for Children (page 70); **Address:** Riley Hosp Children, 702 Barnhill Drive, rm Riley 4340, Indianapolis, IN 46202; **Phone:** 317-274-2143; **Board Cert:** Pediatrics 1987; Pediatric Hematology-Oncology 2004; **Med School:** Johns Hopkins Univ 1983; **Resid:** Pediatrics, UCLA Med Ctr 1986; **Fellow:** Pediatric Hematology-Oncology, Chldns Hosp 1989; **Fac Appt:** Assoc Prof Ped, Indiana Univ

Yaddanapudi, Ravindranath MD [PHO] - **Spec Exp:** Leukemia; **Hospital:** Chldns Hosp of Michigan; **Address:** Children's Hospital Michigan, Div Hem/Onc, 3901 Beaubien Blvd, Detroit, MI 48201; **Phone:** 313-745-5515; **Board Cert:** Pediatrics 1970; Pediatric Hematology-Oncology 1974; **Med School:** India 1964; **Resid:** Pathology, Western Penn Hosp 1967; Pediatrics, Children's Hosp 1969; **Fellow:** Pediatric Hematology-Oncology, Children's Hosp Michigan 1971; **Fac Appt:** Prof Ped, Wayne State Univ

Great Plains and Mountains

Abromowitch, Minnie MD [PHO] - **Hospital:** Children's Hosp - Omaha; **Address:** Children's Hosp-Dept Ped Hem Oncology, 8200 Dodge St, Omaha, NE 68114; **Phone:** 402-955-3950; **Board Cert:** Pediatrics 1980; Pediatric Hematology-Oncology 1982; **Med School:** Canada 1972; **Resid:** Pediatrics, Hospital for Sick Children 1976; **Fellow:** Pediatric Hematology-Oncology, Univ Manitoba 1978; Pediatric Hematology-Oncology, St Jude Chldns Research Hosp 1980; **Fac Appt:** Assoc Prof Ped, Univ Nebr Coll Med

Bruggers, Carol S MD [PHO] - **Spec Exp:** Leukemia; Clinical Trials; **Hospital:** Primary Children's Med Ctr; **Address:** Primary Children's Medical Ctr, 100 N Medical Drive, Salt Lake City, UT 84113; **Phone:** 801-662-4700; **Board Cert:** Pediatrics 2000; Pediatric Hematology-Oncology 2000; **Med School:** Mich State Univ 1984; **Resid:** Pediatrics, Univ Colorado Health Sci Ctr 1987; **Fellow:** Pediatric Hematology-Oncology, Duke Univ Med Ctr 1991; **Fac Appt:** Assoc Prof Med, Univ Utah

Coccia, Peter MD [PHO] - **Spec Exp:** Bone Marrow Transplant; Leukemia & Lymphoma; Solid Tumors; **Hospital:** Nebraska Med Ctr, Children's Hosp - Omaha; **Address:** Univ Nebr Med Ctr, Dept Pediatrics, 982168 Nebraska Med Ctr, Omaha, NE 68198-2168; **Phone:** 402-559-7257; **Board Cert:** Clinical Pathology 1972; Hematology 1975; Pediatrics 1976; Pediatric Hematology-Oncology 1976; **Med School:** SUNY Upstate Med Univ 1968; **Resid:** Pathology, Upstate Med Ctr 1970; Pediatrics, Univ Minn 1973; **Fellow:** Pediatric Hematology-Oncology, Univ Minn 1974; **Fac Appt:** Prof Ped, Univ Nebr Coll Med

Johnston, J Martin MD [PHO] - **Spec Exp:** Leukemia; Lymphoma; **Hospital:** St. Luke's Reg Med Ctr - Boise; **Address:** 100 E Idaho St, Boise, ID 83712; **Phone:** 208-381-2782; **Board Cert:** Pediatric Hematology-Oncology 2002; **Med School:** Duke Univ 1984; **Resid:** Pediatrics, Univ Utah Med Ctr 1988; **Fellow:** Pediatric Hematology-Oncology, Barnes Jewish Hosp 1991

Odom, Lorrie F MD [PHO] - **Spec Exp:** Leukemia; Solid Tumors; Cancer Survivors-Late Effects of Therapy; **Hospital:** Presby - St Luke's Med Ctr, Chldn's Hosp - Denver, The; **Address:** Rocky Mountain Ped Hem Onc, 1601 E 19th Ave, Box 6600, Denver, CO 80218; **Phone:** 303-832-2344; **Board Cert:** Pediatrics 1974; Pediatric Hematology-Oncology 1976; **Med School:** Univ Colorado 1969; **Resid:** Pediatrics, Childrens Hosp 1972; **Fellow:** Pediatric Hematology-Oncology, Dana-Farber Cancer Inst 1974; Pediatric Hematology-Oncology, Univ Colorado Med Ctr 1975; **Fac Appt:** Clin Prof Ped, Univ Colorado

Pediatric Hematology-Oncology

Southwest

Abella, Esteban MD [PHO] - **Spec Exp:** Leukemia; Anemia-Aplastic; Neuroblastoma; Bone Marrow Transplant; **Hospital:** Banner Desert Med Ctr, St Joseph's Hosp & Med Ctr - Phoenix; **Address:** 1432 S Dobson, Ste 107, Mesa, AZ 85202; **Phone:** 480-833-1123; **Board Cert:** Pediatrics 1998; Pediatric Hematology-Oncology 2002; **Med School:** Dominican Republic 1985; **Resid:** Pediatrics, Chldns Hosp Michigan 1988; **Fellow:** Pediatric Hematology-Oncology, Chldns Hosp Michigan/Wayne St Univ 1991

Baranko, Paul MD [PHO] - **Spec Exp:** Leukemia; Kidney Cancer; Wilms' Tumor; **Hospital:** Phoenix Children's Hosp; **Address:** Phoenix Children's Hosp, 1919 E Thomas Rd, Phoenix, AZ 85016; **Phone:** 602-546-0920; **Board Cert:** Pediatrics 1986; Pediatric Hematology-Oncology 1986; **Med School:** Indiana Univ 1965; **Resid:** Pediatrics, Indiana Med Ctr 1967; Pediatrics, St Josephs Hosp 1968; **Fellow:** Pediatric Hematology-Oncology, Los Angeles Chldns Hosp 1971; **Fac Appt:** Clin Prof Ped, Univ Ariz Coll Med

Berg, Stacey MD [PHO] - **Hospital:** Texas Chldns Hosp - Houston; **Address:** Texas Chldns Cancer Ctr, Ped Hem-Onc, 6621 Fannin St, MC 3-3320, Houston, TX 77030; **Phone:** 832-824-4588; **Board Cert:** Pediatrics 2007; Pediatric Hematology-Oncology 2007; **Med School:** Univ Pittsburgh 1985; **Resid:** Pediatrics, Chldns Hosp 1988; **Fellow:** Pediatric Hematology-Oncology, Natl Inst Hlth 1991

Blaney, Susan MD [PHO] - **Spec Exp:** Brain Tumors; Neuro-Oncology; Drug Development; Clinical Trials; **Hospital:** Texas Chldns Hosp - Houston; **Address:** 6621 Fannin St #CC 1410.00, Houston, TX 77030; **Phone:** 832-822-1482; **Board Cert:** Pediatrics 1998; Pediatric Hematology-Oncology 2005; **Med School:** Med Coll OH 1984; **Resid:** Pediatrics, Letterman AMC 1987; **Fellow:** Pediatric Oncology, Walter Reed AMC 1990; **Fac Appt:** Prof Ped, Baylor Coll Med

Corey, Seth MD [PHO] - **Spec Exp:** Bone Marrow Failure Disorders; Leukemia; Myelodysplastic Syndromes; **Hospital:** UT MD Anderson Cancer Ctr (page 81); **Address:** MD Anderson Cancer Ctr, 1515 Holcombe Blvd, Houston, TX 77030; **Phone:** 713-563-5393; **Board Cert:** Pediatrics 1986; Pediatric Hematology-Oncology 2004; **Med School:** Tulane Univ 1982; **Resid:** Pediatrics, St Louis Chldns Hosp 1985; **Fellow:** Hematology & Oncology, Tufts Med Sch 1992; Hematology & Oncology, Boston Chldns-Dana Farber Ctr 1989; **Fac Appt:** Prof Ped, Univ Tex, Houston

Dreyer, ZoAnn E MD [PHO] - **Spec Exp:** Cancer Survivors-Late Effects of Therapy; Leukemia in Infants; **Hospital:** Texas Chldns Hosp - Houston; **Address:** Texas Childrens Hosp, Clinical Care Ctr, 6701 Fannin Fl 14, MC CC1400, Houston, TX 77030; **Phone:** 832-822-4242; **Board Cert:** Pediatrics 1988; Pediatric Hematology-Oncology 1998; **Med School:** UC Davis 1982; **Resid:** Pediatrics, Baylor Affil Hosps 1985; **Fellow:** Pediatric Hematology-Oncology, Baylor Coll Med 1988; **Fac Appt:** Assoc Prof Ped, Baylor Coll Med

Goldman, Stanton C MD [PHO] - **Spec Exp:** Leukemia; Lymphoma; Stem Cell Transplant; **Hospital:** Med City Dallas Hosp; **Address:** 7777 Forest Ln, Ste D400, Dallas, TX 75230; **Phone:** 972-566-6647; **Board Cert:** Pediatrics 2001; Pediatric Hematology-Oncology 2004; **Med School:** Boston Univ 1990; **Resid:** Pediatrics, Chldns Natl Med Ctr; **Fellow:** Pediatric Hematology-Oncology, Johns Hopkins Hosp

Graham, Michael L MD [PHO] - **Spec Exp:** Bone Marrow Transplant; Leukemia; Stem Cell Transplant; **Hospital:** Univ Med Ctr - Tucson; **Address:** Univ Arizona Hlth Science Ctr, 1501 N Campbell Ave, rm 4341, Box 245073, Tucson, AZ 85724-5073; **Phone:** 520-626-6527; **Board Cert:** Pediatrics 1980; Pediatric Hematology-Oncology 1984; **Med School:** Brown Univ 1975; **Resid:** Pediatrics, Johns Hopkins Hosp 1978; Pediatric Hematology-Oncology, Johns Hopkins Hosp 1980; **Fellow:** Medical Oncology, Yale-New Haven Hosp 1982; **Fac Appt:** Assoc Prof Ped, Univ Ariz Coll Med

Murphy, Sharon B MD [PHO] - **Spec Exp:** Lymphoma, Non-Hodgkin's; Leukemia; **Hospital:** Univ Hlth Sys - Univ Hosp; **Address:** UTHSCSA - Children's Cancer Research Inst, 8403 Floyd Curl Drive, MS 7784, San Antonio, TX 78229-3900; **Phone:** 210-562-9000; **Board Cert:** Pediatrics 1990; Pediatric Hematology-Oncology 1990; **Med School:** Harvard Med Sch 1969; **Resid:** Pediatrics, Univ Colorado Med Ctr 1971; **Fellow:** Pediatric Hematology-Oncology, Chldns Hosp 1973; **Fac Appt:** Prof Ped, Univ Tex, San Antonio

Scher, Charles D MD [PHO] - **Spec Exp:** Leukemia; **Hospital:** Tulane Univ Hosp & Clin; **Address:** Tulane Univ Hosp, Dept Pediatrics, 1430 Tulane Ave, Box SL-37, New Orleans, LA 70112; **Phone:** 504-988-5412; **Board Cert:** Pediatrics 1972; **Med School:** Univ Pennsylvania 1965; **Resid:** Pediatrics, Bronx Muni Hosp Ctr 1967; Pediatrics, Chldns Hosp Med Ctr 1972; **Fellow:** Pediatric Hematology-Oncology, Chldns Hosp Med Ctr 1974; **Fac Appt:** Prof Ped, Tulane Univ

Tomlinson, Gail E MD [PHO] - **Spec Exp:** Cancer Survivors-Late Effects of Therapy; Cancer Genetics; Liver Cancer; Kidney Cancer; **Hospital:** Chldns Med Ctr of Dallas, UT Southwestern Med Ctr - Dallas; **Address:** UT Southwestern Med Ctr, 5323 Harry Hines Blvd, Dallas, TX 75390-8593; **Phone:** 214-648-4907; **Board Cert:** Pediatrics 2001; Pediatric Hematology-Oncology 2002; **Med School:** Geo Wash Univ 1984; **Resid:** Pediatrics, Chldns Hosp Natl Med Ctr 1987; **Fellow:** Pediatric Hematology-Oncology, MD Anderson Cancer Ctr 1989; Pediatric Hematology-Oncology, Univ Texas SW Med Ctr 1992; **Fac Appt:** Assoc Prof Ped, Univ Tex SW, Dallas

Wall, Donna A MD [PHO] - **Spec Exp:** Bone Marrow & Stem Cell Transplant; Immunotherapy; **Hospital:** Methodist Chldns Hosp of South Texas, Christus Santa Rosa Children's Hosp; **Address:** Texas Transplant Inst, 7711 Louis Pasteur, Ste 708, San Antonio, TX 78229; **Phone:** 210-575-7268; **Board Cert:** Pediatrics 1986; Pediatric Hematology-Oncology 1987; **Med School:** Canada 1981; **Resid:** Pediatrics, NY Presby-Columbia Med Ctr 1983; Pediatrics, New England Med Ctr 1985; **Fellow:** Pediatric Hematology-Oncology, Dana Farber Cancer Inst 1986

Winick, Naomi J MD [PHO] - **Spec Exp:** Leukemia; **Hospital:** Chldns Med Ctr of Dallas; **Address:** Ctr for Cancer & Blood Disorders, 1935 Motor St, Dallas, TX 75235-7794; **Phone:** 214-456-2382; **Board Cert:** Pediatrics 1984; Pediatric Hematology-Oncology 1987; **Med School:** Northwestern Univ 1978; **Resid:** Pediatrics, Babies Hosp Columbia Presbyterian Med Ctr 1981; **Fellow:** Pediatric Hematology-Oncology, Sloan-Kettering Cancer Ctr 1983; **Fac Appt:** Prof Ped, Univ Tex SW, Dallas

West Coast and Pacific

Andrews, Robert G MD [PHO] - **Spec Exp:** Bone Marrow Transplant; Leukemia; Lymphoma; **Hospital:** Chldns Hosp and Regl Med Ctr - Seattle; **Address:** Fred Hutchinson Cancer Research Ctr, D2-373, 1100 Fairview Ave N, Seattle, WA 98109-1024; **Phone:** 206-288-1024; **Board Cert:** Pediatrics 1984; Pediatric Hematology-Oncology 1984; **Med School:** Univ Minn 1976; **Resid:** Pediatrics, New England Med Ctr 1979; **Fellow:** Pediatric Hematology-Oncology, Children's Hosp Med Ctr 1983; **Fac Appt:** Assoc Prof Ped, Univ Wash

Pediatric Hematology-Oncology

Ducore, Jonathan M MD [PHO] - **Spec Exp:** Brain Tumors; Bone & Soft Tissue Tumors; **Hospital:** UC Davis Med Ctr; **Address:** UC Davis Med Ctr, Dept Pediatrics, Div Pediatric Hematology/Oncology, 2516 Stockton Blvd, Sacramento, CA 95817; **Phone:** 916-734-2781; **Board Cert:** Pediatrics 1978; Pediatric Hematology-Oncology 1978; **Med School:** Duke Univ 1973; **Resid:** Pediatrics, Chldns Med Ctr 1975; **Fellow:** Pediatric Hematology-Oncology, Univ Colorado Med Ctr 1977; Cancer Research, Natl Cancer Inst 1980; **Fac Appt:** Assoc Prof Ped, UC Davis

Finklestein, Jerry Z MD [PHO] - **Hospital:** Long Beach Meml Med Ctr, LAC - Harbor - UCLA Med Ctr; **Address:** 2653 Elm Ave, Ste 200, Long Beach, CA 90806-1652; **Phone:** 562-492-1062; **Board Cert:** Pediatrics 1980; Pediatric Hematology-Oncology 1974; **Med School:** McGill Univ 1963; **Resid:** Pediatrics, Montreal Chldns Hosp 1966; **Fellow:** Pediatric Hematology-Oncology, LA Chldns Hosp 1968; **Fac Appt:** Clin Prof Ped, UCLA

Finlay, Jonathan MD [PHO] - **Spec Exp:** Brain Tumors; **Hospital:** Chldns Hosp - Los Angeles; **Address:** Chldns Hosp-LA, Ped Hematology/Oncology, 4650 Sunset Blvd, MS 54, Los Angeles, CA 90027; **Phone:** 323-906-8147; **Board Cert:** Pediatrics 1984; Pediatric Hematology-Oncology 1987; **Med School:** England 1973; **Resid:** Pediatrics, Univ Birmingham 1975; Pediatrics, Christie Hosp 1976; **Fellow:** Pediatric Allergy & Immunology, Univ Wisconsin Hosp 1978; Pediatric Hematology-Oncology, Univ Wisconsin Hosp 1980; **Fac Appt:** Prof Ped, USC-Keck School of Medicine

Friedman, Debra L MD [PHO] - **Spec Exp:** Cancer Survivors-Late Effects of Therapy; Hodgkin's Disease; Retinoblastoma; **Hospital:** Chldns Hosp and Regl Med Ctr - Seattle, Univ Wash Med Ctr; **Address:** Children's Hosp Regional Med Ctr, 400 Sandpoint Way NE, Box 5371, MS B6553, Seattle, WA 98109; **Phone:** 206-667-5935; **Board Cert:** Pediatric Hematology-Oncology 1998; **Med School:** UMDNJ-RW Johnson Med Sch 1991; **Resid:** Pediatrics, Chldns Hosp 1994; **Fellow:** Pediatric Hematology-Oncology, Chldns Hosp 1997; **Fac Appt:** Asst Prof Ped, Univ Wash

Geyer, J Russell MD [PHO] - **Spec Exp:** Brain Tumors; **Hospital:** Chldns Hosp and Regl Med Ctr - Seattle, Providence Alaska Med Ctr; **Address:** Chldns Hosp & Reg Med Ctr - Div Hem/Onc, 4800 Sands Point Way NE, MS B-6553, Seattle, WA 98105; **Phone:** 206-987-2106; **Board Cert:** Pediatrics 1983; Pediatric Hematology-Oncology 1987; **Med School:** Wayne State Univ 1977; **Resid:** Pediatrics, Chldns Hosp Michigan 1980; **Fellow:** Pediatric Hematology-Oncology, Univ Michigan Med Ctr 1981; **Fac Appt:** Prof Ped, Univ Wash

Hawkins, Douglas MD [PHO] - **Spec Exp:** Bone Tumors; Ewing's Sarcoma; Leukemia; Rhabdomyosarcoma; **Hospital:** Chldns Hosp and Regl Med Ctr - Seattle; **Address:** Children's Hosp & Regl Med Ctr, 4800 Sand Point Way NE, Box 5371, MS B6553, Seattle, WA 98105; **Phone:** 206-987-2106; **Board Cert:** Pediatrics 2001; Pediatric Hematology-Oncology 2004; **Med School:** Harvard Med Sch 1990; **Resid:** Pediatrics, Univ Washington Med Ctr 1993; **Fellow:** Pediatric Hematology-Oncology, Fred Hutchinson Cancer Research Ctr 1996

Horn, Biljana N MD [PHO] - **Spec Exp:** Bone Marrow Transplant; Brain Tumors; Stem Cell Transplant; Immunotherapy; **Hospital:** UCSF Med Ctr; **Address:** UCSF Med Ctr, Pediatric BMT Program, 505 Parnassus Ave, rm M-659, San Francisco, CA 94143; **Phone:** 415-476-2188; **Board Cert:** Pediatrics 2005; Pediatric Hematology-Oncology 2004; **Med School:** Croatia 1983; **Resid:** Pediatrics, Rainbow Babies & Chldns Hosp 1991; **Fellow:** Pediatric Hematology-Oncology, Natl Cancer Inst 1994; Pediatric Neuro-Oncology, UCSF 1998; **Fac Appt:** Assoc Prof Ped, UCSF

Kadota, Richard P MD [PHO] - **Spec Exp:** Bone Marrow Transplant; Brain Tumors; Clinical Trials; **Hospital:** Rady Children's Hosp - San Diego; **Address:** Children's Hospital San Diego, 3020 Children's Way, MC 5035, San Diego, CA 92123; **Phone:** 858-966-5811; **Board Cert:** Pediatrics 1984; Pediatric Hematology-Oncology 1984; **Med School:** Northwestern Univ 1979; **Resid:** Pediatrics, Mayo Clinic 1983; **Fellow:** Pediatric Hematology-Oncology, Mayo Clinic 1985; **Fac Appt:** Clin Prof Ped, UCSD

Kapoor, Neena MD [PHO] - **Spec Exp:** Bone Marrow Transplant; **Hospital:** Chldns Hosp - Los Angeles; **Address:** Chlds Hosp LA-Rsch Immunology/BMT, 4650 Sunset Blvd, MS 62, Los Angeles, CA 90027; **Phone:** 323-669-2546; **Board Cert:** Pediatrics 1978; Pediatric Hematology-Oncology 1996; **Med School:** India 1972; **Resid:** Pediatrics, Rhode Island Hosp 1976; **Fellow:** Pediatric Hematology-Oncology, Meml Sloan-Kettering Cancer Ctr 1978; **Fac Appt:** Prof Ped, USC Sch Med

Kung, Faith MD [PHO] - **Spec Exp:** Leukemia & Lymphoma; Bleeding/Coagulation Disorders; Cancer Survivors-Late Effects of Therapy; **Hospital:** Rady Children's Hosp - San Diego; **Address:** UCSD Med Ctr, Div Ped Hem/Oncology, 200 W Arbor Drive, San Diego, CA 92103-8447; **Phone:** 619-543-6844; **Board Cert:** Pediatrics 1967; Pediatric Hematology-Oncology 1974; **Med School:** Univ VA Sch Med 1957; **Resid:** Pediatrics, NC Meml Hosp 1960; **Fellow:** Pediatric Hematology-Oncology, Chldns Hosp/Babies Hosp 1962; **Fac Appt:** Prof Ped, UCSD

Link, Michael P MD [PHO] - **Spec Exp:** Stem Cell Transplant; **Hospital:** Lucile Packard Chldns Hosp/Stanford Univ Med Ctr, Stanford Univ Med Ctr; **Address:** 1000 Welch Rd, Ste 300, Palo Alto, CA 94304; **Phone:** 650-723-5535; **Board Cert:** Pediatrics 1979; Pediatric Hematology-Oncology 1980; **Med School:** Stanford Univ 1974; **Resid:** Pediatrics, Chldns Hosp Med Ctr 1976; **Fellow:** Hematology & Oncology, Dana Farber Cancer Inst 1979; **Fac Appt:** Prof Ped, Stanford Univ

Marina, Neyssa MD [PHO] - **Spec Exp:** Sarcoma; Cancer Survivors-Late Effects of Therapy; Germ Cell Tumors; **Hospital:** Lucile Packard Chldns Hosp/Stanford Univ Med Ctr; **Address:** Pediatric Hematology & Oncology, 725 Walsh Rd-Clinic E, Palo Alto, CA 94304; **Phone:** 650-497-8953; **Board Cert:** Pediatrics 1987; Pediatric Hematology-Oncology 2005; **Med School:** Puerto Rico 1983; **Resid:** Pediatrics, Univ Pediatric Hosp 1986; **Fellow:** Pediatric Hematology-Oncology, St Jude Children's Hosp 1989; **Fac Appt:** Prof Ped, Stanford Univ

Matthay, Katherine K MD [PHO] - **Spec Exp:** Neuroblastoma; Bone Marrow & Stem Cell Transplant; **Hospital:** UCSF Med Ctr; **Address:** UCSF, Dept Ped Onc, 505 Parnassus Ave, Box 0106, San Francisco, CA 94143; **Phone:** 415-476-0603; **Board Cert:** Pediatrics 1979; Pediatric Hematology-Oncology 1980; **Med School:** Univ Pennsylvania 1973; **Resid:** Pediatrics, Univ Colorado 1976; **Fellow:** Pediatric Hematology-Oncology, UCSF 1979; **Fac Appt:** Prof Ped, UCSF

Nicholson, Henry Stacy MD [PHO] - **Spec Exp:** Brain Tumors; Cancer Survivors-Late Effects of Therapy; **Hospital:** Doernbecher Chldns Hosp/OHSU, OR Hlth & Sci Univ; **Address:** OR Hlth Scis Univ, 709 SW Gaines Rd, Portland, OR 97239; **Phone:** 503-494-4265; **Board Cert:** Pediatrics 2000; Pediatric Hematology-Oncology 2000; **Med School:** Med Coll GA 1985; **Resid:** Pediatrics, Chldns National Med Ctr 1988; **Fellow:** Pediatric Hematology-Oncology, Chldns National Med Ctr 1991; **Fac Appt:** Prof Ped, Oregon Hlth Sci Univ

Pendergrass, Thomas W MD [PHO] - **Spec Exp:** Sarcoma; Leukemia & Lymphoma; Retinoblastoma; **Hospital:** Chldns Hosp and Regl Med Ctr - Seattle, Univ Wash Med Ctr; **Address:** Children's Hosp Regional Med Ctr, 4800 Sandpoint Way NE, Box 5371, MS B6553, Seattle, WA 98105; **Phone:** 206-987-2106; **Board Cert:** Pediatrics 1978; **Med School:** Univ Tenn Coll Med, Memphis 1971; **Resid:** Pediatrics, Children's Memorial Hosp 1973; **Fellow:** Pediatric Hematology-Oncology, Children's Hosp Med Ctr 1977; **Fac Appt:** Prof Ped, Univ Wash

Rosenthal, Joseph MD [PHO] - **Spec Exp:** Bone Marrow Transplant; Clinical Trials; **Hospital:** City of Hope Natl Med Ctr & Beckman Rsch (page 69); **Address:** City of Hope Med Ctr, 1500 E Duarte Rd, Duarte, CA 91010; **Phone:** 626-256-4673 x68442; **Board Cert:** Pediatrics 2003; Pediatric Hematology-Oncology 2004; **Med School:** Israel 1984; **Resid:** Pediatrics, Soroka MC 1988; Pediatrics, Chldrn Hosp 1995; **Fellow:** Pediatric Hematology-Oncology, Univ Colorado 1991; Pediatric Hematology-Oncology, Chldrn Hosp 1994; **Fac Appt:** Assoc Prof Ped, USC-Keck School of Medicine

Russo, Carolyn MD [PHO] - **Spec Exp:** Brain Tumors; Cancer Survivors-Late Effects of Therapy; Palliative Care; **Hospital:** Kaiser Permanente Santa Clara Med Ctr; **Address:** 710 Lawrence Expwy, Dept 190, Santa Clara, CA 95051; **Phone:** 408-554-9810; **Board Cert:** Pediatrics 1988; Pediatric Hematology-Oncology 1998; **Med School:** UCLA 1984; **Resid:** Pediatrics, Harbor-UCLA Med Ctr 1987; **Fellow:** Pediatric Hematology-Oncology, Stanford Med Ctr 1990

Siegel, Stuart E MD [PHO] - **Spec Exp:** Leukemia; Infections in Cancer Patients; Psychiatry in Childhood Cancer; Solid Tumors; **Hospital:** Chldns Hosp - Los Angeles, Ventura Cnty Med Ctr; **Address:** Children's Hospital, 4650 Sunset Blvd, MS 54, Los Angeles, CA 90027-6062; **Phone:** 323-669-2205; **Board Cert:** Pediatrics 1973; Pediatric Hematology-Oncology 1976; **Med School:** Boston Univ 1967; **Resid:** Pediatrics, Univ Minnesota Hosps 1969; **Fellow:** Pediatric Hematology-Oncology, Natl Cancer Inst 1972; **Fac Appt:** Prof Ped, USC Sch Med

Wilkinson, Robert W MD [PHO] - **Hospital:** Kapiolani Med Ctr for Women & Chldn; **Address:** Kapiolani Med Ctr for Women & Children, 1319 Punahou St, Ste 1050, Honolulu, HI 96826; **Phone:** 808-942-8144; **Board Cert:** Pediatrics 1986; Pediatric Hematology-Oncology 1986; **Med School:** Tulane Univ 1967; **Resid:** Pediatrics, Los Angeles Co-USC Med Ctr 1971; **Fellow:** Pediatric Hematology-Oncology, Los Angeles Co-USC Med Ctr 1972; **Fac Appt:** Assoc Prof Ped, Univ Hawaii JA Burns Sch Med

Pediatric Allergy & Immunology

Mid Atlantic

Kamani, Naynesh R MD [PA&I] - **Spec Exp:** Stem Cell Transplant; Immunotherapy; Bone Marrow Transplant; **Hospital:** Chldns Natl Med Ctr; **Address:** Chldns Natl Med Ctr, Div Hematology, 111 Michigan Ave NW, Washington, DC 20010; **Phone:** 202-884-2800; **Board Cert:** Pediatrics 1983; Pediatric Allergy & Immunology 1983; **Med School:** Ethiopia 1975; **Resid:** Pediatrics, Downstate Med Ctr-Kings Co Hosp 1981; **Fellow:** Pediatric Allergy & Immunology, Children's Hosp 1983; **Fac Appt:** Prof Ped, Geo Wash Univ

West Coast and Pacific

Cowan, Morton J MD [PA&I] - **Spec Exp:** Bone Marrow Transplant; **Hospital:** UCSF Med Ctr; **Address:** UCSF Med Ctr, Peds BMT Program, 505 Parnassus Ave, rm R679, San Francisco, CA 94143-1278; **Phone:** 415-476-2188; **Board Cert:** Pediatrics 1981; Allergy & Immunology 1983; **Med School:** Univ Pennsylvania 1970; **Resid:** Surgery, Duke Univ Med Ctr 1972; Pediatrics, UCSF Med Ctr 1977; **Fellow:** Research, Natl Inst Hlth 1975; Immunology, UCSF Med Ctr; **Fac Appt:** Prof Ped, UCSF

Pediatric Endocrinology

Mid Atlantic

Sklar, Charles A MD [PEn] - **Spec Exp:** Cancer Survivors-Late Effects of Therapy; Growth Disorders in Childhood Cancer; **Hospital:** Meml Sloan Kettering Cancer Ctr (page 76); **Address:** 1275 York Ave, Box 151, New York, NY 10021; **Phone:** 212-639-8138; **Board Cert:** Pediatrics 1979; Pediatric Endocrinology 1980; **Med School:** USC Sch Med 1974; **Resid:** Pediatrics, Childrens Hosp 1976; **Fellow:** Pediatric Endocrinology, UCSF Med Ctr 1979; **Fac Appt:** Assoc Prof Ped, Cornell Univ-Weill Med Coll

Southeast

Meacham, Lillian R MD [PEn] - **Spec Exp:** Growth Disorders in Childhood Cancer; Cancer Survivors-Late Effects of Therapy; **Hospital:** Emory Univ Hosp; **Address:** Emory Childrens Ctr, 2015 Uppergate Drive, Altanta, GA 30322; **Phone:** 404-727-5753; **Board Cert:** Pediatrics 2006; Pediatric Endocrinology 2006; **Med School:** Emory Univ 1984; **Resid:** Pediatrics, Emory Univ Hosp 1987; **Fellow:** Pediatric Endocrinology, Emory Univ Hosp 1990; **Fac Appt:** Assoc Prof Ped, Emory Univ

Midwest

Zimmerman, Donald MD [PEn] - **Spec Exp:** Growth Disorders in Childhood Cancer; Thyroid Cancer; Thyroid Disorders; **Hospital:** Children's Mem Hosp; **Address:** Children's Memorial Hosp, 2300 Children's Plaza, Box 54, Chicago, IL 60614; **Phone:** 773-327-7740; **Board Cert:** Internal Medicine 1977; Endocrinology 1979; Pediatrics 1983; Pediatric Endocrinology 1983; **Med School:** Univ IL Coll Med 1974; **Resid:** Internal Medicine, Johns Hopkins Hosp 1977; Pediatrics, Mayo Grad Sch Med 1981; **Fellow:** Endocrinology, Diabetes & Metabolism, Mayo Grad Sch Med 1980; **Fac Appt:** Prof Ped, Northwestern Univ

Pediatric Otolaryngology

New England

McGill, Trevor MD [PO] - **Spec Exp:** Head & Neck Tumors; **Hospital:** Children's Hospital - Boston; **Address:** Childrens Hosp, Dept Otolaryngology, 333 Longwood Ave, Boston, MA 02115; **Phone:** 617-355-6460; **Board Cert:** Otolaryngology 1988; **Med School:** Ireland 1967; **Resid:** Otolaryngology, Royal Natl Throat Nose & Ear Hosp 1974; **Fellow:** Otolaryngology, Mass Eye & Ear Infirmary 1976; **Fac Appt:** Prof Oto, Harvard Med Sch

Mid Atlantic

Potsic, William P MD [PO] - **Spec Exp:** Ear Tumors; **Hospital:** Chldns Hosp of Philadelphia, The; **Address:** Childrens Hosp of Philadelphia, 34 St & Civic Center Blvd, Wood Bldg, Fl 1, Philadelphia, PA 19104; **Phone:** 215-590-3440; **Board Cert:** Otolaryngology 1974; **Med School:** Emory Univ 1969; **Resid:** Otolaryngology, Univ Chicago Hosps 1974; **Fac Appt:** Prof Oto, Univ Pennsylvania

Pediatric Otolaryngology

West Coast and Pacific

Crockett, Dennis M MD [PO] - **Spec Exp:** Head & Neck Cancer; **Hospital:** Chldns Hosp - Los Angeles, USC Univ Hosp - R K Eamer Med Plz; **Address:** USC Health Consultation Ctr #2, 1450 San Pablo St, Ste 4600, Los Angeles, CA 90033; **Phone:** 323-442-5790; **Board Cert:** Otolaryngology 1985; **Med School:** USC Sch Med 1979; **Resid:** Otolaryngology, LAC-USC Med Ctr 1984; **Fellow:** Pediatrics, Boston Chldns Hosp 1985; **Fac Appt:** Assoc Prof Oto, USC Sch Med

Geller, Kenneth Allen MD [PO] - **Spec Exp:** Head & Neck Cancer; **Hospital:** Chldns Hosp - Los Angeles, Huntington Memorial Hosp; **Address:** Chldns Hosp, Div Otolaryngology, 4650 Sunset Blvd, MS 58, Los Angeles, CA 90027; **Phone:** 323-669-2145; **Board Cert:** Otolaryngology 1978; **Med School:** USC Sch Med 1972; **Resid:** Surgery, Wadsworth VA Hosp 1975; Otolaryngology, UCLA Hlth Scis Ctr 1978; **Fellow:** Pediatric Otolaryngology, Chldns Hosp 1979; **Fac Appt:** Assoc Clin Prof Oto, USC Sch Med

Pediatric Surgery

New England

Latchaw, Laurie MD [PS] - **Spec Exp:** Thoracic Surgery; Cancer Surgery; Neonatal Surgery; **Hospital:** Dartmouth - Hitchcock Med Ctr; **Address:** Dartmouth-Hitchcock Med Ctr, Dept Ped Surg, One Medical Center Drive, Labanon, NH 03756; **Phone:** 603-653-9883; **Board Cert:** Surgery 2001; Pediatric Surgery 2003; **Med School:** Rush Med Coll 1976; **Resid:** Surgery, Univ Texas 1981; **Fellow:** Pediatric Surgery, Montreal Chldns Hosp 1983; **Fac Appt:** Assoc Prof S, Dartmouth Med Sch

Shamberger, Robert MD [PS] - **Spec Exp:** Cancer Surgery; **Hospital:** Children's Hospital - Boston; **Address:** Children's Hosp-Dept Surgery, 300 Longwood Ave, Fegan - 3, Boston, MA 02115; **Phone:** 617-355-8326; **Board Cert:** Surgery 2002; Surgical Critical Care 1999; Pediatric Surgery 2003; **Med School:** Harvard Med Sch 1975; **Resid:** Surgery, Massachusetts Genl Hosp 1978; Pediatric Surgery, Children's Hosp 1985; **Fellow:** Surgical Oncology, NCI-Surgical Branch 1980; **Fac Appt:** Prof S, Harvard Med Sch

Mid Atlantic

Alexander, Frederick MD [PS] - **Spec Exp:** Solid Tumors; **Hospital:** Hackensack Univ Med Ctr (page 74); **Address:** Joseph M Sanzari Chldns Hosp-HUMC, 30 Prospect Ave, Ste PC331, Hackensack, NJ 07601; **Phone:** 201-996-2921; **Board Cert:** Pediatric Surgery 1999; **Med School:** Columbia P&S 1976; **Resid:** Surgery, Brigham-Womens Hosp 1984; **Fellow:** Pediatric Surgery, Chldns Hosp 1986; **Fac Appt:** Clin Prof S

Colombani, Paul M MD [PS] - **Spec Exp:** Thoracic Surgery; Transplant-Kidney; Transplant-Liver; Cancer Surgery; **Hospital:** Johns Hopkins Hosp - Baltimore; **Address:** 600 N Wolfe St Harvey 319 Bldg, Baltimore, MD 21287; **Phone:** 410-955-2717; **Board Cert:** Surgery 2003; Pediatric Surgery 2003; **Med School:** Univ KY Coll Med 1976; **Resid:** Surgery, Geo Wash Univ Hosp 1981; **Fellow:** Pediatric Surgery, Johns Hopkins Hosp 1983; **Fac Appt:** Prof S, Johns Hopkins Univ

Ginsburg, Howard B MD [PS] - **Spec Exp:** Neonatal Surgery; Tumor Surgery; Pediatric Urology; Gastrointestinal Surgery; **Hospital:** NYU Med Ctr (page 80), Bellevue Hosp Ctr; **Address:** NYU Medical Ctr, Div Pediatric Surgery, 530 1st Ave, Ste 10W, New York, NY 10016-6402; **Phone:** 212-263-7391; **Board Cert:** Surgery 1978; Pediatric Surgery 2001; **Med School:** Univ Cincinnati 1972; **Resid:** Surgery, NYU-Bellvue Hosp 1977; Pediatric Surgery, Columbia-Presby Med Ctr 1979; **Fellow:** Pediatric Surgery, Mass Genl Hosp 1980; **Fac Appt:** Assoc Prof S, NYU Sch Med

La Quaglia, Michael MD [PS] - **Spec Exp:** Cancer Surgery; Neuroblastoma; Liver Tumors; Colon & Rectal Cancer; **Hospital:** Meml Sloan Kettering Cancer Ctr (page 76), NY-Presby Hosp (page 79); **Address:** 1275 York Ave, Box 325, New York, NY 10021-6007; **Phone:** 212-639-7002; **Board Cert:** Surgery 2003; Pediatric Surgery 1997; **Med School:** UMDNJ-NJ Med Sch, Newark 1976; **Resid:** Surgery, Mass Genl Hosp 1983; **Fellow:** Cardiothoracic Surgery, Broadgreen Ctr 1984; Pediatric Surgery, Chldns Hosp 1985; **Fac Appt:** Prof S, Cornell Univ-Weill Med Coll

Stolar, Charles J H MD [PS] - **Spec Exp:** Pediatric Cancers; Neonatal Surgery; **Hospital:** NY-Presby Hosp (page 79); **Address:** Morgan Stanley Chldns Hosp NY-Presby, 3959 Broadway, Fl 2 - rm 215 North, New York, NY 10032; **Phone:** 212-342-8586; **Board Cert:** Surgery 2001; Pediatric Surgery 1996; **Med School:** Georgetown Univ 1974; **Resid:** Surgery, Univ Illinois Hosp 1980; **Fellow:** Pediatric Surgery, Chldns Hosp Natl Med Ctr 1982; **Fac Appt:** Prof S, Columbia P&S

Southeast

Davidoff, Andrew M MD [PS] - **Spec Exp:** Neuroblastoma; Cancer Surgery; **Hospital:** St Jude Children's Research Hosp, Le Bonheur Chldns Med Ctr; **Address:** St Jude Chldns Rsch Hosp, Dept Surg, 332 N Lauderdale St, Memphis, TN 38105; **Phone:** 901-495-4060; **Board Cert:** Surgery 1995; Pediatric Surgery 1998; **Med School:** Univ Pennsylvania 1987; **Resid:** Surgery, Duke Med Ctr 1994; **Fellow:** Pediatric Surgery, Chldns Hosp 1996; **Fac Appt:** Assoc Prof S, Univ Tenn Coll Med, Memphis

Drucker, David E MD [PS] - **Spec Exp:** Thoracic Surgery; Cancer Surgery; Gastrointestinal Surgery; **Hospital:** Meml Regl Hosp - Hollywood; **Address:** 1150 N 35th Ave, Ste 555, Hollywood, FL 33021-5431; **Phone:** 954-981-0072; **Board Cert:** Surgery 1997; Pediatric Surgery 1999; Surgical Critical Care 2001; **Med School:** Brown Univ 1982; **Resid:** Surgery, Med Coll Virginia Hosps 1988; **Fellow:** Pediatric Surgery, Chldns Hosp 1990

Morgan III, Walter M MD [PS] - **Spec Exp:** Germ Cell Tumors; Neuroblastoma; Bone Cancer; **Hospital:** Vanderbilt Univ Med Ctr; **Address:** Vanderbilt Children's Hosp-Dept Ped Surgery, 2200 Children's Way, Ste 4150, Nashville, TN 37232; **Phone:** 615-936-1050; **Board Cert:** Pediatric Surgery 2001; **Med School:** Vanderbilt Univ 1982; **Resid:** Surgery, Johns Hopkins Hosp 1988; **Fellow:** Pediatric Surgery, Johns Hopkins Hosp 1990; **Fac Appt:** Asst Prof S, Vanderbilt Univ

Paidas, Charles N MD [PS] - **Spec Exp:** Pediatric Cancers; **Hospital:** Tampa Genl Hosp, Univ of S FL - Tampa; **Address:** Tampa Genl Hosp, Div Ped Surgery, 2 Columbia Drive, rm 6441, Tampa, FL 33606; **Phone:** 813-259-0929; **Board Cert:** Surgery 1999; Pediatric Surgery 2001; Surgical Critical Care 2002; **Med School:** NY Med Coll 1981; **Resid:** Surgery, NY Med Coll Affil Hosps 1987; **Fellow:** Pediatric Surgery, Johns Hopkins Hosp 1991; **Fac Appt:** Prof S, Univ S Fla Coll Med

Pediatric Surgery

Rice, Henry MD [PS] - **Spec Exp:** Neonatal Surgery; Cancer Surgery; **Hospital:** Duke Univ Med Ctr; **Address:** Duke Univ Med Ctr, Dept Ped Surg, Box 3815, Durham, NC 27710; **Phone:** 919-681-5077; **Board Cert:** Surgery 1997; Pediatric Surgery 2000; **Med School:** Yale Univ 1988; **Resid:** Surgery, Univ Wash Affil Hosps 1996; **Fellow:** Pediatric Surgery, Chldns Hosp of Buffalo 1998; **Fac Appt:** Assoc Prof S, Duke Univ

Ricketts, Richard R MD [PS] - **Spec Exp:** Neonatal Surgery; Cancer Surgery; Gastrointestinal Surgery; **Hospital:** Chldns Hlthcare Atlanta - Egleston; **Address:** 1975 Century Blvd, Ste 6, Atlanta, GA 30345; **Phone:** 404-982-9938; **Board Cert:** Surgery 2004; Pediatric Surgery 2001; **Med School:** Northwestern Univ 1973; **Resid:** Surgery, LAC-USC Med Ctr 1978; **Fellow:** Pediatric Surgery, Chldns Meml Hosp 1980; **Fac Appt:** Prof S, Emory Univ

Shochat, Stephen J MD [PS] - **Spec Exp:** Cancer Surgery; **Hospital:** St Jude Children's Research Hosp; **Address:** St Jude Childrens Research Hosp, Dept Surgery, 332 N Lauderdale St, Memphis, TN 38105; **Phone:** 901-495-2911; **Board Cert:** Surgery 1969; Thoracic Surgery 1975; Pediatric Surgery 2005; **Med School:** Med Coll VA 1963; **Resid:** Surgery, Barnes Hosp 1964; Pediatric Surgery, Boston Children's Hosp 1968; **Fellow:** Thoracic Surgery, George Washington Univ Med Ctr 1974; **Fac Appt:** Prof S, Univ Tenn Coll Med, Memphis

Skinner, Michael A MD [PS] - **Spec Exp:** Endocrine Cancers; Thyroid Cancer; **Hospital:** Duke Univ Med Ctr; **Address:** Duke Univ Med Ctr, Box 3815, Durham, NC 27710; **Phone:** 919-681-5077; **Board Cert:** Surgery 2000; Pediatric Surgery 2003; **Med School:** Rush Med Coll 1984; **Resid:** Surgery, Duke Univ Med Ctr 1991; **Fellow:** Pediatric Surgery, Indiana Univ 1993; **Fac Appt:** Assoc Prof S, Duke Univ

Weinberger, Malvin MD [PS] - **Spec Exp:** Neonatal Surgery; Cancer Surgery; **Hospital:** Miami Children's Hosp, Baptist Hosp of Miami; **Address:** 3200 SW 60th Ct, Ste 201, Miami, FL 33155-4070; **Phone:** 305-662-8320; **Board Cert:** Surgery 1970; Pediatric Surgery 1995; **Med School:** Temple Univ 1962; **Resid:** Surgery, Temple Univ Hosp 1969; Pediatric Surgery, Chldns Hosp/Ohio St Univ Hosp 1971; **Fac Appt:** Assoc Clin Prof S, Univ Miami Sch Med

Midwest

Aiken, John Judson MD [PS] - **Spec Exp:** Tumor Surgery; **Hospital:** Chldns Hosp - Wisconsin; **Address:** 999 N 92nd St, Ste C-320, Milwaukee, WI 53226; **Phone:** 414-266-6550; **Board Cert:** Surgery 2004; Pediatric Surgery 2000; **Med School:** Univ Cincinnati 1984; **Resid:** Surgery, Mass Genl Hosp 1991; **Fellow:** Pediatric Surgery, Chldns Hosp; **Fac Appt:** Assoc Prof S, Med Coll Wisc

Ehrlich, Peter F MD [PS] - **Spec Exp:** Pediatric Cancers; Wilms' Tumor; Thyroid Cancer; **Hospital:** Mott Chldns Hosp, Mich State Univ-Hurley Med Ctr; **Address:** Mott Children's Hospital, 1500 E Medical Center Drive, rm F3970, Ann Arbor, MI 48109-0245; **Phone:** 734-764-4151; **Board Cert:** Surgery 1997; Pediatric Surgery 2000; **Med School:** Canada 1989; **Resid:** Surgery, Univ Toronto Med Ctr 1996; **Fellow:** Pediatric Surgery, Children's Natl Med Ctr 1998; **Fac Appt:** Assoc Clin Prof S, Univ Mich Med Sch

Grosfeld, Jay L MD [PS] - **Spec Exp:** Cancer Surgery; **Hospital:** Riley Hosp for Children (page 70); **Address:** 702 Barnhill Drive, Ste 2500, Indianapolis, IN 46202-5200; **Phone:** 317-274-5716; **Board Cert:** Surgery 1989; Pediatric Surgery 2000; **Med School:** NYU Sch Med 1961; **Resid:** Surgery, Bellevue-NYU Hosp 1966; Pediatric Surgery, Ohio State Univ 1970; **Fellow:** Surgical Oncology, Chldns Hosp 1970; **Fac Appt:** Prof S, Indiana Univ

Warner, Brad MD [PS] - Spec Exp: Gastrointestinal Surgery; Neonatal Surgery; Cancer Surgery; **Hospital:** Cincinnati Chldns Hosp Med Ctr; **Address:** Cincinnati Chlds Hosp, Div Ped Surg, 3333 Burnet Ave, MLC 2023, Cincinnati, OH 45229; **Phone:** 513-636-4371; **Board Cert:** Surgery 1998; Pediatric Surgery 2001; **Med School:** Univ MO-Kansas City 1982; **Resid:** Surgery, Univ Cincinnati Med Ctr 1989; **Fellow:** Pediatric Surgery, Chldns Hosp Med Ctr 1991; **Fac Appt:** Prof S, Univ Cincinnati

Great Plains and Mountains

Meyers, Rebecka L MD [PS] - Spec Exp: Transplant-Liver; Tumor Surgery-Pediatric; Biliary Surgery; Pancreatic Surgery; **Hospital:** Univ Utah Hosps and Clins; **Address:** Primary Chlds Med Ctr, Dept Ped Surg, 100 N Medical Drive, Ste 2600, Salt Lake City, UT 84113; **Phone:** 801-588-3350; **Board Cert:** Surgery 2003; Pediatric Surgery 1996; **Med School:** Oregon Hlth Sci Univ 1985; **Resid:** Surgery, UCSF 1990; **Fellow:** Research, Cardio Rsch Inst-UCSF 1992; Pediatric Surgery, St Christopher's Hosp for Chldn 1994; **Fac Appt:** Assoc Prof S, Univ Utah

Ziegler, Moritz M MD [PS] - Spec Exp: Gastrointestinal Surgery; Neuroblastoma; Tumor Surgery-Pediatric; **Hospital:** Chldn's Hosp - Denver, The; **Address:** Chldns Hosp, Dept Surgery, 1056 E 19th Ave, Box 323, Denver, CO 80218; **Phone:** 303-861-6524; **Board Cert:** Surgery 1975; Pediatric Surgery 1995; **Med School:** Univ Mich Med Sch 1968; **Resid:** Surgery, Univ Penn Hosp 1975; Pediatric Surgery, Chldns Hosp 1977; **Fellow:** Surgical Oncology, Amer Oncologic Hosp 1975; **Fac Appt:** Prof S, Univ Colorado

Southwest

Jackson, Richard J MD [PS] - Spec Exp: Cancer Surgery; Neonatal Surgery; Robotic Surgery; **Hospital:** Arkansas Chldns Hosp; **Address:** Arkansas Chldns Hosp - Ped Surgery, 800 Marshall St, MS 837, Little Rock, AR 72202; **Phone:** 501-364-1446; **Board Cert:** Surgery 1997; Pediatric Surgery 2001; Surgical Critical Care 1998; **Med School:** W VA Univ 1983; **Resid:** Surgery, W Va Univ Hosps 1988; Pediatric Surgery, Chldns Hosp 1989; **Fellow:** Pediatric Critical Care Medicine, Chldns Hosp-Univ Pittsburgh 1990; Pediatric Surgery, Chldns Hosp-Univ Pittsburgh 1992; **Fac Appt:** Assoc Prof S, Univ Ark

Nuchtern, Jed MD [PS] - Spec Exp: Thoracic Surgery; Cancer Surgery; Laparoscopic Surgery; **Hospital:** Texas Chldns Hosp - Houston, Ben Taub General Hosp; **Address:** Texas Children's Hosp, 6621 Fannin St, MC CC650, Houston, TX 77030; **Phone:** 832-822-3135; **Board Cert:** Surgery 2003; Surgical Critical Care 2002; Pediatric Surgery 1998; **Med School:** Harvard Med Sch 1985; **Resid:** Surgery, Univ Washington 1992; Pediatric Surgery, Baylor Coll Med 1995; **Fellow:** Cellular Molecular Biology, Natl Inst Hlth 1990; **Fac Appt:** Assoc Prof S, Baylor Coll Med

West Coast and Pacific

Atkinson, James B MD [PS] - Spec Exp: Laparoscopic Surgery; Cancer Surgery; **Hospital:** UCLA Med Ctr (page 83), Northridge Hosp Med Ctr - Roscoe Campus; **Address:** 10833 LeConte Ave, Box 709818, Los Angeles, CA 90095; **Phone:** 310-206-2429; **Board Cert:** Surgery 2001; Pediatric Surgery 2003; **Med School:** Wake Forest Univ 1976; **Resid:** Surgery, UCLA Med Ctr 1981; **Fellow:** Pediatric Surgery, Chldns Hosp 1983; **Fac Appt:** Prof S, UCLA

Pediatric Surgery

Sawin, Robert S MD [PS] - **Spec Exp:** Pediatric Cancers; Thoracic Surgery; **Hospital:** Chldns Hosp and Regl Med Ctr - Seattle; **Address:** Chldns Hosp & Regl Med Ctr, PO Box 5371, MS W7724, Seattle, WA 98105; **Phone:** 206-987-2039; **Board Cert:** Surgery 1998; Surgical Critical Care 2001; Pediatric Surgery 1999; **Med School:** Univ Pittsburgh 1982; **Resid:** Surgery, Brigham Women's Hosp 1987; **Fellow:** Pediatric Surgery, Chldns Hosp 1989; **Fac Appt:** Prof S, Univ Wash

Pediatrics

New England

Sallan, Stephen MD [Ped] - **Spec Exp:** Pediatric Cancers; Leukemia; **Hospital:** Children's Hospital - Boston; **Address:** Dana Farber Cancer Inst, Dept Ped Oncology, 44 Binney St, Ste 1642, Boston, MA 02115; **Phone:** 617-632-3316; **Board Cert:** Pediatrics 1972; **Med School:** Wayne State Univ 1967; **Resid:** Pediatrics, Chldns Hosp 1969; Pediatrics, Hosp Sick Chldn 1970; **Fellow:** Pediatric Oncology, Chldns Hosp Med Ctr 1975; **Fac Appt:** Prof Ped, Harvard Med Sch

Schechter, Neil L MD [Ped] - **Spec Exp:** Pain Management; Pain-Cancer; **Hospital:** CT Chldns Med Ctr, St Francis Hosp & Med Ctr; **Address:** St Francis Hosp, Dept Pediatrics, 114 Woodland St, Hartford, CT 06105; **Phone:** 860-714-4931; **Board Cert:** Pediatrics 1979; **Med School:** Mich State Univ 1973; **Resid:** Pediatrics, Univ Conn Hlth Ctr 1977; **Fellow:** Developmental-Behavioral Pediatrics, Chldns Hosp Med Ctr/Harvard 1979; **Fac Appt:** Prof Ped, Univ Conn

Mid Atlantic

Oeffinger, Kevin MD [Ped] - **Spec Exp:** Cancer Survivors-Late Effects of Therapy; **Hospital:** Meml Sloan Kettering Cancer Ctr (page 76); **Address:** 1275 York Ave, New York, NY 10021; **Phone:** 212-639-8469; **Board Cert:** Family Medicine 2000; **Med School:** Univ Tex, San Antonio 1984; **Resid:** Family Medicine, Baylor Coll Med 1985; **Fellow:** Family Medicine, Fam Practice Faculty Dev Ctr 1999; Natl Cancer Inst 2000

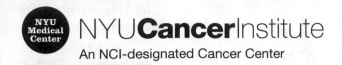

NYU**Cancer**Institute
An NCI-designated Cancer Center

NYU Clinical Cancer Center
160 East 34th Street
New York, New York 10016
www.nyuci.org/atcd

NYU Medical Center
550 First Avenue
(at 31st Street)
New York, New York 10016
www.nyumc.org/atcd

**Stephen D. Hassenfeld
Children's Center
for Cancer and Blood
Disorders**
160 East 32nd Street
New York, New York 10016
www.nyumc.org/hassenfeld

A Collaborative Approach
The NYU Cancer Institute, an NCI designated center, is a "matrix cancer center" without walls operating within the larger NYU Medical Center. With over 200 members and a research funding base of over $81 million, this structure strengthens our capabilities to forge collaborations across medical and scientific disciplines, which translates to comprehensive care for our patients and discoveries that will influence the future of this disease.

Renowned Expertise
Our highly skilled Magnet™ nursing team not only plays a pivotal role in coordinating direct patient care, but is also a source of invaluable patient education. Team members' compassion and expertise help patients better manage the symptoms of their disease as well as their special needs.

A Patient-Focused Setting
The NYU Clinical Cancer Center, with over 70 faculty members from various disciplines at the New York University School of Medicine, is the principal outpatient facility of the Cancer Institute and serves as home for our patients and their caregivers. The center and its multidisciplinary team of experts provide access to the latest treatment options and clinical trials along with a variety of programs in cancer prevention, screening, diagnostics, genetic counseling, and supportive services. When it comes to kids and cancer, the Stephen D. Hassenfeld Children's Center for Cancer and Blood Disorders offers not just innovation but insight. As a leading member of the NCI-sponsored Children's Oncology Group, our physicians are known for developing new ways to treat childhood cancer. Our affiliation with Bellevue Hospital, the oldest public hospital in the country, affords clinically distinctive opportunities to learn and care for patients with cancer by observing its presentation and behavior in a variety of patient groups.

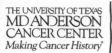
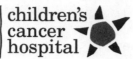

**Children's Cancer Center at
The University of Texas
M. D. Anderson Cancer Center**

1515 Holcombe Blvd.
Houston, Texas 77030-4095
Tel. 713-792-6161 Toll Free 877-MDA-6789
www.mdanderson.org/children

THE CHILDRENS CANCER HOSPITAL AT M. D. ANDERSON CANCER CENTER

At M. D. Anderson, hope is real. We've helped thousands of children survive cancer with the best possible outcomes and quality of life. Unlike most children's hospitals, we do only one thing — treat cancer. Every patient benefits from our extensive knowledge of both common and rare tumors, as well as a strong research program that works to find new pediatric treatments.

At the Children's Cancer Hospital, kids rule — not cancer. At M. D. Anderson, we treat the whole child, not just the cancer. Each patient has a team of specialists to address medical, psychological and developmental issues related to cancer or its treatments. Counseling and support groups help both you and your child overcome fears and concerns. Our in-house classroom allows them to keep up with schoolwork. Even after treatment is finished, follow-up programs will monitor and manage any long-term side effects.

PROTON THERAPY

M. D. Anderson's Proton Therapy Center opened in May 2006 as the largest and most sophisticated center of its type. Proton therapy radiation is one of the most advanced technologies available for treating children's cancer. It allows for the most aggressive cancer therapy possible, while keeping the harm to growing bodies and side effects to a minimum.

MORE INFORMATION

For more information or to make an appointment, call 877-MDA-6789, or visit us onlinc at http://www.mdanderson.org/children.

At M. D. Anderson Cancer Center, our mission is simple – to eliminate cancer. Achieving that goal begins with integrated programs in cancer treatment, clinical trials, education programs and cancer prevention.

We focus exclusively on cancer and have seen cases of every kind. That means you receive expert care no matter what your diagnosis.

Choosing the right partner for cancer care really does make a difference. The fact is, people who choose M. D. Anderson over other hospitals and clinics often have better results. That is how we've been making cancer history for over sixty years.

840

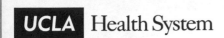

Mattel Children's Hospital at UCLA

1-800-UCLA-MD1 (825-2631)
www.uclahealth.org

For more than 40 years, UCLA's Pediatric Hematology & Oncology Program at Mattel Children's Hospital at UCLA has provided leading-edge treatments for children with leukemia, aplastic anemia, solid tumors, blood diseases, and various genetic disorders.

The program — part of UCLA's Jonsson Cancer Center — has pioneered clinical research in countless arenas, including: bone marrow and stem cell transplantation, pediatric sarcomas (including innovative limb-saving technology), optimal tumor resection using brain mapping and PET scan technology; recognition of the effects of cancer on family members, and recognition and treatment of pain in children with cancer.

UCLA is leading the way in designing new drugs specifically for children with cancer. Children typically get access to new drugs via clinical trials only after they have been available to adults for several years. UCLA researchers are currently testing newly developed therapies on childhood leukemia and tumor cell lines, to bring the most promising ones to clinical trials for children.

When children are diagnosed with cancer, it affects the whole family. At UCLA, Child Life Specialists and dedicated Clinical Social Workers collaborate with the doctors and nurses to help children and their families understand and cope with the illness — from initial diagnosis through treatment, recovery and beyond.

UCLA's Jonsson Cancer Center

Designated by the National Cancer Institute as one of only 39 comprehensive cancer centers in the United States, UCLA's Jonsson Cancer Center has earned an international reputation for developing new cancer therapies, providing the best in experimental and traditional treatments, and expertly guiding and training the next generation of medical researchers. The center's 250 physicians and scientists treat upwards of 20,000 patient visits per year and offer hundreds of clinical trials that provide the latest in experimental cancer treatments (www.cancer.mednet.ucla.edu). The center also offers patients and families complete psychological and support services.

UCLA's Jonsson Cancer Center has been ranked the best cancer center in California by *U.S.News & World Report*'s Annual Best Hospitals survey for the seventh year. UCLA Medical Center, of which the Cancer Center is a part, has ranked best in the West for the past 17 years.

Call 1-800-UCLA-MD1 (825-2631)
for a referral to a UCLA doctor.

LIFE AFTER CANCER

Prior to 1970, most children and young adults under 20 who were diagnosed with cancer had little hope of being cured. Today, nearly 75 percent of all pediatric cancer patients have a chance of surviving to that magic five-year mark and beyond thanks to remarkable advances in treatment. Estimates show that one in every 640 adults aged 20 to 39 has a history of childhood cancer.

The Life After Cancer Clinic at UCLA was created to address the medical and quality-of-life issues of childhood cancer survivors. The unique program provides a comprehensive health evaluation, a psychosocial assessment, targeted sub-specialty referrals, and offers information on the risks for late effects, cancer prevention, and opportunities for participation in research studies.

Plastic Surgery

A plastic surgeon deals with the repair, reconstruction or replacement of physical defects of form or function involving the skin, musculoskeletal system, craniomaxillofacial structures, hand, extremities, breast and trunk and external genitalia. He/she uses aesthetic surgical principles not only to improve undesirable qualities of normal structures (commonly called "cosmetic surgery") but in all reconstructive procedures as well.

A plastic surgeon possesses special knowledge and skill in the design and surgery of grafts, flaps, free tissue transfer and replantation. Competence in the management of complex wounds, the use of implantable materials, and in tumor surgery is required.

Trainging Required: Five to seven years

Plastic Surgery within the Head and Neck: A plastic surgeon with additional training in plastic and reconstructive procedures within the head, face, neck and associated structures, including cutaneous head and neck oncology and reconstruction, management of maxillofacial trauma, soft tissue repair and neural surgery.

The field is diverse and involved a wide range of patients, from the newborn to the aged. While both cosmetic and reconstructive surgery are practiced, there are many additional procedures which interface with them.

Surgery of the Hand:
(See Hand Surgery under Orthopaedic Surgery)

Plastic Surgery

New England

Ariyan, Stephan MD [PlS] - **Spec Exp:** Melanoma; **Hospital:** Yale - New Haven Hosp; **Address:** New Haven Hospital, 60 Temple St, Ste 7C, New Haven, CT 06510-2716; **Phone:** 203-786-3000; **Board Cert:** Plastic Surgery 1978; **Med School:** NY Med Coll 1966; **Resid:** Surgery, Yale-New Haven Hosp 1975; Plastic Surgery, Yale-New Haven Hosp 1976; **Fellow:** Surgical Oncology, Yale-New Haven Hosp 1971; **Fac Appt:** Clin Prof S, Yale Univ

Collins, Eva Dale MD [PlS] - **Spec Exp:** Breast Cancer; Breast Reconstruction; **Hospital:** Dartmouth - Hitchcock Med Ctr; **Address:** Darthmouth-Hitchcock Med Ctr, Div Plas Surgery, One Medical Center Drive, Lebanon, NH 03756; **Phone:** 603-650-5148; **Board Cert:** Plastic Surgery 1997; **Med School:** Emory Univ 1989; **Resid:** Plastic Surgery, Washington Univ Med Ctr 1994; **Fellow:** Microsurgery, Washington Univ Med Ctr 1995; **Fac Appt:** Assoc Prof S, Dartmouth Med Sch

May Jr, James W MD [PlS] - **Spec Exp:** Breast Reconstruction; **Hospital:** Mass Genl Hosp; **Address:** Mass Genl Hosp, 15 Parkman St, WACC 453, Boston, MA 02114; **Phone:** 617-726-8220; **Board Cert:** Surgery 1975; Plastic Surgery 1977; **Med School:** Northwestern Univ 1969; **Resid:** Plastic Surgery, Mass Genl Hosp 1975; **Fellow:** Hand Surgery, Univ Louisville 1975; **Fac Appt:** Prof S, Harvard Med Sch

Stadelmann, Wayne K MD [PlS] - **Spec Exp:** Melanoma-Head & Neck; Breast Reconstruction; **Hospital:** Concord Hospital, Elliot Hosp; **Address:** 248 Pleasant St, Ste 201, Concord, NH 03301; **Phone:** 603-224-5200; **Board Cert:** Plastic Surgery 1999; **Med School:** Univ Chicago-Pritzker Sch Med 1990; **Resid:** Surgery, Univ Chicago Hosps 1994; Plastic Surgery, Univ S Florida/H Lee Moffit Cancer Ctr 1997

Stahl, Richard S MD [PlS] - **Spec Exp:** Breast Reconstruction; Chest Wall Tumors; Chest Wall Reconstruction; Abdominal Wall Reconstruction; **Hospital:** Yale - New Haven Hosp, Hosp of St Raphael; **Address:** 5 Durham Rd, Guilford, CT 06437; **Phone:** 203-458-4440; **Board Cert:** Surgery 2001; Plastic Surgery 1984; **Med School:** Vanderbilt Univ 1976; **Resid:** Surgery, Yale New Haven Hosp 1981; Plastic Surgery, Emory Univ Med Ctr 1983; **Fac Appt:** Clin Prof S, Yale Univ

Mid Atlantic

Bartlett, Scott P MD [PlS] - **Spec Exp:** Craniofacial Surgery/Reconstruction; Pediatric Plastic Surgery; Facial Plastic & Reconstructive Surgery; **Hospital:** Hosp Univ Penn - UPHS (page 84), Chldns Hosp of Philadelphia, The; **Address:** Hosp Univ Penn, 3400 Spruce St, Philadelphia, PA 19104-4227; **Phone:** 215-662-2096; **Board Cert:** Plastic Surgery 1987; **Med School:** Washington Univ, St Louis 1975; **Resid:** Surgery, Mass Genl Hosp 1983; Plastic Surgery, Mass Genl Hosp 1985; **Fellow:** Craniofacial Surgery, Hosp Univ Penn 1986; **Fac Appt:** Prof PlS, Univ Pennsylvania

Cordeiro, Peter G MD [PlS] - **Spec Exp:** Reconstructive Surgery; Breast Reconstruction; Facial Plastic & Reconstructive Surgery; **Hospital:** Meml Sloan Kettering Cancer Ctr (page 76), Manhattan Eye, Ear & Throat Hosp; **Address:** Meml Sloan Kettering Cancer Ctr, 1275 York Ave, rm C1193, New York, NY 10021-6007; **Phone:** 212-639-2521; **Board Cert:** Surgery 1998; Plastic Surgery 1994; **Med School:** Harvard Med Sch 1983; **Resid:** Surgery, New Eng Deaconess Hosp-Harvard 1989; Plastic Surgery, NYU Med Ctr 1991; **Fellow:** Microsurgery, Meml Sloan-Kettering Cancer Ctr. 1992; Craniofacial Surgery, Univ Miami 1992; **Fac Appt:** Prof S, Cornell Univ-Weill Med Coll

Hoffman, Lloyd MD [PlS] - **Spec Exp:** Breast Reconstruction; **Hospital:** NY-Presby Hosp (page 79), Lenox Hill Hosp; **Address:** 12 E 68th St, New York, NY 10021; **Phone:** 212-861-1640; **Board Cert:** Plastic Surgery 1989; **Med School:** Northwestern Univ 1978; **Resid:** Surgery, New York Hosp 1983; Plastic Surgery, NYU Med Ctr 1986; **Fellow:** Hand Surgery, NYU Med Ctr 1987; **Fac Appt:** Assoc Prof PlS, Cornell Univ-Weill Med Coll

Loree, Thom R MD [PlS] - **Spec Exp:** Head & Neck Cancer; Thyroid Cancer; Reconstructive Surgery; **Hospital:** Roswell Park Cancer Inst; **Address:** Roswell Park Cancer Inst, Div Head & Neck Surgery, Elm & Carlton Sts, Buffalo, NY 14263; **Phone:** 716-845-3158; **Board Cert:** Surgery 1997; Plastic Surgery 2004; **Med School:** Geo Wash Univ 1982; **Resid:** Surgery, St Lukes-Roosevelt Hosp 1987; Plastic Surgery, St Lukes-Roosevelt Hosp 1989; **Fellow:** Head & Neck Surgical Oncology, Meml Sloan-Kettering Cancer Ctr 1990; **Fac Appt:** Assoc Prof S, SUNY Buffalo

Noone, R Barrett MD [PlS] - **Spec Exp:** Breast Reconstruction; **Hospital:** Bryn Mawr Hosp, Lankenau Hosp; **Address:** 888 Glenbrook Ave, Bryn Mawr, PA 19010-2506; **Phone:** 610-527-4833; **Board Cert:** Surgery 1972; Plastic Surgery 1974; **Med School:** Univ Pennsylvania 1965; **Resid:** Surgery, Hosp Univ Penn 1971; Plastic Surgery, Hosp Univ Penn 1973; **Fac Appt:** Clin Prof S, Univ Pennsylvania

Serletti, Joseph M MD [PlS] - **Spec Exp:** Breast Reconstruction; Reconstructive Surgery; **Hospital:** Hosp Univ Penn - UPHS (page 84); **Address:** Hosp Univ Penn, 3400 Spruce St, 10 Penn Tower, Philadelphia, PA 19104; **Phone:** 215-662-3743; **Board Cert:** Plastic Surgery 2003; **Med School:** Univ Rochester 1982; **Resid:** Surgery, U Rochester Med Ctr 1986; Plastic Surgery, U Rochester Med Ctr 1988; **Fellow:** Reconstructive Surgery, Johns Hopkins Hosp 1990; **Fac Appt:** Prof PlS, Univ Pennsylvania

Slezak, Sheri MD [PlS] - **Spec Exp:** Breast Reconstruction; **Hospital:** Univ of MD Med Sys; **Address:** Univ Maryland, Dept Plastic Surgery, 22 S Greene St, rm S8D12, Baltimore, MD 21201; **Phone:** 410-328-2360; **Board Cert:** Plastic Surgery 1991; **Med School:** Harvard Med Sch 1980; **Resid:** Surgery, Columbia-Presby Med Ctr 1985; Plastic Surgery, Johns Hopkins Hosp 1989; **Fac Appt:** Assoc Prof PlS, Univ MD Sch Med

Spear, Scott L MD [PlS] - **Spec Exp:** Breast Reconstruction; **Hospital:** Georgetown Univ Hosp; **Address:** Georgetown Univ Hosp, Div Plastic Surg, 3800 Reservoir Rd NW, 1 PHC, Washington, DC 20007; **Phone:** 202-444-8612; **Board Cert:** Plastic Surgery 1981; **Med School:** Univ Chicago-Pritzker Sch Med 1972; **Resid:** Surgery, Beth Israel Hosp 1978; Plastic Surgery, Univ Miami Hosps 1980; **Fellow:** Plastic Surgery, Hosp St Louis 1981; **Fac Appt:** Prof PlS, Georgetown Univ

Sultan, Mark MD [PlS] - **Spec Exp:** Breast Reconstruction; **Hospital:** St Luke's - Roosevelt Hosp Ctr - Roosevelt Div (page 72), Beth Israel Med Ctr - Petrie Division (page 72); **Address:** 1100 Park Ave, New York, NY 10128; **Phone:** 212-360-0700; **Board Cert:** Plastic Surgery 1992; **Med School:** Columbia P&S 1982; **Resid:** Surgery, Columbia-Presby Hosp 1987; Plastic Surgery, Columbia-Presby Hosp 1990; **Fellow:** Head and Neck Surgery, Emory Univ Hosp 1989; **Fac Appt:** Assoc Prof S, Columbia P&S

Plastic Surgery

Whitaker, Linton A MD [PlS] - Spec Exp: Craniofacial Surgery/Reconstruction; Facial Tumors; **Hospital:** Hosp Univ Penn - UPHS (page 84), Chldns Hosp of Philadelphia, The; **Address:** Hosp Univ Penn -10 Penn Tower, 3400 Spruce St, Philadelphia, PA 19104; **Phone:** 215-662-2048; **Board Cert:** Surgery 1970; Plastic Surgery 1978; **Med School:** Tulane Univ 1962; **Resid:** Surgery, Dartmouth Affl Hosp 1969; Plastic Surgery, Hosp Univ Penn 1971; **Fac Appt:** Prof PlS, Univ Pennsylvania

Southeast

Allen, Robert J MD [PlS] - Spec Exp: Breast Reconstruction; **Hospital:** E Cooper Reg Med Ctr, Ochsner Baptist Med Ctr; **Address:** 125 Doughty St, Ste 480, Charleston, SC 29403; **Phone:** 888-890-3437; **Board Cert:** Plastic Surgery 1985; **Med School:** Med Univ SC 1976; **Resid:** Surgery, LSU Med Ctr 1982; Plastic Surgery, LSU Med Ctr 1981; **Fellow:** Microsurgery, NYU Med Ctr 1983; **Fac Appt:** Assoc Clin Prof PlS, Louisiana State Univ

Fix, R Jobe MD [PlS] - Spec Exp: Breast Reconstruction; Microsurgery; **Hospital:** Univ of Ala Hosp at Birmingham, Children's Hospital - Birmingham; **Address:** Univ of Alabama Hosp, Div Plastic Surg, 510 S 20th St, FOT-Ste 1102, Birmingham, AL 35294; **Phone:** 205-934-3358; **Board Cert:** Surgery 1997; Hand Surgery 2001; Plastic Surgery 1991; **Med School:** Univ Nebr Coll Med 1982; **Resid:** Surgery, Valley Med Ctr 1987; Plastic Surgery, Univ Ala Hosp 1989; **Fac Appt:** Prof PlS, Univ Ala

Georgiade, Gregory MD [PlS] - Spec Exp: Breast Reconstruction; **Hospital:** Duke Univ Med Ctr; **Address:** Duke Univ Med Ctr, Box 3960, Durham, NC 27710; **Phone:** 919-684-3039; **Board Cert:** Plastic Surgery 1981; Surgery 1990; **Med School:** Duke Univ 1973; **Resid:** Surgery, Duke Univ Med Ctr 1978; Plastic Surgery, Duke Univ Med Ctr 1980; **Fac Appt:** Prof S, Duke Univ

Hester Jr, T Roderick MD [PlS] - Spec Exp: Breast Reconstruction; **Hospital:** Emory Univ Hosp; **Address:** 3200 Downwood Cir, Ste 6340, Atlanta, GA 30327-1624; **Phone:** 404-351-0051; **Board Cert:** Plastic Surgery 1980; Surgery 1973; **Med School:** Emory Univ 1967; **Resid:** Surgery, Emory Affil Hosps 1972; Plastic Reconstructive Surgery, Emory Affil Hosps 1978

Maxwell, G Patrick MD [PlS] - Spec Exp: Breast Reconstruction; **Hospital:** Baptist Hosp - Nashville, Centennial Med Ctr; **Address:** 2021 Church St, Ste 310, Baptist Medical Plaza Two, Nashville, TN 37203; **Phone:** 615-284-8200; **Board Cert:** Plastic Surgery 1981; **Med School:** Vanderbilt Univ 1972; **Resid:** Surgery, Johns Hopkins Hosp 1976; Plastic Surgery, Johns Hopkins Hosp 1979; **Fellow:** Microsurgery, Davies Med Ctr 1975; **Fac Appt:** Asst Clin Prof PlS, Vanderbilt Univ

McCraw, John MD [PlS] - Spec Exp: Breast Reconstruction; **Hospital:** Univ Hosps & Clins - Jackson; **Address:** Univ Mississippi Med Ctr, Div Plastic Surg, 2500 N State St, Jackson, MS 39216; **Phone:** 601-815-1343; **Board Cert:** Surgery 1972; Plastic Surgery 1974; **Med School:** Univ MO-Columbia Sch Med 1966; **Resid:** Orthopaedic Surgery, Duke U Med Ctr 1969; Surgery, Univ Florida Med Ctr 1972; **Fellow:** Plastic Surgery, Univ Florida Med Ctr 1973; **Fac Appt:** Prof PlS, Univ Miss

Smith Jr, David J MD [PlS] - Spec Exp: Breast Reconstruction; **Hospital:** Univ of S FL - Tampa; **Address:** Univ South Florida, Div Plastic Surg, 4 Columbia Drive, Ste 650, Tampa, FL 33606; **Phone:** 813-259-0929; **Board Cert:** Plastic Surgery 1981; **Med School:** Indiana Univ 1973; **Resid:** Plastic Surgery, Ind Univ 1980; Surgery, Emory Univ-Grady Hosp 1978; **Fellow:** Hand Surgery, Univ Louisville 1979; **Fac Appt:** Prof S, Univ S Fla Coll Med

Vasconez, Luis O MD [PlS] - **Spec Exp:** Breast Reconstruction; **Hospital:** Univ of Ala Hosp at Birmingham; **Address:** 510 20th St S, FOT 1102, Birmingham, AL 35294-3411; **Phone:** 205-934-3245; **Board Cert:** Surgery 1970; Plastic Surgery 1971; **Med School:** Washington Univ, St Louis 1962; **Resid:** Surgery, Strong Meml Hosp 1970; Plastic Surgery, Shands Hosp-Univ FL 1969; **Fac Appt:** Prof S, Univ Ala

Midwest

Brandt, Keith MD [PlS] - **Spec Exp:** Breast Reconstruction; Reconstructive Surgery; Microsurgery; **Hospital:** Barnes-Jewish Hosp, St Louis Chldns Hosp; **Address:** 660 S Euclid, Box 8238, St Louis, MO 63110-1010; **Phone:** 314-747-0541; **Board Cert:** Surgery 1999; Plastic Surgery 2003; Hand Surgery 2005; **Med School:** Univ Tex, Houston 1983; **Resid:** Surgery, Univ Nebraska Med Ctr 1989; Plastic Surgery, Univ Tennessee 1991; **Fellow:** Hand Surgery, Wash Univ 1992; Microsurgery, Wash Univ 1993; **Fac Appt:** Prof S, Washington Univ, St Louis

Coleman, John J MD [PlS] - **Spec Exp:** Cancer Reconstruction; Breast Reconstruction; Head & Neck Surgery; **Hospital:** Indiana Univ Hosp (page 70); **Address:** 545 Barnhill Dr, Emerson Hall, Ste 232, Indianapolis, IN 46202-5120; **Phone:** 317-274-8106; **Board Cert:** Surgery 1998; Plastic Surgery 1981; **Med School:** Harvard Med Sch 1973; **Resid:** Surgery, Emory Univ Affil Hosp 1978; Plastic Surgery, Emory Univ Affil Hosp 1979; **Fellow:** Surgical Oncology, Univ Maryland Med Ctr; **Fac Appt:** Prof S, Indiana Univ

Walton Jr, Robert Lee MD [PlS] - **Spec Exp:** Nasal Reconstruction; Breast Reconstruction; **Hospital:** Univ of Chicago Hosps, Resurrection Hlth Care St Joseph Hosp; **Address:** 60 E Delaware, Ste 1430, Chicago, IL 60611; **Phone:** 312-337-7795; **Board Cert:** Plastic Surgery 1980; **Med School:** Univ Kans 1972; **Resid:** Surgery, Johns Hopkins Hosp 1974; Plastic Surgery, Yale-New Haven Hosp 1978; **Fellow:** Hand Surgery, Hartford Hosp 1978; **Fac Appt:** Prof PlS, Univ Chicago-Pritzker Sch Med

Wilkins, Edwin G MD [PlS] - **Spec Exp:** Breast Reconstruction; Microsurgery; **Hospital:** Univ Michigan Hlth Sys; **Address:** Univ Mich, Div Plastic Surg, 1500 E Med Ctr Drive, rm 2130 Taubman Ctr, Ann Arbor, MI 48109-0340; **Phone:** 734-998-6022; **Board Cert:** Plastic Surgery 1991; **Med School:** Wake Forest Univ 1981; **Resid:** Surgery, Charlotte Meml Hosp 1986; Plastic Surgery, Vanderbilt Univ Med Ctr 1988; **Fellow:** Reconstructive Microsurgery, Univ Louisville Sch Med 1989; **Fac Appt:** Assoc Prof PlS, Univ Mich Med Sch

Yetman, Randall John MD [PlS] - **Spec Exp:** Breast Reconstruction; Melanoma; **Hospital:** Cleveland Clin Fdn (page 71); **Address:** 9500 Euclid Ave, Desk A60, Cleveland, OH 44195; **Phone:** 216-444-6908; **Board Cert:** Plastic Surgery 1984; **Med School:** Univ Miami Sch Med 1975; **Resid:** Surgery, Montefiore Med Ctr 1979; Plastic Surgery, NY Cornell Med Ctr 1981; **Fellow:** Plastic Surgery, Cleveland Clin Fdn 1982

Southwest

Menick, Frederick J MD [PlS] - **Spec Exp:** Reconstructive Surgery-Face; Breast Reconstruction; Cancer Reconstruction; **Hospital:** St Joseph's Hosp - Tucson; **Address:** 1102 N Eldorado Pl, Tucson, AZ 85712; **Phone:** 520-881-4525; **Board Cert:** Plastic Surgery 1983; **Med School:** Yale Univ 1970; **Resid:** Surgery, Stanford Med Ctr; Surgery, Univ Ariz Med Ctr 1979; **Fellow:** Plastic Surgery, Queen Victoria Hosp/UC Irvine 1982; **Fac Appt:** Assoc Clin Prof S, Univ Ariz Coll Med

Plastic Surgery

Robb, Geoffrey L MD [PlS] - **Spec Exp:** Breast Reconstruction; Head & Neck Cancer Reconstruction; Facial Plastic & Reconstructive Surgery; **Hospital:** UT MD Anderson Cancer Ctr (page 81), St Luke's Episcopal Hosp - Houston; **Address:** 1515 Holcombe Blvd, Unit 443, Houston, TX 77030; **Phone:** 713-794-1247; **Board Cert:** Otolaryngology 1979; Plastic Surgery 1986; **Med School:** Univ Miami Sch Med 1974; **Resid:** Otolaryngology, Naval Reg Med Ctr 1979; Plastic Surgery, Univ Pittsburgh 1985; **Fellow:** Microvascular Surgery, Univ Pittsburgh; **Fac Appt:** Prof PlS, Univ Tex, Houston

Rohrich, Rod J MD [PlS] - **Spec Exp:** Breast Reconstruction; **Hospital:** UT Southwestern Med Ctr - Dallas, Baylor Univ Medical Ctr; **Address:** Univ Tex SW Med Ctr, Plastic Surgery, 5323 Harry Hines Blvd, Dallas, TX 75390-9132; **Phone:** 214-648-3119; **Board Cert:** Plastic Surgery 1987; Hand Surgery 1990; **Med School:** Baylor Coll Med 1979; **Resid:** Plastic Surgery, Univ Mich Hosp 1985; Plastic Surgery, Radcliffe Infirm/Oxford 1983; **Fellow:** Hand Surgery, Mass Genl Hosp-Harvard 1987; **Fac Appt:** Prof PlS, Univ Tex SW, Dallas

Schusterman, Mark A MD [PlS] - **Spec Exp:** Breast Reconstruction; Cancer Reconstruction; **Hospital:** St Luke's Episcopal Hosp - Houston, Park Plaza Hosp; **Address:** 6624 Fannin St, Ste 1420, Houston, TX 77030; **Phone:** 713-794-0368; **Board Cert:** Plastic Surgery 1989; **Med School:** Univ Louisville Sch Med 1980; **Resid:** Surgery, Univ Hosp 1985; Pediatric Surgery, Univ Pittsburgh Med Ctr 1987; **Fellow:** Microsurgery, Univ Pittsburgh Med Ctr 1988; **Fac Appt:** Clin Prof PlS, Baylor Coll Med

Yuen, James C MD [PlS] - **Spec Exp:** Breast Reconstruction; Head & Neck Cancer Reconstruction; Chest Wall Reconstruction; Limb Sparing Surgery; **Hospital:** UAMS Med Ctr; **Address:** Univ Aransas for Med Scis, Plastic Surgery, 4301 W Markham, Ste 720, Little Rock, AR 72212; **Phone:** 501-686-8711; **Board Cert:** Surgery 1991; Plastic Surgery 1995; **Med School:** Med Coll VA 1985; **Resid:** Surgery, W Virginia Med Ctr 1990; Plastic Reconstructive Surgery, Duke Univ Med Ctr 1993; **Fellow:** Hand & Microvascular Surgery, Kleinert Inst of Hand & Microsurgery 1991; **Fac Appt:** Assoc Prof S, Univ Ark

West Coast and Pacific

Andersen, James S MD [PlS] - **Spec Exp:** Cancer Reconstruction; Breast Reconstruction; Head & Neck Reconstruction; **Hospital:** City of Hope Natl Med Ctr & Beckman Rsch (page 69); **Address:** City of Hope National Cancer Ctr, Div Plastic Surgery, 1500 E Duarte Rd, Duarte, CA 91010; **Phone:** 626-301-8278; **Board Cert:** Plastic Surgery 1994; **Med School:** Jefferson Med Coll 1983; **Resid:** Surgery, Hosp U Penn 1989; Plastic Surgery, Hosp U Penn 1991; **Fellow:** Microsurgery, USC Med Ctr 1992; **Fac Appt:** Assoc Clin Prof S, USC Sch Med

Isik, F Frank MD [PlS] - **Spec Exp:** Cancer Reconstruction; Breast Reconstruction; **Hospital:** Swedish Med Ctr - Seattle; **Address:** The Polyclinic, 1145 Broadway, Seattle, WA 98122; **Phone:** 206-860-4566; **Board Cert:** Surgery 2001; Plastic Surgery 1997; **Med School:** Mount Sinai Sch Med 1985; **Resid:** Surgery, Boston Univ Hosps 1990; Plastic Surgery, Univ Wash 1995; **Fellow:** Pathology, NIH / Univ Wash 1992

Jewell, Mark L MD [PlS] - **Spec Exp:** Breast Reconstruction; **Hospital:** Sacred Heart Med Ctr; **Address:** 630 E 13th Ave, Eugene, OR 97401; **Phone:** 541-683-3234; **Board Cert:** Plastic Surgery 1981; **Med School:** Univ Kans 1973; **Resid:** Surgery, LAC-Harbor Med Ctr 1976; Plastic Surgery, Erlanger Hosp 1979; **Fellow:** Burn Surgery, LAC-USC Med Ctr 1977; **Fac Appt:** Asst Clin Prof PlS, Oregon Hlth Sci Univ

Miller, Timothy A MD [PlS] - **Spec Exp:** Eyelid Cancer & Reconstruction; Skin Cancer; Nasal Reconstruction; **Hospital:** UCLA Med Ctr (page 83); **Address:** UCLA Med Ctr, Div Plastic Surg, 200 UCLA Med Plaza, Ste 465, Los Angeles, CA 90095-8344; **Phone:** 310-825-5644; **Board Cert:** Surgery 1971; Plastic Surgery 1973; **Med School:** UCLA 1963; **Resid:** Surgery, Johns Hopkins Hosp; Thoracic Surgery, UCLA Med Ctr 1969; **Fellow:** Plastic Surgery, Univ Pittsburgh 1971; **Fac Appt:** Prof S, UCLA

Sherman, Randolph MD [PlS] - **Spec Exp:** Breast Reconstruction; **Hospital:** USC Univ Hosp - R K Eamer Med Plz, Cedars-Sinai Med Ctr; **Address:** 1450 San Pablo St, Ste 2000, Los Angeles, CA 90033; **Phone:** 323-442-6482; **Board Cert:** Surgery 2004; Plastic Surgery 1986; Hand Surgery 2000; **Med School:** Univ MO-Columbia Sch Med 1977; **Resid:** Surgery, UCSF Hosps 1981; Surgery, State Univ of New York 1983; **Fellow:** Plastic Surgery, USC Med Ctr 1985; **Fac Appt:** Prof S, USC Sch Med

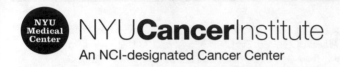

NYU**Cancer**Institute
An NCI-designated Cancer Center

NYU Clinical Cancer Center
160 East 34th Street
New York, New York 10016
www.nyuci.org/atcd

NYU Medical Center
550 First Avenue
(at 31st Street)
New York, New York 10016
www.nyumc.org/atcd

Stephen D. Hassenfeld
Children's Center
for Cancer and Blood
Disorders
160 East 32nd Street
New York, New York 10016
www.nyumc.org/hassenfeld

A Collaborative Approach

The NYU Cancer Institute, an NCI designated center, is a "matrix cancer center" without walls operating within the larger NYU Medical Center. With over 200 members and a research funding base of over $81 million, this structure strengthens our capabilities to forge collaborations across medical and scientific disciplines, which translates to comprehensive care for our patients and discoveries that will influence the future of this disease.

Renowned Expertise

Our highly skilled Magnet™ nursing team not only plays a pivotal role in coordinating direct patient care, but is also a source of invaluable patient education. Team members' compassion and expertise help patients better manage the symptoms of their disease as well as their special needs.

A Patient-Focused Setting

The NYU Clinical Cancer Center, with over 70 faculty members from various disciplines at the New York University School of Medicine, is the principal outpatient facility of the Cancer Institute and serves as home for our patients and their caregivers. The center and its multidisciplinary team of experts provide access to the latest treatment options and clinical trials along with a variety of programs in cancer prevention, screening, diagnostics, genetic counseling, and supportive services. When it comes to kids and cancer, the Stephen D. Hassenfeld Children's Center for Cancer and Blood Disorders offers not just innovation but insight. As a leading member of the NCI-sponsored Children's Oncology Group, our physicians are known for developing new ways to treat childhood cancer. Our affiliation with Bellevue Hospital, the oldest public hospital in the country, affords clinically distinctive opportunities to learn and care for patients with cancer by observing its presentation and behavior in a variety of patient groups.

Psychiatry

A psychiatrist specializes in the prevention, diagnosis and treatment of mental, addictive and emotional disorders such as schizophrenia and other psychotic disorders, mood disorders, anxiety disorders, substance-related disorders, sexual and gender identity disorders and adjustment disorders. The psychiatrist is able to understand the biologic, psychologic and social components of illness, and therefore is uniquely prepared to treat the whole person. A psychiatrist is qualified to order diagnostic laboratory tests and to prescribe medications, evaluate and treat psychologic and interpersonal problems and to intervene with families who are coping with stress, crises and other problems in living.

Training Required: Four years

Certification in one of the following subspecialties requires additional training and examination.

Addiction Psychiatry: A psychiatrist who focuses on the evaluation and treatment of individuals with alcohol, drug, or other substance-related disorders and of individuals with the dual diagnosis of substance-related and other psychiatric disorders.

Child & Adolescent Psychiatry: A psychiatrist with additional training in the diagnosis and treatment of developmental, behavioral, emotional and mental disorders of childhood and adolescence.

Geriatric Psychiatry: A psychiatrist with expertise in the prevention, evaluation, diagnosis and treatment of mental and emotional disorders in the elderly. The geriatric psychiatrist seeks to improve the psychiatric care of the elderly both in health and in disease.

Psychiatry

New England

Block, Susan D MD [Psyc] - **Spec Exp:** Psychiatry in Cancer; **Hospital:** Dana-Farber Cancer Inst; **Address:** Dana Farber Cancer Inst, 44 Binney St, Ste SW411, Boston, MA 02115; **Phone:** 617-632-6181; **Board Cert:** Psychiatry 1984; **Med School:** Case West Res Univ 1977; **Resid:** Internal Medicine, Beth Israel Hosp 1980; Psychiatry, Beth Israel Hosp 1982; **Fac Appt:** Assoc Prof Psyc, Harvard Med Sch

Greenberg, Donna B MD [Psyc] - **Spec Exp:** Psychiatry in Cancer; **Hospital:** Mass Genl Hosp; **Address:** Mass General Hospital, Warren 605, 55 Fruit St, Boston, MA 02114-2696; **Phone:** 617-726-2984; **Board Cert:** Internal Medicine 1978; Psychiatry 1990; **Med School:** Univ Rochester 1975; **Resid:** Internal Medicine, Boston City Hosp 1978; Psychiatry, Mass Genl Hosp 1989; **Fellow:** Psychiatry, Mass Genl Hosp 1979; **Fac Appt:** Assoc Prof Psyc, Harvard Med Sch

Rauch, Paula K MD [Psyc] - **Spec Exp:** Psychiatry in Childhood Cancer; Children/Families facing Severe Illness; Parent Guidance in Parental Cancer; **Hospital:** Mass Genl Hosp; **Address:** Mass General Hosp, Dept Child Psychiatry, 32 Fruit St, Yawkey 6, Boston, MA 02114; **Phone:** 617-724-5600; **Board Cert:** Psychiatry 1990; Child & Adolescent Psychiatry 1991; **Med School:** Univ Cincinnati 1981; **Resid:** Psychiatry, Mass Genl Hosp 1984; **Fac Appt:** Asst Prof Psyc, Harvard Med Sch

Mid Atlantic

Basch, Samuel MD [Psyc] - **Spec Exp:** Psychiatry in Cancer; Psychiatry in Physical Illness; **Hospital:** Mount Sinai Med Ctr (page 77); **Address:** 10 E 85th St, Ste 1B, New York, NY 10028-0412; **Phone:** 212-427-0344; **Board Cert:** Psychiatry 1970; **Med School:** Hahnemann Univ 1961; **Resid:** Psychiatry, Mount Sinai Hosp 1965; **Fellow:** Psychoanalysis, Columbia Presby Hosp 1976; **Fac Appt:** Clin Prof Psyc, Mount Sinai Sch Med

Breitbart, William MD [Psyc] - **Spec Exp:** Psychiatry in Cancer; AIDS Related Cancers; Pain-Cancer; Palliative Care; **Hospital:** Meml Sloan Kettering Cancer Ctr (page 76); **Address:** Meml Sloan Kettering Cancer Center, 641 Lexington Ave Fl 7, New York, NY 10021; **Phone:** 646-888-0020; **Board Cert:** Internal Medicine 1982; Psychiatry 1986; Psychosomatic Medicine 2005; **Med School:** Albert Einstein Coll Med 1978; **Resid:** Internal Medicine, Bronx Muni Hosp Ctr 1982; Psychiatry, Bronx Muni Hosp Ctr 1984; **Fellow:** Psychiatric Oncology, Meml Sloan Kettering Cancer Ctr 1986; **Fac Appt:** Prof Psyc, Cornell Univ-Weill Med Coll

Klagsbrun, Samuel C MD [Psyc] - **Spec Exp:** Psychiatry in Cancer; Psychiatry in Terminal Illness; **Hospital:** Four Winds Hosp; **Address:** Four Winds Hospital, 800 Cross River Rd, Katonah, NY 10536; **Phone:** 914-763-8151; **Board Cert:** Psychiatry 1977; **Med School:** Ros Franklin Univ/Chicago Med Sch 1962; **Resid:** Psychiatry, Yale-New Haven Hosp 1966; **Fac Appt:** Clin Prof Psyc, Albert Einstein Coll Med

Kunkel, Elisabeth J MD [Psyc] - **Spec Exp:** Psychiatry in Cancer; Psychiatry in Physical Illness; **Hospital:** Thomas Jefferson Univ Hosp (page 82); **Address:** Thomas Jefferson Univ, 1020 Samson St, Thompson Bldg, Ste 1652, Philadelphia, PA 19107; **Phone:** 215-955-9545; **Board Cert:** Psychiatry 1989; Geriatric Psychiatry 1994; Addiction Psychiatry 1998; Psychosomatic Medicine 2005; **Med School:** McGill Univ 1983; **Resid:** Psychiatry, NYU Med Ctr 1987; **Fellow:** Liaison Psychiatry, Meml Sloan Kettering Cancer Ctr 1989; **Fac Appt:** Prof Psyc, Jefferson Med Coll

Midwest

Riba, Michelle MD [Psyc] - **Spec Exp:** Psychiatry in Cancer; **Hospital:** Univ Michigan Hlth Sys; **Address:** Univ Mich Med Ctr, Dept Psychiatry, 1500 E Medical Center Dr, MCHC, rm F6236, Ann Arbor, MI 48109-0295; **Phone:** 734-764-6879; **Board Cert:** Psychiatry 1991; Psychosomatic Medicine 2005; **Med School:** Univ Conn 1985; **Resid:** Psychiatry, Univ Connecticut 1988; **Fac Appt:** Clin Prof Psyc, Univ Mich Med Sch

Great Plains and Mountains

Greiner, Carl B MD [Psyc] - **Spec Exp:** Psychiatry in Cancer; Psychiatry in Physical Illness; Palliative Care; Ethics; **Hospital:** Nebraska Med Ctr; **Address:** Dept of Psychiatry, 2626 St Mary's Ave, Omaha, NE 68105; **Phone:** 402-354-6360; **Board Cert:** Psychiatry 1984; Forensic Psychiatry 1999; **Med School:** Univ Cincinnati 1978; **Resid:** Psychiatry, Univ Cincinnati Med Ctr 1982; **Fac Appt:** Prof Psyc, Univ Nebr Coll Med

Southwest

Valentine, Alan D MD [Psyc] - **Spec Exp:** Psychiatry in Cancer; Palliative Care; **Hospital:** UT MD Anderson Cancer Ctr (page 81); **Address:** MD Anderson Cancer Center, Neuro-Oncology Unit 453, PO Box 301402, Houston, TX 77230-1402; **Phone:** 713-745-3344; **Board Cert:** Psychiatry 1992; Geriatric Psychiatry 2006; Psychosomatic Medicine 2005; **Med School:** Univ Tex, Houston 1986; **Resid:** Psychiatry, Univ Texas Affil Hosps; **Fac Appt:** Assoc Prof Psyc, Univ Tex, Houston

West Coast and Pacific

Fann, Jesse R MD [Psyc] - **Spec Exp:** Psychiatry in Physical Illness; Psychiatry in Cancer; **Hospital:** Univ Wash Med Ctr, Harborview Med Ctr; **Address:** Univ Washington Med Ctr, Psychiatry-Box 356560, 1959 NE Pacific St, Seattle, WA 98195-0001; **Phone:** 206-685-3925; **Board Cert:** Psychiatry 2005; **Med School:** Northwestern Univ 1989; **Resid:** Psychiatry, Univ Washington Med Ctr 1993; **Fellow:** Liaison Psychiatry, Univ Washington Med Ctr 1995; **Fac Appt:** Asst Prof Psyc, Univ Wash

Spiegel, David MD [Psyc] - **Spec Exp:** Psychiatry in Cancer; **Hospital:** Stanford Univ Med Ctr; **Address:** Stanford Univ Sch Medicine, Dept Psychiatry & Behavioral Sciences, 401 Quarry Rd, rm 2325, Stanford, CA 94305-5718; **Phone:** 650-723-6421; **Board Cert:** Psychiatry 1976; **Med School:** Harvard Med Sch 1971; **Resid:** Psychiatry, Mass Mental Hlth Ctr 1974; Psychiatry, Cambridge Hosp-Harvard Med Sch 1974; **Fellow:** Community Psychiatry, Harvard Med Sch 1974; **Fac Appt:** Prof Psyc, Stanford Univ

Strouse, Thomas B MD [Psyc] - **Spec Exp:** Psychiatry in Cancer; Pain-Cancer; Psychiatry in Physical Illness; **Hospital:** Cedars-Sinai Med Ctr, UCLA Med Ctr (page 83); **Address:** Cedars-Sinai Outpatient Cancer Ctr, 8700 Beverly Blvd, Ste C2000, Los Angeles, CA 90048-1804; **Phone:** 310-423-0637; **Board Cert:** Psychiatry 1993; Pain Medicine 2000; **Med School:** Case West Res Univ 1987; **Resid:** Psychiatry, UCLA Med Ctr 1991; **Fac Appt:** Assoc Clin Prof Psyc, UCLA

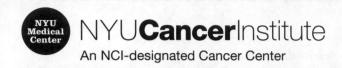

NYU**Cancer**Institute
An NCI-designated Cancer Center

A Collaborative Approach
The NYU Cancer Institute, an NCI designated center, is a "matrix cancer center" without walls operating within the larger NYU Medical Center. With over 200 members and a research funding base of over $81 million, this structure strengthens our capabilities to forge collaborations across medical and scientific disciplines, which translates to comprehensive care for our patients and discoveries that will influence the future of this disease.

Renowned Expertise
Our highly skilled Magnet™ nursing team not only plays a pivotal role in coordinating direct patient care, but is also a source of invaluable patient education. Team members' compassion and expertise help patients better manage the symptoms of their disease as well as their special needs.

A Patient-Focused Setting
The NYU Clinical Cancer Center, with over 70 faculty members from various disciplines at the New York University School of Medicine, is the principal outpatient facility of the Cancer Institute and serves as home for our patients and their caregivers. The center and its multidisciplinary team of experts provide access to the latest treatment options and clinical trials along with a variety of programs in cancer prevention, screening, diagnostics, genetic counseling, and supportive services. When it comes to kids and cancer, the Stephen D. Hassenfeld Children's Center for Cancer and Blood Disorders offers not just innovation but insight. As a leading member of the NCI-sponsored Children's Oncology Group, our physicians are known for developing new ways to treat childhood cancer. Our affiliation with Bellevue Hospital, the oldest public hospital in the country, affords clinically distinctive opportunities to learn and care for patients with cancer by observing its presentation and behavior in a variety of patient groups.

Pulmonary Disease

a subspecialty of Internal Medicine

An internist who treats diseases of the lungs and airways. The pulmonologist diagnoses and treats cancer, pneumonia, pleurisy, asthma, occupational diseases, bronchitis, sleep disorders, emphysema and other complex disorders of the lungs.

Training Required: Three years in internal medicine plus additional training and examination for certification in pulmonary disease.

Pulmonary Disease

New England

Matthay, Richard MD [Pul] - **Spec Exp:** Lung Cancer; **Hospital:** Yale - New Haven Hosp; **Address:** 333 Cedar St, rm 105-LCI, Box 208057, New Haven, CT 06520-3206; **Phone:** 203-785-4198; **Board Cert:** Internal Medicine 1973; Pulmonary Disease 1976; Critical Care Medicine 1997; **Med School:** Tufts Univ 1970; **Resid:** Internal Medicine, Univ Colorado Med Ctr 1973; **Fellow:** Pulmonary Critical Care Medicine, Univ Colorado Med Ctr 1975; **Fac Appt:** Prof Med, Yale Univ

Mid Atlantic

Libby, Daniel MD [Pul] - **Spec Exp:** Lung Cancer; **Hospital:** NY-Presby Hosp (page 79); **Address:** 635 Madison Ave, 11th Fl, New York, NY 10021; **Phone:** 212-628-6611; **Board Cert:** Internal Medicine 1977; Pulmonary Disease 1980; **Med School:** Baylor Coll Med 1974; **Resid:** Internal Medicine, New York Hosp 1977; **Fellow:** Pulmonary Disease, New York Hosp 1979; **Fac Appt:** Clin Prof Med, Cornell Univ-Weill Med Coll

Steinberg, Harry MD [Pul] - **Spec Exp:** Lung Cancer; **Hospital:** Long Island Jewish Med Ctr, N Shore Univ Hosp at Manhasset; **Address:** LI Jewish Med Ctr, Dept Med, 270-05 76th Ave, New Hyde Park, NY 11040-1433; **Phone:** 718-465-5400; **Med School:** Temple Univ 1966; **Resid:** Internal Medicine, LI Jewish Med Ctr 1969; Pulmonary Critical Care Medicine, LI Jewish Med Ctr 1970; **Fellow:** Pulmonary Disease, Hosp U Penn 1974; **Fac Appt:** Clin Prof Med, Albert Einstein Coll Med

Teirstein, Alvin MD [Pul] - **Spec Exp:** Lung Cancer; **Hospital:** Mount Sinai Med Ctr (page 77), VA Med Ctr - Bronx; **Address:** Mount Sinai Med Ctr, 1 Gustave Levy Pl, Box 1232, New York, NY 10029; **Phone:** 212-241-5656; **Board Cert:** Internal Medicine 1961; Pulmonary Disease 1969; **Med School:** SUNY Downstate 1953; **Resid:** Internal Medicine, Mt Sinai Med Ctr 1957; **Fellow:** Pulmonary Disease, Mt Sinai Med Ctr 1954; Pulmonary Disease, VA Med Ctr 1956; **Fac Appt:** Prof Med, Mount Sinai Sch Med

Unger, Michael MD [Pul] - **Spec Exp:** Lung Cancer; Cancer Prevention; **Hospital:** Fox Chase Cancer Ctr (page 73); **Address:** Fox Chase Cancer Center, 7701 Burholme Ave, Philadelphia, PA 19111; **Phone:** 215-728-6900; **Board Cert:** Internal Medicine 1977; Pulmonary Disease 1978; **Med School:** France 1971; **Resid:** Internal Medicine, Mt Sinai Hosp 1974; **Fellow:** Pulmonary Disease, New York Hosp-Cornell 1976; **Fac Appt:** Clin Prof Med, Thomas Jefferson Univ

White, Dorothy MD [Pul] - **Spec Exp:** Lung Cancer; AIDS Related Cancers; **Hospital:** Meml Sloan Kettering Cancer Ctr (page 76); **Address:** 1275 York Ave, rm H803, Box 13, New York, NY 10021; **Phone:** 212-639-8022; **Board Cert:** Internal Medicine 1980; Pulmonary Disease 1984; **Med School:** SUNY Hlth Sci Ctr 1977; **Resid:** Internal Medicine, New York Hosp 1980; Internal Medicine, Meml Sloan Kettering Inst 1981; **Fellow:** Pulmonary Disease, Yale-New Haven Hosp 1984; **Fac Appt:** Prof Med, Cornell Univ-Weill Med Coll

Southeast

Alberts, W Michael MD [Pul] - **Spec Exp:** Lung Cancer; **Hospital:** H Lee Moffitt Cancer Ctr & Research Inst; **Address:** H Lee Moffitt Cancer Ctr, Thoracic Onc, 12902 Magnolia Drive, Tampa, FL 33612; **Phone:** 813-903-4679; **Board Cert:** Internal Medicine 1980; Pulmonary Disease 1982; **Med School:** Univ IL Coll Med 1977; **Resid:** Internal Medicine, Ohio State Univ Hosp 1980; **Fellow:** Pulmonary Critical Care Medicine, UCSD Med Ctr 1983; **Fac Appt:** Prof Med, Univ S Fla Coll Med

Downie, Gordon H MD/PhD [Pul] - **Spec Exp:** Lung Cancer; Photodynamic Therapy; Clinical Trials; **Hospital:** Pitt Cty Mem Hosp - Univ Med Ctr East Carolina; **Address:** The Brody School of Medicine, Ste 3E-149, Greenville, NC 27858-4354; **Phone:** 252-744-4653; **Board Cert:** Pulmonary Disease 2004; **Med School:** Northwestern Univ 1986; **Resid:** Internal Medicine, Univ North Carolina 1989; **Fellow:** Pulmonary Intensive Care, Univ North Carolina 1992; **Fac Appt:** Assoc Prof Med, E Carolina Univ

Garver Jr, Robert MD [Pul] - **Spec Exp:** Lung Cancer; **Hospital:** Univ of Ala Hosp at Birmingham; **Address:** 1900 University Blvd, THT 215, Birmingham, AL 35294; **Phone:** 205-934-7556; **Board Cert:** Internal Medicine 1984; Pulmonary Disease 1986; **Med School:** Johns Hopkins Univ 1981; **Resid:** Internal Medicine, Johns Hopkins Hosp 1984; **Fellow:** Pulmonary Disease, NHLBI 1985; **Fac Appt:** Prof Med, Univ Ala

Goldman, Allan L MD [Pul] - **Spec Exp:** Lung Cancer; **Hospital:** Tampa Genl Hosp, James A Haley VA Hosp; **Address:** USF Coll Med, Dept Internal Medicine, 12901 Bruce B Downs Blvd, Box MDC19, Tampa, FL 33612-4742; **Phone:** 813-974-2271; **Board Cert:** Internal Medicine 1972; Pulmonary Disease 1972; **Med School:** Univ Minn 1968; **Resid:** Internal Medicine, Brooke Army Hosp 1970; **Fellow:** Pulmonary Disease, Walter Reed Army Hosp 1972; **Fac Appt:** Prof Med, Univ S Fla Coll Med

Midwest

Jett, James R MD [Pul] - **Spec Exp:** Lung Cancer; Mesothelioma; Thymoma; **Hospital:** Mayo Med Ctr & Clin - Rochester; **Address:** Mayo Clinic, Thoracic Diseases, 200 First St SW, Rochester, MN 55905; **Phone:** 507-284-3764; **Board Cert:** Internal Medicine 1976; Pulmonary Disease 1978; **Med School:** Univ MO-Columbia Sch Med 1973; **Resid:** Internal Medicine, Mayo Clinic 1976; **Fellow:** Pulmonary Disease, Mayo Clinic 1978; **Fac Appt:** Prof Med, Mayo Med Sch

McLennan, Geoffrey MD [Pul] - **Spec Exp:** Lung Cancer; **Hospital:** Univ Iowa Hosp & Clinics; **Address:** Univ Iowa Hosp, 200 Hawkins Drive, Ste 4900JPP, Iowa City, IA 52242; **Phone:** 319-353-8201; **Med School:** Australia ; **Resid:** Internal Medicine, Royal Adelaide Medical Sch; **Fellow:** Pulmonary Disease, Queen Elizabeth Hosp; **Fac Appt:** Prof Med, Univ Iowa Coll Med

Silver, Michael R MD [Pul] - **Spec Exp:** Lung Cancer; **Hospital:** Rush Univ Med Ctr, Rush Oak Park Hosp; **Address:** 1725 W Harrison St, Prof Bldg 3, Ste 054, Chicago, IL 60612; **Phone:** 312-942-6744; **Board Cert:** Internal Medicine 1984; Pulmonary Disease 1988; Critical Care Medicine 1999; **Med School:** Albany Med Coll 1981; **Resid:** Internal Medicine, Rush-Presby-St Luke's Med Ctr 1985; **Fellow:** Pulmonary Critical Care Medicine, Rush-Presby-St Luke's Med Ctr 1987; **Fac Appt:** Assoc Prof Med, Rush Med Coll

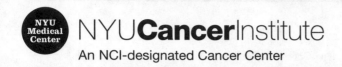

NYU**Cancer**Institute
An NCI-designated Cancer Center

Radiology

A radiologist utilizes radiologic methodologies to diagnose and treat disease. Physicians practicing in the field of radiology most often specialize in radiology, diagnostic radiology, radiation oncology or radiological physics.

Training Required: Four years in radiology plus additional training and examination.

Radiation Oncology: A subspecialist in radiation oncology deals with the therapeutic applications of radiant energy and its modifiers and the study and management of disease, especially malignant tumors.

Diagnostic Radiology: A radiologist who utilizes X-ray, radionuclides, ultrasound and electromagnetic radiation to diagnose and treat disease.

Interventional Radiology: A radiologist who diagnoses and treats diseases by various radiologic imaging modalities. These include fluoroscopy, digital radiography, computed tomography, sonography and magnetic resonance imaging.

Neuroradiology: A radiologist who diagnoses and treats diseases utilizing imaging procedures as they relate to the brain, spine and spinal cord, head, neck and organs of special sense in adults and children.

Training Required: Four years

Additional certification in subspecialties such as Pediatric Radiology and Interventional Radiology require additional training and examination.

Nuclear Medicine: A nuclear medicine specialist employs the properties of radioactive atoms and molecules in the diagnosis and treatment of disease, and in research. Radiation detection and imaging instrument systems are used to detect disease as it changes the function and metabolism of normal cells, tissues and organs. A wide variety of diseases can be found in this way, usually before the structure of the organ involved by the disease can be seen to be abnormal by any other techniques. Early detection of coronary artery disease (including acute heart attack); early cancer detection and evaluation of the effect of tumor treatment; diagnosis of infection and inflammation anywhere in the body; and early detection of blood clot in the lungs, are all possible with these techniques. Unique forms or radioactive molecules can attack and kill cancer cells (e.g., lymphoma, thyroid cancer) or can relieve the severe pain of cancer that has spread to bone.

The nuclear medicine specialist has special knowledge in the biologic effects of radiation exposure, the fundamentals of the physical sciences and the principles and operation of radiation detection and imaging instrumentation systems.

Training Required: Three years

Radiation Oncology

New England

Choi, Noah C MD [RadRO] - **Spec Exp:** Lung Cancer; Esophageal Cancer; **Hospital:** Mass Genl Hosp; **Address:** Mass Genl Hosp, Dept Rad Oncology, 100 Blossom St, Cox 307, Boston, MA 02114; **Phone:** 617-726-6050; **Board Cert:** Therapeutic Radiology 1970; **Med School:** South Korea 1963; **Resid:** Radiation Oncology, Princess Margaret Hosp 1970; **Fac Appt:** Assoc Prof, Harvard Med Sch

D'Amico, Anthony V MD/PhD [RadRO] - **Spec Exp:** Prostate Cancer; Brachytherapy; **Hospital:** Brigham & Women's Hosp, Dana-Farber Cancer Inst; **Address:** Brigham & Women's Hosp, Dept Rad Onc, 75 Francis St, Ste L2, Boston, MA 02115; **Phone:** 617-732-7936; **Board Cert:** Radiation Oncology 1999; **Med School:** Univ Pennsylvania 1990; **Resid:** Radiation Oncology, Hosp Univ Penn 1994; **Fac Appt:** Prof RadRO, Harvard Med Sch

DeLaney, Thomas Francis MD [RadRO] - **Spec Exp:** Sarcoma; Proton Beam Therapy; **Hospital:** Mass Genl Hosp; **Address:** Francis H. Burr Proton Therapy Ctr, 30 Fruit St, Bosont, MA 02114; **Phone:** 617-726-6876; **Board Cert:** Therapeutic Radiology 1986; Radiation Oncology 1999; **Med School:** Harvard Med Sch 1982; **Resid:** Therapeutic Radiology, Mass Gen Hosp 1986; **Fac Appt:** Assoc Prof RadRO, Harvard Med Sch

Harris, Jay R MD [RadRO] - **Spec Exp:** Breast Cancer; **Hospital:** Brigham & Women's Hosp, Dana-Farber Cancer Inst; **Address:** Dana Farber Cancer Inst, 44 Binney St, rm 1622, Boston, MA 02115; **Phone:** 617-632-2291; **Board Cert:** Therapeutic Radiology 1999; **Med School:** Stanford Univ 1970; **Resid:** Radiation Oncology, Joint Ctr Rad Ther 1976; **Fellow:** Radiation Therapy, Harvard Med Sch 1977; **Fac Appt:** Prof RadRO, Harvard Med Sch

Knisely, Jonathan MD [RadRO] - **Spec Exp:** Brain Tumors; Stereotactic Radiosurgery; Gastrointestinal Cancer; **Hospital:** Yale - New Haven Hosp; **Address:** Yale Univ Sch Med, Dept Therapeutic Radiology, 15 York St Bldg Hunter - Ste HRT 1, New Haven, CT 06520-8040; **Phone:** 203-785-2960; **Board Cert:** Internal Medicine 1989; Radiation Oncology 1993; **Med School:** Univ Pennsylvania 1986; **Resid:** Internal Medicine, Michael Reese Hosp 1989; Radiation Oncology, Univ Toronto Med Ctr 1992; **Fac Appt:** Assoc Prof DR, Yale Univ

Mauch, Peter M MD [RadRO] - **Spec Exp:** Lymphoma; Hodgkin's Disease; **Hospital:** Dana-Farber Cancer Inst; **Address:** Dana Farber Cancer Inst, 75 Francis St, Ste RadOnc L2, Boston, MA 02115; **Phone:** 617-632-4116; **Board Cert:** Therapeutic Radiology 1978; **Med School:** St Louis Univ 1974; **Resid:** Radiation Therapy, Harvard Joint Ctr 1978; **Fac Appt:** Prof, Harvard Med Sch

Peschel, Richard E MD [RadRO] - **Spec Exp:** Prostate Cancer; **Hospital:** Yale - New Haven Hosp; **Address:** Yale-New Haven Hosp, Dept Radiology, 15 York St, rm HRT 142, New Haven, CT 06510; **Phone:** 203-785-2958; **Board Cert:** Therapeutic Radiology 1982; **Med School:** Yale Univ 1977; **Resid:** Radiation Oncology, Yale-New Haven Hosp 1981; **Fac Appt:** Prof RadRO, Yale Univ

Recht, Abram MD [RadRO] - **Spec Exp:** Breast Cancer; Gastrointestinal Cancer; Gynecologic Cancer; **Hospital:** Beth Israel Deaconess Med Ctr - Boston; **Address:** Beth Israel Deaconess Med Ctr, 330 Brookline Ave, Boston, MA 02215; **Phone:** 617-667-2345; **Board Cert:** Therapeutic Radiology 1984; **Med School:** Johns Hopkins Univ 1980; **Resid:** Radiation Oncology, Joint Ctr RadiationTherapy 1984; **Fac Appt:** Assoc Prof RadRO, Harvard Med Sch

Radiation Oncology

Roberts, Kenneth MD [RadRO] - **Spec Exp:** Pediatric Cancers; Lymphoma; Hodgkin's Disease; **Hospital:** Yale - New Haven Hosp, Backus Hosp, Norwich; **Address:** Yale Univ School of Medicine, Dept Radiation Therapy, 15 York St, New Haven, CT 06520-8040; **Phone:** 203-785-2957; **Board Cert:** Internal Medicine 1987; Medical Oncology 1989; Radiation Oncology 1995; **Med School:** Duke Univ 1984; **Resid:** Internal Medicine, Ohio State Univ Hosps 1987; Radiation Oncology, Duke Univ Med Ctr 1992; **Fellow:** Hematology & Oncology, Duke Univ Med Ctr 1989; **Fac Appt:** Assoc Prof DR, Yale Univ

Shipley, William U MD [RadRO] - **Spec Exp:** Bladder Cancer; Prostate Cancer; **Hospital:** Mass Genl Hosp; **Address:** Mass Genl Hosp, Dept Rad Oncology, 100 Blossom St, Cox 347, Boston, MA 02114; **Phone:** 617-726-8146; **Board Cert:** Therapeutic Radiology 1975; **Med School:** Harvard Med Sch 1966; **Resid:** Surgery, Mass Genl Hosp 1971; Radiation Therapy, Harvard Joint Ctr Rad Therapy 1973; **Fellow:** Radiation Therapy, Royal Marsden Hosp 1974; **Fac Appt:** Prof RadRO, Harvard Med Sch

Tarbell, Nancy MD [RadRO] - **Spec Exp:** Brain Tumors-Pediatric; Proton Beam Therapy; **Hospital:** Mass Genl Hosp; **Address:** Massachusetts Genl Hosp BPTC107, 55 Fruit St Yawkey Bldg, Boston, MA 02114; **Phone:** 617-724-1836; **Board Cert:** Therapeutic Radiology 1983; **Med School:** SUNY Upstate Med Univ 1979; **Resid:** Radiation Therapy, Harvard Med School 1983; **Fac Appt:** Prof RadRO, Harvard Med Sch

Wazer, David E MD [RadRO] - **Spec Exp:** Breast Cancer; Melanoma; **Hospital:** Rhode Island Hosp, Tufts-New England Med Ctr; **Address:** 593 Eddy St, Providence, RI 02903; **Phone:** 401-444-8311; **Board Cert:** Radiation Oncology 1988; **Med School:** NYU Sch Med 1982; **Resid:** Radiation Oncology, Tufts New England Med Ctr 1988; **Fellow:** Neurological Chemistry, NYU Med Ctr 1984; **Fac Appt:** Prof RadRO, Tufts Univ

Wilson, Lynn D MD [RadRO] - **Spec Exp:** Lymphoma, Cutaneous T Cell (CTCL); Lymphoma, Cutaneous B Cell (CBCL); Lung Cancer; Head & Neck Cancer; **Hospital:** Yale - New Haven Hosp; **Address:** Yale Univ Sch Med, Dept Therapeutic Rad, PO Box 208040, New Haven, CT 06520-8040; **Phone:** 203-688-1861; **Board Cert:** Radiation Oncology 2004; **Med School:** Geo Wash Univ 1990; **Resid:** Therapeutic Radiology, Yale-New Haven Hosp 1994; **Fac Appt:** Prof RadRO, Yale Univ

Zietman, Anthony L MD [RadRO] - **Spec Exp:** Prostate Cancer; Urologic Cancer; **Hospital:** Mass Genl Hosp; **Address:** Mass Genl Hosp Cancer Ctr, Dept Radiation Oncology, 55 Fruit St, Boston, MA 02114; **Phone:** 617-724-4000; **Board Cert:** Radiation Oncology 1994; **Med School:** England 1983; **Resid:** Internal Medicine, St Stephens & Westminster Hosp 1986; Radiation Oncology, Mass Genl Hosp 1989; **Fellow:** Radiation Oncology, Middlesex/Mt Vernon Hosps 1991; **Fac Appt:** Prof RadRO, Harvard Med Sch

Mid Atlantic

Berg, Christine D MD [RadRO] - **Spec Exp:** Breast Cancer; **Hospital:** Natl Inst of Hlth - Clin Ctr; **Address:** 6130 Executive Blvd, Bethesda, MD 20892-7346; **Phone:** 301-496-8544; **Board Cert:** Internal Medicine 1980; Medical Oncology 1983; Therapeutic Radiology 1999; **Med School:** Northwestern Univ 1977; **Resid:** Internal Medicine, Northwestern Meml Hosp 1981; Radiation Oncology, Georgetown Univ Hosp 1986; **Fellow:** Medical Oncology, Natl Cancer Inst-NIH 1984

Berson, Anthony M MD [RadRO] - **Spec Exp:** Prostate Cancer; Breast Cancer; Lung Cancer; **Hospital:** St Vincent Cath Med Ctrs - Manhattan; **Address:** 325 W 15th St, New York, NY 10011-5903; **Phone:** 212-604-6081; **Board Cert:** Radiation Oncology 1990; **Med School:** Hahnemann Univ 1984; **Resid:** Radiation Oncology, UCSF Med Ctr 1989; **Fellow:** Neoplastic Diseases, Lawrence Berkeley Lab 1987; **Fac Appt:** Assoc Prof RadRO, NY Med Coll

Coia, Lawrence R MD [RadRO] - **Spec Exp:** Gastrointestinal Cancer; Prostate Cancer; Breast Cancer; Brachytherapy; **Hospital:** Comm Med Ctr - Toms River (page 73), Southern Ocean County Hosp; **Address:** Community Medical Center, Dept Rad Oncology, 99 Route 37 W, Toms River, NJ 08755-6498; **Phone:** 732-557-8148; **Board Cert:** Therapeutic Radiology 1982; **Med School:** Temple Univ 1976, **Resid:** Radiation Oncology, Thos Jefferson Univ Hosp 1981; **Fac Appt:** Assoc Clin Prof, Univ Pennsylvania

Constine III, Louis S MD [RadRO] - **Spec Exp:** Pediatric Cancers; Lymphoma; Cancer Survivors-Late Effects of Therapy; Sarcoma; **Hospital:** Univ of Rochester Strong Meml Hosp; **Address:** 601 Elmwood Ave, Box 647, Rochester, NY 14642; **Phone:** 585-275-5622; **Board Cert:** Pediatrics 1978; Therapeutic Radiology 1981; Pediatric Hematology-Oncology 1978; **Med School:** Johns Hopkins Univ 1973; **Resid:** Pediatrics, Moffitt Hosp-UCSF Med Ctr 1975; Pediatrics, Stanford Hosp Med Ctr 1976; **Fellow:** Stanford Hosp Med Ctr 1981; Pediatric Hematology-Oncology, Univ Wash/Chldns Ortho Hosp 1978; **Fac Appt:** Prof RadRO, Univ Rochester

Cooper, Jay MD [RadRO] - **Spec Exp:** Head & Neck Cancer; Skin Cancer; Chemo-Radiation Combined Therapy; **Hospital:** Maimonides Med Ctr (page 75); **Address:** Maimonides Cancer Ctr, 6300 8th Ave, Brooklyn, NY 11220; **Phone:** 718-765-2700; **Board Cert:** Therapeutic Radiology 1977; **Med School:** NYU Sch Med 1973; **Resid:** Radiation Oncology, NYU Med Ctr 1977

Curran Jr, Walter J MD [RadRO] - **Spec Exp:** Lung Cancer; Brain Tumors; Gastrointestinal Cancer; Esophageal Cancer; **Hospital:** Thomas Jefferson Univ Hosp (page 82); **Address:** Thomas Jefferson Univ Hosp, Dept Rad Onc, 111 S 11th St, Bodine Ctr, Philadelphia, PA 19107; **Phone:** 215-955-6701; **Board Cert:** Therapeutic Radiology 1986; **Med School:** Med Coll GA 1982; **Resid:** Radiation Therapy, Hosp Univ Penn 1986; **Fac Appt:** Prof RadRO, Jefferson Med Coll

DeWeese, Theodore L MD [RadRO] - **Spec Exp:** Urologic Cancer; Prostate Cancer; Testicular Cancer; **Hospital:** Johns Hopkins Hosp - Baltimore; **Address:** Johns Hopkins Medicine, Dept Rad Oncology, 401 N Broadway, rm 1343, Baltimore, MD 21231; **Phone:** 410-502-8000; **Board Cert:** Radiation Oncology 1995; **Med School:** Univ Colorado 1990; **Resid:** Radiation Oncology, Johns Hopkins Hosp 1994; **Fellow:** Urologic Oncology, Johns Hopkins Hosp 1995; **Fac Appt:** Prof RadRO, Johns Hopkins Univ

Dicker, Adam P MD/PhD [RadRO] - **Spec Exp:** Prostate Cancer; **Hospital:** Thomas Jefferson Univ Hosp (page 82); **Address:** Bodine Cancer Treatment Ctr, 111 South 11th St, Philadelphia, PA 19107-5097; **Phone:** 215-955-6527; **Board Cert:** Radiation Oncology 2000; **Med School:** Cornell Univ-Weill Med Coll 1992; **Resid:** Surgery, Lenox Hill Hosp 1994; Radiation Oncology, Meml Sloan Kettering Cancer Ctr 1997; **Fac Appt:** Assoc Prof RadRO, Thomas Jefferson Univ

Radiation Oncology

Dritschilo, Anatoly MD [RadRO] - Spec Exp: Breast Cancer; Prostate Cancer; **Hospital:** Georgetown Univ Hosp; **Address:** Georgetown Univ Hosp, Dept Radiation Medicine, 3800 Reservoir Rd NW, Washington, DC 20007; **Phone:** 202-687-2144; **Board Cert:** Therapeutic Radiology 1977; **Med School:** UMDNJ-NJ Med Sch, Newark 1973; **Resid:** Radiation Therapy, Harvard Joint Rad Ther Ctr 1977; **Fac Appt:** Prof Med, Georgetown Univ

Ennis, Ronald D MD [RadRO] - Spec Exp: Prostate Cancer; Brachytherapy; Gynecologic Cancer; **Hospital:** St Luke's - Roosevelt Hosp Ctr - Roosevelt Div (page 72), Beth Israel Med Ctr - Petrie Division (page 72); **Address:** St Luke's Roosevelt Hosp, Dept Rad Oncol, 1000 10th Ave, Lower Level, New York, NY 10019; **Phone:** 212-523-7165; **Board Cert:** Radiation Oncology 2005; **Med School:** Yale Univ 1990; **Resid:** Therapeutic Radiology, Yale-New Haven Hosp 1994

Flickinger, John C MD [RadRO] - Spec Exp: Neuro-Oncology; Brain & Spinal Tumors; **Hospital:** UPMC Presby, Pittsburgh; **Address:** UPMC Cancer Ctr, Radiation Oncology, 200 Lothrop St, Ste B 300, Pittsburgh, PA 15213; **Phone:** 412-647-3600; **Board Cert:** Therapeutic Radiology 1985; **Med School:** Univ Chicago-Pritzker Sch Med 1981; **Resid:** Radiation Therapy, Mass General Hosp 1985; **Fac Appt:** Prof RadRO, Univ Pittsburgh

Formenti, Silvia C MD [RadRO] - Spec Exp: Breast Cancer; Prostate Cancer; Chemo-Radiation Combined Therapy; **Hospital:** NYU Med Ctr (page 80); **Address:** NYU Med Ctr, Dept Radiation Oncology, 160 E 34th St, New York, NY 10016; **Phone:** 212-263-2601; **Board Cert:** Radiation Oncology 1991; **Med School:** Italy 1980; **Resid:** Internal Medicine, San Carlo Borromeo Hosp 1983; Medical Oncology, Univ of Pavia Med Ctr 1985; **Fellow:** Radiation Oncology, USC Med Ctr 1990; **Fac Appt:** Asst Prof RadRO, NYU Sch Med

Glassburn, John R MD [RadRO] - Spec Exp: Gynecologic Cancer; Prostate Cancer; Breast Cancer; **Hospital:** Pennsylvania Hosp (page 84); **Address:** Pennsylvania Hosp, Dept Radiation Oncology, 800 Spruce St, Philadelphia, PA 19107; **Phone:** 215-829-3873; **Board Cert:** Therapeutic Radiology 1973; **Med School:** Hahnemann Univ 1966; **Resid:** Radiation Oncology, Hahnemann Hosp 1972; **Fac Appt:** Clin Prof RadRO, Univ Pennsylvania

Glatstein, Eli MD [RadRO] - Spec Exp: Lymphoma; Lung Cancer; Photodynamic Therapy; Sarcoma; **Hospital:** Hosp Univ Penn - UPHS (page 84); **Address:** Hosp Univ Penn, Dept Rad Oncology, 3400 Spruce St, Donner Bldg Fl 2, Philadelphia, PA 19104; **Phone:** 215-662-3383; **Board Cert:** Therapeutic Radiology 1972; **Med School:** Stanford Univ 1964; **Resid:** Radiation Therapy, Stanford Med Ctr 1970; **Fellow:** Radiological Biology, Hammersmith Hosp 1972; **Fac Appt:** Prof RadRO, Univ Pennsylvania

Goodman, Robert L MD [RadRO] - Spec Exp: Breast Cancer; Lymphoma; Prostate Cancer; **Hospital:** St Barnabas Med Ctr; **Address:** St Barnabas Med Ctr, Dept Rad Oncology, 94 Old Short Hills Rd, Livingston, NJ 07039; **Phone:** 973-322-5133; **Board Cert:** Internal Medicine 1971; Therapeutic Radiology 1974; Medical Oncology 1975; **Med School:** Columbia P&S 1966; **Resid:** Internal Medicine, Beth Israel Hosp 1970; Radiation Therapy, Harvard Joint Ctr Rad Therapy 1974; **Fellow:** Hematology, Presby Hosp 1969

Greenberger, Joel S MD [RadRO] - Spec Exp: Lung Cancer; Esophageal Cancer; **Hospital:** UPMC Presby, Pittsburgh; **Address:** UPMC Cancer Ctr, Radiation Oncology, 200 Lothrop St, Ste B300, Pittsburgh, PA 15232; **Phone:** 412-647-3600; **Board Cert:** Therapeutic Radiology 1977; **Med School:** Harvard Med Sch 1971; **Resid:** Radiation Therapy, Mass General Hosp 1977; **Fac Appt:** Prof RadRO, Univ Pittsburgh

Haffty, Bruce MD [RadRO] - Spec Exp: Breast Cancer; Head & Neck Cancer; Lung Cancer; **Hospital:** Robert Wood Johnson Univ Hosp - New Brunswick, Robert Wood Johnson Univ Hosp Hamilton; **Address:** The Cancer Institute of New Jersey, 195 Little Albany St, New Brunswick, NJ 08903; **Phone:** 732-253-3939; **Board Cert:** Radiation Oncology 1988; **Med School:** Yale Univ 1984; **Resid:** Radiation Oncology, Yale-New Haven Hosp 1988; **Fac Appt:** Prof RadRO, Robert W Johnson Med Sch

Hahn, Stephen M MD [RadRO] - Spec Exp: Lung Cancer; Prostate Cancer; Sarcoma; **Hospital:** Hosp Univ Penn - UPHS (page 84), Penn Presby Med Ctr - UPHS (page 84); **Address:** Hosp of the Univ of Penn, 3400 Spruce St 2 Donner Bldg, Philadelphia, PA 19104; **Phone:** 215-662-7296; **Board Cert:** Radiation Oncology 2004; Internal Medicine 1987; Medical Oncology 2001; **Med School:** Temple Univ 1984; **Resid:** Internal Medicine, UCSF Med Ctr 1988; Medical Oncology, Natl Inst Hlth 1991; **Fellow:** Radiation Oncology, Natl Inst Hlth 1994; **Fac Appt:** Prof RadRO, Univ Pennsylvania

Harrison, Louis MD [RadRO] - Spec Exp: Brachytherapy; Head & Neck Cancer; Radiation Therapy-Intraoperative; **Hospital:** Beth Israel Med Ctr - Petrie Division (page 72), St Luke's - Roosevelt Hosp Ctr - Roosevelt Div (page 72); **Address:** Beth Israel Med Ctr, Dept Rad Onc, 10 Union Square East, Ste 4G, New York, NY 10003-3314; **Phone:** 212-844-8087; **Board Cert:** Therapeutic Radiology 1986; **Med School:** SUNY Downstate 1982; **Resid:** Therapeutic Radiology, Yale-New Haven Hosp 1986; **Fac Appt:** Prof RadRO, Albert Einstein Coll Med

Horwitz, Eric MD [RadRO] - Spec Exp: Prostate Cancer; Intensity Modulated Radiotherapy (IMRT); Brachytherapy; **Hospital:** Fox Chase Cancer Ctr (page 73); **Address:** Fox Chase Cancer Ctr, Dept Radiation Oncology, 333 Cottman Ave, Philadelphia, PA 19111; **Phone:** 215-728-2995; **Board Cert:** Radiation Oncology 1999; **Med School:** Albany Med Coll 1992; **Resid:** Radiation Oncology, William Beaumont Hosp 1997

Isaacson, Steven MD [RadRO] - Spec Exp: Brain Tumors; Neuro-Oncology; **Hospital:** NY-Presby Hosp (page 79); **Address:** Columbia Presby Med Ctr, Dept Rad Oncol, 622 W 168th St BHN Bldg - rm B11, New York, NY 10032-3720; **Phone:** 212-305-2611; **Board Cert:** Radiation Oncology 1988; Otolaryngology 1978; **Med School:** Jefferson Med Coll 1973; **Resid:** Otolaryngology, Hosp Univ Penn 1978; Radiation Oncology, SUNY Hlth Sci Ctr 1988; **Fac Appt:** Clin Prof RadRO, Columbia P&S

Kleinberg, Lawrence MD [RadRO] - Spec Exp: Brain & Spinal Cord Tumors; Brain Tumors-Metastatic; Stereotactic Radiosurgery; Esophageal Cancer; **Hospital:** Johns Hopkins Hosp - Baltimore; **Address:** Johns Hopkins Univ, Dept of Radiation Oncology, 401 N Broadway Weinberg Bldg - Ste 1440, Baltimore, MD 21231; **Phone:** 410-614-2597; **Board Cert:** Radiation Oncology 1994; **Med School:** Yale Univ 1989; **Resid:** Radiation Oncology, Meml Sloan-Kettering Canc Ctr 1993; **Fac Appt:** Assoc Prof RadRO, Johns Hopkins Univ

Konski, Andre MD [RadRO] - Spec Exp: Esophageal Cancer; Rectal Cancer; Pancreatic Cancer; Gastrointestinal Cancer; **Hospital:** Fox Chase Cancer Ctr (page 73); **Address:** Fox Chase Cancer Ctr, Dept Rad Onc, 333 Cottman Ave, Philadelphia, PA 19111; **Phone:** 215-728-2916; **Board Cert:** Radiation Oncology 2000; **Med School:** NY Med Coll 1984; **Resid:** Radiation Oncology, Stong Meml/Genesee Hosps 1988

Kuettel, Michael MD/PhD [RadRO] - Spec Exp: Prostate Cancer; **Hospital:** Roswell Park Cancer Inst; **Address:** Roswell Park Cancer Inst, Rad Med Dept, Elm and Carlton St, Buffalo, NY 14263; **Phone:** 716-845-1562; **Board Cert:** Radiation Oncology 1992; **Med School:** Med Coll Wisc ; **Resid:** Internal Medicine, Northwestern Hosp; Radiation Oncology, Johns Hopkins Hosp; **Fac Appt:** Prof Med, SUNY Buffalo

Radiation Oncology

Lepanto, Philip B MD [RadRO] - **Hospital:** St Mary's Med Ctr - Huntington, Cabell Huntington Hosp; **Address:** St Mary's Med Ctr, Dept Radiation Oncology, 2900 First Ave, Huntington, WV 25702; **Phone:** 304-526-1143; **Board Cert:** Therapeutic Radiology 1975; **Med School:** Univ Louisville Sch Med 1970; **Resid:** Diagnostic Radiology, Graduate Hosp 1972; Radiation Therapy, Hosp Univ Penn 1975; **Fac Appt:** Clin Prof Rad, Marshall Univ

Machtay, Mitchell MD [RadRO] - **Spec Exp:** Head & Neck Cancer; Ear Tumors; Eye Tumors/Cancer; **Hospital:** Thomas Jefferson Univ Hosp (page 82); **Address:** Bodine Ctr for Cancer Treatment, Dept Rad Onc, 111 S 11 St, Bodine Ctr, Philadelphia, PA 19107-5097; **Phone:** 215-955-6706; **Board Cert:** Radiation Oncology 1994; **Med School:** NYU Sch Med 1989; **Resid:** Radiation Oncology, Hosp Univ Penn 1993; **Fac Appt:** Assoc Prof RadRO, Jefferson Med Coll

McCormick, Beryl MD [RadRO] - **Spec Exp:** Breast Cancer; Eye Tumors/Cancer; **Hospital:** Meml Sloan Kettering Cancer Ctr (page 76), NY-Presby Hosp (page 79); **Address:** Meml Sloan Kettering - Radiation Oncology, 1275 York Ave, rm SM 04, New York, NY 10021-6007; **Phone:** 212-639-6828; **Board Cert:** Therapeutic Radiology 1977; **Med School:** UMDNJ-NJ Med Sch, Newark 1973; **Resid:** Therapeutic Radiology, Meml Sloan Kettering Cancer Ctr 1977; **Fac Appt:** Prof RadRO, Cornell Univ-Weill Med Coll

Nori, Dattatreyudu MD [RadRO] - **Spec Exp:** Breast Cancer; Prostate Cancer; Gynecologic Cancer; **Hospital:** NY-Presby Hosp (page 79), NY Hosp Queens; **Address:** 525 E 68th St, Box 575, New York, NY 10021-4870; **Phone:** 212-746-3679; **Board Cert:** Therapeutic Radiology 1979; **Med School:** India 1970; **Resid:** Radiation Oncology, Meml Sloan Kettering Cancer Ctr 1975; **Fellow:** Radiation Oncology, Meml Sloan Kettering Cancer Ctr 1978; **Fac Appt:** Prof RadRO, Cornell Univ-Weill Med Coll

Pollack, Alan MD/PhD [RadRO] - **Spec Exp:** Prostate Cancer; Genitourinary Cancer; Sarcoma; **Hospital:** Fox Chase Cancer Ctr (page 73); **Address:** Fox Chase Cancer Ctr, Dept Rad Oncol, 333 Cottman Ave, Philadelphia, PA 19111; **Phone:** 215-728-2940; **Board Cert:** Radiation Oncology 1993; **Med School:** Univ Miami Sch Med 1987; **Resid:** Radiation Oncology, MD Anderson Cancer Ctr 1992; **Fac Appt:** Prof RadRO, Temple Univ

Pollack, Jed MD [RadRO] - **Spec Exp:** Head & Neck Cancer; Prostate Cancer; Brain Tumors; **Address:** Long Island Radiation Therapy, 6 Ohio Drive, Ste 103, Lake Success, NY 11042; **Phone:** 516-394-8100; **Board Cert:** Therapeutic Radiology 1985; **Med School:** Univ New Mexico 1981; **Resid:** Therapeutic Radiology, Meml Sloan-Kettering Cancer Ctr 1985

Regine, William F MD [RadRO] - **Spec Exp:** Stereotactic Radiosurgery; Brain & Spinal Tumors; Gastrointestinal Cancer; **Hospital:** Univ of MD Med Sys; **Address:** Univ MD Med System-Greenbaum Cancer Ctr, 22 S Green St Guldelsky Bldg, Baltimore, MD 21201; **Phone:** 410-328-6080; **Board Cert:** Radiation Oncology 1992; **Med School:** SUNY Upstate Med Univ 1987; **Resid:** Radiation Oncology, Thomas Jefferson Univ Hosp 1991; **Fellow:** Radiation Oncology, Thomas Jefferson Univ Hosp 1992; **Fac Appt:** Prof RadRO, Univ MD Sch Med

Rotman, Marvin MD [RadRO] - **Spec Exp:** Bladder Cancer; Gynecologic Cancer; Breast Cancer; Prostate Cancer; **Hospital:** SUNY Downstate Med Ctr, Long Island Coll Hosp (page 72); **Address:** 450 Clarkson Ave, Box 1211, Brooklyn, NY 11203-2056; **Phone:** 718-270-2181; **Board Cert:** Diagnostic Radiology 1966; Radiation Oncology 1999; **Med School:** Jefferson Med Coll 1958; **Resid:** Internal Medicine, Albert Einstein Med Ctr 1960; Radiation Oncology, Montefiore Hosp Med Ctr 1965; **Fac Appt:** Prof RadRO, SUNY Downstate

Schiff, Peter B MD/PhD [RadRO] - **Spec Exp:** Prostate Cancer; Gynecologic Cancer; Breast Cancer; **Hospital:** NY-Presby Hosp (page 79); **Address:** Columbia Univ Med Ctr, Dept Rad Oncology, 622 W 168th St, New York, NY 10032-3720; **Phone:** 212-305-2991; **Board Cert:** Radiation Oncology 1990; **Med School:** Albert Einstein Coll Med 1984; **Resid:** Radiation Oncology, Meml Sloan Kettering Cancer Ctr 1988; **Fac Appt:** Prof RadRO, Columbia P&S

Solin, Lawrence J MD [RadRO] - **Spec Exp:** Breast Cancer; **Hospital:** Hosp Univ Penn - UPHS (page 84); **Address:** Univ Penn Med Ctr, Dept Rad Oncology, 3400 Spruce St, 2 Donner Bldg, Philadelphia, PA 19104; **Phone:** 215-662-7267; **Board Cert:** Radiation Oncology 1999; **Med School:** Brown Univ 1978; **Resid:** Surgery, Jefferson Univ Hosp 1981; Radiation Oncology, Jefferson Univ Hosp/Hosp Univ Penn 1984; **Fac Appt:** Prof RadRO, Univ Pennsylvania

Stock, Richard MD [RadRO] - **Spec Exp:** Prostate Cancer; **Hospital:** Mount Sinai Med Ctr (page 77); **Address:** 1184 5th Ave Fl 1 - rm PA-34, New York, NY 10029; **Phone:** 212-241-7502; **Board Cert:** Radiation Oncology 1993; **Med School:** Mount Sinai Sch Med 1988; **Resid:** Radiation Oncology, Meml Sloan Kettering Cancer Ctr 1992; **Fac Appt:** Prof RadRO, Mount Sinai Sch Med

Weiss, Marisa C MD [RadRO] - **Spec Exp:** Breast Cancer; **Hospital:** Lankenau Hosp; **Address:** Lankenau Hospital, Dept Radiation Oncology, 100 Lancaster Ave, Wynnewood, PA 19096; **Phone:** 610-645-2433; **Board Cert:** Radiation Oncology 1988; **Med School:** Univ Pennsylvania 1984; **Resid:** Radiation Oncology, Hosp Univ Penn 1988; **Fellow:** Radiological Biology, Hosp Univ Penn 1990

Wharam Jr, Moody D MD [RadRO] - **Spec Exp:** Pediatric Cancers; Brain Tumors; Sarcoma-Soft Tissue; **Hospital:** Johns Hopkins Hosp - Baltimore; **Address:** Kimmel Cancer Ctr, Dept Rad Oncology, 401 N Broadway St, Ste 1440, Baltimore, MD 21231-1146; **Phone:** 410-955-7312; **Board Cert:** Therapeutic Radiology 1974; **Med School:** Univ VA Sch Med 1969; **Resid:** Radiation Oncology, UCSF Medical Ctr 1973; **Fac Appt:** Prof RadRO, Johns Hopkins Univ

Yahalom, Joachim MD [RadRO] - **Spec Exp:** Lymphoma; Hodgkin's Disease; Multiple Myeloma; **Hospital:** Meml Sloan Kettering Cancer Ctr (page 76); **Address:** Meml Sloan Kettering Cancer Ctr, Dept Radiation Oncology, 1275 York Ave, New York, NY 10021-6007; **Phone:** 212-639-5999; **Board Cert:** Radiation Oncology 1988; **Med School:** Israel 1976; **Resid:** Internal Medicine, Hadassah Hosp 1979; Radiation Oncology, Hadassah Hosp 1984; **Fellow:** Radiation Oncology, Meml Sloan Kettering Canc Ctr 1986; **Fac Appt:** Prof RadRO, Cornell Univ-Weill Med Coll

Zelefsky, Michael J MD [RadRO] - **Spec Exp:** Prostate Cancer; Brachytherapy; Genitourinary Cancer; **Hospital:** Meml Sloan Kettering Cancer Ctr (page 76); **Address:** Meml Sloan-Kettering Cancer Ctr, 1275 York Ave, New York, NY 10021-6094; **Phone:** 212-639-6802; **Board Cert:** Radiation Oncology 1991; **Med School:** Albert Einstein Coll Med 1986; **Resid:** Radiation Oncology, Meml Sloan Kettering Cancer Ctr 1990; **Fac Appt:** Prof RadRO, Cornell Univ-Weill Med Coll

Radiation Oncology

Southeast

Anscher, Mitchell MD [RadRO] - **Spec Exp:** Prostate Cancer; Brachytherapy; **Hospital:** Med Coll of VA Hosp, Henrico Doctors Hosp; **Address:** Virginia Commonwealth Univ, Department of Radiation Oncology, Box 980058, Richmond, VA 23298-0058; **Phone:** 804-828-7238; **Board Cert:** Radiation Oncology 1987; Internal Medicine 1984; **Med School:** Med Coll VA 1981; **Resid:** Internal Medicine, St Marys Hosp 1984; Radiation Oncology, Duke Univ Med Ctr 1987; **Fac Appt:** Prof RadRO, Duke Univ

Bonner, James Alan MD [RadRO] - **Spec Exp:** Head & Neck Cancer; Lung Cancer; **Hospital:** Univ of Ala Hosp at Birmingham; **Address:** 1824 6th Ave S, WTI, rm 105, Birmingham, AL 35294; **Phone:** 205-934-2761; **Board Cert:** Radiation Oncology 1990; **Med School:** Wayne State Univ 1985; **Resid:** Radiation Oncology, Univ Michigan Med Ctr 1989; **Fac Appt:** Prof RadRO, Univ Ala

Brizel, David M MD [RadRO] - **Spec Exp:** Head & Neck Cancer; Sarcoma; Lymphoma; **Hospital:** Duke Univ Med Ctr; **Address:** Duke Univ Med Ctr, Dept Rad Onc, Box 3085, Durham, NC 27710-0001; **Phone:** 919-668-5637; **Board Cert:** Radiation Oncology 1987; **Med School:** Northwestern Univ 1983; **Resid:** Radiation Oncology, Harvard Joint Center 1987; **Fac Appt:** Prof RadRO, Duke Univ

Chakravarthy, Anuradha MD [RadRO] - **Spec Exp:** Breast Cancer; Gastrointestinal Cancer; **Hospital:** Vanderbilt Univ Med Ctr; **Address:** Vanderbilt Univ Med Ctr, Dept Rad Onc, 1301 22nd Ave S, Preston Research Bldg, Ste 1003, Nashville, TN 37232; **Phone:** 615-322-2555; **Board Cert:** Radiation Oncology 1994; Internal Medicine 1986; Medical Oncology 1989; **Med School:** Geo Wash Univ 1983; **Resid:** Internal Medicine, Mayo Clinic 1986; Medical Oncology, Univ MD Cancer Ctr 1989; **Fellow:** Radiation Oncology, Johns Hopkins Hosp; **Fac Appt:** Asst Prof RadRO, Vanderbilt Univ

Crocker, Ian MD [RadRO] - **Spec Exp:** Brain Tumors; Eye Tumors/Cancer; Vascular Brachytherapy; **Hospital:** Emory Univ Hosp, Crawford Long Hosp of Emory Univ; **Address:** Emory Univ Hosp - Dept Radiation Oncology, 1365 Clifton Rd NE, T Ste 104, Atlanta, GA 30322; **Phone:** 404-778-3473; **Board Cert:** Therapeutic Radiology 1999; Internal Medicine 1980; **Med School:** Univ Saskatchewan 1976; **Resid:** Internal Medicine, Univ Hosp-Univ West Ontario 1980; **Fellow:** Radiation Oncology, Princess Margaret Hosp-Univ Toronto 1983; **Fac Appt:** Prof RadRO, Emory Univ

Halle, Jan MD [RadRO] - **Spec Exp:** Breast Cancer; Lung Cancer; **Hospital:** Univ NC Hosps; **Address:** Univ North Carolina Sch Med, Dept Rad Onc, CB 7512, 101 Manning Drive, Chapel Hill, NC 27599; **Phone:** 919-966-7700; **Board Cert:** Therapeutic Radiology 1982; **Med School:** Tufts Univ 1975; **Resid:** Radiation Oncology, North Carolina Meml Hosp 1981; **Fac Appt:** Assoc Prof RadRO, Univ NC Sch Med

Jose, Baby Oliapuram MD [RadRO] - **Spec Exp:** Head & Neck Cancer; Lung Cancer; Gynecologic Cancer; Prostate Cancer; **Hospital:** Univ of Louisville Hosp; **Address:** 529 S Jackson St Fl 4, Louisville, KY 40202; **Phone:** 502-561-2700; **Board Cert:** Therapeutic Radiology 1978; **Med School:** India 1971; **Resid:** Surgery, CMC Hosp 1974; Radiation Oncology, CMC Hosp 1976; **Fellow:** Radiation Oncology, Brown Univ-RI Hosp 1979; **Fac Appt:** Prof RadRO, Univ Louisville Sch Med

Kun, Larry E MD [RadRO] - **Spec Exp:** Brain Tumors; Pediatric Cancers; **Hospital:** St Jude Children's Research Hosp, Le Bonheur Chldns Med Ctr; **Address:** St Jude Chldns Research Hosp-Dept Rad Onc, 332 N Lauderdale St, rm C2002F, MS 220, Memphis, TN 38105; **Phone:** 901-495-3565; **Board Cert:** Therapeutic Radiology 1973; **Med School:** Jefferson Med Coll 1968; **Resid:** Therapeutic Radiology, Penrose Cancer Hosp 1972; **Fellow:** Radiation Oncology, Natl Cancer Inst 1974; Radiation Oncology, Rotterdam Radiotherapy Inst 1975; **Fac Appt:** Prof, Univ Tenn Coll Med, Memphis

Landry, Jerome C MD [RadRO] - **Spec Exp:** Gastrointestinal Cancer; Stomach Cancer; Sarcoma; Breast Cancer; **Hospital:** Emory Univ Hosp, Grady Hlth Sys; **Address:** Emory Clinic, 1365 Clifton Rd NE, Ste A-1313, Atlanta, GA 30322; **Phone:** 404-778-3651; **Board Cert:** Radiation Oncology 1988; **Med School:** Harvard Med Sch 1983; **Resid:** Radiation Oncology, Mass Genl Hosp 1987; **Fac Appt:** Prof RadRO, Emory Univ

Larner, James MD [RadRO] - **Spec Exp:** Neuro-Oncology; Brain Tumors; **Hospital:** Univ Virginia Med Ctr; **Address:** Univ Virginia Medical Ctr, Dept Radiation Oncology, PO Box 800383, Charlottesville, VA 22908; **Phone:** 434-924-5191; **Board Cert:** Radiation Oncology 1989; Internal Medicine 1983; Hematology 1988; Medical Oncology 1987; **Med School:** Univ VA Sch Med 1980; **Resid:** Internal Medicine, Thos Jefferson Univ Hosp 1983; Radiation Oncology, Montefiore-Einstein Med Ctr 1989; **Fellow:** Hematology & Oncology, Thos Jefferson Univ Hosp 1986; **Fac Appt:** Assoc Prof Med, Univ VA Sch Med

Lee, W Robert MD [RadRO] - **Spec Exp:** Prostate Cancer; **Hospital:** Duke Univ Med Ctr; **Address:** Duke Univ Med Ctr, Div Radiation Oncology, Box 3085, Durham, NC 27710; **Phone:** 919-668-7342; **Board Cert:** Radiation Oncology 1994; **Med School:** Univ VA Sch Med 1989; **Resid:** Radiation Oncology, Univ Florida 1993; **Fac Appt:** Prof RadRO, Duke Univ

Lewin, Alan A MD [RadRO] - **Spec Exp:** Breast Cancer; Lung Cancer; Brain & Spinal Cord Tumors; **Hospital:** Baptist Hosp of Miami; **Address:** Baptist Hosp Cancer Treatment Ctr, Dept Rad Onc, 8900 N Kendall Drive, Miami, FL 33176-2118; **Phone:** 786-596-6566; **Board Cert:** Therapeutic Radiology 1982; Medical Oncology 1981; Hematology 1978; Internal Medicine 1976; **Med School:** Geo Wash Univ 1973; **Resid:** Internal Medicine, Mt Sinai Hosp 1976; **Fellow:** Hematology & Oncology, Beth Israel Med Ctr 1978; Radiation Oncology, Joint Ctr Radiation Therapy 1980; **Fac Appt:** Clin Prof RadRO, Univ Miami Sch Med

Marcus Jr, Robert B MD [RadRO] - **Spec Exp:** Pediatric Cancers; Sarcoma; Bone Cancer; Brain Tumors; **Hospital:** Emory Univ Hosp; **Address:** Emory Clinic, Dept Rad Oncology, 1365 Clifton Rd NE, Ste A1300, Atlanta, GA 30322; **Phone:** 404-778-5751; **Board Cert:** Therapeutic Radiology 1980; **Med School:** Univ Fla Coll Med 1975; **Resid:** Radiation Oncology, Shands Hosp 1979; **Fac Appt:** Prof RadRO, Emory Univ

Marks, Lawrence MD [RadRO] - **Spec Exp:** Breast Cancer; Lung Cancer; **Hospital:** Duke Univ Med Ctr; **Address:** Duke Univ Med Ctr, Box 3085, Durham, NC 27710; **Phone:** 919-668-5640; **Board Cert:** Radiation Oncology 1989; **Med School:** Univ Rochester 1985; **Resid:** Radiation Oncology, Mass Genl Hosp 1989; **Fac Appt:** Prof RadRO, Duke Univ

Mendenhall, Nancy P MD [RadRO] - **Spec Exp:** Breast Cancer; Lymphoma; Hodgkin's Disease; **Hospital:** Shands Hlthcre at Univ of FL; **Address:** Univ Florida, Dept Radiation Oncology, Box 100385, Gainesville, FL 32610-0385; **Phone:** 352-265-0287; **Board Cert:** Therapeutic Radiology 1985; **Med School:** Univ Fla Coll Med 1980; **Resid:** Diagnostic Radiology, Shands-Univ of Florida 1984; **Fac Appt:** Prof RadRO, Univ Fla Coll Med

Mendenhall, William M MD [RadRO] - **Spec Exp:** Head & Neck Cancer; Stereotactic Radiosurgery; Colon Cancer; **Hospital:** Shands Hlthcre at Univ of FL; **Address:** Univ Florida, Dept Radiation Oncology, Box 100385, Gainesville, FL 32610-0385; **Phone:** 352-265-0287; **Board Cert:** Therapeutic Radiology 1983; **Med School:** Univ S Fla Coll Med 1978; **Resid:** Radiation Oncology, University of Florida 1983; **Fac Appt:** Prof RadRO, Univ Fla Coll Med

Merchant, Thomas DO [RadRO] - **Spec Exp:** Brain Tumors-Pediatric; **Hospital:** St Jude Children's Research Hosp; **Address:** St Jude Children's Research Hosp, 332 N Lauderdale St, Ste 2002, MS 220, Memphis, TN 38105; **Phone:** 901-495-3604; **Board Cert:** Radiation Oncology 1995; **Med School:** Chicago Coll Osteo Med 1989; **Resid:** Radiation Oncology, Meml Sloan Kettering Cancer Ctr 1994

Meredith, Ruby F MD [RadRO] - **Spec Exp:** Multiple Myeloma; Breast Cancer; **Hospital:** Univ of Ala Hosp at Birmingham; **Address:** Univ Alabama Hosps-Radiation Oncology, 619 19th St S, Birmingham, AL 35233; **Phone:** 205-934-2763; **Board Cert:** Radiation Oncology 1987; **Med School:** Ohio State Univ 1983; **Resid:** Radiation Oncology, Med Coll Va 1987; **Fac Appt:** Prof RadRO, Univ Ala

Prosnitz, Leonard MD [RadRO] - **Spec Exp:** Lymphoma; Breast Cancer; Hyperthermia Treatment of Cancer; Sarcoma; **Hospital:** Duke Univ Med Ctr; **Address:** Duke Univ Med Ctr, Dept Rad Onc, Box 3085, Durham, NC 27710; **Phone:** 919-668-5637; **Board Cert:** Therapeutic Radiology 1970; **Med School:** SUNY Downstate 1961; **Resid:** Internal Medicine, Dartmouth Affil Hosps 1963; Radiation Oncology, Yale-New Haven Hosp 1969; **Fellow:** Hematology & Oncology, Yale-New Haven Hosp 1967; **Fac Appt:** Prof RadRO, Duke Univ

Randall, Marcus MD [RadRO] - **Spec Exp:** Gynecologic Cancer; **Hospital:** Univ of Kentucky Chandler Hosp; **Address:** Univ Kentucky Medical Ctr, 800 Rose St, rm N-14, Lexington, KY 40536; **Phone:** 252-744-2900; **Board Cert:** Therapeutic Radiology 1986; **Med School:** Univ NC Sch Med 1982; **Resid:** Radiation Oncology, Univ Va Med Ctr 1986; **Fellow:** Radiation Oncology, Univ Va Med Ctr 1986; **Fac Appt:** Prof RadRO, Univ KY Coll Med

Rich, Tyvin Andrew MD [RadRO] - **Spec Exp:** Colon & Rectal Cancer; Chemo-Radiation Combined Therapy; Esophageal Cancer; **Hospital:** Univ Virginia Med Ctr; **Address:** Univ Va Hlth Sys, Dept Rad Onc, Box 800383, Charlottesville, VA 22908-0383; **Phone:** 434-924-5191; **Board Cert:** Radiation Oncology 1978; **Med School:** Univ VA Sch Med 1973; **Resid:** Mass Genl Hosp 1978; **Fellow:** Radiation Oncology, Mt Vernon Hosp/Gray Lab; **Fac Appt:** Prof RadRO, Univ VA Sch Med

Rosenman, Julian MD [RadRO] - **Spec Exp:** Lung Cancer; Breast Cancer; Prostate Cancer; **Hospital:** Univ NC Hosps; **Address:** Univ North Carolina, Dept Rad Onc, CB 7512, 101 Manning Drive, Chapel Hill, NC 27599-7512; **Phone:** 919-966-7700; **Board Cert:** Therapeutic Radiology 1981; **Med School:** Univ Tex SW, Dallas 1977; **Resid:** Therapeutic Radiology, Mass Genl Hosp 1981; **Fac Appt:** Prof RadRO, Univ NC Sch Med

Sailer, Scott MD [RadRO] - **Spec Exp:** Head & Neck Cancer; Genitourinary Cancer; Pediatric Cancers; **Hospital:** WakeMed Cary, WakeMed New Bern; **Address:** 300 Ashville Ave, Ste 110, Cary, NC 27511; **Phone:** 919-854-4588; **Board Cert:** Radiation Oncology 1988; **Med School:** Harvard Med Sch 1984; **Resid:** Radiation Therapy, Mass Genl Hosp 1988

Shaw, Edward G MD [RadRO] - **Spec Exp:** Stereotactic Radiosurgery; Brain Tumors; **Hospital:** Wake Forest Univ Baptist Med Ctr (page 85); **Address:** Wake Forest Med Ctr, Dept Rad Onc, Medical Center Blvd, Comp Cancer Ctr, Winston Salem, NC 27157-1029; **Phone:** 336-713-6506; **Board Cert:** Radiation Oncology 1987; **Med School:** Rush Med Coll 1983; **Resid:** Radiation Oncology, Mayo Grad Sch Med 1987; **Fac Appt:** Prof RadRO, Wake Forest Univ

Tepper, Joel MD [RadRO] - **Spec Exp:** Gastrointestinal Cancer; Sarcoma; Rectal Cancer; **Hospital:** Univ NC Hosps; **Address:** North Carolina Clin Cancer Ctr, Dept Rad Onc - CB#7512, Chapel Hill, NC 27599-7512; **Phone:** 919-966-0400; **Board Cert:** Therapeutic Radiology 1976; **Med School:** Washington Univ, St Louis 1972; **Resid:** Therapeutic Radiology, Mass Genl Hosp 1976; **Fellow:** Therapeutic Radiology, Mass Genl Hosp 1977; **Fac Appt:** Prof RadRO, Univ NC Sch Med

Toonkel, Leonard M MD [RadRO] - **Spec Exp:** Prostate Cancer; Breast Cancer; Brachytherapy; **Hospital:** Mount Sinai Med Ctr - Miami; **Address:** Dept Rad Onc, 4300 Alton Rd, Miami Beach, FL 33140; **Phone:** 305-535-3400; **Board Cert:** Therapeutic Radiology 1979; **Med School:** Univ Miami Sch Med 1975; **Resid:** Radiation Therapy, Jackson Meml Hosp 1977; Diagnostic Radiology, MD Anderson Hosp 1978; **Fellow:** Radiation Oncology, MD Anderson Hosp 1979; **Fac Appt:** Assoc Clin Prof DR, Univ Miami Sch Med

Trotti III, Andrea MD [RadRO] - **Spec Exp:** Head & Neck Cancer; Gastrointestinal Cancer; Skin Cancer; **Hospital:** H Lee Moffitt Cancer Ctr & Research Inst; **Address:** H Lee Moffitt Cancer Ctr, Dept Rad Onc, 12902 Magnolia Drive, Tampa, FL 33612-9416; **Phone:** 813-972-8424; **Board Cert:** Radiation Oncology 1988; **Med School:** Univ Fla Coll Med 1984; **Resid:** Radiation Oncology, Univ Alabama 1988; **Fac Appt:** Prof RadRO, Univ S Fla Coll Med

Willett, Christopher MD [RadRO] - **Spec Exp:** Gastrointestinal Cancer; Clinical Trials; **Hospital:** Duke Univ Med Ctr; **Address:** Duke Univ Med Ctr, PO Box 3085, Durham, NC 27710; **Phone:** 919-668-5640; **Board Cert:** Therapeutic Radiology 1985; **Med School:** Tufts Univ 1981; **Resid:** Radiation Oncology, Mass Genl Hosp 1986; **Fac Appt:** Prof, Duke Univ

Midwest

Abrams, Ross A MD [RadRO] - **Spec Exp:** Gastrointestinal Cancer; Lymphoma; **Hospital:** Rush Univ Med Ctr; **Address:** Rush Univ Med Ctr, Dept Radiation Oncology, 1653 W Congress Pkwy Atrium Bldg, Chicago, IL 60612; **Phone:** 312-942-5751; **Board Cert:** Internal Medicine 1976; Medical Oncology 1979; Hematology 1982; Radiation Oncology 1987; **Med School:** Univ Pennsylvania 1973; **Resid:** Internal Medicine, Pennsylvania Hosp 1975; Hematology & Oncology, Hosp Univ Penn 1976; **Fellow:** Hematology & Oncology, Natl Cancer Inst 1978; Radiation Oncology, Med Coll Wisconsin 1987; **Fac Appt:** Prof RadRO, Rush Med Coll

Ben-Josef, Edgar MD [RadRO] - **Spec Exp:** Bone Cancer; Gastrointestinal Cancer; Pancreatic Cancer; Intensity Modulated Radiotherapy (IMRT); **Hospital:** Univ Michigan Hlth Sys; **Address:** University Hospital, 1500 E Medical Ctr Drive, rm UH B2C490, Ann Arbor, MI 48109-0010; **Phone:** 734-936-8207; **Board Cert:** Radiation Oncology 1994; **Med School:** Israel 1986; **Resid:** Radiation Oncology, Wayne State Univ Hosp 1994; **Fellow:** Cancer Biology, Wayne State Univ Hosp 1995; **Fac Appt:** Assoc Prof RadRO, Univ Mich Med Sch

Charboneau, J William MD [RadRO] - **Spec Exp:** Radiofrequency Tumor Ablation; Liver Cancer; Thyroid Cancer; **Hospital:** Mayo Med Ctr & Clin - Rochester; **Address:** 200 First St SW, Mayo Clinic, Rochester, MN 55905-0002; **Phone:** 507-284-2097; **Board Cert:** Diagnostic Radiology 1980; **Med School:** Univ Wisc 1976; **Resid:** Diagnostic Radiology, Mayo Clinic 1980; **Fac Appt:** Prof, Mayo Med Sch

Emami, Bahman MD [RadRO] - **Spec Exp:** Head & Neck Cancer; Lung Cancer; **Hospital:** Loyola Univ Med Ctr, Hines VA Hosp; **Address:** Loyola Univ Med Ctr, Dept Rad Onc, 2160 S First Ave Bldg 105 - rm 2932, Maywood, IL 60153-3328; **Phone:** 708-216-2729; **Board Cert:** Therapeutic Radiology 1976; **Med School:** Iran 1968; **Resid:** Radiation Therapy, Tufts Univ-New Eng Med Ctr 1976; **Fellow:** Radiation Therapy, Tufts Univ-New Eng Med Ctr 1977; **Fac Appt:** Prof RadRO, Loyola Univ-Stritch Sch Med

Forman, Jeffrey D MD [RadRO] - **Spec Exp:** Neutron Therapy for Advanced Cancer; Genitourinary Cancer; Prostate Cancer; **Hospital:** Karmanos Cancer Inst; **Address:** BA Karmanos Cancer Institute, 31995 Northwestern Hwy, Farmington Hills, MI 48334; **Phone:** 248-538-6545; **Board Cert:** Radiation Oncology 1986; **Med School:** NYU Sch Med 1982; **Resid:** Radiation Oncology, Johns Hopkins Hosp 1986; **Fellow:** Therapeutic Radiology, Johns Hopkins Hosp 1987; **Fac Appt:** Prof RadRO, Wayne State Univ

Grigsby, Perry W MD [RadRO] - **Spec Exp:** Gynecologic Cancer; Thyroid Cancer; **Hospital:** Barnes-Jewish Hosp, St Louis Chldns Hosp; **Address:** Washington Univ School of Med, 4921 Parkview Pl, Box 9038635, St Louis, MO 63110; **Phone:** 314-747-7236; **Board Cert:** Radiation Oncology 1987; **Med School:** Univ KY Coll Med 1982; **Resid:** Radiation Oncology, Barnes Jewish Hosp 1985; **Fac Appt:** Prof DR, Washington Univ, St Louis

Halpern, Howard MD/PhD [RadRO] - **Spec Exp:** Breast Cancer; Esophageal Cancer; Gynecologic Cancer; **Hospital:** Univ of Chicago Hosps, Univ of IL Med Ctr at Chicago; **Address:** 1801 W Taylor St, rm C400, MC-933, Chicago, IL 60612; **Phone:** 312-996-3630; **Board Cert:** Therapeutic Radiology 1984; **Med School:** Univ Miami Sch Med 1980; **Resid:** Therapeutic Radiology, Jnt Ctr Rad Ther Harvard 1984; **Fellow:** Therapeutic Radiology, Jnt Ctr Rad Ther Harvard 1985; **Fac Appt:** Prof DR, Univ Chicago-Pritzker Sch Med

Haraf, Daniel MD [RadRO] - **Spec Exp:** Head & Neck Cancer; Lung Cancer; Prostate Cancer; **Hospital:** Univ of Chicago Hosps; **Address:** Univ Chicago Hosps, Dept Rad Oncology, 5758 S Maryland, MS 9006, Chicago, IL 60637; **Phone:** 773-702-6870; **Board Cert:** Internal Medicine 1985; Radiation Oncology 1990; **Med School:** Ros Franklin Univ/Chicago Med Sch 1982; **Resid:** Internal Medicine, Michael Reese Hosp 1985; **Fellow:** Radiation Oncology, Michael Reese Hosp/Univ Chicago 1988; **Fac Appt:** Clin Prof RadRO, Univ Chicago-Pritzker Sch Med

Hayman, James A MD [RadRO] - **Spec Exp:** Breast Cancer; Stomach Cancer; Lung Cancer; Brain Tumors; **Hospital:** Univ Michigan Hlth Sys; **Address:** University Hospital, 1500 E Medical Ctr Drive, rm UH B2C490, Ann Arbor, MI 48109-0010; **Phone:** 734-936-4288; **Board Cert:** Radiation Oncology 2004; **Med School:** Univ Chicago-Pritzker Sch Med 1991; **Resid:** Radiation Therapy, Joint Ctr for Radiation Therapy 1996; **Fac Appt:** Assoc Prof RadRO, Univ Mich Med Sch

Kiel, Krystyna D MD [RadRO] - **Spec Exp:** Breast Cancer; Sarcoma; Gastrointestinal Cancer; Colon & Rectal Cancer; **Hospital:** Northwestern Meml Hosp; **Address:** Northwestern Meml Hosp, Radiation Oncology, 251 E Huron St Galter Bldg - Ste L178, Chicago, IL 60611-2914; **Phone:** 312-926-2520; **Board Cert:** Therapeutic Radiology 2000; **Med School:** Univ Mass Sch Med 1977; **Resid:** Radiation Oncology, Mass Genl Hosp 1982; **Fac Appt:** Assoc Prof DR, Northwestern Univ

Kim, Jae Ho MD [RadRO] - **Spec Exp:** Brain Tumors; Spinal Cord Tumors; Breast Cancer; **Hospital:** Henry Ford Hosp; **Address:** Radiation Oncology, 2799 W Grand Blvd, Detroit, MI 48202; **Phone:** 313-916-1029; **Board Cert:** Therapeutic Radiology 1973; **Med School:** Korea 1959; **Resid:** Therapeutic Radiology, Meml-Sloan-Kettering 1972; **Fellow:** Diagnostic Radiology, Meml-Sloan-Kettering 1968; **Fac Appt:** Prof RadRO, Wayne State Univ

Kinsella, Timothy J MD [RadRO] - **Spec Exp:** Brain Tumors; Sarcoma; Gastrointestinal Cancer; **Hospital:** Univ Hosps Case Med Ctr; **Address:** Univ Hosps - Dept Radiation Oncology, 11100 Euclid Ave Fl BSMT - rm B181, MC LT6068, Cleveland, OH 44106-6068; **Phone:** 216-844-2530; **Board Cert:** Internal Medicine 1977; Medical Oncology 1979; Therapeutic Radiology 1980; **Med School:** Univ Rochester 1974; **Resid:** Internal Medicine, Mayo Clinic 1976; Radiation Oncology, Joint Ctr for Rad Therapy 1980; **Fellow:** Medical Oncology, Dana Farber Cancer Ctr 1977; **Fac Appt:** Prof RadRO, Case West Res Univ

Lawrence, Theodore S MD/PhD [RadRO] - **Spec Exp:** Gastrointestinal Cancer; Liver Cancer; Pancreatic Cancer; **Hospital:** Univ Michigan Hlth Sys; **Address:** Univ Hosp, Dept Radiation Oncology, 1500 E Med Ctr Dr, B2C502, Box 0010, Ann Arbor, MI 48109-0010; **Phone:** 734-936-4300; **Board Cert:** Internal Medicine 1983; Medical Oncology 1985; Radiation Oncology 1987; **Med School:** Cornell Univ-Weill Med Coll 1980; **Resid:** Internal Medicine, Stanford Univ Hosp 1983; Radiation Oncology, Natl Cancer Inst 1987; **Fellow:** Medical Oncology, Natl Cancer Inst 1986; **Fac Appt:** Prof RadRO, Univ Mich Med Sch

Lee, Chung K MD [RadRO] - **Spec Exp:** Head & Neck Cancer; Breast Cancer; Lymphoma; Gastrointestinal Cancer; **Hospital:** Univ Minn Med Ctr, Fairview - Univ Campus; **Address:** Dept of Radiation Oncology, 420 Delaware St SE, MC 400, Minneapolis, MN 55455; **Phone:** 612-273-6700; **Board Cert:** Therapeutic Radiology 1976; **Med School:** Korea 1965; **Resid:** Therapeutic Radiology, Univ of Minn Hosp 1976; Diagnostic Radiology, Yonsei Univ Hosp 1971; **Fac Appt:** Prof, Univ Minn

Macklis, Roger M MD [RadRO] - **Spec Exp:** Radioimmunotherapy of Cancer; Breast Cancer; Lymphoma; **Hospital:** Cleveland Clin Fdn (page 71); **Address:** Cleveland Cin Fdn, Dept Rad Onc T18, 9500 Euclid Ave, Cleveland, OH 44195; **Phone:** 216-444-5576; **Board Cert:** Radiation Oncology 1989; **Med School:** Harvard Med Sch 1983; **Resid:** Radiation Oncology, Joint Ctr Radiotherapy Inst 1987; **Fellow:** Research, Dana Farber Cancer Inst 1987; **Fac Appt:** Prof RadRO, Case West Res Univ

Martenson Jr, James A MD [RadRO] - **Spec Exp:** Mucositis; Esophageal Cancer; **Hospital:** Mayo Med Ctr & Clin - Rochester; **Address:** Mayo Clinic, Dept Rad/Onc, 200 First St SW, Rochester, MN 55905; **Phone:** 507 284-4561; **Board Cert:** Therapeutic Radiology 1985; **Med School:** Univ Wash 1981; **Resid:** Radiation Oncology, Mayo Clinic 1985; **Fac Appt:** Assoc Prof, Mayo Med Sch

Mehta, Minesh P MD [RadRO] - **Spec Exp:** Brain Tumors; Lung Cancer; Pediatric Cancers; **Hospital:** Univ WI Hosp & Clins; **Address:** Univ Wisconsin, Dept Rad Oncology, 600 Highland Ave, K4B-100, Madison, WI 53792, **Phone:** 608-263-8500; **Board Cert:** Radiation Oncology 1988; **Med School:** Zambia 1981; **Resid:** Internal Medicine, Ndola Central Hosp 1983; Radiation Oncology, Ndola Central Hosp 1988; **Fac Appt:** Prof RadRO, Univ Wisc

Radiation Oncology

Michalski, Jeff M MD [RadRO] - **Spec Exp:** Prostate Cancer; Sarcoma; Pediatric Cancers; **Hospital:** Barnes-Jewish Hosp, St Louis Chldns Hosp; **Address:** Washington Univ Sch Med, Dept Rad Oncology, 4921 Parkview Place, Lower Level, Box 8224, St Louis, MO 63110; **Phone:** 314-362-8566; **Board Cert:** Radiation Oncology 1991; **Med School:** Med Coll Wisc 1986; **Resid:** Radiation Oncology, Columbia Presbyterian Med Ctr 1988; Radiation Oncology, Mallinckrodt Inst of Radiology 1990; **Fellow:** Radiation Oncology, Mallinckrodt Inst of Radiology 1991; **Fac Appt:** Assoc Prof RadRO, Washington Univ, St Louis

Mittal, Bharat MD [RadRO] - **Spec Exp:** Head & Neck Cancer; Lymphoma; Skin Cancer; **Hospital:** Northwestern Meml Hosp; **Address:** 251 E Huron St, Bldg LC-178, Chicago, IL 60611; **Phone:** 312-926-2520; **Board Cert:** Radiation Oncology 1981; **Med School:** India 1973; **Resid:** Internal Medicine, Christian Med Coll 1976; Radiation Oncology, Northwestern Meml Hosp 1980; **Fellow:** Radiation Oncology, Mallinckrodt Inst 1981; **Fac Appt:** Prof RadRO, Northwestern Univ

Movsas, Benjamin MD [RadRO] - **Spec Exp:** Lung Cancer; Brain Tumors; Prostate Cancer; Stereotactic Radiosurgery; **Hospital:** Henry Ford Hosp; **Address:** Henry Ford Health System, Radiation Oncology, 2799 W Grand Blvd, Detroit, MI 48202; **Phone:** 313-916-5188; **Board Cert:** Radiation Oncology 1999; **Med School:** Washington Univ, St Louis 1990; **Resid:** Radiation Oncology, National Cancer Inst 1995

Myerson, Robert J MD [RadRO] - **Spec Exp:** Gastrointestinal Cancer; Breast Cancer; Hyperthermia Treatment of Cancer; **Hospital:** Barnes-Jewish Hosp; **Address:** Ctr for Advanced Med-Siteman Cancer Ctr, 4921 Parkview Pl, Box 9038635, St Louis, MO 63110; **Phone:** 314-747-7236; **Board Cert:** Therapeutic Radiology 1985; **Med School:** Univ Miami Sch Med 1980; **Resid:** Radiation Therapy, Hosp Univ Penn 1984; **Fac Appt:** Prof RadRO, Washington Univ, St Louis

Pierce, Lori J MD [RadRO] - **Spec Exp:** Breast Cancer; **Hospital:** Univ Michigan Hlth Sys; **Address:** Univ Hosp, Dept Rad Onc, 1500 E Med Ctr Dr, rm B2C440, Box 0010, Ann Arbor, MI 48109-0999; **Phone:** 734-936-4300; **Board Cert:** Radiation Oncology 1989; **Med School:** Duke Univ 1985; **Resid:** Radiation Oncology, Hosp Univ Penn 1989; **Fac Appt:** Prof RadRO, Univ Mich Med Sch

Sandler, Howard M MD [RadRO] - **Spec Exp:** Prostate Cancer; Genitourinary Cancer; Brain Tumors; **Hospital:** Univ Michigan Hlth Sys; **Address:** Univ Michigan Med Ctr, Dept Rad Onc, 1500 E Medical Ctr Dr. UH B2C502, Box 0010, Ann Arbor, MI 48109-0010; **Phone:** 734-936-9338; **Board Cert:** Radiation Oncology 1989; **Med School:** Univ Conn 1985; **Resid:** Radiation Oncology, Hosp Univ Penn 1989; **Fac Appt:** Prof RadRO, Univ Mich Med Sch

Schomberg, Paula J MD [RadRO] - **Spec Exp:** Brain Tumors; Pediatric Cancers; **Hospital:** Mayo Med Ctr & Clin - Rochester; **Address:** Mayo Clinic - Charlton Bldg, Desk R, 200 1st St SW, Rochester, MN 55905; **Phone:** 507-284-3551; **Board Cert:** Therapeutic Radiology 1984; **Med School:** Med Coll Wisc 1979; **Resid:** Radiation Therapy, Mayo Clinic 1983; **Fac Appt:** Prof RadRO, Mayo Med Sch

Small Jr, William MD [RadRO] - **Spec Exp:** Gynecologic Cancer; Gastrointestinal Cancer; Breast Cancer; Pancreatic Cancer; **Hospital:** Northwestern Meml Hosp; **Address:** Northwestern Meml Hosp, Rad Oncology, 251 E Huron St Galter Bldg - Ste L178, Chicago, IL 60611; **Phone:** 312-926-2520; **Board Cert:** Radiation Oncology 2004; **Med School:** Northwestern Univ 1990; **Resid:** Radiation Oncology, Northwestern Univ 1994; **Fac Appt:** Assoc Prof RadRO, Northwestern Univ

Suh, John H MD [RadRO] - **Spec Exp:** Brain Tumors-Adult & Pediatric; Clinical Trials; Gamma Knife Surgery; **Hospital:** Cleveland Clin Fdn (page 71); **Address:** Cleveland Clinic, Dept Rad/Onc, Desk T28, 9500 Euclid Ave, Cleveland, OH 44195; **Phone:** 216-444-5574; **Board Cert:** Radiation Oncology 2000; **Med School:** Univ Miami Sch Med 1990; **Resid:** Radiation Oncology, Cleveland Clinic 1994; **Fellow:** Radiation Oncology, Cleveland Clinic 1995

Taylor, Marie E MD [RadRO] - **Spec Exp:** Breast Cancer; **Hospital:** Barnes-Jewish Hosp, Barnes-Jewish West County Hosp; **Address:** Center for Advanced Med-Siteman Cancer Ctr, 4921 Parkview Pl, Box 9038635, St Louis, MO 63110; **Phone:** 314-747-7236; **Board Cert:** Radiation Oncology 1987; **Med School:** Univ Wash 1982; **Resid:** Radiation Oncology, Univ Wash Med Ctr 1986

Thornton Jr, Allan F MD [RadRO] - **Spec Exp:** Proton Beam Therapy; **Address:** Midwest Proton Radiotherapy Institute, 2425 N Milo Sampson Ln, Bloomington, IN 47408; **Phone:** 812-349-5074; **Board Cert:** Radiation Oncology 1999; **Med School:** Univ VA Sch Med 1981; **Resid:** Radiation Oncology, Princess Margaret Hosp 1986

Vicini, Frank A MD [RadRO] - **Spec Exp:** Breast Cancer; Prostate Cancer; Brachytherapy; **Hospital:** William Beaumont Hosp; **Address:** William Beaumont Hospital, 3601 W 13 Mile Rd, Royal Oak, MI 48073; **Phone:** 248-551-1219; **Board Cert:** Radiation Oncology 1999; **Med School:** Wayne State Univ 1985; **Resid:** Radiation Oncology, William Beaumont Hosp 1989; **Fellow:** Radiation Oncology, Harvard Med Sch/Joint Ctr for Rad Ther 1990; **Fac Appt:** Clin Prof RadRO, Univ Mich Med Sch

Weichselbaum, Ralph R MD [RadRO] - **Spec Exp:** Gene Targeted Radiotherapy; Head & Neck Cancer; Esophageal Cancer; **Hospital:** Univ of Chicago Hosps; **Address:** Univ Chicago, Dept Rad Onc, 5758 S Maryland Ave, MC-9006-DCAM-1D, Chicago, IL 60637; **Phone:** 773-702-0817; **Board Cert:** Therapeutic Radiology 1975; **Med School:** Univ IL Coll Med 1971; **Resid:** Therapeutic Radiology, Harvard Jt Ctr Rad Therapy 1975; **Fellow:** Diagnostic Radiology, Harvard Med Sch 1976; **Fac Appt:** Prof DR, Univ Chicago-Pritzker Sch Med

Wilson, J Frank MD [RadRO] - **Spec Exp:** Breast Cancer; Skin Cancer; **Hospital:** Froedtert Meml Lutheran Hosp; **Address:** Dept Radiation Oncology, 9200 W Wisconsin Ave, Milwaukee, WI 53226; **Phone:** 414-805-4400; **Board Cert:** Therapeutic Radiology 1971; **Med School:** Univ MO-Columbia Sch Med 1965; **Resid:** Radiation Oncology, Penrose Cancer Hosp 1969; **Fellow:** Radiation Oncology, Natl Cancer Inst/NIH 1971; **Fac Appt:** Prof RadRO, Med Coll Wisc

Radiation Oncology

Great Plains and Mountains

Gaffney, David K MD/PhD [RadRO] - **Spec Exp:** Breast Cancer; Gynecologic Cancer; **Hospital:** Univ Utah Hosps and Clins; **Address:** Huntsman Cancer Hosp, Dept Rad Oncology, 1950 Circle of Hope, rm 1440, Salt Lake City, UT 84112-5560; **Phone:** 801-581-2396; **Board Cert:** Radiation Oncology 1997; **Med School:** Med Coll Wisc 1992; **Resid:** Radiation Oncology, Univ Utah Hosps 1996; **Fac Appt:** Assoc Prof, Univ Utah

Rabinovitch, Rachel A MD [RadRO] - **Spec Exp:** Breast Cancer; Lymphoma; **Hospital:** Univ Colorado Hosp; **Address:** Anschutz Cancer Pavilion, Dept Rad Oncology, 1665 N Ursula St, PO Box 6510, MS F-706, Aurora, CO 80045; **Phone:** 720-848-0156; **Board Cert:** Radiation Oncology 1994; **Med School:** Albert Einstein Coll Med 1989; **Resid:** Radiation Oncology, Meml Sloan Kettering Cancer Ctr 1993; **Fac Appt:** Assoc Prof RadRO, Univ Colorado

Shrieve, Dennis C MD [RadRO] - **Spec Exp:** Brain Tumors-Adult & Pediatric; Genitourinary Cancer; Gastrointestinal Cancer; **Hospital:** Univ Utah Hosps and Clins, Primary Children's Med Ctr; **Address:** Huntsman Cancer Inst, Dept Rad Oncology, 1950 Circle of Hope, Salt Lake City, UT 84112; **Phone:** 801-581-2396; **Board Cert:** Radiation Oncology 1993; **Med School:** Univ Miami Sch Med ; **Resid:** Radiation Oncology, UCSF Med Ctr; **Fac Appt:** Prof RadRO, Univ Utah

Smalley, Stephen R MD [RadRO] - **Spec Exp:** Colon Cancer; Gastrointestinal Cancer; **Hospital:** Olathe Med Ctr; **Address:** Olathe Med Ctr, 20375 W 151st St, Doctors Bldg, Ste 180, Olathe, KS 66061-4575; **Phone:** 913-768-7200; **Board Cert:** Internal Medicine 1982; Radiation Oncology 1987; Medical Oncology 1985; **Med School:** Univ MO-Kansas City 1979; **Resid:** Internal Medicine, Mayo Clinic 1982; Radiation Oncology, Mayo Clinic 1986; **Fellow:** Medical Oncology, Mayo Clinic 1984; **Fac Appt:** Prof RadRO, Univ Kans

Southwest

Ang, Kie-Kian MD/PhD [RadRO] - **Spec Exp:** Head & Neck Cancer; **Hospital:** UT MD Anderson Cancer Ctr (page 81); **Address:** UT MD Anderson Cancer Ctr, 1515 Holcombe Blvd, Box 97, Houston, TX 77030; **Phone:** 713-563-8400; **Board Cert:** Radiation Oncology 1987; **Med School:** Belgium 1975; **Resid:** Radiation Oncology, Univ Hosp Louvian 1980; **Fac Appt:** Prof, Univ Tex, Houston

Buchholz, Thomas A MD [RadRO] - **Spec Exp:** Breast Cancer; **Hospital:** UT MD Anderson Cancer Ctr (page 81); **Address:** Univ Texas MD Anderson Cancer Ctr, 1515 Holcombe Blvd, Unit 1202, Houston, TX 77030; **Phone:** 713-794-4892; **Board Cert:** Radiation Oncology 1993; **Med School:** Tufts Univ 1988; **Resid:** Radiation Oncology, Univ Washington Med Ctr 1993; **Fellow:** Research, Univ Washington Med Ctr 1994; **Fac Appt:** Prof RadRO, Univ Tex, Houston

Choy, Hak MD [RadRO] - **Spec Exp:** Lung Cancer; **Hospital:** UT Southwestern Med Ctr - Dallas; **Address:** UT SW Med Ctr - Dallas, Dept Rad-Onc, 5801 Forest Park Rd, Dallas, TX 75390-9183; **Phone:** 214-645-7600; **Board Cert:** Radiation Oncology 1993; **Med School:** Univ Tex Med Br, Galveston 1987; **Resid:** Radiation Oncology, Ohio State Univ Hosp 1989; Radiation Oncology, Univ Texas Hlth Sci Ctr 1991; **Fac Appt:** Prof RadRO, Univ Tex SW, Dallas

Cox, James D MD [RadRO] - **Spec Exp:** Lymphoma; Lung Cancer; Gynecologic Cancer; **Hospital:** UT MD Anderson Cancer Ctr (page 81); **Address:** Univ Tex MD Anderson Cancer Ctr, 1515 Holcombe Blvd, Unit 97, Houston, TX 77030; **Phone:** 713-563-2316; **Board Cert:** Radiation Oncology 1999; **Med School:** Univ Rochester 1965; **Resid:** Diagnostic Radiology, Penrose Cancer Hosp 1969; **Fellow:** Therapeutic Radiology, Inst Gustave-Roussy 1970; **Fac Appt:** Prof RadRO, Univ Tex, Houston

Eifel, Patricia J MD [RadRO] - **Spec Exp:** Cervical Cancer; Uterine Cancer; Vulvar Disease/Cancer; Vaginal Cancer; **Hospital:** UT MD Anderson Cancer Ctr (page 81); **Address:** MD Anderson Cancer Ctr, Dept Rad Onc, 1515 Holcombe Blvd, Unit 1202, Houston, TX 77030-4009; **Phone:** 713-563-6830; **Board Cert:** Therapeutic Radiology 1983; **Med School:** Stanford Univ 1977; **Resid:** Radiation Oncology, Stanford Univ Med Ctr 1981; **Fellow:** Therapeutic Radiology, Stanford Univ Med Ctr 1982

Grado, Gordon L MD [RadRO] - **Spec Exp:** Prostate Cancer; Brachytherapy; **Hospital:** Scottsdale Hlthcare - Shea; **Address:** 2926 N Civic Center Plaza, Scottsdale, AZ 85251; **Phone:** 480-614-6300; **Board Cert:** Therapeutic Radiology 1981; Radiation Oncology 1999; **Med School:** Southern IL Univ 1977; **Resid:** Therapeutic Radiology, Mayo Clinic 1981

Gunderson, Leonard MD [RadRO] - **Spec Exp:** Gastrointestinal Cancer; Brachytherapy; Sarcoma; **Hospital:** Mayo Clin Hosp - Scottsdale; **Address:** Mayo Clinic, Dept Radiation Oncol, 13400 E Shea Blvd, Scottsdale, AZ 85259-5404; **Phone:** 480-342-1262; **Board Cert:** Therapeutic Radiology 1975; **Med School:** Univ KY Coll Med 1969; **Resid:** Radiation Oncology, Latter Day Saints Hosp 1974; **Fac Appt:** Prof RadRO, Mayo Med Sch

Herman, Terence Spencer MD [RadRO] - **Spec Exp:** Breast Cancer; Sarcoma; Brain Tumors; **Hospital:** OU Med Ctr; **Address:** Oklahoma Univ Health Sci Ctr, 825 NE 10th St, OUPB 1430, Oklahoma City, OK 73104-5417; **Phone:** 405-271-5641; **Board Cert:** Internal Medicine 1975; Medical Oncology 1977; Therapeutic Radiology 1985; **Med School:** Univ Conn 1972; **Resid:** Internal Medicine, Univ Arizona 1975; Radiation Oncology, Stanford Univ 1985; **Fellow:** Medical Oncology, Univ Arizona 1977; **Fac Appt:** Prof RadRO, Univ Okla Coll Med

Janjan, Nora Anita MD [RadRO] - **Spec Exp:** Gastrointestinal Cancer; Palliative Care; **Hospital:** UT MD Anderson Cancer Ctr (page 81); **Address:** Univ TX MD Anderson Cancer Ctr, 1515 Holcombe Blvd, Box 97, Houston, TX 77030; **Phone:** 713-563-2326; **Board Cert:** Radiation Oncology 2000; **Med School:** Univ Ariz Coll Med 1979; **Resid:** Internal Medicine, Baylor Affil Hosps 1981; Radiation Oncology, Baylor Affil Hosps 1984; **Fac Appt:** Prof RadRO, Univ Tex, Houston

Jhingran, Anuja MD [RadRO] - **Spec Exp:** Gynecologic Cancer; Brachytherapy; **Hospital:** UT MD Anderson Cancer Ctr (page 81); **Address:** MD Anderson Cancer Ctr, 1515 Holcombe Ave, Box 1202, Houston, TX 77030; **Phone:** 713-563-2300; **Board Cert:** Radiation Oncology 1993; **Med School:** Texas Tech Univ 1988; **Resid:** Radiation Oncology, Baylor College Med 1993; **Fac Appt:** Assoc Prof RadRO, Univ Tex, Houston

Komaki, Ritsuko MD [RadRO] - **Spec Exp:** Lung Cancer; Thymoma; Esophageal Cancer; **Hospital:** UT MD Anderson Cancer Ctr (page 81); **Address:** UT-MD Anderson Cancer Ctr, Dept Rad Onc, 1515 Holcombe Blvd, Unit 97, Houston, TX 77030; **Phone:** 713-563-2300; **Board Cert:** Therapeutic Radiology 1977; Radiation Oncology 2001; **Med School:** Japan 1969; **Resid:** Radiation Oncology, Med Coll Wisc 1978; **Fac Appt:** Prof RadRO, Univ Tex, Houston

Radiation Oncology

Kuske, Robert R MD [RadRO] - **Spec Exp:** Breast Cancer; **Hospital:** Scottsdale Hlthcare - Shea; **Address:** 8994 E Desert Cove Ave, Ste 100, Scottsdale, AZ 85260; **Phone:** 602-274-4484; **Board Cert:** Therapeutic Radiology 1985; **Med School:** Univ Cincinnati 1980; **Resid:** Radiation Oncology, Univ Cincinnati Med Ctr 1984

Medbery, Clinton A MD [RadRO] - **Spec Exp:** Breast Cancer; Gynecologic Cancer; **Hospital:** St Anthony Hosp; **Address:** Frank C Love Cancer Institute, 1000 N Lee St, Oklahoma City, OK 73102; **Phone:** 405-272-7311; **Board Cert:** Internal Medicine 1980; Medical Oncology 1983; Radiation Oncology 1987; **Med School:** Med Univ SC 1976; **Resid:** Internal Medicine, Naval Hosp 1980; Radiation Oncology, Natl Cancer Inst 1987; **Fellow:** Medical Oncology, Naval Hosp 1982

Pistenmaa, David A MD/PhD [RadRO] - **Spec Exp:** Stereotactic Radiosurgery; Prostate Cancer; Breast Cancer; **Hospital:** UT Southwestern Med Ctr - Dallas, Parkland Meml Hosp - Dallas; **Address:** UTSW Med Ctr, Dept Rad Oncology, 5801 Forest Park Rd, Dallas, TX 75390; **Phone:** 214-645-8525; **Board Cert:** Therapeutic Radiology 1974; **Med School:** Stanford Univ 1969; **Resid:** Radiation Oncology, Stanford Univ Med Ctr 1973; **Fac Appt:** Prof RadRO, Univ Tex SW, Dallas

Senzer, Neil N MD [RadRO] - **Spec Exp:** Clinical Trials; Gene Targeted Radiotherapy; Gene Therapy; **Hospital:** Baylor Univ Medical Ctr; **Address:** Morg Crowley Medical Research Ctr, 3535 Worth St, Ste 302, Dallas, TX 75246-2044; **Phone:** 214-370-1400; **Board Cert:** Pediatrics 1976; Pediatric Hematology-Oncology 1978; Therapeutic Radiology 1985; **Med School:** SUNY Buffalo 1971; **Resid:** Pediatrics, Johns Hopkins Hosp 1974; Radiation Oncology, St Barnabas Med Ctr 1985; **Fellow:** Pediatric Hematology-Oncology, St Jude Chldns Rsch Hosp 1978

Shina, Donald C MD [RadRO] - **Spec Exp:** Breast Cancer; **Hospital:** St Vincent Hosp - Santa Fe; **Address:** Santa Fe Cancer Ctr at St Vincent Hosp, 455 Saint Michael's Drive, Santa Fe, NM 87505; **Phone:** 505-820-5233; **Board Cert:** Internal Medicine 1977; Medical Oncology 1979; Therapeutic Radiology 1981; **Med School:** Case West Res Univ 1974; **Resid:** Internal Medicine, Univ Hosps 1977; **Fellow:** Radiation Oncology, Univ Hosps 1980; Medical Oncology, Univ Hosps 1980

Stea, Baldassarre MD/PhD [RadRO] - **Spec Exp:** Brain Tumors; Stereotactic Radiosurgery; Pediatric Cancers; **Hospital:** Univ Med Ctr - Tucson; **Address:** Univ Hlth Scis Ctr, Dept Rad Onc, 1501 N Campbell Ave, Tucson, AZ 85724-0001; **Phone:** 520-626-6724; **Board Cert:** Radiation Oncology 1987; **Med School:** Geo Wash Univ 1983; **Resid:** Radiation Oncology, Natl Cancer Inst 1987; **Fac Appt:** Prof RadRO, Univ Ariz Coll Med

West Coast and Pacific

Blasko, John C MD [RadRO] - **Spec Exp:** Prostate Cancer; **Hospital:** Swedish Med Ctr - Seattle; **Address:** 1101 Madison, Ste 1101, Seattle, WA 98104; **Phone:** 206-215-2480; **Board Cert:** Therapeutic Radiology 1976; **Med School:** Univ MD Sch Med 1969; **Resid:** Diagnostic Radiology, Maine Med Ctr 1974; Radiation Therapy, Univ Washington 1976; **Fac Appt:** Prof, Univ Wash

Donaldson, Sarah S MD [RadRO] - **Spec Exp:** Pediatric Cancers; Hodgkin's Disease; **Hospital:** Stanford Univ Med Ctr; **Address:** 875 Blake Wilbur Drive, CC Bldg Fl G - rm 226, MC 5847, Stanford, CA 94305-5847; **Phone:** 650-723-6195; **Board Cert:** Therapeutic Radiology 1974; **Med School:** Harvard Med Sch 1968; **Resid:** Radiation Oncology, Stanford Univ Med Ctr 1972; **Fellow:** Pediatric Hematology-Oncology, Inst Gustave-Roussy 1973; Pediatric Hematology-Oncology, MD Anderson Cancer Ctr 1971; **Fac Appt:** Prof RadRO, Stanford Univ

Douglas, James G MD [RadRO] - **Spec Exp:** Pediatric Cancers; Head & Neck Cancer; Brain Tumors; **Hospital:** Univ Wash Med Ctr, Chldns Hosp and Regl Med Ctr - Seattle; **Address:** Univ Washington Med Ctr, Dept Radiation Onc, 1959 NE Pacific St, Box 356043, Seattle, WA 98195-6043; **Phone:** 206-598-4100; **Board Cert:** Pediatrics 1986; Radiation Oncology 1997; **Med School:** Case West Res Univ 1980; **Resid:** Pediatrics, Children's Hosp Med Ctr 1983; Radiation Oncology, Univ Washington Med Ctr 1996; **Fellow:** Pediatric Hematology-Oncology, Natl Inst Hlth 1986; **Fac Appt:** Assoc Prof RadRO, Univ Wash

Halberg, Francine MD [RadRO] - **Spec Exp:** Breast Cancer; **Hospital:** Marin Genl Hosp, UCSF Med Ctr; **Address:** Marin Cancer Inst-Dept of Rad.Oncology, 1350 S Eliseo Drive, Ste 100, Greenbrae, CA 94904; **Phone:** 415-925-7326; **Board Cert:** Internal Medicine 1981; Therapeutic Radiology 1984; **Med School:** Cornell Univ-Weill Med Coll 1978; **Resid:** Internal Medicine, USPHS Hosp 1981; **Fellow:** Radiation Oncology, Stanford Univ Med Ctr 1984; **Fac Appt:** Assoc Prof RadRO, UCSF

Hancock, Steven MD [RadRO] - **Spec Exp:** Prostate Cancer; Breast Cancer; Cancer Survivors-Late Effects of Therapy; **Hospital:** Stanford Univ Med Ctr; **Address:** Stanford Cancer Center-Dept Rad Onc, 875 Blake Wilber Drive, MC 5847, Stanford, CA 94305; **Phone:** 650-723-6440; **Board Cert:** Therapeutic Radiology 1982; Internal Medicine 1980; **Med School:** Stanford Univ 1976; **Resid:** Radiation Therapy, Stanford Univ Med Ctr 1981; Internal Medicine, Stanford Univ Med Ctr 1979; **Fac Appt:** Prof RadRO, Stanford Univ

Hoppe, Richard T MD [RadRO] - **Spec Exp:** Lymphoma; Hodgkin's Disease; **Hospital:** Stanford Univ Med Ctr; **Address:** Stanford Med Ctr, Dept Rad Onc, 875 Blake Wilbur, MC 5847, Stanford, CA 94305-5847; **Phone:** 650-723-5510; **Board Cert:** Therapeutic Radiology 1976; **Med School:** Cornell Univ-Weill Med Coll 1971; **Resid:** Radiation Therapy, Stanford Univ Med Ctr 1976; **Fac Appt:** Prof DR, Stanford Univ

Koh, Wui-Jin MD [RadRO] - **Spec Exp:** Gynecologic Cancer; Brachytherapy; Clinical Trials; **Hospital:** Univ Wash Med Ctr; **Address:** Univ Washington Med Ctr, Dept of Radiation Oncology, Box 356043, Seattle, WA 98195; **Phone:** 206-598-4121; **Board Cert:** Radiation Oncology 1988; **Med School:** Loma Linda Univ 1984; **Resid:** Radiation Oncology, Univ Washington Med Ctr 1988; **Fellow:** Tumor Imaging, Univ Washington Med Ctr 1988; **Fac Appt:** Prof RadRO, Univ Wash

Laramore, George E MD [RadRO] - **Spec Exp:** Neutron Therapy for Advanced Cancer; Salivary Gland Tumors; Head & Neck Cancer; Skin Cancer; **Hospital:** Univ Wash Med Ctr; **Address:** Univ Washington Med Ctr, Dept Rad Onc Box 356043, Seattle, WA 98195; **Phone:** 206-598-4110, **Board Cert:** Therapeutic Radiology 1980; Radiation Oncology 2000; **Med School:** Univ Miami Sch Med 1976; **Resid:** Radiation Oncology, Univ Washington 1980; **Fac Appt:** Prof RadRO, Univ Wash

Larson, David Andrew MD/PhD [RadRO] - **Spec Exp:** Neuro-Oncology; Brain Tumors; Stereotactic Radiosurgery; **Hospital:** UCSF Med Ctr; **Address:** UCSF Med Ctr, Dept Rad Onc, 505 Parnassus Ave, rm L-75, San Francisco, CA 94143-0226; **Phone:** 415-353-8900; **Board Cert:** Therapeutic Radiology 1986; **Med School:** Univ Miami Sch Med 1981; **Resid:** Radiation Therapy, Joint Ctr RadTherapy 1985; **Fac Appt:** Prof RadRO, UCSF

Le, Quynh-Thu Xuan MD [RadRO] - **Spec Exp:** Head & Neck Cancer; Lung Cancer; Thoracic Cancers; Clinical Trials; **Hospital:** Stanford Univ Med Ctr; **Address:** Stanford Univ, Dept Rad Oncology, 875 Blake Wilbur Drive, MC 5847, Stanford, CA 94305; **Phone:** 650-498-5032; **Board Cert:** Radiation Oncology 1998; **Med School:** UCSF 1993; **Resid:** Radiation Oncology, UCSF Med Ctr 1997; **Fac Appt:** Assoc Prof RadRO, Stanford Univ

Radiation Oncology

Leibel, Steven A MD [RadRO] - **Spec Exp:** Prostate Cancer; **Hospital:** Stanford Univ Med Ctr; **Address:** Stanford Univ Med Ctr, 875 Blake Wilber Dr, MC5827, Stanford, CA 94305-5827; **Phone:** 650-723-4250; **Board Cert:** Therapeutic Radiology 1976; Radiation Oncology 1999; **Med School:** UCSF 1972; **Resid:** Radiation Oncology, UCSF Med Ctr 1976; **Fac Appt:** Prof RadRO, Stanford Univ

Mundt, Arno J MD [RadRO] - **Spec Exp:** Gynecologic Cancer; Intensity Modulated Radiotherapy (IMRT); **Hospital:** UCSD Med Ctr; **Address:** Moores UCSD Cancer Center, 3855 Health Sciences Drive, MC 0843, La Jolla, CA 92093; **Phone:** 858-822-6040; **Board Cert:** Radiation Oncology 1994; **Med School:** Univ Mich Med Sch 1987; **Resid:** Physical Medicine & Rehabilitation, George Washington Univ Hosp 1990; Radiation Oncology, Univ Chicago Hosps 1993; **Fac Appt:** Assoc Prof RadRO, Univ Chicago-Pritzker Sch Med

Pezner, Richard D MD [RadRO] - **Spec Exp:** Brain Tumors; Gastrointestinal Cancer; Stereotactic Radiosurgery; **Hospital:** City of Hope Natl Med Ctr & Beckman Rsch (page 69); **Address:** City of Hope Med Ctr-Div Radiation Onc, 1500 E Duarte Rd, Duarte, CA 91010-3000; **Phone:** 626-301-8247; **Board Cert:** Diagnostic Radiology 1979; **Med School:** Northwestern Univ 1975; **Resid:** Radiation Oncology, Oregon Health Sci Ctr 1979; **Fac Appt:** Assoc Clin Prof DR, UC Irvine

Quivey, Jeanne Marie MD [RadRO] - **Spec Exp:** Head & Neck Cancer; Breast Cancer; Eye Tumors/Cancer; Intensity Modulated Radiotherapy (IMRT); **Hospital:** UCSF Med Ctr; **Address:** 1600 Divisadero St, Ste H1031, San Francisco, CA 94115-3010; **Phone:** 415-353-7175; **Board Cert:** Therapeutic Radiology 1974; **Med School:** UCSF 1970; **Resid:** Radiation Therapy, UCSF Med Ctr 1974; **Fac Appt:** Prof RadRO, UCSF

Roach III, Mack MD [RadRO] - **Spec Exp:** Prostate Cancer; Genitourinary Cancer; Lung Cancer; **Hospital:** UCSF - Mt Zion Med Ctr, UCSF Med Ctr; **Address:** UCSF Mt Zion Cancer Ctr, Div Rad Oncol, 1600 Divisadero St, Ste H1031, San Francisco, CA 94115; **Phone:** 415-353-7175; **Board Cert:** Medical Oncology 1985; Radiation Oncology 1987; Internal Medicine 1984; **Med School:** Stanford Univ 1979; **Resid:** Internal Medicine, ML King Genl Hosp 1981; Radiation Oncology, Stanford Univ Med Ctr 1987; **Fellow:** Medical Oncology, UCSF Med Ctr 1983; **Fac Appt:** Prof RadRO, UCSF

Rose, Christopher M MD [RadRO] - **Spec Exp:** Prostate Cancer; Breast Cancer; Intensity Modulated Radiotherapy (IMRT); **Address:** Santa Fe Radiation Therapy, 9229 Wilshire Blvd, Beverly Hills, CA 90210; **Phone:** 310-205-5700; **Board Cert:** Radiation Oncology 1999; **Med School:** Harvard Med Sch 1974; **Resid:** Internal Medicine, Beth Israel Deaconess 1976; Radiation Oncology, Joint Ctr Rad Therapy 1979; **Fellow:** Research, British Inst Cancer Rsch 1979; **Fac Appt:** Assoc Clin Prof RadRO, UCLA

Rossi, Carl John MD [RadRO] - **Spec Exp:** Prostate Cancer; Proton Beam Therapy; **Hospital:** Loma Linda Univ Med Ctr; **Address:** Loma Linda Univ Med Ctr, 11234 Anderson St, rm B121, Loma Linda, CA 92354; **Phone:** 909-558-4280; **Board Cert:** Radiation Oncology 1994; **Med School:** Loyola Univ-Stritch Sch Med 1988; **Resid:** Radiation Oncology, Loma Linda Univ Med Ctr 1992; **Fac Appt:** Asst Prof RadRO, Loma Linda Univ

Russell, Kenneth J MD [RadRO] - **Spec Exp:** Prostate Cancer; Lymphoma; Genitourinary Cancer; **Hospital:** Univ Wash Med Ctr; **Address:** Seattle Cancer Care Alliance, G1101, 825 Eastlake Ave E, Seattle, WA 98109; **Phone:** 206-288-7100; **Board Cert:** Therapeutic Radiology 1984; **Med School:** Harvard Med Sch 1979; **Resid:** Radiation Therapy, Stanford Univ Med Ctr 1983; **Fellow:** Radiological Biology, Stanford Univ Med Ctr 1985; **Fac Appt:** Prof, Univ Wash

Streeter Jr, Oscar E MD [RadRO] - **Spec Exp:** Lung Cancer; Head & Neck Cancer; **Hospital:** USC Norris Comp Cancer Ctr, USC Univ Hosp - R K Eamer Med Plz; **Address:** Norris Comp Cancer Ctr-Dept Rad Onc, 1441 Eastlake Ave Fl Ground, Los Angeles, CA 90033; **Phone:** 323-865-3051; **Board Cert:** Radiation Oncology 1989; **Med School:** Howard Univ 1982; **Resid:** Radiation Oncology, Howard Univ 1986; **Fac Appt:** Assoc Prof RadRO, USC Sch Med

Tripuraneni, Prabhakar MD [RadRO] - **Spec Exp:** Prostate Cancer; Head & Neck Cancer; Lymphoma; **Hospital:** Scripps Green Hosp, Scripps Meml Hosp - La Jolla; **Address:** Scripps Clinic, Div Radiation Oncology, 10666 N Torrey Pines Rd, MSB 1, La Jolla, CA 92037; **Phone:** 858-554-2000; **Board Cert:** Therapeutic Radiology 1983; **Med School:** India 1976; **Resid:** Radiation Oncology, Univ Alberta 1981; Radiation Oncology, UCSF Med Ctr 1983; **Fac Appt:** Clin Prof DR, UCSD

Underhill, Kelly J MD [RadRO] - **Spec Exp:** Brachytherapy; Breast Cancer; Gynecologic Cancer; **Hospital:** Providence St Vincent Med Ctr, Providence Portland Med Ctr; **Address:** Providence St Vincent Med Ctr, 9205 SW Barnes Rd, Dept of Radiation Oncology, Portland, OR 97225; **Phone:** 503-216-2195; **Board Cert:** Radiation Oncology 1998; **Med School:** Queens Univ 1992; **Resid:** Radiation Oncology, Queens Univ 1997; **Fellow:** Brachytherapy, Meml Sloan Kettering Med Ctr 1998

Vijayakumar, Srinivasan MD [RadRO] - **Spec Exp:** Brachytherapy; Prostate Cancer; **Hospital:** UC Davis Med Ctr; **Address:** UC Davis Med Ctr, Cancer Ctr, 4501 X St, Ste G140, Sacramento, CA 95817; **Phone:** 916-734-8252; **Board Cert:** Therapeutic Radiology 1986; **Med School:** India 1978; **Resid:** Radiation Oncology, Madras Univ Med Ctr 1981; Radiation Oncology, Michael Reese Hosp 1984; **Fellow:** Brachytherapy, Univ Chicago Hosps 1985; **Fac Appt:** Prof, UC Davis

Wong, Jeffrey Y C MD [RadRO] - **Spec Exp:** Radioimmunotherapy of Cancer; Prostate Cancer; **Hospital:** City of Hope Natl Med Ctr & Beckman Rsch (page 69); **Address:** City of Hope Med Ctr-Dept Radiation Onc, 1500 E Duarte Rd, Duarte, CA 91768-3000; **Phone:** 626-359-8111 x62969; **Board Cert:** Therapeutic Radiology 1985; **Med School:** Johns Hopkins Univ 1981; **Resid:** Radiation Oncology, UCSF Med Ctr 1985; **Fac Appt:** Clin Prof, UC Irvine

Diagnostic Radiology

New England

Kopans, Daniel B MD [DR] - **Spec Exp:** Breast Imaging; **Hospital:** Mass Genl Hosp; **Address:** Mass Genl Hosp - Avon Comprehensive Breast Ctr, 15 Parkman St, WAC 240, Boston, MA 02114-3117; **Phone:** 617-724-9729; **Board Cert:** Diagnostic Radiology 1977; **Med School:** Harvard Med Sch 1973; **Resid:** Diagnostic Radiology, Mass Genl Hosp 1977; **Fac Appt:** Prof, Harvard Med Sch

McCarthy, Shirley M MD/PhD [DR] - **Spec Exp:** Gynecologic Cancer; Pelvic Imaging; **Hospital:** Yale - New Haven Hosp; **Address:** Yale-New Haven Hosp, 333 Cedar St, Ste TE2, New Haven, CT 06520; **Phone:** 203-785-2384; **Board Cert:** Diagnostic Radiology 1983; **Med School:** Yale Univ 1979; **Resid:** Diagnostic Radiology, Yale-New Haven Hosp 1983; **Fellow:** Cross Sectional Imaging, UCSF Med Ctr 1984; **Fac Appt:** Prof Rad, Yale Univ

Schepps, Barbara MD [DR] - **Spec Exp:** Breast Imaging; **Hospital:** Rhode Island Hosp; **Address:** Anne C Pappas Breast Imaging Ctr, 2 Dudley St, Ste G85, Providence, RI 02903; **Phone:** 401-444-6266; **Board Cert:** Diagnostic Radiology 1973; **Med School:** Hahnemann Univ 1968; **Resid:** Diagnostic Radiology, Boston City Hosp 1972; **Fac Appt:** Clin Prof, Brown Univ

Weinreb, Jeffrey C MD [DR] - **Spec Exp:** Breast Cancer; Abdominal Imaging; Prostate Cancer; **Hospital:** Yale - New Haven Hosp; **Address:** Yale Univ Sch Medicine, Dept Radiology, 333 Cedar St, rm MRC147, Box 208042, New Haven, CT 06520-8042; **Phone:** 203-785-5913; **Board Cert:** Diagnostic Radiology 1983; **Med School:** Mount Sinai Sch Med 1978; **Resid:** Diagnostic Radiology, LI Jewish Med Ctr 1982; **Fellow:** Ultrasound/CT, Hosp Univ Penn 1983; **Fac Appt:** Prof Rad, Yale Univ

Mid Atlantic

Austin, John H M MD [DR] - **Spec Exp:** Lung Cancer; **Hospital:** NY-Presby Hosp (page 79); **Address:** Columbia Presby Hosp, Dept Radiology, 622 W 168th St, MHB 3-202C, New York, NY 10032-3784; **Phone:** 212-305-2986; **Board Cert:** Diagnostic Radiology 1970; **Med School:** Yale Univ 1965; **Resid:** Diagnostic Radiology, UCSF Med Ctr 1968; **Fellow:** Diagnostic Radiology, UCSF Med Ctr 1970; **Fac Appt:** Prof Rad, Columbia P&S

Berg, Wendie A MD/PhD [DR] - **Spec Exp:** Breast Imaging; Breast Cancer; **Hospital:** Johns Hopkins Hosp - Baltimore; **Address:** Johns Hopkins - Greenspring Station Breast Ctr, 10755 Falls Rd, Pav 1, Ste 440, Lutherville, MD 21093; **Phone:** 410-583-2888; **Board Cert:** Diagnostic Radiology 1992; **Med School:** Johns Hopkins Univ 1987; **Resid:** Diagnostic Radiology, Johns Hopkins Hosp 1992; **Fellow:** Abdominal Imaging, Johns Hopkins Univ 1992

Conant, Emily F MD [DR] - **Spec Exp:** Breast Cancer; Breast Imaging; **Hospital:** Hosp Univ Penn - UPHS (page 84); **Address:** Hosp U Penn, Dept Radiology (Breast Imaging), 3400 Spruce St, 1 Silverstein, Philadelphia, PA 19104; **Phone:** 215-662-4032; **Board Cert:** Diagnostic Radiology 1989; **Med School:** Univ Pennsylvania 1983; **Resid:** Diagnostic Radiology, Hosp Univ Penn 1986; **Fellow:** Breast Imaging, Hosp Univ Penn 1989; **Fac Appt:** Prof Rad, Univ Pennsylvania

Dershaw, D David MD [DR] - **Spec Exp:** Breast Imaging; Breast Cancer; **Hospital:** Meml Sloan Kettering Cancer Ctr (page 76); **Address:** 1275 York Ave, New York, NY 10021-6007; **Phone:** 212-639-7295; **Board Cert:** Diagnostic Radiology 1978; **Med School:** Jefferson Med Coll 1974; **Resid:** Diagnostic Radiology, New York Hosp 1978; **Fellow:** Ultrasound, Thos Jefferson Univ Hosp 1979; **Fac Appt:** Prof Rad, Cornell Univ-Weill Med Coll

Edelstein, Barbara A MD [DR] - **Spec Exp:** Breast Cancer; **Address:** 1045 Park Ave, New York, NY 10028; **Phone:** 212-860-7700; **Board Cert:** Diagnostic Radiology 1983; **Med School:** NY Med Coll 1977; **Resid:** Diagnostic Radiology, Montefiore Hosp 1982

Evers, Kathryn MD [DR] - **Spec Exp:** Breast Cancer; Mammography; **Hospital:** Fox Chase Cancer Ctr (page 73); **Address:** Fox Chase Cancer Ctr, Diagnostic Imaging, 333 Cottman Ave, Philadelphia, PA 19111; **Phone:** 215-728-3024; **Board Cert:** Diagnostic Radiology 1980; **Med School:** NYU Sch Med 1975; **Resid:** Diagnostic Radiology, Hosp Univ Penn 1980; **Fellow:** Gastrointestinal Radiology, Hosp Univ Penn 1981; **Fac Appt:** Assoc Clin Prof Rad, Temple Univ

Fishman, Elliot MD [DR] - **Spec Exp:** CT Body Scan; Abdominal Imaging; CT Cardiac Scan; **Hospital:** Johns Hopkins Hosp - Baltimore; **Address:** Johns Hopkins Hosp, Dept Radiology, 601 N Caroline St, JHOC 3254, Baltimore, MD 21287-0006; **Phone:** 410-955-5173; **Board Cert:** Diagnostic Radiology 1981; **Med School:** Univ MD Sch Med 1977; **Resid:** Diagnostic Radiology, Sinai Hosp 1980; **Fellow:** Computerized Tomography, Johns Hopkins Hosp 1981; **Fac Appt:** Prof Rad, Johns Hopkins Univ

Hann, Lucy MD [DR] - **Spec Exp:** Liver & Biliary Cancer Ultrasound; Ovarian Cancer Ultrasound Diagnosis; Thyroid Ultrasound; **Hospital:** Meml Sloan Kettering Cancer Ctr (page 76); **Address:** Memorial Sloan-Kettering Cancer Ctr, 1275 York Ave, rm C278, New York, NY 10021; **Phone:** 212-639-2179; **Board Cert:** Diagnostic Radiology 1977; **Med School:** Harvard Med Sch 1971; **Resid:** Diagnostic Radiology, Hosp Univ Penn 1974; Diagnostic Radiology, Mass General Hosp 1977; **Fellow:** Body Imaging, Mass General Hosp 1978; **Fac Appt:** Prof Rad, Cornell Univ-Weill Med Coll

Henschke, Claudia L MD/PhD [DR] - **Spec Exp:** Lung Cancer; Lung Disease Imaging; Thoracic Imaging; **Hospital:** NY-Presby Hosp (page 79); **Address:** NY Weill Medical College, Dept Radiology, 525 E 68th St, Box 586, New York, NY 10021; **Phone:** 212-746-1325; **Board Cert:** Diagnostic Radiology 1981; **Med School:** Howard Univ 1977; **Resid:** Diagnostic Radiology, Brigham & Womens Hosp 1983; **Fac Appt:** Prof, Cornell Univ-Weill Med Coll

Hricak, Hedvig MD/PhD [DR] - **Spec Exp:** Prostate Cancer-MR Spectroscopy (MRSI); Breast Imaging; Breast Cancer; **Hospital:** Meml Sloan Kettering Cancer Ctr (page 76); **Address:** Meml Sloan Kettering Cancer Ctr, Dept Radiology, 1275 York Ave, New York, NY 10021-6007; **Phone:** 212-639-7284; **Board Cert:** Diagnostic Radiology 1978; **Med School:** Yugoslavia 1970; **Resid:** Diagnostic Radiology, St Joseph Mercy Hosp 1977; **Fellow:** Ultrasound/CT, Henry Ford Hosp 1978; **Fac Appt:** Prof Rad, Cornell Univ-Weill Med Coll

Levy, Angela D MD [DR] - **Spec Exp:** Gastrointestinal Cancer; **Hospital:** Unif Serv Univ of the Hlth Sci, Armed Forces Inst of Path; **Address:** Uniformed Services Univ of the Hlth Scis, Dept Radiology, 4301 Jones Bridge Rd, Bethesda, MD 20814; **Phone:** 301-295-3145; **Board Cert:** Diagnostic Radiology 1993; **Med School:** Uniformed Srvs Univ, Bethesda 1988; **Resid:** Diagnostic Radiology, Walter Reed Army Hosp 1992; **Fac Appt:** Assoc Prof Rad, Uniformed Srvs Univ, Bethesda

Mitnick, Julie MD [DR] - **Spec Exp:** Mammography; Breast Cancer; **Address:** 650 1st Ave, New York, NY 10016; **Phone:** 212-686-4440; **Board Cert:** Diagnostic Radiology 1977; **Med School:** NYU Sch Med 1973; **Resid:** Diagnostic Radiology, NYU Med Ctr 1977; **Fellow:** Pediatric Radiology, NYU Med Ctr 1978; **Fac Appt:** Assoc Clin Prof Rad, NYU Sch Med

Orel, Susan G MD [DR] - **Spec Exp:** Breast Imaging; Breast Cancer; **Hospital:** Hosp Univ Penn - UPHS (page 84); **Address:** Hosp Univ Penn, Dept Radiology, 3400 Spruce St, 1 Silverstein, Philadelphia, PA 19104; **Phone:** 215-662-3016; **Board Cert:** Diagnostic Radiology 1989; **Med School:** Univ Pennsylvania 1986; **Resid:** Diagnostic Radiology, Johns Hopkins Hosp 1989; **Fac Appt:** Prof Rad, Univ Pennsylvania

Panicek, David MD [DR] - **Spec Exp:** Bone Cancer; Soft Tissue Tumors; **Hospital:** Meml Sloan Kettering Cancer Ctr (page 76); **Address:** Memorial Hosp - Dept Radiology, 1275 York Ave, rm C276G, New York, NY 10021; **Phone:** 212-639-5825; **Board Cert:** Diagnostic Radiology 1984; **Med School:** Cornell Univ-Weill Med Coll 1980; **Resid:** Diagnostic Radiology, New York Hosp-Cornell 1984; **Fac Appt:** Prof Rad, Cornell Univ-Weill Med Coll

Diagnostic Radiology

Rao, Vijay M MD [DR] - **Spec Exp:** Head & Neck Tumors Imaging; **Hospital:** Thomas Jefferson Univ Hosp (page 82); **Address:** 132 S 10th St, 1087, Main Bldg, Philadelphia, PA 19107-4824; **Phone:** 215-955-4804; **Board Cert:** Diagnostic Radiology 1978; Neuroradiology 1997; **Med School:** India 1973; **Resid:** Diagnostic Radiology, Thomas Jefferson Univ Hosp 1978; **Fac Appt:** Prof Rad, Thomas Jefferson Univ

Southeast

Abbitt, Patricia L MD [DR] - **Spec Exp:** Breast Imaging; Breast Cancer; **Hospital:** Shands Hlthcare at Univ of FL; **Address:** Shands Healthcare, Dept Radiology, 1600 SW Archer Rd, PO Box 100374, Gainesville, FL 32610; **Phone:** 352-265-0291; **Board Cert:** Diagnostic Radiology 1986; **Med School:** Tufts Univ 1981; **Resid:** Diagnostic Radiology, Univ VA Med Ctr 1986; **Fellow:** Breast Imaging, Univ VA Med Ctr 1987; **Fac Appt:** Prof DR, Univ Fla Coll Med

Patz, Edward F MD [DR] - **Spec Exp:** Thoracic Imaging; PET Imaging; Lung Cancer; **Hospital:** Duke Univ Med Ctr; **Address:** Duke Univ Med Ctr, Dept Radiology, Box 3808, Durham, NC 27710; **Phone:** 919-684-7311; **Board Cert:** Diagnostic Radiology 1990; **Med School:** Univ MD Sch Med 1985; **Resid:** Diagnostic Radiology, Brigham & Womens Hosp 1990; **Fellow:** Thoracic Radiology, Brigham & Womens Hosp 1990; **Fac Appt:** Prof, Duke Univ

Pisano, Etta D MD [DR] - **Spec Exp:** Breast Imaging; **Hospital:** Univ NC Hosps; **Address:** UNC Health Care, 101 Manning Dr, Box 7510, Chapel Hill, NC 27299-7510; **Phone:** 919-966-1081; **Board Cert:** Diagnostic Radiology 1988; **Med School:** Duke Univ 1983; **Resid:** Diagnostic Radiology, Beth Israel Hosp 1988; **Fac Appt:** Prof, Univ NC Sch Med

Midwest

Helvie, Mark A MD [DR] - **Spec Exp:** Breast Imaging; Breast Cancer; Mammography; **Hospital:** Univ Michigan Hlth Sys; **Address:** 2910N Taubman Univ Michigan Health Ctr, 1500 E Medical Ctr Drive, Ann Arbor, MI 48109-0326; **Phone:** 734-936-4367; **Board Cert:** Internal Medicine 1983; Diagnostic Radiology 1986; **Med School:** Univ NC Sch Med 1980; **Resid:** Internal Medicine, Univ Michigan Hosps 1983; Diagnostic Radiology, Univ Michigan Hosps 1986; **Fellow:** Ultrasound/CT, Univ Michigan Hosps 1987; **Fac Appt:** Prof, Univ Mich Med Sch

Jackson, Valerie P MD [DR] - **Spec Exp:** Breast Imaging; **Hospital:** Indiana Univ Hosp (page 70); **Address:** Indiana Univ Hosp, Dept Radiology, 550 N University Blvd, #0663, Indianapolis, IN 46202; **Phone:** 317-274-1866; **Board Cert:** Diagnostic Radiology 1982; **Med School:** Indiana Univ 1978; **Resid:** Diagnostic Radiology, Indiana Univ Med Ctr 1982; **Fac Appt:** Prof DR, Indiana Univ

Monsees, Barbara MD [DR] - **Spec Exp:** Mammography; Breast Cancer; **Hospital:** Barnes-Jewish Hosp; **Address:** Ctr for Advanced Med, Campus Box 8131, 510 S Kingshighway Blvd, St Louis, MO 63110; **Phone:** 314-454-7500; **Board Cert:** Diagnostic Radiology 1980; **Med School:** Washington Univ, St Louis 1975; **Resid:** Pediatrics, St Louis Chldns Hosp 1977; Diagnostic Radiology, Mallinckrodt Inst Radiology 1980; **Fac Appt:** Prof DR, Washington Univ, St Louis

Sagel, Stuart S MD [DR] - **Spec Exp:** Lung Cancer; **Hospital:** Barnes-Jewish Hosp; **Address:** Mallinckrodt Inst Rad-Barnes Hosp, 510 S Kingshighway Blvd, Box 8131, St Louis, MO 63110-1016; **Phone:** 314-362-2927; **Board Cert:** Diagnostic Radiology 1970; **Med School:** Temple Univ 1965; **Resid:** Diagnostic Radiology, Yale New Haven Hosp 1968; Diagnostic Radiology, UCSF Med Ctr 1970; **Fac Appt:** Prof, Washington Univ, St Louis

Swensen, Stephen J MD [DR] - **Spec Exp:** Lung Cancer; Lung Disease Imaging; **Hospital:** Mayo Med Ctr & Clin - Rochester; **Address:** Mayo Clinic - Diagnostic Radiology, 200 1st St SW, Rochester, MN 55905; **Phone:** 507-538-3270; **Board Cert:** Diagnostic Radiology 1986; **Med School:** Univ Wisc 1981; **Resid:** Diagnostic Radiology, Mayo Clinic 1986; **Fellow:** Pulmonary Radiology, Brigham & Womens Hosp 1987; **Fac Appt:** Prof Rad, Mayo Med Sch

Southwest

Huynh, Phan Tuong MD [DR] - **Spec Exp:** Mammography; Breast Cancer; **Hospital:** St Luke's Episcopal Hosp - Houston; **Address:** 6624 Fannin St, St Luke's Tower, Women's Ctr Fl 10, Houston, TX 77030; **Phone:** 832-355-8130; **Board Cert:** Diagnostic Radiology 1994; **Med School:** Univ VA Sch Med 1989; **Resid:** Diagnostic Radiology, Univ Virginia Med Ctr 1994; **Fellow:** Mammography, Univ Virginia 1995; **Fac Appt:** Assoc Clin Prof Rad, Baylor Coll Med

Otto, Pamela MD [DR] - **Spec Exp:** Breast Imaging; **Hospital:** Univ Hlth Sys - Univ Hosp, Audie L Murphy Meml Vets Hosp; **Address:** 7703 Floyd Curl Drive, MC 7800, San Antonio, TX 78229-3900; **Phone:** 210-567-3448; **Board Cert:** Diagnostic Radiology 1993; **Med School:** Univ MO-Columbia Sch Med 1988; **Resid:** Diagnostic Radiology, Univ Texas Hlth Sci Ctr 1993; **Fellow:** Breast Imaging, Univ Texas Hlth Sci Ctr 1993; **Fac Appt:** Assoc Prof Rad, Univ Tex, San Antonio

West Coast and Pacific

Bassett, Lawrence W MD [DR] - **Spec Exp:** Breast Imaging; **Hospital:** UCLA Med Ctr (page 83); **Address:** 200 UCLA Med Plaza, rm 165-47, Los Angeles, CA 90095; **Phone:** 310-206-9608; **Board Cert:** Diagnostic Radiology 1975; **Med School:** UC Irvine 1968; **Resid:** Diagnostic Radiology, UCLA Med Ctr 1972; **Fac Appt:** Prof DR, UCLA

Lehman, Constance D MD/PhD [DR] - **Spec Exp:** Breast Imaging; **Hospital:** Univ Wash Med Ctr; **Address:** Seattle Cancer Care Alliance, 825 Eastlake Ave E, rm G3200, Seattle, WA 98109-1023; **Phone:** 206-288-2046; **Board Cert:** Diagnostic Radiology 1995; **Med School:** Yale Univ 1990; **Resid:** Diagnostic Radiology, Univ Wash Med Ctr 1995; **Fellow:** Diagnostic Radiology, Univ Wash Med Ctr 1996; **Fac Appt:** Assoc Prof Rad, Univ Wash

Neuroradiology

Mid Atlantic

Vezina, L Gilbert MD [NRad] - Spec Exp: Pediatric Neuroradiology; Brain Tumors; **Hospital:** Chldns Natl Med Ctr; **Address:** Chldns Natl Med Ctr, Dept Radiology, 111 Michigan Ave NW, Washington, DC 20010-2970; **Phone:** 202-884-3651; **Board Cert:** Diagnostic Radiology 1987; Neuroradiology 1998; **Med School:** McGill Univ 1983; **Resid:** Diagnostic Radiology, Mass Genl Hosp 1987; **Fellow:** Neurological Radiology, Mass Genl Hosp 1989; Pediatric Neuroradiology, Chldns Natl Med Ctr 1991; **Fac Appt:** Prof DR, Geo Wash Univ

Southeast

Murtagh, F Reed MD [NRad] - Spec Exp: Neuro-Oncology; Brain Tumor Imaging; Spinal Tumor Imaging; **Hospital:** H Lee Moffitt Cancer Ctr & Research Inst; **Address:** Univ Diagnostic Institute-USF, 3301 Alumni Drive, Tampa, FL 33612; **Phone:** 813-975-0725; **Board Cert:** Diagnostic Radiology 1978; Neuroradiology 1995; **Med School:** Temple Univ 1971; **Resid:** Diagnostic Radiology, Jackson Meml Hosp 1978; **Fellow:** Neurological Radiology, Univ Miami; **Fac Appt:** Prof, Univ S Fla Coll Med

Provenzale, James M MD [NRad] - Spec Exp: Brain Tumor Imaging; **Hospital:** Duke Univ Med Ctr; **Address:** Duke University Medical Ctr, Dept Radiology, Box 3808, Durham, NC 27710; **Phone:** 919-684-7218; **Board Cert:** Neurology 1988; Diagnostic Radiology 1991; Neuroradiology 2001; **Med School:** Albany Med Coll 1983; **Resid:** Neurology, NC Memorial Hosp 1987; Diagnostic Radiology, Mass General Hosp 1991; **Fellow:** Neuroradiology, Mass General Hosp 1992; **Fac Appt:** Prof DR, Duke Univ

Midwest

Koeller, Kelly K MD [NRad] - Spec Exp: Brain Tumor Imaging; Head & Neck Tumors; Spinal Tumor Imaging; **Hospital:** Mayo Med Ctr & Clin - Rochester; **Address:** Mayo Clinic, 200 First St SW Charlton Bldg - rm 2-290, Rochester, MN 55905; **Phone:** 507-266-3412; **Board Cert:** Diagnostic Radiology 1990; Neuroradiology 2004; **Med School:** Univ Tenn Coll Med, Memphis 1982; **Resid:** Diagnostic Radiology, Naval Hosp 1990; **Fellow:** Neuroradiology, UCSF Med Ctr 1992

West Coast and Pacific

Atlas, Scott W MD [NRad] - Spec Exp: Brain Tumors; **Hospital:** Stanford Univ Med Ctr; **Address:** Stanford Univ Med Ctr, Dept Rad, 300 Pasteur Drive, rm S-047, Stanford, CA 94304-2204; **Phone:** 650-498-7152; **Board Cert:** Diagnostic Radiology 1985; Neuroradiology 2005; **Med School:** Univ Chicago-Pritzker Sch Med 1981; **Resid:** Diagnostic Radiology, Northwestern Univ Med Ctr 1985; **Fellow:** Neuroradiology, Hosp U Penn 1987; **Fac Appt:** Prof, Stanford Univ

Dillon, William P MD [NRad] - Spec Exp: Brain Tumors; **Hospital:** UCSF Med Ctr; **Address:** 505 Parnassus Ave, rm L 371, San Francisco, CA 94143-0628; **Phone:** 415-353-1668; **Board Cert:** Diagnostic Radiology 1982; Neuroradiology 1996; **Med School:** Loyola Univ-Stritch Sch Med 1978; **Resid:** Diagnostic Radiology, Univ Utah Hosp 1982; **Fellow:** Neuroradiology, UCSF Med Ctr 1983; **Fac Appt:** Prof, UCSF

Vascular & Interventional Radiology

New England

Hallisey, Michael J MD [VIR] - **Spec Exp:** Liver Cancer/Chemoembolization; **Hospital:** Hartford Hosp; **Address:** 85 Seymour St, Ste 200, Hartford, CT 06106; **Phone:** 860-246-6589; **Board Cert:** Diagnostic Radiology 1991; Vascular & Interventional Radiology 1998; **Med School:** Univ Conn 1987; **Resid:** Diagnostic Radiology, Hospital of St Raphael 1991

Mid Atlantic

Geschwind, Jean Francois H MD [VIR] - **Spec Exp:** Liver Cancer/Chemoembolization; Cancer Chemoembolization; Cancer Radiotherapy; **Hospital:** Johns Hopkins Hosp - Baltimore; **Address:** Interventional Radiology, 600 N Wolfe St Blalock Bldg - rm 545, Baltimore, MD 21287; **Phone:** 410-955-6358; **Board Cert:** Diagnostic Radiology 1998; **Med School:** Boston Univ 1991; **Resid:** Diagnostic Radiology, UCSF Med Ctr 1996; **Fellow:** Interventional Radiology, Johns Hopkins Hosp 1998; **Fac Appt:** Assoc Prof DR, Johns Hopkins Univ

Haskal, Ziv MD [VIR] - **Spec Exp:** Liver Cancer/Chemoembolization; **Hospital:** NY-Presby Hosp (page 79); **Address:** Director, Div Interventional Radiology, 177 Fort Washington Ave, Ste MHB 4-100, New York, NY 10032; **Phone:** 212-305-8070; **Board Cert:** Diagnostic Radiology 1991; Vascular & Interventional Radiology 1999; **Med School:** Boston Univ 1986; **Resid:** Diagnostic Radiology, UCSF Med Ctr 1991; **Fellow:** Vascular & Interventional Radiology, UCSF Med Ctr 1992; **Fac Appt:** Prof, Columbia P&S

Soulen, Michael C MD [VIR] - **Spec Exp:** Liver Cancer/Chemoembolization; Kidney Cancer; Radiofrequency Tumor Ablation; **Hospital:** Hosp Univ Penn - UPHS (page 84); **Address:** Hosp U Penn, Interventional Radiology, 3400 Spruce St, Philadelphia, PA 19104; **Phone:** 215-662-6839; **Board Cert:** Diagnostic Radiology 1989; Vascular & Interventional Radiology 1995; **Med School:** Univ Pennsylvania 1984; **Resid:** Diagnostic Radiology, Johns Hopkins Med Inst 1989; **Fellow:** Vascular & Interventional Radiology, Thomas Jefferson Univ Hosp 1991; **Fac Appt:** Prof Rad, Univ Pennsylvania

Wood, Bradford J MD [VIR] - **Spec Exp:** Radiofrequency Tumor Ablation; Liver Cancer; Kidney Cancer; Gene Therapy Delivery Systems; **Hospital:** Natl Inst of Hlth - Clin Ctr; **Address:** National Inst Health, Bldg D, 9000 Rockville Pike, rm 1C-660, Bethesda, MD 20892; **Phone:** 301-594-4511; **Board Cert:** Diagnostic Radiology 1996; Vascular & Interventional Radiology 2000; **Med School:** Univ VA Sch Med 1991; **Resid:** Diagnostic Radiology, Georgetown Univ Med Ctr 1996; **Fellow:** Abdominal/Interventional Radiology, Mass General Hosp 1997; **Fac Appt:** Asst Clin Prof, Georgetown Univ

Southeast

Mauro, Matthew MD [VIR] - **Spec Exp:** Cancer Chemoembolization; Cancer Radiotherapy; Gastrointestinal Cancer; **Hospital:** Univ NC Hosps; **Address:** University NC Hosps, Dept Radiology, CB 7510, 2006 Old Clinic Bldg, Chapel Hill, NC 27514; **Phone:** 919-966-4400; **Board Cert:** Diagnostic Radiology 1981; Vascular & Interventional Radiology 2003; **Med School:** Cornell Univ-Weill Med Coll 1977; **Resid:** Diagnostic Radiology, Univ NC Hosps 1981; **Fellow:** Interventional Radiology, Mallinckrodt Inst 1982; **Fac Appt:** Prof, Univ NC Sch Med

Midwest

Rilling, William S MD [VIR] - **Spec Exp:** Liver Cancer/Chemoembolization; **Hospital:** Froedtert Meml Lutheran Hosp; **Address:** Froedtert & Med Coll Clinics, Interventional Radiology, 9200 W Wisconsin Ave, Milwaukee, WI 53226; **Phone:** 414-805-3028; **Board Cert:** Diagnostic Radiology 1995; Vascular & Interventional Radiology 1997; **Med School:** Univ Wisc 1990; **Resid:** Diagnostic Radiology, Univ Wisc Affil Hosps 1995; **Fellow:** Vascular & Interventional Radiology, Northwestern Meml Hosp 1996; **Fac Appt:** Assoc Prof DR, Univ Wisc

Salem, Riad MD [VIR] - **Spec Exp:** Cancer Radiotherapy; Cancer Chemoembolization; Liver Cancer/Chemoembolization; **Hospital:** Northwestern Meml Hosp; **Address:** Northwestern Univ Med Sch - Dept Radiology, 676 N St Clair St, Ste 800, Chicago, IL 60611; **Phone:** 312-695-0517; **Board Cert:** Diagnostic Radiology 1997; Vascular & Interventional Radiology 1999; **Med School:** McGill Univ 1993; **Resid:** Diagnostic Radiology, Geo Washington Univ Hosp 1997; **Fellow:** Interventional Radiology, Childrens Hosp 1998; Interventional Radiology, Hosp Univ Penn 1998; **Fac Appt:** Asst Prof, Northwestern Univ

West Coast and Pacific

Goodwin, Scott C MD [VIR] - **Spec Exp:** Liver Cancer/Chemoembolization; **Hospital:** VA Med Ctr - W Los Angeles; **Address:** VA Hosp-Dept Radiology, 11301 Wilshire Blvd, MC 114, Los Angeles, CA 90073; **Phone:** 310-268-3478; **Board Cert:** Diagnostic Radiology 1989; Vascular & Interventional Radiology 1996; **Med School:** Harvard Med Sch 1984; **Resid:** Diagnostic Radiology, UCLA Medical Ctr 1988; **Fellow:** Vascular & Interventional Radiology, UCLA Medical Ctr 1989; **Fac Appt:** Prof DR, UCLA

McGahan, John P MD [VIR] - **Spec Exp:** Radiofrequency Tumor Ablation; Liver Cancer; Kidney Cancer; **Hospital:** UC Davis Med Ctr; **Address:** UC Davis Medical Ctr, Dept Radiology, 4860 Y St, Ste 3100, Sacramento, CA 95817; **Phone:** 916-734-3606; **Board Cert:** Diagnostic Radiology 1979; Vascular & Interventional Radiology 1995; **Med School:** Oregon Hlth Sci Univ 1974; **Resid:** Surgery, UC Davis Med Ctr 1976; Diagnostic Radiology, UC Davis Med Ctr 1979; **Fac Appt:** Prof DR, UC Davis

Nuclear Medicine

Mid Atlantic

Alavi, Abass MD [NuM] - **Spec Exp:** Neurologic Imaging; Brain Tumors; PET Imaging-Brain; **Hospital:** Hosp Univ Penn - UPHS (page 84), Chldns Hosp of Philadelphia, The; **Address:** Hosp Univ Penn, Div Nuclear Med, 3400 Spruce St, Donner Bldg rm 110, Philadelphia, PA 19104; **Phone:** 215-662-3014; **Board Cert:** Nuclear Medicine 1973; Internal Medicine 1972; **Med School:** Iran 1964; **Resid:** Internal Medicine, Albert Einstein Med Ctr/Phila VA Hosp 1969; Hematology, Hosp Univ Penn 1970; **Fellow:** Nuclear Medicine, Hosp Univ Penn 1973; **Fac Appt:** Prof Rad, Univ Pennsylvania

Carrasquillo, Jorge A MD [NuM] - **Spec Exp:** Radioimmunotherapy of Cancer; PET Imaging; **Hospital:** Meml Sloan Kettering Cancer Ctr (page 76); **Address:** Memorial Sloan Kettering Cancer Ctr, 1275 York Ave, New York, NY 10021; **Phone:** 212-639-2459; **Board Cert:** Internal Medicine 1977; Nuclear Medicine 1982; **Med School:** Univ Puerto Rico 1974; **Resid:** Internal Medicine, Univ Dist Hosp 1977; Nuclear Medicine, Univ Wash Hosp 1982

Goldsmith, Stanley J MD [NuM] - **Spec Exp:** Thyroid Cancer; Neuroendocrine Tumors; PET Imaging; Lymphoma; **Hospital:** NY-Presby Hosp (page 79); **Address:** 525 E 68th St Starr Bldg - rm 2-21, New York, NY 10021-9800; **Phone:** 212-746-4588; **Board Cert:** Internal Medicine 1969; Nuclear Medicine 1972; Endocrinology 1972; **Med School:** SUNY Downstate 1962; **Resid:** Internal Medicine, Kings Co Hosp 1967; **Fellow:** Endocrinology, Diabetes & Metabolism, Mt Sinai Hosp 1968; Nuclear Medicine, Bronx VA Hosp 1969; **Fac Appt:** Prof Rad, Cornell Univ-Weill Med Coll

Kramer, Elissa MD [NuM] - **Spec Exp:** Cancer Detection & Staging; Lymphedema Imaging; Radioimmunotherapy of Cancer; **Hospital:** NYU Med Ctr (page 80), Bellevue Hosp Ctr; **Address:** 560 1st Ave, rm HW231, New York, NY 10016-6402; **Phone:** 212-263-7410; **Board Cert:** Nuclear Medicine 1982; Diagnostic Radiology 1982; **Med School:** NYU Sch Med 1977; **Resid:** Diagnostic Radiology, Bellevue Hosp/NYU 1980; **Fellow:** Nuclear Medicine, Bellevue Hosp/NYU 1982; **Fac Appt:** Prof Rad, NYU Sch Med

Lamonica, Dominick M MD [NuM] - **Spec Exp:** Thyroid Cancer; **Hospital:** Roswell Park Cancer Inst; **Address:** Roswell Park Cancer Inst, Elm & Carlton St, Dept of Nuclear Medicine, Buffalo, NY 14263; **Phone:** 716-845-3282; **Board Cert:** Internal Medicine 2005; **Med School:** Mount Sinai Sch Med 1987; **Resid:** Internal Medicine, Univ Hosp-SUNY Stony Brook 1991; Diagnostic Radiology, Nassau City Med Ctr 1992; **Fellow:** Nuclear Medicine, DVAMC North Port-SUNY Stony Brook 1994; Nuclear Medicine, SUNY Buffalo-RPCI 1995; **Fac Appt:** Asst Prof, SUNY Buffalo

Larson, Steven M MD [NuM] - **Spec Exp:** Thyroid Cancer; PET Imaging; **Hospital:** Meml Sloan Kettering Cancer Ctr (page 76); **Address:** Meml Sloan Kettering Cancer Ctr, Dept Nuclear Medicine, 1275 York Ave, Box 77, New York, NY 10021; **Phone:** 212-639-7373; **Board Cert:** Nuclear Medicine 1972; Internal Medicine 1973; **Med School:** Univ Wash 1965; **Resid:** Internal Medicine, Virginia Mason Hosp 1970; Nuclear Medicine, Natl Inst Hlth 1972; **Fac Appt:** Prof NuM, Cornell Univ-Weill Med Coll

Strauss, H William MD [NuM] - **Spec Exp:** Cardiac Imaging in Cancer Therapy; Thyroid Disorders; **Hospital:** Meml Sloan Kettering Cancer Ctr (page 76); **Address:** Meml Sloan Kettering Cancer Ctr, 1275 York Ave, S-212, Box 77, Nw York, NY 10021; **Phone:** 212-639-7238; **Board Cert:** Nuclear Medicine 1988; **Med School:** SUNY Downstate 1965; **Resid:** Internal Medicine, Downstate Med Ctr 1967; Internal Medicine, Bellevue Hosp 1968; **Fellow:** Nuclear Medicine, Johns Hopkins Hosp 1970; **Fac Appt:** Prof NuM, Cornell Univ-Weill Med Coll

Wahl, Richard L MD [NuM] - **Spec Exp:** Radioimmunotherapy of Cancer; PET Imaging; PET Imaging-Breast; **Hospital:** Johns Hopkins Hosp - Baltimore; **Address:** Johns Hopkins Hosp, Div Nuclear Medicine, 601 N Caroline St, JHOC-3223, Baltimore, MD 21287; **Phone:** 410-955-7226; **Board Cert:** Diagnostic Radiology 1982; Nuclear Radiology 1983; Nuclear Medicine 1985; **Med School:** Washington Univ, St Louis 1978; **Resid:** Diagnostic Radiology, Mallinckrodt Inst 1982; **Fellow:** Nuclear Radiology, Mallinckrodt Inst 1983; **Fac Appt:** Prof Rad, Johns Hopkins Univ

Southeast

Alazraki, Naomi P MD [NuM] - **Spec Exp:** Nuclear Oncology; **Hospital:** VA Med Ctr - Atlanta, Emory Univ Hosp; **Address:** VA Medical Ctr - Atlanta, 1670 Clairmont Rd, MC 115, Decatur, GA 30033; **Phone:** 404-728-7629; **Board Cert:** Nuclear Medicine 1972; Diagnostic Radiology 1972; **Med School:** Albert Einstein Coll Med 1966; **Resid:** Diagnostic Radiology, Univ Hospital 1971; **Fac Appt:** Prof DR, Emory Univ

Nuclear Medicine

Coleman, Ralph E MD [NuM] - **Spec Exp:** PET Imaging; Tumor Imaging; **Hospital:** Duke Univ Med Ctr; **Address:** Duke Univ Med Ctr, Erwin Rd, Box 3949, Durham, NC 27710; **Phone:** 919-684-7244; **Board Cert:** Nuclear Medicine 1974; Internal Medicine 1973; **Med School:** Washington Univ, St Louis 1968; **Resid:** Internal Medicine, Royal Victoria Hosp 1970; **Fellow:** Nuclear Medicine, Mallinckrodt Inst Radiology 1974; **Fac Appt:** Prof DR, Duke Univ

Midwest

Dillehay, Gary MD [NuM] - **Spec Exp:** Lymphoma; PET Imaging; **Hospital:** Northwestern Meml Hosp; **Address:** Northwestern Meml Hosp, Dept Nuclear Medicine, 675 N St Clair St, Galter 8-104, Chicago, IL 60611; **Phone:** 312-926-0411; **Board Cert:** Nuclear Medicine 1985; Nuclear Radiology 1987; **Med School:** Mayo Med Sch 1979; **Resid:** Diagnostic Radiology, Northwestern Meml Hosp 1983; Nuclear Medicine, Northwestern Meml Hosp 1984

Neumann, Donald R MD [NuM] - **Spec Exp:** Nuclear Oncology; **Hospital:** Cleveland Clin Fdn (page 71); **Address:** Cleveland Clinic, MFI Dept, 9500 Euclid Ave, MS Gb3, Cleveland, OH 44195; **Phone:** 216-444-2193; **Board Cert:** Diagnostic Radiology 1987; Nuclear Radiology 1990; **Med School:** Wright State Univ 1980; **Resid:** Diagnostic Radiology, Mount Sinai Med Ctr 1987; **Fellow:** Magnetic Resonance Imaging, Mount Sinai Med Ctr 1987

Siegel, Barry A MD [NuM] - **Spec Exp:** Cancer Detection & Staging; PET Imaging; **Hospital:** Barnes-Jewish Hosp, St Louis Chldns Hosp; **Address:** Mallinckrodt Inst of Radiology, 510 S Kingshighway Blvd, St Louis, MO 63110-1016; **Phone:** 314-362-2809; **Board Cert:** Diagnostic Radiology 1977; Nuclear Medicine 1973; Nuclear Radiology 1981; **Med School:** Washington Univ, St Louis 1969; **Resid:** Diagnostic Radiology, Mallinckrodt Inst Radiology 1973; **Fellow:** Nuclear Medicine, Mallinckrodt Inst Radiology 1973; **Fac Appt:** Prof, Washington Univ, St Louis

Silberstein, Edward B MD [NuM] - **Spec Exp:** Thyroid Cancer; Prostate Cancer Pain; Lymphoma; **Hospital:** Univ Hosp - Cincinnati, Jewish Hosp - Kenwood - Cincinnati; **Address:** Univ Hosp, 234 Goodman Ave, G026 Mont Reid Pav, Cincinnati, OH 45219-2364; **Phone:** 513-584-9032; **Board Cert:** Internal Medicine 1980; Nuclear Medicine 1972; Hematology 1972; Medical Oncology 1981; **Med School:** Harvard Med Sch 1962; **Resid:** Internal Medicine, Univ Cincinnati Hosp 1964; Internal Medicine, Univ Hosps-Case Western Reserve 1967; **Fellow:** Hematology, New England Med Ctr 1968; **Fac Appt:** Prof Emeritus Med, Univ Cincinnati

Wiseman, Gregory MD [NuM] - **Spec Exp:** Lymphoma, Non-Hodgkin's; Multiple Myeloma; Radioimmunotherapy of Cancer; **Hospital:** Mayo Med Ctr & Clin - Rochester; **Address:** Mayo Clinic, Dept Nuc Med, 200 First St SW, Charlton Bldg, Rochester, MN 55905; **Phone:** 507-284-9599; **Board Cert:** Internal Medicine 1986; Hematology 1988; Nuclear Medicine 2002; **Med School:** Univ Utah 1983; **Resid:** Internal Medicine, Mayo Clinic 1986; Nuclear Medicine, Univ Washington Med Ctr 1992; **Fellow:** Hematology, Mayo Clinic 1989; Medical Oncology, Univ Washington 1991; **Fac Appt:** Asst Prof, Mayo Med Sch

Southwest

Podoloff, Donald MD [NuM] - **Spec Exp:** Prostate Cancer; Breast Cancer; Lymphoma; **Hospital:** UT MD Anderson Cancer Ctr (page 81); **Address:** UT MD Anderson Cancer Ctr, 1515 Holcombe Blvd, Box 57, Houston, TX 77030; **Phone:** 713-745-1160; **Board Cert:** Diagnostic Radiology 1973; Nuclear Medicine 1975; Nuclear Radiology 1975; **Med School:** SUNY Downstate 1964; **Resid:** Internal Medicine, Beth Israel Med Ctr 1968; Diagnostic Radiology, Wilford Hall USAF Med Ctr 1973; **Fac Appt:** Prof Rad, Univ Tex, Houston

West Coast and Pacific

Scheff, Alice M MD [NuM] - **Spec Exp:** PET Imaging; Thyroid Imaging; **Hospital:** Santa Clara Vly Med Ctr; **Address:** 751 S Bascom Ave, San Jose, CA 95128; **Phone:** 408-885-6970; **Board Cert:** Nuclear Medicine 1982; Nuclear Radiology 1983; **Med School:** Penn State Univ-Hershey Med Ctr 1978; **Resid:** Diagnostic Radiology, Penn State-Hershey Med Ctr 1982; Nuclear Medicine, Penn State-Hershey Med Ctr 1982; **Fellow:** Magnetic Resonance Imaging, Long Beach Meml Med Ctr 1993

Waxman, Alan D MD [NuM] - **Spec Exp:** PET Imaging-Brain; Thyroid Cancer; Cancer Detection & Staging; **Hospital:** Cedars-Sinai Med Ctr, USC Univ Hosp - R K Eamer Med Plz; **Address:** Cedars-Sinai Med Ctr, Taper Imaging, 8700 Beverly Blvd, rm 1251, Los Angeles, CA 90048-1804; **Phone:** 310-423-2981; **Board Cert:** Nuclear Medicine 1972; **Med School:** USC Sch Med 1963; **Resid:** Nuclear Medicine, Wadsworth VA Hosp 1965; **Fellow:** Internal Medicine, Natl Inst Hlth 1967; **Fac Appt:** Clin Prof DR, USC Sch Med

What is TomoTherapy and how can it save your life?

cANSWEr.

TomoTherapy is the most precise form of radiation therapy. For many cancer patients unable to have surgery, this could be a lifesaver. It offers unprecedented accuracy in targeting cancerous tumors while preserving healthy tissue. The result is fewer side effects and a faster recovery. At City of Hope, our team of nationally recognized experts is the first in the Western U.S. to offer TomoTherapy to patients with many forms of cancer including lung, brain, head and neck, and prostate cancers. To learn more, call City of Hope Radiation Oncology at 800-341-HOPE. We accept most insurance. At City of Hope, we have answers to cancer.

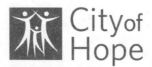

City of Hope

Science saving lives.
cityofhope.org/topdoctors

FOX CHASE
CANCER CENTER

333 Cottman Avenue
Philadelphia, PA 19111-2497
Phone: 1-888-FOX CHASE • Fax: 215-728-2702
www.fccc.edu

RADIATION ONCOLOGY

Fox Chase Cancer Center has one of the country's largest, most experienced programs in radiation oncology. Recognized as international leaders in developing the most advanced treatment technologies, our radiation oncologists include nationally and internationally known experts in prostate, breast, lung and gastrointestinal cancers. Other major treatment interests include central nervous system and head and neck cancers and sarcomas.

We treat patients with radiation therapy alone, in combination with surgery and/or chemotherapy and through Fox Chase and national clinical trials offering the newest treatments. We also conduct research in medical physics and radiation biology to enhance the effectiveness of therapy.

- Fox Chase physicians are among the nation's most experienced in treating patients with intensity-modulated radiation therapy (IMRT) and are developing the image-guided radiation therapies of the future.
- Advances in brachytherapy such as real-time intraoperative planning mean our patients receive the most precise prostate implants, either permanent low-dose-rate or temporary high-dose-rate.
- Stereotactic radiosurgery and radiation therapy permits sub-millimeter precision for brain and lung cancers.

We offer treatment with radiation alone, as part of a multidisciplinary regimen or through clinical trials to determine the most effective approaches for specific cancers. Fox Chase uses sophisticated imaging tools during treatment planning and daily treatment sessions to target the cancer better and spare any healthy surrounding tissue undue exposure to radiation.

Because of our outstanding reputation as a leader in cancer therapy, we frequently work with the world's foremost makers of medical equipment to test prototypes and develop the best applications—long before they are available elsewhere.

For example, Fox Chase has the first high-intensity focused ultrasound (HIFU) dedicated for cancer treatment in North America. This allows us to deliver hyperthermia treatment in conjunction with radiation to treat patients with certain primary and recurrent tumors.

The Most Precise Treatment

- Fox Chase has been first in the region to offer these advanced tools for the most targeted radiation therapy.
- The Calypso 4-D Localization System is brand-new four-dimensional monitoring technology to localize and track the prostate throughout treatment for more accurate radiation delivery.
- Magnetic resonance spectroscopy (MRS, or functional MRI) aids treatment planning to tailor radiation therapy for some prostate and brain cancers by identifying the metabolic activity of the tumor.
- The Trilogy Stereotactic System for image-guided radiation therapy and stereotactic radiosurgery is the world's premier image-guided system for delivering all forms of external radiation. It automatically adjusts the treatment table position as needed and tailors treatment to phases in the patient's breathing cycle.
- A 4-D CT treatment simulator helps doctors plan treatment to correlate with patient motion such as breathing—especially important for patients with lung, breast or some gastrointestinal cancers.

For more about Fox Chase physicians and services, visit our web site, www.fccc.edu, or call 1-888-FOX CHASE.

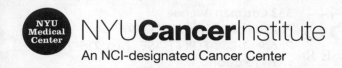

THE UNIVERSITY OF TEXAS
MD ANDERSON
CANCER CENTER
Making Cancer History®

**The University of Texas
M. D. Anderson Cancer Center**

1515 Holcombe Blvd.
Houston, Texas 77030-4095
Tel. 713-792-6161
Toll Free 877-MDA-6789
http://www.mdanderson.org

RADIATION ONCOLOGY

The Radiation Treatment Center at M. D. Anderson is the most comprehensive facility of its kind in the world. We offer the latest, most advanced technology, and provide the broadest range of radiation treatment options available anywhere. We hold ourselves to quality standards that are higher than the industry requires, and provide a rare breadth of technology, expertise, and experience, all which translate into personalized care and the best outcomes for the over 5,000 new patients we treat a year.

M. D. Anderson radiation oncologists are specially trained, board-certified, and skilled in both standard and unique radiation therapies. We are constantly seeking innovative ways to use existing technology, and developing new therapies to help our patients have the best outcomes possible.

PROTON THERAPY

M. D. Anderson's Proton Therapy Center opened in May 2006 as the largest and most sophisticated center of its type. Proton therapy allows for the most aggressive cancer therapy possible, deriving its advantage over traditional forms of radiation treatment from its ability to deliver targeted radiation doses to the tumor with remarkable precision. Proton therapy radiation avoids the surrounding tissue, generates fewer side effects, and improves tumor control. It is used to treat cancers of the prostate, lung, brain and skull base, head and neck, eye, and various forms of pediatric cancer.

Combined with M. D. Anderson's more than 60 years of expertise and pioneering research in radiation therapy, the Proton Therapy Center is the premier destination for cancer patients seeking the best treatment by the most experienced radiation oncologists.

MORE INFORMATION

For more information or to make an appointment, call 877-MDA-6789, or visit us online at http://www.mdanderson.org.

At M. D. Anderson Cancer Center, our mission is simple – to eliminate cancer. Achieving that goal begins with integrated programs in cancer treatment, clinical trials, education programs and cancer prevention.

We focus exclusively on cancer and have seen cases of every kind. That means you receive expert care no matter what your diagnosis.

Choosing the right partner for cancer care really does make a difference. The fact is, people who choose M. D. Anderson over other hospitals and clinics often have better results. That is how we've been making cancer history for over sixty years.

841

Surgery

A surgeon manages a broad spectrum of surgical conditions affecting almost any area of the body. The surgeon establishes the diagnosis and provides the preoperative, operative and postoperative care to surgical patients and is usually responsible for the comprehensive management of the trauma victim and the critically ill surgical patient.

The surgeon uses a variety of diagnostic techniques, including endoscopy, for observing internal structures and may use specialized instruments during operative procedures. A general surgeon is expected to be familiar with the salient features of other surgical specialties in order to recognize problems in those areas and to know when to refer a patient to another specialist.

Training Required: Five years

Surgery

New England

Becker, James MD [S] - **Spec Exp:** Gastrointestinal Cancer; Gastrointestinal Surgery; **Hospital:** Boston Med Ctr, Qunicy Med Ctr; **Address:** Boston Med Ctr, Dept Surg, 88 E Newton St, rm C500, Boston, MA 02118-2393; **Phone:** 617-638-8600; **Board Cert:** Surgery 1999; **Med School:** Case West Res Univ 1975; **Resid:** Surgery, Univ Utah Med Ctr 1980; **Fellow:** Research, Mayo Clinic 1982; **Fac Appt:** Prof S, Boston Univ

Cady, Blake MD [S] - **Spec Exp:** Breast Cancer; Thyroid Cancer; **Hospital:** Rhode Island Hosp, Women & Infants Hosp - Rhode Island; **Address:** 503 Eddy St, APC 435, Providence, RI 02903; **Phone:** 401-444-6158; **Board Cert:** Surgery 1966; **Med School:** Cornell Univ-Weill Med Coll 1957; **Resid:** Surgery, Boston City Hosp/Tufts 1959; Surgery, Boston City Hosp/Harvard 1965; **Fellow:** Surgery, NY Meml Cancer Hosp 1967; **Fac Appt:** Prof S, Brown Univ

Cioffi, William MD [S] - **Spec Exp:** Cancer Surgery; **Hospital:** Rhode Island Hosp; **Address:** Rhode Island Hosp, Dept Surg, 2 Dudley St, Ste 470, Providence, RI 02905; **Phone:** 401-553-8348; **Board Cert:** Surgery 1995; Surgical Critical Care 1997; **Med School:** Univ VT Coll Med 1981; **Resid:** Surgery, Med Ctr Hosp VT 1986; **Fac Appt:** Prof S, Brown Univ

Eisenberg, Burton L MD [S] - **Spec Exp:** Breast Cancer; Melanoma; Sarcoma; **Hospital:** Dartmouth - Hitchcock Med Ctr; **Address:** Dartmouth-Hitchcock Med Ctr, Dept Surgery, One Medical Center Drive, Lebanon, NH 03756; **Phone:** 603-650-9479; **Board Cert:** Surgery 1999; **Med School:** Univ Tenn Coll Med, Memphis 1974; **Resid:** Surgery, Wilford Hall USAF Med Ctr 1979; **Fellow:** Surgical Oncology, Meml Sloan-Kettering Cancer Ctr 1981; **Fac Appt:** Prof S, Dartmouth Med Sch

Hughes, Kevin S MD [S] - **Spec Exp:** Breast Cancer; Ovarian Cancer; **Hospital:** Mass Genl Hosp; **Address:** Massachusetts General Hosp, Dept Surgery, Wang Bldg Fl 2 - rm 240, Boston, MA 02114; **Phone:** 617-724-4800; **Board Cert:** Surgery 1993; **Med School:** Dartmouth Med Sch 1979; **Resid:** Surgery, Mercy Hosp 1984; **Fellow:** Surgical Oncology, National Cancer Inst 1985; **Fac Appt:** Assoc Prof S, Harvard Med Sch

Iglehart, J Dirk MD [S] - **Spec Exp:** Breast Cancer; **Hospital:** Brigham & Women's Hosp, Dana-Farber Cancer Inst; **Address:** Brigham & Women's Hospital, 75 Francis St, Surgical Oncology, Smith 822, Boston, MA 02115; **Phone:** 617-632-5178; **Board Cert:** Surgery 2005; **Med School:** Harvard Med Sch 1975; **Resid:** Surgery, Duke Univ Med Ctr 1981; Thoracic Surgery, Duke Univ Med Ctr 1984; **Fac Appt:** Prof S, Harvard Med Sch

Jenkins, Roger L MD [S] - **Spec Exp:** Transplant-Liver; Liver & Biliary Cancer; Biliary Surgery; **Hospital:** Lahey Clin, Children's Hospital - Boston; **Address:** Lahey Clin, Dept Hepatobiliary Surg, 41 Mall Rd, Burlington, MA 01805; **Phone:** 781-744-2500; **Board Cert:** Surgery 2005; **Med School:** Univ VT Coll Med 1977; **Resid:** Surgery, New Eng Deaconess Hosp 1982; **Fellow:** Cardiovascular Surgery, Deaconess Hosp 1983; Transplant Surgery, Univ Pittsburgh Hosp 1983; **Fac Appt:** Prof S, Tufts Univ

Kavanah, Maureen MD [S] - **Spec Exp:** Breast Cancer; Gynecologic Cancer; Melanoma; **Hospital:** Boston Med Ctr; **Address:** Boston Medical Ctr, 88 E Newton St, rm D510, Boston, MA 02118; **Phone:** 617-638-8473; **Board Cert:** Surgery 1999; **Med School:** Tufts Univ 1975; **Resid:** Surgery, St Elizabeths Hosp 1979; **Fellow:** Surgical Oncology, Boston Univ Med Ctr 1981; **Fac Appt:** Assoc Prof S, Boston Univ

Krag, David MD [S] - Spec Exp: Sentinel Node Surgery; Breast Cancer; **Hospital:** FAHC - UHC Campus; **Address:** Univ Vermont Coll Med, Dept Surgery, 89 Beaumont Ave, Given Bldg - E309C, Burlington, VT 05405; **Phone:** 802-656-5830; **Board Cert:** Surgery 1996; **Med School:** Loyola Univ-Stritch Sch Med 1980; **Resid:** Surgery, UC Davis Med Ctr 1983; **Fellow:** Surgical Oncology, UCLA Med Ctr 1984; **Fac Appt:** Assoc Prof S, Univ VT Coll Med

Ponn, Teresa MD [S] - Spec Exp: Breast Cancer; Breast Disease; **Hospital:** Elliot Hosp; **Address:** Elliot Breast Health Center, 275 Mammoth Rd, Ste 1, Manchester, NH 03109; **Phone:** 603-668-3067; **Board Cert:** Surgery 2000; **Med School:** Univ Fla Coll Med 1976; **Resid:** Surgery, Stanford Univ Med Ctr 1982

Salem, Ronald R MD [S] - Spec Exp: Cancer Surgery; Liver & Biliary Surgery; Gastrointestinal Cancer; **Hospital:** Yale - New Haven Hosp; **Address:** Yale Univ Sch Med, Dept Surg, 330 Cedar St, TMP 202, New Haven, CT 06520-8062; **Phone:** 203-785-3577; **Board Cert:** Surgery 2000; **Med School:** Zimbabwe 1978; **Resid:** Surgery, Hammersmith Hosp 1985; Surgery, New Eng-Deaconess Hosp 1989; **Fac Appt:** Assoc Prof S, Yale Univ

Smith, Barbara Lynn MD/PhD [S] - Spec Exp: Breast Cancer; **Hospital:** Mass Genl Hosp; **Address:** Mass Genl Hosp, 55 Fruit St, Yawkey - 9A, Boston, MA 02114; **Phone:** 617-724-4800; **Board Cert:** Surgery 2000; **Med School:** Harvard Med Sch 1983; **Resid:** Surgery, Brigham & Women's Hosp 1989; **Fac Appt:** Asst Prof S, Harvard Med Sch

Sutton, John E MD [S] - Spec Exp: Esophageal Cancer; Liver & Biliary Surgery; Pancreatic Cancer; **Hospital:** Dartmouth - Hitchcock Med Ctr; **Address:** One Medical Center Drive, Lebanon, NH 03756; **Phone:** 603-650-8022; **Board Cert:** Surgery 2001; Surgical Critical Care 1995; **Med School:** Georgetown Univ 1974; **Resid:** Surgery, Dartmouth-Hitchcock Med Ctr 1981; **Fellow:** Surgical Critical Care, Dartmouth-Hitchcock Med Ctr 1983; **Fac Appt:** Prof S, Dartmouth Med Sch

Tanabe, Kenneth K MD [S] - Spec Exp: Liver Cancer; Colon & Rectal Cancer; Melanoma; **Hospital:** Mass Genl Hosp, Newton - Wellesley Hosp; **Address:** Mass General Hosp, Div Surgical Oncology, 55 Fruit St, Yawkey 7.924, Boston, MA 02114; **Phone:** 617-724-3868; **Board Cert:** Surgery 2000; **Med School:** UCSD 1985; **Resid:** Surgery, New York Hosp-Cornell 1990; **Fellow:** Surgical Oncology, MD Anderson Cancer Ctr 1993; **Fac Appt:** Assoc Prof S, Harvard Med Sch

Udelsman, Robert MD [S] - Spec Exp: Parathyroid Cancer; Adrenal Tumors; Thyroid Cancer; **Hospital:** Yale - New Haven Hosp; **Address:** Yale School Medicine, Chair of Surgery, 789 Howard Ave FMB Bldg - rm 102, New Haven, CT 06511; **Phone:** 203-785-2697; **Board Cert:** Surgery 1999; **Med School:** Geo Wash Univ 1981; **Resid:** Surgery, Natl Inst Hlth 1986; Surgery, Johns Hopkins Hosp 1989; **Fellow:** Gastrointestinal Surgery, Johns Hopkins Hosp 1990; **Fac Appt:** Prof S, Yale Univ

Ward, Barbara MD [S] - Spec Exp: Breast Cancer; Breast Disease; **Hospital:** Greenwich Hosp; **Address:** 77 Lafayette Pl, Ste 301, Greenwich, CT 06830-5426; **Phone:** 203-863-4250; **Board Cert:** Surgery 2002; **Med School:** Temple Univ 1983; **Resid:** Surgery, Yale-New Haven Hosp 1990; **Fellow:** Surgical Oncology, Natl Cancer Inst 1987; **Fac Appt:** Assoc Clin Prof S, Yale Univ

Warshaw, Andrew L MD [S] - **Spec Exp:** Pancreatic Cancer; Pancreatic Surgery; Liver Cancer; **Hospital:** Mass Genl Hosp; **Address:** Mass Genl Hosp, Dept Surg, 55 Fruit St, WHT 506, Boston, MA 02114-2696; **Phone:** 617-726-8254; **Board Cert:** Surgery 1971; **Med School:** Harvard Med Sch 1963; **Resid:** Surgery, Mass Genl Hosp 1971; **Fellow:** Internal Medicine, Mass Genl Hosp 1970; **Fac Appt:** Prof S, Harvard Med Sch

Zinner, Michael MD [S] - **Spec Exp:** Colon & Rectal Cancer; Gastrointestinal Surgery; Pancreatic Cancer; **Hospital:** Brigham & Women's Hosp, Dana-Farber Cancer Inst; **Address:** Brigham & Women's Hosp, Dept Surg, 75 Francis St, Twr 1, Ste 220, Boston, MA 02115; **Phone:** 617-732-8181; **Board Cert:** Surgery 2000; **Med School:** Univ Fla Coll Med 1971; **Resid:** Surgery, Johns Hopkins Hosp 1974; Surgery, Johns Hopkins Hosp 1979; **Fac Appt:** Prof S, Harvard Med Sch

Mid Atlantic

Alfonso, Antonio MD [S] - **Spec Exp:** Breast Cancer; Head & Neck Surgery; Thyroid Cancer; **Hospital:** Long Island Coll Hosp (page 72), SUNY Downstate Med Ctr; **Address:** Long Island Coll Hosp, 339 Hicks St, Brooklyn, NY 11201; **Phone:** 718-875-3244; **Board Cert:** Surgery 1973; **Med School:** Philippines 1968; **Resid:** Surgery, Temple Univ Hosp 1972; **Fellow:** Surgical Oncology, Meml Sloan Kettering Cancer Ctr 1974; **Fac Appt:** Prof S, SUNY Downstate

August, David MD [S] - **Spec Exp:** Cancer Surgery; Gastrointestinal Cancer; Breast Cancer; Sarcoma-Soft Tissue; **Hospital:** Robert Wood Johnson Univ Hosp - New Brunswick; **Address:** Canc Inst NJ, 195 Little Albany St, New Brunswick, NJ 08903-1914; **Phone:** 732-235-7701; **Board Cert:** Surgery 2005; **Med School:** Yale Univ 1980; **Resid:** Surgery, Yale-New Haven Hosp 1986; **Fellow:** Surgical Oncology, Natl Cancer Inst 1984; **Fac Appt:** Prof S, UMDNJ-RW Johnson Med Sch

Axelrod, Deborah MD [S] - **Spec Exp:** Breast Cancer; Breast Disease; **Hospital:** NYU Med Ctr (page 80), St Vincent Cath Med Ctrs - Manhattan; **Address:** NYU Clinical Cancer Ctr, 160 E 34th St, New York, NY 10016; **Phone:** 212-731-5366; **Board Cert:** Surgery 1998; **Med School:** Israel 1982; **Resid:** Surgery, Beth Israel Med Ctr 1988; **Fellow:** Surgical Oncology, Meml Sloan Kettering Cancer Ctr 1986; **Fac Appt:** Assoc Prof S, NYU Sch Med

Balch, Charles MD [S] - **Spec Exp:** Sentinel Node Surgery; Melanoma; Cancer Surgery; **Hospital:** Johns Hopkins Hosp - Baltimore; **Address:** 600 N Wolfe St Osler Bldg - Ste 624, Baltimore, MD 21287; **Phone:** 410-502-5977; **Board Cert:** Surgery 1997; **Med School:** Columbia P&S 1967; **Resid:** Surgery, Univ Alabama Med Ctr 1971; Surgery, Univ Alabama Med Ctr 1975; **Fellow:** Immunology, Scripps Clin-Rsch Fdn 1973; **Fac Appt:** Prof Surg & Onc, Johns Hopkins Univ

Ballantyne, Garth MD [S] - **Spec Exp:** Laparoscopic Surgery; Colon Cancer; **Hospital:** Hackensack Univ Med Ctr (page 74); **Address:** 20 Prospect Ave, Ste 901, Hackensack, NJ 07601-1974; **Phone:** 201-996-2959; **Board Cert:** Surgery 1984; Colon & Rectal Surgery 1985; **Med School:** Columbia P&S 1977; **Resid:** Surgery, UCLA Med Ctr 1980; Surgery, Northwestern Univ 1982; **Fellow:** Colon & Rectal Surgery, Mayo Clinic 1984; **Fac Appt:** Prof S, UMDNJ-NJ Med Sch, Newark

Bartlett, David L MD [S] - **Spec Exp:** Peritoneal Carcinomatosis; Pancreatic Cancer; Liver Cancer; Appendix Cancer; **Hospital:** UPMC Shadyside; **Address:** UPMC Cancer Ctr, 5150 Centre Ave Fl 4 - rm 415, Pittsburgh, PA 15232; **Phone:** 412-692-2852; **Board Cert:** Surgery 2004; **Med School:** Univ Tex, Houston 1987; **Resid:** Surgery, Hosp Univ Penn 1993; **Fellow:** Surgical Oncology, Meml Sloan-Kettering Cancer Ctr 1995; **Fac Appt:** Assoc Prof S, Univ Pittsburgh

Borgen, Patrick I MD [S] - **Spec Exp:** Breast Cancer; **Hospital:** Maimonides Med Ctr (page 75); **Address:** Maimonides Cancer Ctr, 6300 8th Ave, Brooklyn, NY 11220; **Phone:** 718-765-2570; **Board Cert:** Surgery 1991; **Med School:** Louisiana State Univ 1984; **Resid:** Surgery, Ochsner Fdn Hosp 1989; **Fellow:** Surgical Oncology, Meml Sloan Kettering Canc Ctr 1990; **Fac Appt:** Prof S, Cornell Univ-Weill Med Coll

Brennan, Murray MD [S] - **Spec Exp:** Sarcoma; Pancreatic Cancer; Cancer Surgery; **Hospital:** Meml Sloan Kettering Cancer Ctr (page 76); **Address:** 1275 York Ave, rm H1203, New York, NY 10021; **Phone:** 212-639-6586; **Board Cert:** Surgery 1975; **Med School:** New Zealand 1964; **Resid:** Surgery, Univ Otago Hosp 1969; **Fellow:** Surgery, Harvard Med Sch 1972; Surgery, Peter Bent Brigham Hosp 1975; **Fac Appt:** Prof S, Cornell Univ-Weill Med Coll

Cameron, John MD [S] - **Spec Exp:** Pancreatic Cancer; Pancreatic Surgery; Biliary Cancer; **Hospital:** Johns Hopkins Hosp - Baltimore; **Address:** 600 N Wolfe St Blalock Bldg - Ste 679, Baltimore, MD 21287; **Phone:** 410-955-5166; **Board Cert:** Surgery 1970; Thoracic Surgery 1971; **Med School:** Johns Hopkins Univ 1962; **Resid:** Surgery, Johns Hopkins Hosp 1970; **Fellow:** Thoracic Surgery, Johns Hopkins Hosp 1971; **Fac Appt:** Prof S, Johns Hopkins Univ

Chabot, John A MD [S] - **Spec Exp:** Liver & Biliary Surgery; Pancreatic Cancer; Thyroid & Parathyroid Surgery; **Hospital:** NY-Presby Hosp (page 79), Lawrence Hosp Ctr; **Address:** 161 Ft Washington Ave, Fl 8, New York, NY 10032; **Phone:** 212-305-9468; **Board Cert:** Surgery 2000; **Med School:** Dartmouth Med Sch 1983; **Resid:** Surgery, Columbia-Presby Med Ctr 1990; **Fac Appt:** Assoc Prof S, Columbia P&S

Choti, Michael A MD [S] - **Spec Exp:** Gastrointestinal Cancer; Colon & Rectal Cancer; Carcinoid Tumors; Palliative Care; **Hospital:** Johns Hopkins Hosp - Baltimore; **Address:** Johns Hopkins Hosp., 600 N Wolfe St Blalock Bldg - rm 665, Baltimore, MD 21287; **Phone:** 410-955-7113; **Board Cert:** Surgery 1991; **Med School:** Yale Univ 1983; **Resid:** Surgery, Hosp Univ Penn 1990; **Fellow:** Surgical Oncology, Meml Sloan-Kettering Canc Ctr 1992; **Fac Appt:** Prof S, Johns Hopkins Univ

Coit, Daniel G MD [S] - **Spec Exp:** Melanoma; Pancreatic Cancer; Stomach Cancer; **Hospital:** Meml Sloan Kettering Cancer Ctr (page 76); **Address:** 1275 York Ave, New York, NY 10021-6007; **Phone:** 212-639-8411; **Board Cert:** Surgery 2004; **Med School:** Univ Cincinnati 1976; **Resid:** Internal Medicine, New England Deaconess Hosp 1978; Surgery, New England Deaconess Hosp 1983; **Fellow:** Surgical Oncology, Meml Sloan Kettering Canc Ctr 1985; **Fac Appt:** Assoc Prof S, Cornell Univ-Weill Med Coll

Drebin, Jeffrey A MD/PhD [S] - **Spec Exp:** Pancreatic Cancer; Liver Cancer; Biliary Cancer; Stomach Cancer; **Hospital:** Hosp Univ Penn - UPHS (page 84); **Address:** Hosp Univ of Pennsylvania, 3400 Spruce St, 4 Silverstein Pavilion, Fl 4, Philadelphia, PA 19104; **Phone:** 215-662-2165; **Board Cert:** Surgery 2004; **Med School:** Harvard Med Sch 1987; **Resid:** Surgery, Johns Hopkins Hosp 1994; **Fellow:** Medical Oncology, Johns Hopkins Hosp 1991; Surgical Oncology, Johns Hopkins Hosp 1995; **Fac Appt:** Prof S, Univ Pennsylvania

Edge, Stephen B MD [S] - **Spec Exp:** Breast Cancer; **Hospital:** Roswell Park Cancer Inst; **Address:** Roswell Park Cancer Inst, Dept Surg Onc, Elm & Carlton Streets, Buffalo, NY 14263; **Phone:** 716-845-5789; **Board Cert:** Surgery 1996; **Med School:** Case West Res Univ 1979; **Resid:** Surgery, Univ Hosp 1986; **Fellow:** Surgical Oncology, Natl Cancer Inst 1984; **Fac Appt:** Prof S, SUNY Buffalo

Edington, Howard D MD [S] - **Spec Exp:** Breast Cancer; Melanoma; Reconstructive Surgery; **Hospital:** UPMC Presby, Pittsburgh, Magee-Womens Hosp - UPMC; **Address:** Magee-Women's Hospital, Dept Surgery, 300 Halket St, rm 2502, Pittsburgh, PA 15213; **Phone:** 412-641-1342; **Board Cert:** Surgery 1998; Plastic Surgery 1993; **Med School:** Temple Univ 1983; **Resid:** Surgery, Univ Pittsburgh Med Ctr 1989; Plastic Surgery, Univ Pittsburgh Med Ctr 1990; **Fellow:** Hand Surgery, Univ Pittsburgh Med Ctr 1991; Surgical Oncology, National Cancer Inst 1993; **Fac Appt:** Assoc Prof S, Univ Pittsburgh

Emond, Jean C MD [S] - **Spec Exp:** Transplant-Liver; Liver Cancer; **Hospital:** NY-Presby Hosp (page 79); **Address:** 622 W 168th St, PH - Fl 14, New York, NY 10032; **Phone:** 212-305-0914; **Board Cert:** Surgery 1994; **Med School:** Univ Chicago-Pritzker Sch Med 1979; **Resid:** Surgery, Cook Cty Hosp 1984; **Fellow:** Surgery, Hopital P Brousse/Univ de Paris Sud 1985; Transplant Surgery, Univ Chicago Hosps 1987; **Fac Appt:** Prof S, Columbia P&S

Eng, Kenneth MD [S] - **Spec Exp:** Colon & Rectal Cancer & Surgery; Pancreatic Cancer; **Hospital:** NYU Med Ctr (page 80); **Address:** 530 1st Ave, Ste 6B, New York, NY 10016-6402; **Phone:** 212-263-7301; **Board Cert:** Surgery 1982; **Med School:** NYU Sch Med 1967; **Resid:** Surgery, NYU Med Ctr 1972; **Fac Appt:** Prof S, NYU Sch Med

Estabrook, Alison MD [S] - **Spec Exp:** Breast Cancer; Breast Cancer-High Risk Women; **Hospital:** St Luke's - Roosevelt Hosp Ctr - Roosevelt Div (page 72); **Address:** 425 W 59th St, Ste 7A, New York, NY 10019-1104; **Phone:** 212-523-7500; **Board Cert:** Surgery 2004; **Med School:** NYU Sch Med 1978; **Resid:** Surgery, Columbia Presby Med Ctr 1984; **Fellow:** Surgical Oncology, Columbia Presby Med Ctr 1982; **Fac Appt:** Prof S, Columbia P&S

Fong, Yuman MD [S] - **Spec Exp:** Pancreatic Cancer; Liver & Biliary Cancer; Stomach Cancer; **Hospital:** Meml Sloan Kettering Cancer Ctr (page 76), NY-Presby Hosp (page 79); **Address:** Memorial Sloan-Kettering Cancer Ctr, 1275 York Ave, New York, NY 10021; **Phone:** 212-639-2016; **Board Cert:** Surgery 2002; **Med School:** Cornell Univ-Weill Med Coll 1986; **Resid:** Surgery, New York Hosp-Cornell Med Ctr 1992; **Fellow:** Surgical Oncology, Meml Sloan-Kettering Cancer Ctr 1994; **Fac Appt:** Prof S, Cornell Univ-Weill Med Coll

Fraker, Douglas L MD [S] - **Spec Exp:** Melanoma; Endocrine Tumors; Liver Cancer; Sarcoma; **Hospital:** Hosp Univ Penn - UPHS (page 84); **Address:** Hosp Univ Penn, Dept Surgery, 3400 Spruce St, 4 Silverstein Pavilion, Philadelphia, PA 19104; **Phone:** 215-662-7866; **Board Cert:** Surgery 2002; **Med School:** Harvard Med Sch 1983; **Resid:** Surgery, UCSF Med Ctr 1986; Surgery, UCSF Med Ctr 1991; **Fellow:** Surgical Oncology, National Cancer Inst 1989; **Fac Appt:** Prof S, Univ Pennsylvania

Frazier, Thomas MD [S] - **Spec Exp:** Breast Cancer; Breast Disease; **Hospital:** Bryn Mawr Hosp; **Address:** 101 S Bryn Mawr Ave, Ste 201, Bryn Mawr, PA 19010; **Phone:** 610-520-0700; **Board Cert:** Surgery 2004; **Med School:** Univ Pennsylvania 1968; **Resid:** Surgery, Hosp Univ Penn 1975; **Fellow:** Surgical Oncology, MD Anderson Cancer Ctr 1976; **Fac Appt:** Clin Prof S, Jefferson Med Coll

Gibbs, John F MD [S] - **Spec Exp:** Liver Cancer; Liver & Biliary Surgery; Pancreatic Cancer; **Hospital:** Roswell Park Cancer Inst; **Address:** Roswell Park Cancer Inst, Dept Surg Onc, Elm & Carlton Sts, Buffalo, NY 14263-0001; **Phone:** 716-845-5807; **Board Cert:** Surgery 2000; **Med School:** UCSD 1985; **Resid:** Surgery, Rush Presby-St Luke's Med Ctr 1990; **Fellow:** Transplant Surgery, Baylor Univ Med Ctr 1992; Surgical Oncology, Roswell Park Cancer Inst 1996; **Fac Appt:** Assoc Prof S, SUNY Buffalo

Hoffman, John P MD [S] - **Spec Exp:** Pancreatic Cancer; Gastrointestinal Cancer; Breast Cancer; Pancreatic Surgery; **Hospital:** Fox Chase Cancer Ctr (page 73); **Address:** Fox Chase Cancer Ctr, 333 Cottman Ave, Philadelphia, PA 19111-2497; **Phone:** 215-728-3518; **Board Cert:** Surgery 1998; **Med School:** Case West Res Univ 1970; **Resid:** Surgery, Virginia Mason Hosp 1977; **Fellow:** Surgical Oncology, Meml Sloan Kettering Cancer Ctr 1980; **Fac Appt:** Prof S, Temple Univ

Johnson, Ronald R MD [S] - **Spec Exp:** Breast Cancer; **Hospital:** Magee-Womens Hosp - UPMC; **Address:** Magee-Womens Hosp - UPMC, 300 Halket St, Ste 2601, Pittsburgh, PA 15213; **Phone:** 412-641-1225; **Board Cert:** Surgery 1999; **Med School:** Univ Pittsburgh 1983; **Resid:** Surgery, Univ Pittsburgh Med Ctr 1989; **Fac Appt:** Asst Prof S, Univ Pittsburgh

Julian, Thomas B MD [S] - **Spec Exp:** Breast Cancer; Clinical Trials; **Hospital:** Allegheny General Hosp; **Address:** Allegheny Cancer Center, 320 E North Ave Fl 5, Pittsburgh, PA 15212; **Phone:** 412-359-8229; **Board Cert:** Surgery 2001; **Med School:** Univ Pittsburgh 1976; **Resid:** Surgery, Univ Pittsburgh Med Ctr 1982; **Fac Appt:** Assoc Prof S, Drexel Univ Coll Med

Karpeh Jr, Martin S MD [S] - **Spec Exp:** Gastrointestinal Cancer; Esophageal Cancer; Colon & Rectal Cancer; **Hospital:** Stony Brook Univ Med Ctr; **Address:** Stony Brook Univ Hosp, Hlth Science Ctr, Fl 18 - rm 060, Stony Brook, NY 11794-8191; **Phone:** 631-444-1793; **Board Cert:** Surgery 1998; **Med School:** Penn State Univ-Hershey Med Ctr 1983; **Resid:** Surgery, Hosp Univ Penn 1989; **Fellow:** Surgical Oncology, Memorial Sloan Kettering Cancer Ctr 1991; **Fac Appt:** Prof S, SUNY Stony Brook

Kaufman, Howard L MD [S] - **Spec Exp:** Cancer Surgery; Vaccine Therapy; Melanoma; Immunotherapy; **Hospital:** NY-Presby Hosp (page 79); **Address:** Columbia University, MHB-7SK, 177 Fort Washington Ave, New York, NY 10032-3733; **Phone:** 212-342-6042; **Board Cert:** Surgery 1996; **Med School:** Loyola Univ-Stritch Sch Med 1986; **Resid:** Surgery, Boston Univ Hosp 1995; **Fellow:** Surgical Oncology, Natl Cancer Inst 1996; **Fac Appt:** Assoc Prof S, Columbia P&S

Lee, Kenneth K W MD [S] - **Spec Exp:** Pancreatic Cancer; Gastrointestinal Cancer & Surgery; **Hospital:** UPMC Presby, Pittsburgh, UPMC Shadyside; **Address:** Univ Pittsburgh, 497 Scaife Hall, Pittsburgh, PA 15261; **Phone:** 412-647-0457; **Board Cert:** Surgery 1998; **Med School:** Univ Chicago-Pritzker Sch Med 1981; **Resid:** Surgery, Univ Chicago Hosps 1988; **Fac Appt:** Assoc Prof S, Univ Pittsburgh

Libutti, Steven K MD [S] - **Spec Exp:** Liver Cancer; Pancreatic Cancer; Endocrine Tumors; Gastrointestinal Cancer; **Hospital:** Natl Inst of Hlth - Clin Ctr; **Address:** National Cancer Institute, Surgery Branch, 10 Center Drive Bldg 10 - rm 4W-5940, Bethesda, MD 20892-1201; **Phone:** 301-496-5049; **Board Cert:** Surgery 1996; **Med School:** Columbia P&S 1990; **Resid:** Surgery, Columbia Presby Med Ctr 1995; **Fellow:** Surgical Oncology, Natl Cancer Inst 1996

Lotze, Michael T MD/PhD [S] - **Spec Exp:** Melanoma; Gene Therapy; Immunotherapy; **Hospital:** UPMC Presby, Pittsburgh; **Address:** Hillman Cancer Ctr, Research Pavilion Fl 1 - Ste G21, 5117 Center Ave, Pittsburgh, PA 15213; **Phone:** 412-623-7732; **Board Cert:** Surgery 1983; **Med School:** Northwestern Univ 1974; **Resid:** Surgery, Strong Meml Hosp 1977; **Fellow:** Surgical Oncology, Natl Cancer Institute 1980; **Fac Appt:** Prof S, Univ Pittsburgh

Marsh Jr, James W MD [S] - **Spec Exp:** Transplant-Liver; Liver Cancer; **Hospital:** UPMC Presby, Pittsburgh; **Address:** UPMC, Starzl Transplant Inst, 3459 Fifth Ave 7 South, Pittsburgh, PA 15213; **Phone:** 412-692-2001; **Board Cert:** Surgery 2003; **Med School:** Univ Ark 1979; **Resid:** Surgery, St Paul Hosp 1984; **Fellow:** Transplant Surgery, Mayo Clinic 1985; Transplant Surgery, Univ Pittsburgh Hosps 1986; **Fac Appt:** Assoc Prof S, Univ Pittsburgh

Michelassi, Fabrizio MD [S] - **Spec Exp:** Gastrointestinal Cancer; Pancreatic Cancer; Colon & Rectal Cancer; **Hospital:** NY-Presby Hosp (page 79); **Address:** Weill Med College, Dept Surgery, 525 E 68th St, rm F-739, New York, NY 10021; **Phone:** 212-746-6006; **Board Cert:** Surgery 2002; **Med School:** Italy 1975; **Resid:** Surgery, NYU Med Ctr 1981; **Fellow:** Research, Mass Genl Hosp-Harvard 1983; **Fac Appt:** Prof S, Cornell Univ-Weill Med Coll

Morrow, Monica MD [S] - **Spec Exp:** Breast Cancer; **Hospital:** Fox Chase Cancer Ctr (page 73); **Address:** Fox Chase Cancer Ctr, Div Surg Oncology, 333 Cottman Ave, rm C 302, Philadelphia, PA 19111-2497; **Phone:** 215-728-3096; **Board Cert:** Surgery 2001; **Med School:** Jefferson Med Coll 1976; **Resid:** Surgery, Med Ctr Hosp Vermont 1981; **Fellow:** Surgical Oncology, Meml Sloan Kettering Cancer Ctr 1983; **Fac Appt:** Prof S, Temple Univ

Nava-Villarreal, Hector MD [S] - **Spec Exp:** Esophageal Cancer; Stomach Cancer; Barrett's Esophagus; **Hospital:** Roswell Park Cancer Inst; **Address:** Roswell Park Cancer Inst, Elm & Carlton Sts, Buffalo, NY 14263; **Phone:** 716-845-5915; **Board Cert:** Surgery 2001; **Med School:** Mexico 1967; **Resid:** Surgery, Buffalo Genl Hosp 1974; **Fellow:** Surgical Oncology, Roswell Park Cancer Inst 1976; **Fac Appt:** Assoc Prof S, SUNY Buffalo

Niederhuber, John E MD [S] - **Spec Exp:** Breast Cancer; Liver Cancer; Esophageal Cancer; Pancreatic Cancer; **Hospital:** Natl Inst of Hlth - Clin Ctr; **Address:** Natl Cancer Institute, 31 Center Drive Bldg 31, rm 11A48, MS 2590, Bethesda, MD 20892-2590; **Phone:** 301-594-6369; **Board Cert:** Surgery 1974; **Med School:** Ohio State Univ 1964; **Resid:** Surgery, Univ Mich Hosp 1973; **Fellow:** Immunology, Karolinska Inst 1971

O'Hea, Brian MD [S] - **Spec Exp:** Breast Cancer; Sentinel Node Surgery; **Hospital:** Stony Brook Univ Med Ctr; **Address:** SUNY Stony Brook, Dept Surg, HSC T-18, Rm 060, Stony Brook, NY 11794-8191; **Phone:** 631-444-1795; **Board Cert:** Surgery 1992; **Med School:** Georgetown Univ 1986; **Resid:** Surgery, St Vincent's Hosp 1991; **Fellow:** Breast Disease, Meml Sloan-Kettering Cancer Ctr 1996; **Fac Appt:** Asst Prof S, SUNY Stony Brook

Osborne, Michael P MD [S] - **Spec Exp:** Breast Cancer; Breast Cancer-High Risk Women; Breast Disease; **Hospital:** NY-Presby Hosp (page 79); **Address:** 425 E 61 St Fl 8, New York, NY 10021-8722; **Phone:** 212-821-0828; **Med School:** England 1970; **Resid:** Surgery, Charing Cross Hosp 1977; Surgery, Royal Marsden Hosp 1980; **Fellow:** Surgical Oncology, Meml Sloan-Kettering Canc Ctr 1981; **Fac Appt:** Prof S, Cornell Univ-Weill Med Coll

Paty, Philip B MD [S] - **Spec Exp:** Colon & Rectal Cancer; Pelvic Tumors; Appendix Cancer; **Hospital:** Meml Sloan Kettering Cancer Ctr (page 76); **Address:** Memorial Sloan Kettering Cancer Ctr, 1275 York Ave, rm C1081, New York, NY 10021; **Phone:** 212-639-6703; **Board Cert:** Surgery 2001; **Med School:** Stanford Univ 1983; **Resid:** Surgery, UCSF Med Ctr 1990; **Fellow:** Surgical Oncology, Memorial Sloan Kettering Cancer Ctr 1992; **Fac Appt:** Prof S, Cornell Univ-Weill Med Coll

Petrelli, Nicholas J MD [S] - **Spec Exp:** Cancer Surgery; Gastrointestinal Cancer; **Hospital:** Christiana Care Hlth Svs; **Address:** Helen F Graham Cancer Ctr, 4701 Ogletown-Stanton Rd, Ste 1213, Newark, DE 19713; **Phone:** 302-623-4550; **Board Cert:** Surgery 1997; **Med School:** Tulane Univ 1973; **Resid:** Surgery, St Mary's Hosp-Med Ctr 1978; **Fellow:** Surgical Oncology, Roswell Park Cancer Inst 1980; **Fac Appt:** Prof S, Thomas Jefferson Univ

Ridge, John A MD/PhD [S] - **Spec Exp:** Head & Neck Cancer & Surgery; Thyroid Cancer & Surgery; Laryngeal Cancer; **Hospital:** Fox Chase Cancer Ctr (page 73); **Address:** Fox Chase Cancer Ctr, Dept Surgical Oncology, 333 Cottman Ave, Philadelphia, PA 19111; **Phone:** 215-728-3517; **Board Cert:** Surgery 1997; **Med School:** Stanford Univ 1981; **Resid:** Surgery, Univ Colorado Med Ctr 1987; **Fellow:** Surgical Oncology, Meml Sloan-Kettering Cancer Ctr 1989

Roh, Mark S MD [S] - **Spec Exp:** Liver Cancer; Cancer Surgery; **Hospital:** Allegheny General Hosp; **Address:** Allegheny General Hospital, Dept Surgery, 320 E North Ave, Pittsburgh, PA 15212; **Phone:** 412-359-6738; **Board Cert:** Surgery 1996; **Med School:** Ohio State Univ 1979; **Resid:** Surgery, Univ Pittsburgh Med Ctr 1982; Surgery, Univ Pittsburgh Med Ctr 1986; **Fellow:** Surgical Oncology, Meml Sloan-Kettering Cancer Ctr 1984; Surgical Oncology, Meml Sloan-Kettering Cancer Ctr 1987; **Fac Appt:** Prof S, Drexel Univ Coll Med

Rosato, Ernest F MD [S] - **Spec Exp:** Gastrointestinal Cancer & Surgery; Esophageal Cancer; Pancreatic Cancer; **Hospital:** Hosp Univ Penn - UPHS (page 84); **Address:** Hosp Univ Penn, Dept Surg, 3400 Spruce St, 4 Silverstein, Philadelphia, PA 19104; **Phone:** 215-662-2033; **Board Cert:** Surgery 1969; **Med School:** Univ Pennsylvania 1962; **Resid:** Surgery, Hosp Univ Penn 1968; **Fac Appt:** Prof S, Univ Pennsylvania

Rosenberg, Steven MD [S] - **Spec Exp:** Melanoma; Kidney Cancer; **Hospital:** Natl Inst of Hlth - Clin Ctr; **Address:** National Cancer Institute, 9000 Rockville Pike CRC Bldg, rm 3W-3940, Bethesda, MD 20892; **Phone:** 301-496-4164; **Board Cert:** Surgery 1975; **Med School:** Johns Hopkins Univ 1964; **Resid:** Surgery, Peter Bent Brigham Hosp 1974

Roses, Daniel F MD [S] - **Spec Exp:** Breast Cancer; Melanoma; Thyroid & Parathyroid Cancer & Surgery; **Hospital:** NYU Med Ctr (page 80); **Address:** 530 First Ave, Ste 6E, New York, NY 10016-6402; **Phone:** 212-263-7329; **Board Cert:** Surgery 1975; **Med School:** NYU Sch Med 1969; **Resid:** Surgery, NYU-Bellevue Hosp 1974; **Fellow:** Surgical Oncology, NYU-Bellevue Hosp 1978; **Fac Appt:** Prof Surg & Onc, NYU Sch Med

Schnabel, Freya MD [S] - **Spec Exp:** Breast Cancer; Breast Cancer-High Risk Women; **Hospital:** NY-Presby Hosp (page 79); **Address:** 161 Fort Washington Ave H 10 - Ste 1011, New York, NY 10032; **Phone:** 212-305-1534; **Board Cert:** Surgery 1998; **Med School:** NYU Sch Med 1982; **Resid:** Surgery, NYU Med Ctr 1987; **Fellow:** Research, SUNY Hlth Sci Ctr 1988; **Fac Appt:** Assoc Clin Prof S, Columbia P&S

Schraut, Wolfgang H MD [S] - Spec Exp: Gastrointestinal Surgery; Colon & Rectal Cancer & Surgery; Laparoscopic Surgery; **Hospital:** UPMC Presby, Pittsburgh, Magee-Womens Hosp - UPMC; **Address:** Univ Pittsburgh Med Ctr, Dept Surgery, 497 Scaife Hall, 3550 Terrace St, Pittsburgh, PA 15261; **Phone:** 412-647-0311; **Board Cert:** Surgery 1999; **Med School:** Germany 1970; **Resid:** Surgery, Univ Chicago Hosps 1978; **Fac Appt:** Prof S, Univ Pittsburgh

Schwartz, Gordon F MD [S] - Spec Exp: Breast Cancer; Breast Disease; **Hospital:** Thomas Jefferson Univ Hosp (page 82), Pennsylvania Hosp (page 84); **Address:** 1015 Chestnut St, Ste 510, Philadelphia, PA 19107-4305; **Phone:** 215-627-8487; **Board Cert:** Surgery 1970; **Med School:** Harvard Med Sch 1960; **Resid:** Surgery, Columbia-Presby Med Ctr 1968; **Fellow:** Oncology, Univ Penn 1969; **Fac Appt:** Prof S, Jefferson Med Coll

Shah, Jatin P MD [S] - Spec Exp: Head & Neck Cancer; Thyroid Cancer; Skull Base Tumors; **Hospital:** Meml Sloan Kettering Cancer Ctr (page 76); **Address:** 1275 York Ave, Ste C1061, New York, NY 10021-6007; **Phone:** 212-639-7604; **Board Cert:** Surgery 1975; **Med School:** India 1964; **Resid:** Surgery, SSG Hosp 1967; Surgery, New York Infirm 1974; **Fellow:** Head & Neck Surgical Oncology, Meml Sloan-Kettering Hosp 1972; **Fac Appt:** Prof S, Cornell Univ-Weill Med Coll

Shaha, Ashok MD [S] - Spec Exp: Head & Neck Cancer; Thyroid Cancer; Parathyroid Cancer; **Hospital:** Meml Sloan Kettering Cancer Ctr (page 76); **Address:** 1275 York Ave, Dept of Head & Neck Surgery, New York, NY 10021-6007; **Phone:** 212-639-7649; **Board Cert:** Surgery 1992; **Med School:** India 1970; **Resid:** Surgery, Downstate Med Ctr 1981; **Fellow:** Surgical Oncology, Meml Sloan Kettering Cancer Ctr 1976; Head and Neck Surgery, Meml Sloan Kettering Cancer Ctr 1982; **Fac Appt:** Prof S, Cornell Univ-Weill Med Coll

Sigurdson, Elin Ruth MD [S] - Spec Exp: Breast Cancer; Colon & Rectal Cancer; Melanoma; Gastrointestinal Cancer; **Hospital:** Fox Chase Cancer Ctr (page 73); **Address:** 333 Cottman Ave, Philadelphia, PA 19111-2412; **Phone:** 215-728-3519; **Board Cert:** Surgery 1997; **Med School:** Canada 1980; **Resid:** Surgery, Univ Toronto Med Ctr 1984; **Fellow:** Surgical Oncology, Meml Sloan-Kettering Cancer Ctr 1987; **Fac Appt:** Assoc Prof S

Singer, Samuel MD [S] - Spec Exp: Sarcoma-Soft Tissue; **Hospital:** Meml Sloan Kettering Cancer Ctr (page 76); **Address:** Meml Sloan Kettering Cancer Ctr, 1275 York Ave, rm 1210, New York, NY 10021; **Phone:** 212-639-2940; **Board Cert:** Surgery 1998; **Med School:** Harvard Med Sch 1982; **Resid:** Surgery, Brigham & Women's Hosp 1988; **Fellow:** Surgical Oncology, Dana Farber Cancer Inst 1990; **Fac Appt:** Assoc Prof S, Cornell Univ-Weill Med Coll

Skinner, Kristin A MD [S] - Spec Exp: Breast Cancer; Gastrointestinal Cancer; Melanoma; **Hospital:** Univ of Rochester Strong Meml Hosp; **Address:** Univ Rochester Med Ctr, 601 Elmwood Ave, Box SURG, Rochester, NY 14642; **Phone:** 585-276-3332; **Board Cert:** Surgery 1996; **Med School:** Johns Hopkins Univ 1988; **Resid:** Surgery, UCLA Med Ctr 1995; **Fellow:** Surgical Oncology, UCLA Med Ctr 1994; **Fac Appt:** Assoc Prof S, NYU Sch Med

Sugarbaker, Paul H MD [S] - Spec Exp: Peritoneal Carcinomatosis; Cystadenocarcinoma; Ovarian Cancer; Appendix Cancer; **Hospital:** Washington Hosp Ctr; **Address:** Washington Hosp Ctr, 106 Irving St NW, Ste 3900N, Washington, DC 20010; **Phone:** 202-877-3908; **Board Cert:** Surgery 1973; **Med School:** Cornell Univ-Weill Med Coll 1967; **Resid:** Surgery, Peter Bent Brigham Hosp 1973; **Fellow:** Surgical Oncology, Mass Genl Hosp 1976; **Fac Appt:** Prof S, Univ Wash

Swistel, Alexander MD [S] - **Spec Exp:** Breast Cancer; Breast Disease; Sentinel Node Surgery; **Hospital:** NY-Presby Hosp (page 79), St Luke's - Roosevelt Hosp Ctr - Roosevelt Div (page 72); **Address:** 425 E 61st St Fl 8, New York, NY 10021; **Phone:** 212-821-0602; **Board Cert:** Surgery 2005; **Med School:** Brown Univ 1975; **Resid:** Surgery, St Luke's Roosevelt Hosp Ctr 1981; **Fellow:** Surgical Oncology, Meml Sloan Kettering Canc Ctr 1983; **Fac Appt:** Asst Prof S, Cornell Univ-Weill Med Coll

Tafra, Lorraine MD [S] - **Spec Exp:** Breast Cancer; **Hospital:** Anne Arundel Med Ctr; **Address:** 2002 Medical Parkway, Ste 120, Annapolis, MD 21401; **Phone:** 443-481-5300; **Board Cert:** Surgery 2005; **Med School:** Case West Res Univ 1986; **Resid:** Surgery, Rhode Island Hosp 1988; Surgery, Hosp Univ Penn 1992; **Fellow:** Surgical Oncology, John Wayne Cancer Inst 1994

Tartter, Paul MD [S] - **Spec Exp:** Breast Cancer; Breast Cancer in Elderly; Sentinel Node Surgery; **Hospital:** St Luke's - Roosevelt Hosp Ctr - Roosevelt Div (page 72), Mount Sinai Med Ctr (page 77); **Address:** 425 W 59th St, Ste 7A, New York, NY 10019; **Phone:** 212-523-7500; **Board Cert:** Surgery 2003; **Med School:** Brown Univ 1977; **Resid:** Surgery, Mount Sinai Hosp 1982; **Fac Appt:** Assoc Prof S, Columbia P&S

Tsangaris, Theodore N MD [S] - **Spec Exp:** Breast Cancer; **Hospital:** Johns Hopkins Hosp - Baltimore; **Address:** Johns Hopkins Hospital, 600 N Wolfe St, Carnegie 686, Baltimore, MD 21287; **Phone:** 410-955-2615; **Board Cert:** Surgery 2005; **Med School:** Geo Wash Univ 1983; **Resid:** Surgery, Geo Washington Univ Med Ctr 1989; **Fellow:** Surgical Oncology, Baylor Univ Med Ctr 1990; **Fac Appt:** Assoc Prof S, Johns Hopkins Univ

Willey, Shawna C MD [S] - **Spec Exp:** Breast Cancer; Clinical Trials; **Hospital:** Georgetown Univ Hosp; **Address:** 3800 Reservoir Rd NW, PHC Bldg Fl 4, Washington, DC 20007; **Phone:** 202-444-0241; **Board Cert:** Surgery 1998; **Med School:** Univ Iowa Coll Med 1982; **Resid:** Surgery, George Washington U Med Ctr 1988; **Fac Appt:** Asst Prof S, Georgetown Univ

Yang, James C MD [S] - **Spec Exp:** Kidney Cancer; Kidney Cancer Clinical Trials; Clinical Trials; Immunotherapy; **Hospital:** Natl Inst of Hlth - Clin Ctr; **Address:** National Cancer Institute, 9000 Rockville Pike CRC Bldg - rm 3-5952, Bethesda, MD 20892; **Phone:** 301-496-1574; **Board Cert:** Surgery 1995; **Med School:** UCSD 1978; **Resid:** Surgery, UCSD Med Ctr 1984; **Fellow:** Surgical Oncology, Natl Cancer Inst 1986

Southeast

Adams, Reid MD [S] - **Spec Exp:** Gastrointestinal Cancer; Liver Cancer; Pancreatic & Biliary Surgery; **Hospital:** Univ Virginia Med Ctr; **Address:** UVa Health System, Dept Surgery, PO Box 800709, Charlottesville, VA 22908; **Phone:** 434-924-2839; **Board Cert:** Surgery 2003; **Med School:** Univ VA Sch Med 1987; **Resid:** Surgery, Univ Va Hlth Sci Ctr 1994; **Fellow:** Hepatopancreatobiliary Surgery, Univ Toronto Med Ctr 1995; **Fac Appt:** Assoc Prof S, Univ VA Sch Med

Beauchamp, Robert Daniel MD [S] - **Spec Exp:** Breast Cancer; Colon & Rectal Cancer; Pancreatic Cancer; Cancer Surgery; **Hospital:** Vanderbilt Univ Med Ctr; **Address:** Medical Center North, rm D4316, 1161 21st Ave S, Nashville, TN 37232; **Phone:** 615-322-2363; **Board Cert:** Surgery 1997; **Med School:** Univ Tex Med Br, Galveston 1982; **Resid:** Surgery, Univ Tex Med Br 1987; **Fellow:** Cellular Molecular Biology, Vanderbilt Univ 1989; **Fac Appt:** Prof S, Vanderbilt Univ

Behrns, Kevin E MD [S] - **Spec Exp:** Pancreatic Cancer; Gastrointestinal Cancer & Surgery; **Hospital:** Shands Hlthcre at Univ of FL; **Address:** Shands Healthcare at Univ Florida, PO Box 100286, Gainesville, FL 32610-0286; **Phone:** 352-265-0761; **Board Cert:** Surgery 2005; **Med School:** Mayo Med Sch 1988; **Resid:** Surgery, Mayo Clinic 1995; **Fac Appt:** Prof S, Univ Fla Coll Med

Bland, Kirby MD [S] - **Spec Exp:** Breast Cancer; Colon Cancer; Thyroid & Parathyroid Cancer & Surgery; **Hospital:** Univ of Ala Hosp at Birmingham; **Address:** University of Alabama, Dept Surgery, 1530 3rd Ave S, BDB 502, Birmingham, AL 35294-0002; **Phone:** 205-975-2193; **Board Cert:** Surgery 2000; **Med School:** Univ Ala 1968; **Resid:** Surgery, Univ Fla Hosp 1970; Surgery, Univ Fla Hosp 1976; **Fellow:** Surgical Oncology, MD Anderson Cancer Ctr 1977; **Fac Appt:** Prof S, Univ Ala

Calvo, Benjamin MD [S] - **Spec Exp:** Pancreatic Cancer; Endocrine Cancers; Breast Cancer; **Hospital:** Univ NC Hosps; **Address:** Dept Surg CB 7213, Chapel Hill, NC 27599; **Phone:** 919-966-9700; **Board Cert:** Surgery 1999; **Med School:** Univ MD Sch Med 1981; **Resid:** Surgery, G Washington Univ Hosp 1988; Surgery, Natl Inst Hlth 1991; **Fellow:** Surgery, Meml Sloan Kettering Cancer Ctr 1993; **Fac Appt:** Assoc Prof S, Univ NC Sch Med

Cance, William George MD [S] - **Spec Exp:** Pancreatic Cancer; Colon & Rectal Cancer; Endocrine Cancers; **Hospital:** Shands Hlthcre at Univ of FL, VA Med Ctr - Gainesville; **Address:** Shands at Univ Florida-Dept Surgery, 1600 SW Archer Rd, PO Box 100286, Gainesville, FL 32610-0286; **Phone:** 352-265-0622; **Board Cert:** Surgery 1998; **Med School:** Duke Univ 1982; **Resid:** Surgery, Barnes Hosp-Wash Univ 1988; **Fellow:** Surgical Oncology, Meml Sloan Kettering Canc Ctr 1990; **Fac Appt:** Prof S, Univ Fla Coll Med

Chari, Ravi S MD [S] - **Spec Exp:** Liver Cancer; Biliary Cancer; Transplant-Liver; **Hospital:** Vanderbilt Univ Med Ctr; **Address:** Vanderbilt Univ Med Ctr, Hepatobillary Surg, 1313 21st Ave S, Ste 801 Oxford House, Nashville, TN 37232-4753; **Phone:** 615-936-2573; **Board Cert:** Surgery 1997; **Med School:** Canada 1989; **Resid:** Surgery, Duke Univ Med Ctr 1996; **Fellow:** Transplant Surgery, Univ Toronto-Toronto Hosp 1998; **Fac Appt:** Prof S, Vanderbilt Univ

Cole, David J MD [S] - **Spec Exp:** Breast Brachytherapy; Gastrointestinal Cancer; Vaccine Therapy; Gene Therapy; **Hospital:** MUSC Med Ctr; **Address:** 96 Jonathan Lucas St, PO BOX 250613, Charleston, SC 29425; **Phone:** 843-792-4638; **Board Cert:** Surgery 2000; **Med School:** Cornell Univ-Weill Med Coll 1986; **Resid:** Surgery, Emory Univ School Med 1991; **Fellow:** Surgical Oncology, Natl Cancer Institute 1994; **Fac Appt:** Prof S, Med Univ SC

Copeland III, Edward M MD [S] - **Spec Exp:** Breast Cancer; Colon & Rectal Cancer; Melanoma; **Hospital:** Shands Hlthcre at Univ of FL; **Address:** Univ Florida Coll Medicine, Dept Surgery, 1600 SW Archer Rd, Box 100286, Gainesville, FL 32610; **Phone:** 352-265-0169; **Board Cert:** Surgery 1971; **Med School:** Cornell Univ-Weill Med Coll 1963; **Resid:** Surgery, Hosp Univ Penn 1969; Surgical Oncology, Univ TX MD Anderson Cancer Ctr 1972; **Fellow:** Research, Hosp Univ Penn 1967; **Fac Appt:** Prof S, Univ Fla Coll Med

Dilawari, Raza A MD [S] - **Spec Exp:** Skin Cancer; Melanoma; Breast Cancer; Ovarian Cancer; **Hospital:** Methodist Univ Hosp - Memphis, St Francis Hosp - Memphis; **Address:** Methodist Univ Hosp, 1325 Eastmoreland Ave, Ste 410, Memphis, TN 38104; **Phone:** 901-767-7204; **Board Cert:** Surgery 1975; **Med School:** Pakistan 1968; **Resid:** Surgery, SUNY-Upstate Med Ctr 1974; **Fellow:** Surgical Oncology, Roswell Park Meml Hosp 1976; **Fac Appt:** Prof S, Univ Tenn Coll Med, Memphis

Flynn, Michael B MD [S] - Spec Exp: Head & Neck Cancer; Head & Neck Surgery; **Hospital:** Univ of Louisville Hosp, Norton Hosp; **Address:** 601 S Floyd St, Ste 700, Louisville, KY 40202; **Phone:** 502-583-8303; **Board Cert:** Surgery 1972; **Med School:** Ireland 1962; **Resid:** Surgery, Univ Maryland Hosp 1969; **Fellow:** Surgical Oncology, MD Anderson Hosp 1971; **Fac Appt:** Prof S, Univ Louisville Sch Med

Gabram, Sheryl MD [S] - Spec Exp: Breast Cancer; Breast Disease; **Hospital:** Emory Univ Hosp, Grady Hlth Sys; **Address:** Winship Cancer Institute, 1365 Clifton Rd NE C Bldg Fl 2, Atlanta, GA 30322; **Phone:** 404-778-1230; **Board Cert:** Surgery 1996; **Med School:** Georgetown Univ 1982; **Resid:** Surgery, Washington Hosp Ctr 1987; **Fellow:** Trauma, Hartford Hosp 1988; **Fac Appt:** Prof S, Emory Univ

Greene, Frederick L MD [S] - Spec Exp: Gastrointestinal Surgery; Gastrointestinal Cancer; **Hospital:** Carolinas Med Ctr; **Address:** Carolinas Medical Ctr, 1025 Morehead Medical Drive, Ste 275, Charlotte, NC 28203; **Phone:** 704-355-1813; **Board Cert:** Surgery 1998; **Med School:** Univ VA Sch Med 1970; **Resid:** Surgery, Yale-New Haven Hosp 1976; **Fellow:** Surgical Oncology, Yale-New Haven Hosp 1973; **Fac Appt:** Prof S, Univ NC Sch Med

Hanks, John B MD [S] - Spec Exp: Endocrine Cancers; Breast Cancer; Thyroid Cancer & Surgery; **Hospital:** Univ Virginia Med Ctr; **Address:** Univ VA Hlth Sys, Dept Surg, PO Box 800709, Charlottesville, VA 22908-0709; **Phone:** 434-924-0376; **Board Cert:** Surgery 2001; **Med School:** Univ Rochester 1973; **Resid:** Surgery, Duke Univ Med Ctr 1982; **Fac Appt:** Prof S, Univ VA Sch Med

Hemming, Alan W MD [S] - Spec Exp: Liver Cancer; Transplant-Liver; Hepatobiliary Surgery; Pancreatic Cancer; **Hospital:** Shands Hlthcre at Univ of FL; **Address:** University of Florida, Dept Surgery, 1600 SW Archer Rd, rm 6142, Box 100286, Gainsville, FL 32610-3003; **Phone:** 352-265-0606; **Board Cert:** Surgery 2005; **Med School:** Canada 1987; **Resid:** Surgery, Univ British Columbia Med Ctr 1993; **Fellow:** Transplant Surgery, Univ Toronto/Hosp for Sick Children 1995; Hepatobiliary Surgery, Univ Toronto 1996; **Fac Appt:** Prof S, Univ Fla Coll Med

Herrmann, Virginia M MD [S] - Spec Exp: Breast Cancer; Nutrition & Cancer Prevention/Control; **Hospital:** Meml Hlth Univ Med Ctr - Savannah; **Address:** Center for Breast Care, 4700 Waters Ave, Ste 405, Savannah, GA 31404; **Phone:** 912-350-2700; **Board Cert:** Surgery 2000; **Med School:** St Louis Univ 1974; **Resid:** Surgery, St Louis Univ Hosps 1979; **Fellow:** Surgery, Brigham & Women's Hosp/Harvard 1980; **Fac Appt:** Prof S, Mercer Univ Sch Med

Heslin, Martin J MD [S] - Spec Exp: Gastrointestinal Cancer; Pancreatic Cancer; Biliary Cancer; Sarcoma-Soft Tissue; **Hospital:** Univ of Ala Hosp at Birmingham; **Address:** Univ Alabama, 1922 7th Ave S, Ste 321, Birmingham, AL 35294-0016; **Phone:** 205-934-3064; **Board Cert:** Surgery 1995; **Med School:** SUNY Upstate Med Univ 1987; **Resid:** Surgery, NYU Med Ctr 1994; Surgery, Meml Sloan-Kettering Canc Ctr 1991; **Fellow:** Surgical Oncology, Meml Sloan-Kettering Cancer Ctr 1996; **Fac Appt:** Prof S, Univ Ala

Israel, Philip 7 MD [S] - Spec Exp: Breast Cancer; **Hospital:** WellStar Kennestone Hosp; **Address:** 702 Canton Rd, Marietta, GA 30060; **Phone:** 770-428-4486; **Board Cert:** Surgery 1967; **Med School:** Emory Univ 1961; **Resid:** Surgery, Emory Univ Hosp 1966; **Fac Appt:** Prof S, Univ Tenn Coll Med,Chattanooga

Kelley, Mark C MD [S] - **Spec Exp:** Breast Cancer; Melanoma; **Hospital:** Vanderbilt Univ Med Ctr; **Address:** Vanderbilt Univ Med Ctr, Div Surg Oncology, 2220 Pierce Ave, 597 Preston Rsch Bldg, Nashville, TN 37232; **Phone:** 615-322-2391; **Board Cert:** Surgery 2006; **Med School:** Univ Fla Coll Med 1989; **Resid:** Surgery, Univ Fla-Shands Hosp 1995; **Fellow:** Surgical Oncology, John Wayne Cancer Inst-St Johns Hosp 1997; **Fac Appt:** Asst Prof Surg & Onc, Vanderbilt Univ

Leight, George MD [S] - **Spec Exp:** Breast Cancer; Thyroid Cancer; Parathyroid Cancer; **Hospital:** Duke Univ Med Ctr; **Address:** Duke Univ Med Ctr, Dept Surgery, DUMC Box 3513, Durham, NC 27710; **Phone:** 919-684-6849; **Board Cert:** Surgery 1999; **Med School:** Duke Univ 1972; **Resid:** Surgery, Duke Univ Med Ctr 1978; **Fac Appt:** Prof S, Duke Univ

Levi, Joe U MD [S] - **Spec Exp:** Pancreatic Cancer; **Hospital:** Jackson Meml Hosp; **Address:** 1475 NW 12th Ave, Ste 3524, Miami, FL 33136; **Phone:** 305-243-4211; **Board Cert:** Surgery 1975; **Med School:** Univ Fla Coll Med 1967; **Resid:** Surgery, Johns Hopkins Hosp 1969; Surgery, Jackson Meml Hosp 1974; **Fac Appt:** Prof S, Univ Miami Sch Med

Levine, Edward A MD [S] - **Spec Exp:** Breast Cancer; Esophageal Cancer; Peritoneal Carcinomatosis; **Hospital:** Wake Forest Univ Baptist Med Ctr (page 85); **Address:** Wake Forest Univ Baptist Med Ctr, Dept of Surgery, Medical Center Blvd, Winston-Salem, NC 27157; **Phone:** 336-716-4276; **Board Cert:** Surgery 1999; **Med School:** Ros Franklin Univ/Chicago Med Sch 1985; **Resid:** Surgery, Michael Reese Hosp 1990; **Fellow:** Surgical Oncology, Univ Illinois 1992; **Fac Appt:** Prof S, Wake Forest Univ

Lind, David Scott MD [S] - **Spec Exp:** Breast Cancer; Melanoma; Sarcoma; **Hospital:** Med Coll of GA Hosp and Clin; **Address:** MCG Health System-Dept Hem Onc, 1120 15th St, Augusta, GA 30912; **Phone:** 706-721-6744; **Board Cert:** Surgery 2000; **Med School:** Eastern VA Med Sch 1984; **Resid:** Surgery, Univ Texas 1989; **Fellow:** Medical Oncology, Med Coll Virginia 1992; **Fac Appt:** Prof Surg & Onc, Med Coll GA

Livingstone, Alan S MD [S] - **Spec Exp:** Liver & Biliary Cancer; Stomach Cancer; Pancreatic Cancer; Esophageal Cancer; **Hospital:** Jackson Meml Hosp, Univ of Miami Hosp & Clins/Sylvester Comp Canc Ctr; **Address:** Sylvester Comp Cancer Ctr, Dept Surgery (310T), 1475 NW 12th Ave, rm 3550, Miami, FL 33136; **Phone:** 305-243-4902; **Board Cert:** Surgery 1995; **Med School:** McGill Univ 1971; **Resid:** Surgery, Montreal Genl Hosp 1976; Surgery, Jackson Meml Hosp 1975; **Fac Appt:** Prof S, Univ Miami Sch Med

Lyerly, H Kim MD [S] - **Spec Exp:** Breast Cancer; Immunotherapy; **Hospital:** Duke Univ Med Ctr, Durham Regional Hosp; **Address:** Duke Univ Med Ctr, Dept Surg, DUMC Box 2714, Durham, NC 27710; **Phone:** 919-684-5613; **Board Cert:** Surgery 2001; **Med School:** UCLA 1983; **Resid:** Surgery, Duke Univ Med Ctr 1990; **Fac Appt:** Prof S, Duke Univ

Malafa, Mokenge P MD [S] - **Spec Exp:** Pancreatic Cancer; Liver Cancer; Esophageal Cancer; Colon Cancer; **Hospital:** H Lee Moffitt Cancer Ctr & Research Inst; **Address:** H Lee Moffitt Cancer Ctr, 12902 Magnolia Drive, Ste 12507, Tampa, FL 33612; **Phone:** 813-632-1432; **Board Cert:** Surgery 2000; **Med School:** Univ Wisc 1986; **Resid:** Surgery, Medical Coll Ohio 1991; **Fellow:** Surgical Oncology, City of Hope Cancer Ctr 1994

McGrath, Patrick C MD [S] - Spec Exp: Breast Cancer; Cancer Surgery; **Hospital:** Univ of Kentucky Chandler Hosp; **Address:** Univ Kentucky Med Ctr, Dept Genl Surgery, 800 Rose St, rm C224, Lexington, KY 40536-0293; **Phone:** 859-323-6346 x233; **Board Cert:** Surgery 1996; **Med School:** Univ IL Coll Med 1980; **Resid:** Surgery, Med Coll Virginia Hosp 1986; **Fellow:** Surgical Oncology, Med Coll Virginia Hosp 1988; **Fac Appt:** Prof S, Univ KY Coll Med

McMasters, Kelly M MD [S] - Spec Exp: Melanoma; Breast Cancer; Liver Cancer; **Hospital:** Univ of Louisville Hosp; **Address:** 601 S Floyd St, Ste 700, Louisville, KY 40202; **Phone:** 502-583-8303; **Board Cert:** Surgery 1995; **Med School:** UMDNJ-RW Johnson Med Sch ; **Resid:** Surgery, Univ Louisville Sch Med 1994; **Fellow:** Surgical Oncology, Texas-MD Anderson Cancer Ctr 1995; **Fac Appt:** Prof S, Univ Louisville Sch Med

Neifeld, James MD [S] - Spec Exp: Melanoma; Head & Neck Cancer; Gastrointestinal Cancer; **Hospital:** Med Coll of VA Hosp; **Address:** Medical College of Virginia Hospital, PO Box 980645, Richmond, VA 23298-0645; **Phone:** 804-828-9324; **Board Cert:** Surgery 1998; **Med School:** Med Coll VA 1972; **Resid:** Surgery, Med Coll VA Hosp 1978; **Fac Appt:** Prof S, Med Coll VA

Pappas, Theodore N MD [S] - Spec Exp: Pancreatic Surgery; Laparoscopic Surgery; **Hospital:** Duke Univ Med Ctr; **Address:** Duke Univ Med Ctr, Dept Surgery, DUMC Box 3479, Durham, NC 27710-0001; **Phone:** 919-681-3442; **Board Cert:** Surgery 1997; **Med School:** Ohio State Univ 1981; **Resid:** Surgery, Brigham & Womens Hosp 1988; **Fellow:** Research, Wadworth VA Med Ctr 1985; **Fac Appt:** Prof S, Duke Univ

Pinson, C Wright MD [S] - Spec Exp: Transplant-Liver; Liver & Biliary Cancer; Pancreatic Cancer; **Hospital:** Vanderbilt Univ Med Ctr; **Address:** Vanderbilt Transplant Ctr, TVC 3810A, 1301 21st Ave S, Nashville, TN 37232-5545; **Phone:** 615-343-9324; **Board Cert:** Surgery 1996; Surgical Critical Care 1997; **Med School:** Vanderbilt Univ 1980; **Resid:** Surgery, Oregon Health Sci Ctr 1986; **Fellow:** Gastrointestinal Surgery, Lahey Clinic 1987; Transplant Surgery, Deaconess Hosp 1988; **Fac Appt:** Prof S, Vanderbilt Univ

Polk Jr, Hiram C MD [S] - Spec Exp: Melanoma; Colon Cancer; **Hospital:** Univ of Louisville Hosp, Norton Hosp; **Address:** 601 S Floyd St, Ste 700, Louisville, KY 40292; **Phone:** 502-583-8303; **Board Cert:** Surgery 1966; **Med School:** Harvard Med Sch 1960; **Resid:** Surgery, Barnes Hosp 1965; **Fac Appt:** Prof S, Univ Louisville Sch Med

Reintgen, Douglas Scott MD [S] - Spec Exp: Melanoma; Breast Cancer; Cancer Surgery; **Hospital:** Lakeland Regl Med Ctr; **Address:** 3525 Lakeland Hills Blvd, Lakeland, FL 33805-1965; **Phone:** 863-603-6565; **Board Cert:** Surgery 1997; **Med School:** Duke Univ 1979; **Resid:** Surgery, Duke Univ Med Ctr 1987; **Fac Appt:** Prof S, Univ S Fla Coll Med

Rosemurgy, Alexander S MD [S] - Spec Exp: Pancreatic Cancer; Gastrointestinal Surgery; **Hospital:** Tampa Genl Hosp; **Address:** Digestive Disorders Ctr, Tampa General Hospital, 2 Columbia Drive, rm F145, Tampa, FL 33601; **Phone:** 813-844-7393; **Board Cert:** Surgery 2005; **Med School:** Univ Mich Med Sch 1979; **Resid:** Surgery, Univ Chicago Hosps 1984; **Fac Appt:** Prof S, Univ S Fla Coll Med

Salo, Jonathan C MD [S] - Spec Exp: Gastrointestinal Cancer; Immunotherapy; **Hospital:** Carolinas Med Ctr; **Address:** Blumenthal Cancer Center, 1025 Morehead Medical Drive, Ste 600, Charlotte, NC 28204; **Phone:** 704-355-2884; **Board Cert:** Surgery 2005; **Med School:** UCSF 1981; **Resid:** Surgery, UCSF Med Ctr 1993; **Fellow:** Surgical Oncology, Natl Cancer Inst 1991; Surgical Oncology, Meml Sloan-Kettering Cancer Ctr 1998

Slingluff Jr, Craig L MD [S] - **Spec Exp:** Melanoma; Immunotherapy; **Hospital:** Univ Virginia Med Ctr; **Address:** UVA Health System, Dept Surgery, PO Box 800709, Charlottesville, VA 22908; **Phone:** 434-924-1730; **Board Cert:** Surgery 2002; **Med School:** Univ VA Sch Med 1984; **Resid:** Surgery, Duke Univ Med Ctr 1991; **Fellow:** Surgical Research, Duke Univ Med Ctr 1992; **Fac Appt:** Prof S, Univ VA Sch Med

Sondak, Vernon K MD [S] - **Spec Exp:** Cancer Surgery; Melanoma; Sarcoma; **Hospital:** H Lee Moffitt Cancer Ctr & Research Inst; **Address:** H Lee Moffitt Cancer Ctr-Cutaneous Program, 12902 Magnolia Drive, Tampa, FL 33612; **Phone:** 813-745-1968; **Board Cert:** Surgery 1996; **Med School:** Boston Univ 1980; **Resid:** Surgery, UCLA Med Ctr 1987; **Fellow:** Surgical Oncology, UCLA Med Ctr 1984; **Fac Appt:** Prof S, Univ S Fla Coll Med

Tyler, Douglas S MD [S] - **Spec Exp:** Pancreatic Cancer; Colon & Rectal Cancer; Rectal Cancer/Sphincter Preservation; Melanoma; **Hospital:** Duke Univ Med Ctr; **Address:** Duke University Med Ctr, Box 3118, Durham, NC 27710; **Phone:** 919-684-6858; **Board Cert:** Surgery 2000; **Med School:** Dartmouth Med Sch 1985; **Resid:** Surgery, Duke Univ Med Ctr 1992; **Fellow:** Surgical Oncology, MD Anderson Cancer Ctr 1994; **Fac Appt:** Prof S, Duke Univ

Urist, Marshall M MD [S] - **Spec Exp:** Cancer Surgery; Breast Cancer; Melanoma; **Hospital:** Univ of Ala Hosp at Birmingham; **Address:** Univ Alabama Sch Med, Dept Surgery, 1922 7th Ave S, Kracke Bldg, Ste 321, Birmingham, AL 35294; **Phone:** 205-934-3065; **Board Cert:** Surgery 2000; **Med School:** Univ Chicago-Pritzker Sch Med 1971; **Resid:** Surgery, Johns Hopkins Hosp 1978; **Fellow:** Surgical Oncology, UCLA Med Ctr 1976; **Fac Appt:** Prof S, Univ Ala

Vogel, Stephen Burton MD [S] - **Spec Exp:** Esophageal Cancer; Liver Cancer; **Hospital:** Shands Hlthcre at Univ of FL; **Address:** University of Florida, Dept Surgery, PO Box 100286, Gainesville, FL 32610-0286; **Phone:** 352-265-0604; **Board Cert:** Surgery 1976; **Med School:** Univ Fla Coll Med 1967; **Resid:** Surgery, Univ Minn Hosp 1975; **Fac Appt:** Prof S, Univ Fla Coll Med

White Jr, Richard L MD [S] - **Spec Exp:** Breast Cancer; Melanoma; Sarcoma; Immunotherapy; **Hospital:** Carolinas Med Ctr; **Address:** Carolinas Medical Center, 1000 Blythe Blvd, Box 32861, Charlotte, NC 28203; **Phone:** 704-355-2884; **Board Cert:** Surgery 2002; **Med School:** Columbia P&S 1986; **Resid:** Surgery, Georgetown Univ Hosp 1992; **Fellow:** Surgical Oncology, NIH- Natl Cancer Inst 1995; **Fac Appt:** Assoc Clin Prof S, Univ NC Sch Med

Whitworth, Pat W MD [S] - **Spec Exp:** Breast Cancer; **Hospital:** Baptist Hosp - Nashville, Centennial Med Ctr; **Address:** 300 20th Ave N, Ste 401, Nashville, TN 37203; **Phone:** 615-284-8229; **Board Cert:** Surgery 1999; **Med School:** Univ Tenn Coll Med, Memphis 1983; **Resid:** Surgery, Univ Louisville Med Ctr 1988; **Fellow:** Surgical Oncology, MD Anderson Cancer Ctr 1991; **Fac Appt:** Assoc Clin Prof S, Vanderbilt Univ

Willis, Irvin MD [S] - **Spec Exp:** Pancreatic Surgery; Cancer Surgery; Laparoscopic Surgery; **Hospital:** Mount Sinai Med Ctr - Miami; **Address:** 4302 Alton Rd, Ste 630, Miami Beach, FL 33140-2876; **Phone:** 305-534-6050; **Board Cert:** Surgery 1970; **Med School:** Univ Cincinnati 1964; **Resid:** Surgery, Univ Miami-Jackson Meml 1969

Wood, William C MD [S] - Spec Exp: Breast Cancer; **Hospital:** Emory Univ Hosp; **Address:** Emory Univ Hosp, Dept Surgery, 1364 Clifton Rd NE, Ste B206, Atlanta, GA 30322; **Phone:** 404-727-5800; **Board Cert:** Surgery 1974; **Med School:** Harvard Med Sch 1966; **Resid:** Surgery, Mass Genl Hosp 1968; Surgery, Mass Genl Hosp 1974; **Fac Appt:** Prof S, Emory Univ

Yeatman, Timothy J MD [S] - Spec Exp: Colon Cancer; Gastrointestinal Cancer; **Hospital:** H Lee Moffitt Cancer Ctr & Research Inst; **Address:** H Lee Moffitt Cancer Ctr, 12902 Magnolia Drive, Tampa, FL 33612-9497; **Phone:** 813-979-7292; **Board Cert:** Surgery 2000; **Med School:** Emory Univ 1984; **Resid:** Surgery, Univ Florida 1990; **Fellow:** Surgical Oncology, MD Anderson Cancer Ctr 1992; **Fac Appt:** Prof S, Univ S Fla Coll Med

Midwest

Angelos, Peter MD/PhD [S] - Spec Exp: Endocrine Tumors; Carcinoid Tumors; Islet Cell Tumors; Ethics; **Hospital:** Univ of Chicago Hosps; **Address:** Bernard A. Mitchell Hospital, 5841 S Maryland Ave, MC 5031, Chicago, IL 60637; **Phone:** 773-702-4429; **Board Cert:** Surgery 2004; **Med School:** Boston Univ 1989; **Resid:** Surgery, Northwestern Univ 1995; **Fellow:** Medical Ethics, Univ of Chicago-Pritzker Sch Med 1992; Endocrine Surgery, Univ of Michigan Med Sch 1996; **Fac Appt:** Prof S, Univ Chicago-Pritzker Sch Med

Aranha, Gerard MD [S] - Spec Exp: Pancreatic & Biliary Surgery; Stomach Cancer; Esophageal Cancer; **Hospital:** Loyola Univ Med Ctr, Hines VA Hosp; **Address:** Loyola Univ Med Ctr, Dept Surg, 2160 S First Ave Bldg 110 - rm 3236, Maywood, IL 60153-3328; **Phone:** 708-327-3430; **Board Cert:** Surgery 1996; **Med School:** India 1969; **Resid:** Surgery, Loyola Univ Med Ctr 1975; **Fellow:** Surgical Oncology, Univ Minn Hosp 1977; **Fac Appt:** Prof S, Loyola Univ-Stritch Sch Med

Averbook, Bruce J MD [S] - Spec Exp: Melanoma; Clinical Trials; **Hospital:** MetroHealth Med Ctr; **Address:** Metrohealth Medical Ctr, Surgical Oncology, 2500 Metrohealth Drive, Cleveland, OH 44109; **Phone:** 216-778-4795; **Board Cert:** Surgery 2000; **Med School:** Geo Wash Univ 1983; **Resid:** Surgery, UC Irvine Med Ctr 1990; **Fellow:** Surgical Oncology, NCI,NIH Surg Br 1993; **Fac Appt:** Assoc Prof S, Case West Res Univ

Blom, Dennis MD [S] - Spec Exp: Esophageal Cancer; Barrett's Esophagus; Esophageal Disorders; **Hospital:** Indiana Univ Hosp (page 70); **Address:** 545 Barnhill Drive, Emerson Hall 232, Indianapolis, IN 46202; **Phone:** 317-278-7373; **Board Cert:** Surgery 2000; **Med School:** Albany Med Coll 1992; **Resid:** Surgery, Univ Rochester 1999; **Fellow:** Gastrointestinal Surgery, Univ S California 2001; **Fac Appt:** Assoc Prof S, Indiana Univ

Brems, John MD [S] - Spec Exp: Transplant-Liver; Pancreatic Cancer; Liver Cancer; **Hospital:** Loyola Univ Med Ctr; **Address:** 2160 S 1st Ave, MC-EMS-3268, Maywood, IL 60153-3304; **Phone:** 708-327-2539; **Board Cert:** Surgery 2004; Surgical Critical Care 2000; **Med School:** St Louis Univ 1981; **Resid:** Surgery, St Louis Univ 1986; **Fellow:** Transplant Surgery, UCLA Med Ctr 1987; **Fac Appt:** Prof S, Loyola Univ-Stritch Sch Med

Brunt, L Michael MD [S] - Spec Exp: Minimally Invasive Surgery; Adrenal Tumors; **Hospital:** Barnes-Jewish Hosp; **Address:** Washington Univ Sch Medicine, Dept Surg, 660 S Euclid Ave, Box 8109, St Louis, MO 63110; **Phone:** 314-454-7194; **Board Cert:** Surgery 1996; **Med School:** Johns Hopkins Univ 1980; **Resid:** Surgery, Barnes Jewish Hosp 1987; **Fellow:** Surgery, Barnes Jewish Hosp 1984; **Fac Appt:** Prof S, Washington Univ, St Louis

Chang, Alfred E MD [S] - **Spec Exp:** Breast Cancer; Gastrointestinal Cancer; Melanoma; Sarcoma; **Hospital:** Univ Michigan Hlth Sys; **Address:** Univ Mich Comp Cancer Ctr/Geriatric Ctr, 1500 E Med Ctr Dr 3302 CGC, Ann Arbor, MI 48109-0932; **Phone:** 734-936-4392; **Board Cert:** Surgery 2001; **Med School:** Harvard Med Sch 1974; **Resid:** Surgery, Duke Univ Med Ctr 1976; Surgery, Hosp Univ Penn 1982; **Fellow:** Surgical Oncology, Natl Cancer Inst 1979; **Fac Appt:** Prof S, Univ Mich Med Sch

Chapman, William C MD [S] - **Spec Exp:** Transplant-Liver-Adult & Pediatric; Liver Cancer; Liver & Biliary Surgery; **Hospital:** Barnes-Jewish Hosp, St Louis Chldns Hosp; **Address:** Washington Univ Sch Med, 660 S Euclid Ave, Box 8604, St Louis, MO 63110; **Phone:** 314-362-7792; **Board Cert:** Surgery 2001; Surgical Critical Care 2001; **Med School:** Med Univ SC 1984; **Resid:** Surgery, Vanderbilt Univ Med Ctr 1991; **Fellow:** Hepatobiliary Surgery, Kings College Hosp 1992; **Fac Appt:** Prof S, Washington Univ, St Louis

Crowe Jr, Joseph P MD [S] - **Spec Exp:** Breast Cancer; Tumor Surgery; **Hospital:** Cleveland Clin Fdn (page 71); **Address:** Cleveland Clinic Fdn, Dept Surg, 9500 Euclid Ave, Desk A10, Cleveland, OH 44195; **Phone:** 216-444-3024; **Board Cert:** Surgery 2004; **Med School:** Case West Res Univ 1978; **Resid:** Surgery, Univ Hosp-Case West Reserve 1983; **Fellow:** Surgical Oncology, Meml Sloan Kettering Cancer Ctr 1985

Donohue, John H MD [S] - **Spec Exp:** Gastrointestinal Cancer; Breast Cancer; Stomach Cancer; **Hospital:** Mayo Med Ctr & Clin - Rochester; **Address:** Mayo Clinic, Dept Surgery, 200 First St SW, Rochester, MN 55905; **Phone:** 507-284-0362; **Board Cert:** Surgery 2005; **Med School:** Harvard Med Sch 1978; **Resid:** Surgery, UCSF Med Ctr 1981; Surgery, UCSF Med Ctr 1985; **Fellow:** Surgery, Natl Inst Hlth 1983; Surgical Oncology, Meml Sloan-Kettering Canc Ctr 1987; **Fac Appt:** Prof S, Mayo Med Sch

Eberlein, Timothy J MD [S] - **Spec Exp:** Breast Cancer; Melanoma; Immunotherapy; **Hospital:** Barnes-Jewish Hosp, St Louis Chldns Hosp; **Address:** Wash Univ School of Med, Dept Surgery, 660 S Euclid Ave, Box 8109, St Louis, MO 63110-1093; **Phone:** 314-362-8020; **Board Cert:** Surgery 1995; **Med School:** Univ Pittsburgh 1977; **Resid:** Surgery, Peter Bent Brigham Hosp 1979; Surgery, Brigham-Womens Hosp 1985; **Fellow:** Allergy & Immunology, Natl Inst Hlth 1982; **Fac Appt:** Prof S, Washington Univ, St Louis

Ellison, E Christopher MD [S] - **Spec Exp:** Biliary Cancer; Pancreatic Cancer; **Hospital:** Ohio St Univ Med Ctr; **Address:** 1654 Upham Drive, Ste 327 Means Hall, Columbus, OH 43210-1236; **Phone:** 614-293-9722; **Board Cert:** Surgery 2001; **Med School:** Univ Wisc 1975; **Resid:** Surgery, Ohio State Univ 1981; **Fac Appt:** Prof S, Ohio State Univ

Farrar, William B MD [S] - **Spec Exp:** Breast Cancer; Thyroid Cancer; **Hospital:** Arthur G James Cancer Hosp & Research Inst, Ohio St Univ Med Ctr; **Address:** 410 W 10th Ave, N924 Doan Hall, Columbus, OH 43210-1240; **Phone:** 614-293-8890; **Board Cert:** Surgery 2000; **Med School:** Univ VA Sch Med 1975; **Resid:** Surgery, Ohio State Univ Hosps 1980; **Fellow:** Surgical Oncology, Meml Sloan-Kettering Cancer Ctr 1982; **Fac Appt:** Prof S, Ohio State Univ

Fung, John J MD/PhD [S] - **Spec Exp:** Transplant-Liver; Transplant-Kidney; Liver & Biliary Cancer; **Hospital:** Cleveland Clin Fdn (page 71), Euclid Hosp (page 71); **Address:** Cleveland Clinic, Dept Surgery, Desk A80, 9500 Euclid Ave, Cleveland, OH 44195-0001; **Phone:** 216-444-3776; **Board Cert:** Surgery 1997; **Med School:** Univ Chicago-Pritzker Sch Med 1982; **Resid:** Surgery, Strong Memorial Hosp 1988; **Fellow:** Transplant Surgery, Univ Pittsburgh 1986; **Fac Appt:** Prof S, Cleveland Cl Coll Med/Case West Res

Goulet Jr, Robert J MD [S] - Spec Exp: Breast Cancer; **Hospital:** Indiana Univ Hosp (page 70); **Address:** Indiana Univ Hosp, Cancer Pavilion, 535 Barnhill Drive, Ste 431, Indianapolis, IN 46202-5112; **Phone:** 317-274-9800; **Board Cert:** Surgery 1995; **Med School:** SUNY Downstate 1979; **Resid:** Surgery, SUNY-Downstate Med Ctr 1986; **Fellow:** Surgical Research, SUNY-Downstate Med Ctr 1983; **Fac Appt:** Assoc Prof S, Indiana Univ

Grant, Clive S MD [S] - Spec Exp: Thyroid & Parathyroid Cancer & Surgery; Adrenal Tumors; Breast Cancer; **Hospital:** Mayo Med Ctr & Clin - Rochester; **Address:** Mayo Clinic, Dept Surgery, 200 First St SW, Rochester, MN 55905-0001; **Phone:** 507-284-2644; **Board Cert:** Surgery 2001; **Med School:** Univ Colorado 1975; **Resid:** Surgery, Mayo Clinic 1980; **Fac Appt:** Prof S, Mayo Med Sch

Harkema, James M MD [S] - Spec Exp: Breast Cancer; Thyroid Cancer; Parathyroid Cancer; **Hospital:** Mich State Univ-Sparrow Hos, Ingham Regl Med Ctr- Greenlawn Campus; **Address:** Sparrow Professional Bldg, 1200 E Michigan Ave, Ste 655, Lansing, MI 48912; **Phone:** 517-267-2461; **Board Cert:** Surgery 1975; **Med School:** Univ Mich Med Sch 1968; **Resid:** Surgery, Univ Mich Hosp 1974; **Fac Appt:** Prof S, Mich State Univ

Hinshaw, Daniel B MD [S] - Spec Exp: Palliative Care; **Hospital:** VA Med Ctr - Ann Arbor, Univ Michigan Hlth Sys; **Address:** VA Medical Ctr, 2215 Fuller Rd, rm 530, MS 112, Ann Arbor, MI 48105; **Phone:** 734-769-7100 x5939; **Board Cert:** Surgery 2003; **Med School:** Loma Linda Univ 1978; **Resid:** Surgery, Loma Linda U Med Ctr 1983; **Fellow:** Immunology, Scripps Clinic Rsch Fdn 1985; Cleveland Clinic 2001; **Fac Appt:** Clin Prof S, Univ Mich Med Sch

Howe, James MD [S] - Spec Exp: Endocrine Surgery; Gastrointestinal Cancer; Colon & Rectal Cancer; **Hospital:** Univ Iowa Hosp & Clinics; **Address:** Univ Iowa, Dept Surgery, 200 Hawkins Drive, 1504 John Colloton Pavilion, Iowa City, IA 52242-1086; **Phone:** 319-356-1727; **Board Cert:** Surgery 1995; **Med School:** Univ VT Coll Med 1987; **Resid:** Surgery, Barnes Hosp-Wash Univ 1994; **Fellow:** Research, Wash Univ-NCI 1991; Surgical Oncology, Meml Sloan Kettering Cancer Ctr 1996; **Fac Appt:** Prof S, Univ Iowa Coll Med

Kim, Julian A MD [S] - Spec Exp: Melanoma; Breast Cancer; Gastrointestinal Cancer; Immunotherapy; **Hospital:** Univ Hosps Case Med Ctr; **Address:** Univ Hosps of Cleveland, LKS 5047, 11100 Euclid Ave, Cleveland, OH 44106; **Phone:** 216-844-8247; **Board Cert:** Surgery 2002; **Med School:** Med Univ Ohio at Toledo 1986; **Resid:** Surgery, Univ Maryland Hosps 1991; **Fellow:** Surgical Oncology, Arthur James Cancer Hosp & Rsch Inst 1993; Immunotherapy, Ohio State Univ Comp Cancer Ctr 1994; **Fac Appt:** Assoc Prof S, Case West Res Univ

Kraybill Jr, William G MD [S] - Spec Exp: Sarcoma-Soft Tissue; Melanoma; Skin Cancer-Advanced; **Hospital:** St Luke's Hosp of Kansas City; **Address:** Medical Director of Surgical Services, St Luke's Cancer Inst, 4320 Wornall Rd, Ste 420, Kansas City, MO 64111; **Phone:** 816-932-1601; **Board Cert:** Surgery 2005; **Med School:** Univ Cincinnati 1969; **Resid:** Surgery, Univ Oregon Hlth Sci Ctr 1978; **Fellow:** Surgical Oncology, Meml Sloan Kettering Cancer Ctr 1980; **Fac Appt:** Prof S, SUNY Buffalo

Leeming, Rosemary A MD [S] - Spec Exp: Breast Cancer & Surgery; Breast Disease; Clinical Trials; **Hospital:** Univ Hosps Case Med Ctr; **Address:** UH Chagrin Highlands Hlth Ctr, 3909 Orange Pl, Orange Village, OH 44122; **Phone:** 216-591-1909; **Board Cert:** Surgery 2000; **Med School:** Hahnemann Univ 1983; **Resid:** Surgery, Mt Sinai Med Ctr 1989; **Fellow:** Breast Disease, Univ Pitts-Shadyside Hosp 1989; **Fac Appt:** Asst Prof S, Case West Res Univ

Lillemoe, Keith D MD [S] - **Spec Exp:** Pancreatic Cancer; Colon Cancer; Pancreatic & Biliary Surgery; **Hospital:** Indiana Univ Hosp (page 70); **Address:** Indiana Univ, Dept Surgery, 545 Barnhill Drive, EH 203, Indianapolis, IN 46202-5112; **Phone:** 317-274-5707; **Board Cert:** Surgery 1995; **Med School:** Johns Hopkins Univ 1978; **Resid:** Surgery, Johns Hopkins Hosp 1985; **Fac Appt:** Prof S, Indiana Univ

Mamounas, Eleftherios P MD [S] - **Spec Exp:** Breast Cancer; **Hospital:** Aultman Hosp; **Address:** Aultman Cancer Ctr, 2600 6th St SW, Main 1, Clinical Trials Dept, Canton, OH 44710; **Phone:** 330-363-6281; **Board Cert:** Surgery 1999; **Med School:** Greece 1983; **Resid:** Surgery, McKeesport Hosp 1989; **Fellow:** Clinical Oncology, Univ Pittsburgh 1991; Surgical Oncology, Roswell Park Cancer Inst 1992; **Fac Appt:** Asst Clin Prof S, Case West Res Univ

Melvin, W Scott MD [S] - **Spec Exp:** Liver & Biliary Surgery; Pancreatic Cancer; Laparoscopic Surgery; **Hospital:** Ohio St Univ Med Ctr; **Address:** 410 W 10th Ave, Ste N729 Doan Hall, Columbus, OH 43210; **Phone:** 614-293-4499; **Board Cert:** Surgery 1993; **Med School:** Med Coll OH 1987; **Resid:** Surgery, Univ Maryland 1992; **Fellow:** Gastrointestinal Surgery, Grant Med Ctr 1993; **Fac Appt:** Prof S, Ohio State Univ

Merrick III, Hollis W MD [S] - **Spec Exp:** Cancer Surgery; **Hospital:** Univ of Toledo Med Ctr; **Address:** 3065 Arlington Ave, Toledo, OH 43614-2570; **Phone:** 419-383-4421; **Board Cert:** Surgery 1997; **Med School:** McGill Univ 1964; **Resid:** Surgery, Royal Victoria Hosp 1972; **Fac Appt:** Prof S, Med Coll OH

Millis, J Michael MD [S] - **Spec Exp:** Transplant-Liver-Adult & Pediatric; Liver Cancer; Transplant-Pancreas; **Hospital:** Univ of Chicago Hosps; **Address:** Univ Chicago, Dept Surgery, 5841 S Maryland Ave, MC 5027, Chiciago, IL 60637; **Phone:** 773-702-6319; **Board Cert:** Surgery 2001; Surgical Critical Care 2001; **Med School:** Univ Tenn Coll Med, Memphis 1985; **Resid:** Surgery, UCLA Med Ctr 1992; **Fellow:** Transplant Surgery, UCLA Med Ctr 1994; **Fac Appt:** Prof S, Univ Chicago-Pritzker Sch Med

Moley, Jeffrey F MD [S] - **Spec Exp:** Thyroid Cancer & Surgery; Endocrine Cancers; Melanoma; **Hospital:** Barnes-Jewish Hosp; **Address:** Washington Univ School Med, Dept Surgery, 660 S Euclid Ave, Box 8109, St. Louis, MO 63110; **Phone:** 314-362-2280; **Board Cert:** Surgery 1998; **Med School:** Columbia P&S 1980; **Resid:** Surgery, Yale-New Haven Hosp 1985; **Fellow:** Surgical Oncology, National Cancer Inst 1987; **Fac Appt:** Prof S, Washington Univ, St Louis

Nagorney, David M MD [S] - **Spec Exp:** Pancreatic Cancer; Hepatobiliary Surgery; Gastrointestinal Cancer; **Hospital:** Mayo Med Ctr & Clin - Rochester; **Address:** Mayo Clinic, Dept Surgery, 200 1st St SW, Mayo E12, Rochester, MN 55905; **Phone:** 507-284-2644; **Board Cert:** Surgery 2001; **Med School:** Univ Kans 1975; **Resid:** Surgery, Mayo Clinic 1982; **Fellow:** Hepatobiliary Surgery, Hammersmith Hosp 1985; **Fac Appt:** Prof S, Mayo Med Sch

Nathanson, S David MD [S] - **Spec Exp:** Breast Cancer; Breast Cancer Risk Assessment; Melanoma; Sarcoma; **Hospital:** Henry Ford Hosp; **Address:** 2799 W Grand Blvd, Detroit, MI 48202; **Phone:** 313-916-2917; **Board Cert:** Surgery 2002; **Med School:** South Africa 1966; **Resid:** Surgery, Univ Witwaterstrand 1974; Surgical Oncology, UCLA Med Ctr 1980; **Fellow:** Surgery, UC Davis 1982; **Fac Appt:** Prof S, Case West Res Univ

Newman, Lisa A MD [S] - **Spec Exp:** Breast Cancer; **Hospital:** Univ Michigan Hlth Sys; **Address:** Univ Michigan Cancer Center, 1500 E Medical Center Drive, rm 3308-CGC, Ann Arbor, MI 48109; **Phone:** 734-936-8771; **Board Cert:** Surgery 2001; **Med School:** SUNY Downstate 1985; **Resid:** Surgery, Downstate Med Ctr 1990; **Fac Appt:** Assoc Prof S, Univ Mich Med Sch

Onders, Raymond P MD [S] - **Spec Exp:** Laparoscopic Surgery; Gastrointestinal Cancer; **Hospital:** Univ Hosps Case Med Ctr; **Address:** University Hosps Cleveland, 11100 Euclid Ave, LKS 5047, Cleveland, OH 44106; **Phone:** 216-844-5797; **Board Cert:** Surgery 2001; **Med School:** NE Ohio Univ 1988; **Resid:** Surgery, Case Western Reserve Univ 1993; **Fac Appt:** Asst Prof S, Case West Res Univ

Posner, Mitchell C MD [S] - **Spec Exp:** Pancreatic Cancer; Gastrointestinal Cancer; Esophageal Cancer; **Hospital:** Univ of Chicago Hosps; **Address:** Univ of Chicago Hospitals, 5841 S Maryland Ave, Ste G209, MC 5094, Chicago, IL 60637; **Phone:** 773-834-0156; **Board Cert:** Surgery 1997; **Med School:** SUNY Buffalo 1981; **Resid:** Surgery, Univ Colorado Sch Med 1986; **Fellow:** Surgical Oncology, Meml Sloan Kettering 1988; **Fac Appt:** Prof S, Univ Chicago-Pritzker Sch Med

Rikkers, Layton F MD [S] - **Spec Exp:** Pancreatic Cancer; Liver & Biliary Cancer; **Hospital:** Univ WI Hosp & Clins; **Address:** 600 Highland Ave, rm H4-710D, Madison, WI 53792; **Phone:** 608-265-8854; **Board Cert:** Surgery 1996; **Med School:** Stanford Univ 1970; **Resid:** Surgery, Univ Utah Hosp 1973; Surgery, Univ Utah Hosp 1976; **Fellow:** Hepatology, Royal Free Hosp 1974; **Fac Appt:** Prof S, Univ Wisc

Saha, Sukamal MD [S] - **Spec Exp:** Sentinel Node Surgery; Colon Cancer; Head & Neck Cancer & Surgery; **Hospital:** McLaren Reg Med Ctr, Genesys Reg Med Ctr - St Joseph Campus; **Address:** 3500 Calkins Rd, Ste A, Flint, MI 48532; **Phone:** 810-230-9600 x500; **Board Cert:** Surgery 2000; **Med School:** India 1977; **Resid:** Surgery, Hahnemann Univ Hosp 1985; Surgery, Easton Hosp 1987; **Fellow:** Surgical Oncology, Tulane Univ Med Ctr 1989; Head and Neck Surgery, Roswell Park Meml Hosp; **Fac Appt:** Asst Prof S, Mich State Univ

Sarr, Michael G MD [S] - **Spec Exp:** Pancreatic Cancer; Gastrointestinal Cancer; **Hospital:** Mayo Med Ctr & Clin - Rochester; **Address:** Mayo Clinic, Dept Surg, Desk West 6, Rochester, MN 55905; **Phone:** 507-284-2644; **Board Cert:** Surgery 2001; **Med School:** Johns Hopkins Univ 1976; **Resid:** Surgery, Johns Hopkins Hosp 1982; **Fellow:** Surgery, Mayo Clinic 1984; Surgery, Johns Hopkins Hosp 1985; **Fac Appt:** Prof S, Mayo Med Sch

Schwartzentruber, Douglas J MD [S] **Spec Exp:** Cancer Surgery; Melanoma; Kidney Cancer; **Hospital:** Goshen Genl Hosp; **Address:** Cancer Ctr at Goshen Health System, 200 High Park Ave, Goshen, IN 46526; **Phone:** 574-535-2888; **Board Cert:** Surgery 1997; **Med School:** Indiana Univ 1982; **Resid:** Surgery, Indiana Univ Med Ctr 1987; **Fellow:** Surgical Oncology, Natl Cancer Inst 1990; **Fac Appt:** Assoc Clin Prof S, Indiana Univ

Scott-Conner, Carol E.H. MD/PhD [S] - **Spec Exp:** Breast Cancer; Cancer Surgery; Laparoscopic Surgery; **Hospital:** Univ Iowa Hosp & Clinics, VA Med Ctr - Iowa City; **Address:** Univ Iowa, Dept Surg, 200 Hawkins Drive, rm 4601-JCP, Iowa City, IA 52242-1086; **Phone:** 319-356-0330; **Board Cert:** Surgery 2000; Surgical Critical Care 1998; **Med School:** NYU Sch Med 1976; **Resid:** Surgery, NYU Med Ctr 1981; **Fac Appt:** Prof S, Univ Iowa Coll Med

Sener, Stephen MD [S] - **Spec Exp:** Breast Cancer; Pancreatic Cancer; Lymphedema; **Hospital:** Evanston Hosp; **Address:** 2650 Ridge Ave Walgreen, rm 2507, Dept of Surgery, Evanston, IL 60201-1718; **Phone:** 847-570-1328; **Board Cert:** Surgery 2001; **Med School:** Northwestern Univ 1977; **Resid:** Surgery, Northwestern Univ 1982; **Fellow:** Surgery, Meml Sloan Kettering Cancer Ctr 1984; **Fac Appt:** Prof S, Northwestern Univ

Shenk, Robert R MD [S] - **Spec Exp:** Breast Cancer; Melanoma; Pancreatic Cancer; Stomach Cancer; **Hospital:** Univ Hosps Case Med Ctr; **Address:** Univ Hosp Case Med Ctr, 11100 Euclid Ave, Cleveland, OH 44106; **Phone:** 216-844-3026; **Board Cert:** Surgery 2004; **Med School:** Case West Res Univ 1978; **Resid:** Surgery, Univ Hosp 1985; Immunology, Natl Cancer Inst 1982; **Fellow:** Surgical Oncology, Anderson Hosp 1987; **Fac Appt:** Assoc Prof S, Case West Res Univ

Sielaff, Timothy D MD/PhD [S] - **Spec Exp:** Liver Cancer; Pancreatic Cancer; Gallbladder & Biliary Cancer; **Hospital:** Abbott - Northwestern Hosp; **Address:** Virginia Piper Cancer Inst, Liver and Pancreas Clinic, 800 E 28th St, Minneapolis, MN 55407; **Phone:** 612-863-7553; **Board Cert:** Surgery 1998; **Med School:** Med Coll VA 1989; **Resid:** Surgery, Univ Minn Hosps 1997; **Fellow:** Transplant Surgery, Univ Toronto 1998; **Fac Appt:** Assoc Prof S, Univ Minn

Siperstein, Allan E MD [S] - **Spec Exp:** Laparoscopic Surgery; Endocrine Tumors; Thyroid & Parathyroid Cancer & Surgery; **Hospital:** Cleveland Clin Fdn (page 71); **Address:** Cleveland Clinic Fdn, Dept Genl Surg, 9500 Euclid Ave, Desk A80, Cleveland, OH 44195; **Phone:** 216-444-5664; **Board Cert:** Surgery 1997; **Med School:** Univ Tex SW, Dallas 1983; **Resid:** Surgery, UCSF Med Ctr 1990; **Fellow:** Research, UCSF Med Ctr 1988

Staren, Edgar MD/PhD [S] - **Spec Exp:** Breast Cancer; Endocrine Cancers; Liver Cancer; **Hospital:** Cancer Treatment Ctrs of Amer-Midwest Reg Med Ctr; **Address:** Cancer Treatment Centers of America, 2610 Sheridan Rd, Zion, IL 60099; **Phone:** 847-731-5805; **Board Cert:** Surgery 1996; **Med School:** Loyola Univ-Stritch Sch Med 1982; **Resid:** Surgery, Rush-Presby-St Lukes Med Ctr 1987; **Fellow:** Surgical Oncology, Rush-Presby-St Lukes Med Ctr 1988

Strasberg, Steven M MD [S] - **Spec Exp:** Liver & Biliary Cancer; Pancreatic Cancer; Gastrointestinal Cancer; **Hospital:** Barnes-Jewish Hosp; **Address:** Washington University School of Medicine, Dept Surgery, 660 S Euclid Ave, Box 8109, Saint Louis, MO 63110; **Phone:** 314-362-7147; **Board Cert:** Surgery 2005; **Med School:** Canada 1963; **Resid:** Surgery, Toronto General Hosp 1969; **Fellow:** Surgical Research, Toronto General Hosp 1971; **Fac Appt:** Prof S, Washington Univ, St Louis

Talamonti, Mark S MD [S] - **Spec Exp:** Pancreatic Cancer; Liver Cancer; Gastrointestinal Cancer & Surgery; Melanoma; **Hospital:** Northwestern Meml Hosp; **Address:** Northwestern University Hosp, 675 N St Clair Fl 21, Chicago, IL 60611; **Phone:** 312-695-0990; **Board Cert:** Surgery 1999; **Med School:** Northwestern Univ 1983; **Resid:** Surgery, Northwestern Meml Hosp 1989; **Fellow:** Surgical Oncology, MD Anderson Cancer Ctr 1991; **Fac Appt:** Assoc Prof S, Northwestern Univ

Tuttle, Todd M MD [S] - **Spec Exp:** Breast Cancer; Minimally Invasive Surgery; Cancer Surgery; **Hospital:** Univ Minn Med Ctr, Fairview - Univ Campus, Univ Minn Med Ctr, Fairview - Riverside Campus; **Address:** Univ Minn, Dept Surgery, 420 Delaware St SE, MMC 195, Minneapolis, MN 55455; **Phone:** 612-625-2991; **Board Cert:** Surgery 1995; **Med School:** Johns Hopkins Univ 1988; **Resid:** Surgery, Med Coll Virginia Hosps 1994; **Fellow:** Surgical Oncology, MD Anderson Cancer Ctr 1996; **Fac Appt:** Assoc Prof S

Vickers, Selwyn M MD [S] - Spec Exp: Pancreatic Cancer; Liver Tumors; Gastrointestinal Surgery; **Hospital:** Univ Minn Med Ctr, Fairview - Univ Campus; **Address:** University of Minnesota, 420 Delaware St SE, Phillips Wangensteen Bldg, MMC 195, Minneapolis, MN 55455; **Phone:** 612-625-5411; **Board Cert:** Surgery 2003; **Med School:** Johns Hopkins Univ 1986; **Resid:** Surgery, Johns Hopkins Hosp 1992; **Fac Appt:** Prof S, Johns Hopkins Univ

Walker, Alonzo P MD [S] - Spec Exp: Breast Cancer; **Hospital:** Froedtert Meml Lutheran Hosp; **Address:** Dept Surgery, 9200 W Wisconsin Ave, Milwaukee, WI 53226-3522; **Phone:** 414-805-5737; **Board Cert:** Surgery 2004; **Med School:** Univ Fla Coll Med 1976; **Resid:** Surgery, Univ Maryland Hosps 1983; **Fac Appt:** Prof S, Med Coll Wisc

Walsh, R Matthew MD [S] - Spec Exp: Pancreatic Cancer; Gastrointestinal Surgery; Hepatobiliary Surgery; **Hospital:** Cleveland Clin Fdn (page 71); **Address:** Cleveland Clinic, Dept Surgery, Desk A80, 9500 Euclid Ave, Cleveland, OH 44195; **Phone:** 216-445-7576; **Board Cert:** Surgery 1999; **Med School:** Med Coll Wisc 1985; **Resid:** Surgery, Loyola Univ Hosp 1990; **Fellow:** Endoscopy, Mass General Hosp 1991; Hepatopancreatobiliary Surgery, Cleveland Clinic; **Fac Appt:** Assoc Prof S, Cleveland Cl Coll Med/Case West Res

Weigel, Ronald J MD/PhD [S] - Spec Exp: Breast Cancer; Endocrine Surgery; **Hospital:** Univ Iowa Hosp & Clinics; **Address:** Univ Iowa Carver Coll Med - Dept Surgery, 200 Hawkins Drive, 1516 JCP, Iowa City, IA 52242-1086; **Phone:** 319-356-4200; **Board Cert:** Surgery 2001; **Med School:** Yale Univ 1986; **Resid:** Surgery, Duke Univ Med Ctr 1992; **Fellow:** Immunology, Duke Univ Med Ctr; **Fac Appt:** Prof S, Univ Iowa Coll Med

Witt, Thomas MD [S] - Spec Exp: Breast Cancer; Breast Disease; **Hospital:** Rush Univ Med Ctr, Glenbrook Hosp; **Address:** 1725 W Harrison St, Ste 409, Chicago, IL 60612-3828; **Phone:** 312-942-2302; **Board Cert:** Surgery 2000; **Med School:** Northwestern Univ 1975; **Resid:** Surgery, Rush Presby-St Lukes Med Ctr 1980; **Fellow:** Surgical Oncology, Meml Sloan Kettering Cancer Ctr 1982; **Fac Appt:** Assoc Prof S, Rush Med Coll

Great Plains and Mountains

Edney, James A MD [S] - Spec Exp: Breast Cancer; Thyroid & Parathyroid Cancer & Surgery; Cancer Surgery; **Hospital:** Nebraska Med Ctr; **Address:** Univ Nebraska Med Ctr, Dept Surgery, 984030 Nebraska Medical Ctr, Omaha, NE 68198-4030; **Phone:** 402-559-7272; **Board Cert:** Surgery 2001; **Med School:** Univ Nebr Coll Med 1975; **Resid:** Surgery, Univ Nebraska Med Ctr 1980; **Fellow:** Surgical Oncology, Univ Colorado Med Ctr 1981; **Fac Appt:** Prof S, Univ Nebr Coll Med

Mulvihill, Sean J MD [S] - Spec Exp: Gastrointestinal Surgery; Liver & Biliary Cancer; Pancreatic Cancer; **Hospital:** Univ Utah Hosps and Clins; **Address:** Univ Utah, Dept Surgery, 30 N 1900 E, rm 3B110, Salt Lake City, UT 84132; **Phone:** 801-581-7304; **Board Cert:** Surgery 1999; **Med School:** USC Sch Med 1981; **Resid:** Surgery, UCLA Med Ctr 1987; **Fac Appt:** Prof S, Univ Utah

Nelson, Edward W MD [S] - Spec Exp: Breast Cancer; **Hospital:** Univ Utah Hosps and Clins; **Address:** University Utah Medical Ctr, Dept Surgery, 50 N Medical Drive, Salt Lake City, UT 84132; **Phone:** 801-581-7738; **Board Cert:** Surgery 1999; **Med School:** Univ Utah 1974; **Resid:** Surgery, Univ Utah Medical Ctr 1979; **Fac Appt:** Prof S, Univ Utah

Pearlman, Nathan W MD [S] - **Spec Exp:** Gastrointestinal Cancer; Melanoma; Head & Neck Cancer; **Hospital:** Univ Colorado Hosp; **Address:** C313, University Hosp, 4200 E 9th Ave, Denver, CO 80262; **Phone:** 720-848-0168; **Board Cert:** Surgery 1974; **Med School:** Univ IL Coll Med 1966; **Resid:** Surgery, Univ Colorado Med Ctr 1973; **Fellow:** Surgical Oncology, Sloan-Kettering Cancer Ctr 1975; **Fac Appt:** Prof S, Univ Colorado

Sasson, Aaron R MD [S] - **Spec Exp:** Gastrointestinal Cancer; Pancreatic Cancer; Liver Cancer; Biliary Cancer; **Hospital:** Nebraska Med Ctr; **Address:** Univ Nebraska Med Ctr, Box 984030, Omaha, NE 68198-0001; **Phone:** 402-559-8941; **Board Cert:** Surgery 2000; **Med School:** UMDNJ-NJ Med Sch, Newark 1993; **Resid:** Surgery, Univ California-San Diego Med Ctr 1999; **Fellow:** Surgical Oncology, Fox Chase Cancer Ctr 2001; **Fac Appt:** Assoc Prof S, Univ Nebr Coll Med

Southwest

Ames, Frederick C MD [S] - **Spec Exp:** Breast Cancer; **Hospital:** UT MD Anderson Cancer Ctr (page 81); **Address:** MD Anderson Cancer Ctr, Dept Surgery, 1515 Holcombe Blvd, Unit 444, Houston, TX 77030-4009; **Phone:** 713-792-6929; **Board Cert:** Surgery 1975; **Med School:** Univ Tex Med Br, Galveston 1969; **Resid:** Surgery, St Joseph Hosp 1974; **Fellow:** Surgical Oncology, MD Anderson Cancer Ctr 1975; **Fac Appt:** Prof S, Univ Tex, Houston

Beitsch, Peter D MD [S] - **Spec Exp:** Breast Cancer; **Hospital:** Med City Dallas Hosp, Presby Hosp of Dallas; **Address:** 5920 Forrest Park Rd, Ste 500, Dallas, TX 75235; **Phone:** 214-956-6802; **Board Cert:** Surgery 2002; **Med School:** Univ Tex SW, Dallas 1986; **Resid:** Surgery, Univ TX SW Med Ctr 1993; **Fellow:** Surgical Oncology, MD Anderson Cancer Ctr 1990; Surgical Oncology, John Wayne Cancer Inst 1994

Brunicardi, F Charles MD [S] - **Spec Exp:** Pancreatic Cancer; **Hospital:** St Luke's Episcopal Hosp - Houston; **Address:** 1709 Dryden, Ste 1500, Houston, TX 77030; **Phone:** 713-798-8070; **Board Cert:** Surgery 1998; **Med School:** UMDNJ-Rutgers Med Sch 1980; **Resid:** Surgery, SUNY Brooklyn Hlth Sci Ctr 1989; **Fellow:** Pancreatic Physiology, SUNY Brooklyn Hlth Sci Ctr 1986; **Fac Appt:** Prof S, Baylor Coll Med

Curley, Steven A MD [S] - **Spec Exp:** Colon & Rectal Cancer; Liver Cancer; Hepatobiliary Surgery; **Hospital:** UT MD Anderson Cancer Ctr (page 81); **Address:** MD Anderson Cancer Ctr, Dept Surg Oncology, Unit 444, PO Box 301402, Houston, TX 77230-1402; **Phone:** 713-794-4957; **Board Cert:** Surgery 1997; **Med School:** Univ Tex, Houston 1982; **Resid:** Surgery, Univ New Mexico Hosps 1988; **Fellow:** Surgical Oncology, MD Anderson Cancer Ctr 1990; **Fac Appt:** Prof S, Univ Tex, Houston

Dooley, William C MD [S] - **Spec Exp:** Breast Cancer; Tumors-Rare & Multiple; **Hospital:** OU Med Ctr, VA Med Ctr - Oklahoma City; **Address:** 825 NE 10th St, Ste 5200, Oklahoma City, OK 73104; **Phone:** 405-271-7867; **Board Cert:** Surgery 1997; **Med School:** Vanderbilt Univ 1982; **Resid:** Surgical Oncology, Oxford Univ 1986; Surgery, Johns Hopkins Hosp 1987; **Fellow:** Surgical Oncology, Johns Hopkins 1988; **Fac Appt:** Prof S, Univ Okla Coll Med

Edwards, Michael J MD [S] - **Spec Exp:** Breast Cancer; Melanoma; **Hospital:** UAMS Med Ctr; **Address:** 4301 W Markham St Slot 520, Shorey Bldg - Ste S706, Little Rock, AR 72205; **Phone:** 501-686-7874; **Board Cert:** Surgery 1996; **Med School:** Emory Univ 1981; **Resid:** Surgery, Univ Louisville Hosp 1986; **Fellow:** Surgical Oncology, MD Anderson Cancer Ctr 1987; **Fac Appt:** Prof S, Univ Ark

Ellis, Lee M MD [S] - **Spec Exp:** Liver Cancer; Colon & Rectal Cancer; Metastatic Cancer; **Hospital:** UT MD Anderson Cancer Ctr (page 81); **Address:** MD Anderson Cancer Ctr, Dept Surgery, 1515 Holcombe Blvd, Box 444, Houston, TX 77030; **Phone:** 713-792-6926; **Board Cert:** Surgery 1999; **Med School:** Univ VA Sch Med 1983; **Resid:** Surgery, Univ Fla-Shands Hosp 1990; **Fellow:** Surgical Oncology, MD Anderson Cancer Ctr 1992; **Fac Appt:** Prof S, Univ Tex, Houston

Euhus, David M MD [S] - **Spec Exp:** Breast Cancer; **Hospital:** UT Southwestern Med Ctr - Dallas; **Address:** Univ Texas SW Med Ctr - Div Surg Oncology, 5323 Harry Hines Blvd, Dallas, TX 75390-9155; **Phone:** 214-648-6467; **Board Cert:** Surgery 2001; **Med School:** St Louis Univ 1984; **Resid:** Surgery, UCLA Med Ctr 1991; **Fellow:** Surgical Oncology, UCLA Med Ctr 1988; Breast Disease, Queens Med Ctr 1990; **Fac Appt:** Assoc Prof S, Univ Tex SW, Dallas

Evans, Douglas B MD [S] - **Spec Exp:** Pancreatic Cancer; Thyroid Cancer; Endocrine Cancers; **Hospital:** UT MD Anderson Cancer Ctr (page 81); **Address:** Dept Surgery/Oncology, Unit 444, P.O. Box 301402, Houston, TX 77030-4095; **Phone:** 713-794-4324; **Board Cert:** Surgery 1996; **Med School:** Boston Univ 1983; **Resid:** Surgery, Dartmouth-Hitchcock Med Ctr 1988; **Fellow:** Surgical Oncology, MD Anderson Cancer Ctr 1990; **Fac Appt:** Prof S, Univ Tex, Houston

Feig, Barry W MD [S] - **Spec Exp:** Gastrointestinal Cancer; Sarcoma; Breast Cancer; **Hospital:** UT MD Anderson Cancer Ctr (page 81); **Address:** UT MD Anderson Cancer Ctr, Dept Surg Onc, Unit 444, PO Box 301402, Houston, TX 77230-1402; **Phone:** 713-794-1002; **Board Cert:** Surgery 1998; Surgical Critical Care 1996; **Med School:** SUNY Upstate Med Univ 1984; **Resid:** Surgery, Northwestern Univ Med Ctr 1990; **Fellow:** Trauma, Univ Minnesota 1991; Surgical Oncology, UT MD Anderson Cancer Ctr 1994; **Fac Appt:** Prof S, Univ Tex, Houston

Fisher, William E MD [S] - **Spec Exp:** Pancreatic Cancer; **Hospital:** St Luke's Episcopal Hosp - Houston; **Address:** Baylor College of Medicine, Dept Surgery, 1709 Dreyden, Ste 1500, Houston, TX 77030; **Phone:** 713-798-8070; **Board Cert:** Surgery 1999; **Med School:** Univ Cincinnati 1990; **Resid:** Surgery, Ohio State U Hosps 1996; **Fellow:** Cancer Research, Ohio State U Hosps 1998; **Fac Appt:** Asst Prof S, Baylor Coll Med

Grant, Michael D MD [S] - **Spec Exp:** Breast Cancer; **Hospital:** Baylor Univ Medical Ctr; **Address:** 3409 Worth St, Ste 300, Sammons Tower, Dallas, TX 75246; **Phone:** 214-826-7300; **Board Cert:** Surgery 2001; **Med School:** Univ Tex, Houston 1987; **Resid:** Surgery, Baylor Univ Med Ctr 1992; **Fellow:** Breast Cancer, Baylor Univ Med Ctr 1993

Hunt, Kelly K MD [S] - **Spec Exp:** Breast Cancer; Sarcoma-Soft Tissue; Gene Therapy; **Hospital:** UT MD Anderson Cancer Ctr (page 81); **Address:** MD Anderson Cancer Ctr, 1515 Holcombe Blvd, Box 444, Houston, TX 77030; **Phone:** 713-792-7216; **Board Cert:** Surgery 2001; **Med School:** Univ Tenn Coll Med, Memphis 1986; **Resid:** Surgery, UCLA Med Ctr 1993; **Fellow:** Surgical Oncology, MD Anderson Cancer Ctr 1996; **Fac Appt:** Prof S, Univ Tex, Houston

Jackson, Gilchrist MD [S] - **Spec Exp:** Thyroid & Parathyroid Surgery; Head & Neck Cancer & Surgery; Endocrine Tumors; Gastrointestinal Cancer & Surgery; **Hospital:** St Luke's Episcopal Hosp - Houston, Woman's Hosp TX, The; **Address:** 2727 W Holcombe Blvd, MC 3, Houston, TX 77025; **Phone:** 713-442-1132; **Board Cert:** Surgery 1998; **Med School:** Univ Louisville Sch Med 1974; **Resid:** Surgery, Parkland Hosp 1979; **Fellow:** Surgical Oncology, MD Anderson Hosp 1980; **Fac Appt:** Assoc Clin Prof S, Baylor Coll Med

Klimberg, Vicki Suzanne MD [S] - **Spec Exp:** Breast Cancer; Radiofrequency Tumor Ablation; **Hospital:** UAMS Med Ctr; **Address:** Univ Arkansas Medical Sciences, 4301 W Markham, MS 721-7, Little Rock, AR 72205; **Phone:** 501-686-5669; **Board Cert:** Surgery 1999; **Med School:** Univ Fla Coll Med 1984; **Resid:** Surgery, Univ Fla 1990; **Fellow:** Clinical Oncology, Univ Fla 1991; Breast Disease, Univ Arkansas for Med Scis 1991; **Fac Appt:** Prof S, Univ Ark

Krouse, Robert S MD [S] - **Spec Exp:** Cancer Surgery; Gastrointestinal Cancer; Palliative Care; **Hospital:** VA Medical Center - Tucson; **Address:** SAVAHCS-Surg Care Line, 2-112, 3601 S 6th Ave, Tucson, AZ 85723; **Phone:** 520-792-1450 x6145; **Board Cert:** Surgery 1998; **Med School:** Hahnemann Univ 1991; **Resid:** Surgery, Univ Hawaii Integrated Surg Prog 1993; Immunotherapy, Natl Cancer Inst 1994; **Fellow:** Surgery, W Virginia Univ Sch Med 1997; Surgical Oncology, City of Hope Natl Med Ctr 2000; **Fac Appt:** Asst Prof S, Univ Ariz Coll Med

Kuhn, Joseph A MD [S] - **Spec Exp:** Liver Cancer; Peritoneal Carcinomatosis; Melanoma; **Hospital:** Baylor Univ Medical Ctr; **Address:** 3409 Worth St, Ste 420, Sammons Tower, Dallas, TX 75246; **Phone:** 214-824-9963; **Board Cert:** Surgery 1999; Surgical Critical Care 1993; **Med School:** Univ Tex Med Br, Galveston 1984; **Resid:** Surgery, Baylor Univ Med Ctr 1989; **Fellow:** Surgical Oncology, City Hosp Natl Med Ctr 1992

Lee, Jeffrey E MD [S] - **Spec Exp:** Melanoma; Pancreatic Cancer; Endocrine Tumors; **Hospital:** UT MD Anderson Cancer Ctr (page 81); **Address:** UT MD Anderson Cancer Ctr, 1400 Holcombe Blvd, Unit 444 Fl 12, Houston, TX 77030-4009; **Phone:** 713-792-7218; **Board Cert:** Surgery 1999; **Med School:** Stanford Univ 1984; **Resid:** Surgery, Stanford Univ Hosp 1987; Surgery, Stanford Univ Hosp 1991; **Fellow:** Immunology, Stanford Univ Sch Med 1989; Surgical Oncology, Univ Tex-MD Anderson Cancer Ctr 1993; **Fac Appt:** Prof S, Univ Tex, Houston

Leitch, A Marilyn MD [S] - **Spec Exp:** Breast Cancer & Surgery; Melanoma; Sarcoma; **Hospital:** UT Southwestern Med Ctr - Dallas; **Address:** UT Southwestern Med Ctr - Dept Surgery, 5323 Harry Hines Blvd, Dallas, TX 75390-9155; **Phone:** 214-648-3039; **Board Cert:** Surgery 2003; **Med School:** Univ Tex SW, Dallas 1978; **Resid:** Surgery, UCLA Med Ctr 1984; **Fellow:** Surgical Oncology, MD Anderson Cancer Ctr 1985; **Fac Appt:** Prof S, Univ Tex SW, Dallas

Li, Benjamin D L MD [S] - **Spec Exp:** Gastrointestinal Cancer; Sarcoma; Breast Cancer; **Hospital:** Louisiana State Univ Hosp, Willis Knighton Hlth Sys; **Address:** LSU Hlth Scis Ctr, Dept Surg, 1501 Kings Hwy, Shreveport, LA 71130; **Phone:** 318-675-6123; **Board Cert:** Surgery 2002; **Med School:** Yale Univ 1986; **Resid:** Surgery, Northwestern Univ-McGraw Med Ctr 1992; **Fellow:** Surgical Oncology, Roswell Park Cancer Inst 1995; **Fac Appt:** Prof S, Louisiana State Univ

Pisters, Peter MD [S] - **Spec Exp:** Pancreatic Cancer; Sarcoma-Soft Tissue; Gastrointestinal Cancer; **Hospital:** UT MD Anderson Cancer Ctr (page 81); **Address:** MD Anderson Cancer Ctr, PO Box 301402, Unit 444, Houston, TX 77230-1402; **Phone:** 713-794-1572; **Board Cert:** Surgery 2001; **Med School:** Univ Western Ontario 1985; **Resid:** Surgery, NYU/Bellevue Hosp 1992; **Fellow:** Surgical Research, Meml Sloan-Kettering Cancer Ctr 1989; Surgical Oncology, Meml Sloan-Kettering Cancer Ctr 1994; **Fac Appt:** Prof S, Univ Tex, Houston

Pockaj, Barbara A MD [S] - **Spec Exp:** Melanoma; Breast Cancer; Stomach Cancer; Clinical Trials; **Hospital:** Mayo Clin Hosp - Scottsdale; **Address:** Mayo Clinic, Dept Surgery, 5777 E Mayo Blvd, Phoenix, AZ 85054; **Phone:** 480-342-1051; **Board Cert:** Surgery 1996; **Med School:** Vanderbilt Univ 1987; **Resid:** Surgery, Case Western Res Univ Affil Hosps 1995; **Fellow:** Surgical Oncology, Natl Inst Hlth 1992; **Fac Appt:** Assoc Prof S, Mayo Med Sch

Pollock, Raphael E MD/PhD [S] - **Spec Exp:** Sarcoma; **Hospital:** UT MD Anderson Cancer Ctr (page 81); **Address:** MD Anderson Cancer Ctr, Dept Surg Oncology, 1515 Holcombe Blvd, Unit 345, Houston, TX 77230; **Phone:** 713-792-8850; **Board Cert:** Surgery 2003; **Med School:** St Louis Univ 1977; **Resid:** Surgery, Univ Chicago 1979; Surgery, Rush Presby-St Lukes Hosp 1982; **Fellow:** Surgical Oncology, MD Anderson Cancer Ctr 1984; **Fac Appt:** Prof S, Univ Tex, Houston

Postier, Russell MD [S] - **Spec Exp:** Pancreatic Cancer; Biliary Surgery; **Hospital:** OU Med Ctr; **Address:** Univ Oklahoma Dept Surgery, PO Box 26901, WP-2140, Oklahoma City, OK 73190; **Phone:** 405-271-3445; **Board Cert:** Surgery 2000; **Med School:** Univ Okla Coll Med 1975; **Resid:** Surgery, Johns Hopkins Hosp 1981; **Fac Appt:** Prof S, Univ Okla Coll Med

Ross, Merrick I MD [S] - **Spec Exp:** Sentinel Node Surgery; Breast Cancer; Melanoma; **Hospital:** UT MD Anderson Cancer Ctr (page 81); **Address:** UT MD Anderson Cancer Ctr, Dept Surg Onc, PO Box 301402, Unit 444, Houston, TX 77230-1402; **Phone:** 713-792-7217; **Board Cert:** Surgery 1997; **Med School:** Univ IL Coll Med 1980; **Resid:** Surgery, Univ Illinois Hosp & Clin 1982; Surgery, Univ Illinois Hosp & Clin 1987; **Fellow:** Research, Scripps Clin & Rsch 1984; Surgical Oncology, Univ TX-MD Anderson Cancer Ctr 1989; **Fac Appt:** Prof S, Univ Tex, Houston

Singletary, Sonja Eva MD [S] - **Spec Exp:** Breast Cancer; **Hospital:** UT MD Anderson Cancer Ctr (page 81); **Address:** Univ Tex MD Anderson Cancer Ctr, 1515 Holcombe Blvd, Box 444, Houston, TX 77030-4009; **Phone:** 713-792-6937; **Board Cert:** Surgery 2003; **Med School:** Med Univ SC 1977; **Resid:** Surgery, Shands Hosp-Univ Florida 1983; **Fellow:** Surgery, MD Anderson Hosp 1985; **Fac Appt:** Prof S, Univ Tex, Houston

Skibber, John M MD [S] - **Spec Exp:** Rectal Cancer/Sphincter Preservation; Colon & Rectal Cancer-Familial Polyposis; **Hospital:** UT MD Anderson Cancer Ctr (page 81); **Address:** UT MD Anderson Cancer Ctr, Unit 444 PO Box 301402, Houston, TX 77230-1402; **Phone:** 713-792-5165; **Board Cert:** Surgery 1998; **Med School:** Jefferson Med Coll 1981; **Resid:** Surgery, NYU Med Ctr 1989; **Fellow:** Surgical Oncology, Univ Texas-MD Anderson 1991; **Fac Appt:** Prof S, Univ Tex, Houston

Stolier, Alan J MD [S] - **Spec Exp:** Breast Cancer; **Hospital:** Ochsner Baptist Med Ctr, Louisiana State Univ Hosp; **Address:** 2525 Severn Ave, Metairie, LA 70001; **Phone:** 504-832-4200; **Board Cert:** Surgery 1994; **Med School:** Louisiana State Univ 1970; **Resid:** Surgery, Charity Hosp 1974; **Fellow:** Surgical Oncology, MD Anderson Hosp 1976

Vauthey, Jean Nicholas MD [S] - **Spec Exp:** Hepatobiliary Surgery; Liver Cancer; Gallbladder & Biliary Cancer; **Hospital:** UT MD Anderson Cancer Ctr (page 81); **Address:** UT MD Anderson Cancer Ctr -Surg Oncol, 1515 Holcombe Blvd, Unit 444, Houston, TX 77030; **Phone:** 713-792-2022; **Board Cert:** Surgery 2000; **Med School:** Switzerland 1979; **Resid:** Surgery, Ochsner Med Fdn 1989; **Fellow:** Hepatobiliary Surgery, Med Fac Univ Bern 1991; Surgical Oncology, Meml Sloan-Kettering Cancer Ctr 1993; **Fac Appt:** Prof S, Univ Tex, Houston

Surgery

Woltering, Eugene MD [S] - **Spec Exp:** Carcinoid Tumors; **Hospital:** Louisiana State Univ Hosp; **Address:** 3401 North Blvd, Ste 400, Baton Rouge, LA 70806; **Phone:** 225-381-2755; **Board Cert:** Surgery 2002; **Med School:** Ohio State Univ 1975; **Resid:** Surgery, Vanderbilt Med Ctr 1982; Surgical Oncology, Natl Inst Hlth 1979; **Fellow:** Surgical Oncology, Ohio State 1984

Wood, R Patrick MD [S] - **Spec Exp:** Transplant-Liver; Liver Cancer; **Hospital:** St Luke's Episcopal Hosp - Houston; **Address:** 6624 Fannin St, Ste 1200, Houston, TX 77030; **Phone:** 713-795-8994; **Board Cert:** Surgery 2004; **Med School:** Univ Rochester 1979; **Resid:** Surgery, NYU/Bellevue Hosp Ctr 1984; **Fellow:** Transplant Surgery, Univ Pittsburgh 1985; **Fac Appt:** Clin Prof S, Univ Tex, Houston

Zannis, Victor J MD [S] - **Spec Exp:** Breast Cancer; **Hospital:** Phoenix Baptist Hosp & Med Ctr; **Address:** 2525 W Greenway Rd, Ste 130, Phoenix, AZ 85023; **Phone:** 602-942-8000; **Board Cert:** Surgery 2000; **Med School:** UCLA 1976; **Resid:** Surgery, Maricopa Med Ctr 1982

West Coast and Pacific

Anderson, Benjamin O MD [S] - **Spec Exp:** Breast Cancer; International Breast Healthcare; **Hospital:** Univ Wash Med Ctr; **Address:** Univ Washington Dept Surgery, 1959 NE Pacific St, Box 356410, Seattle, WA 98195-6410; **Phone:** 206-598-5500; **Board Cert:** Surgery 2002; **Med School:** Albert Einstein Coll Med 1985; **Resid:** Surgery, Univ Colorado 1992; **Fellow:** Surgical Oncology, Meml Sloan Kettering Cancer Ctr 1994; **Fac Appt:** Prof S, Univ Wash

Bilchik, Anton J MD [S] - **Spec Exp:** Gastrointestinal Cancer; Laparoscopic Surgery; **Hospital:** St John's Hlth Ctr, Santa Monica, Cedars-Sinai Med Ctr; **Address:** John Wayne Cancer Institute, 2200 Santa Monica Blvd, Santa Monica, CA 90404; **Phone:** 310-449-5206; **Board Cert:** Surgery 1997; **Med School:** South Africa 1985; **Resid:** Surgery, UCLA Med Ctr 1996; **Fellow:** John Wayne Cancer Inst. 1998; **Fac Appt:** Asst Clin Prof S, UCLA

Butler, John A MD [S] - **Spec Exp:** Breast Cancer; Thyroid Cancer; Adrenal Tumors; Small Bowel Cancer; **Hospital:** UC Irvine Med Ctr; **Address:** UCI Medical Ctr, 101 City Drive S, Bldg 56 Office 252 Rt 81, Orange, CA 92868-3298; **Phone:** 714-456-8030; **Board Cert:** Surgery 2003; **Med School:** Loyola Univ-Stritch Sch Med 1976; **Resid:** Surgery, LAC-USC Med Ctr 1982; Surgery, Harbor-UCLA Med Ctr 1982; **Fellow:** Surgical Oncology, Meml Sloan-Kettering Cancer Ctr 1984; **Fac Appt:** Assoc Prof S, UC Irvine

Byrd, David MD [S] - **Spec Exp:** Tumor Surgery; Breast Cancer; Melanoma; **Hospital:** Univ Wash Med Ctr; **Address:** Univ Washington Med Ctr, Dept Surgical Specialites Center, 1959 NE Pacific St, Box 356165, Seattle, WA 98195; **Phone:** 206-598-4477; **Board Cert:** Surgery 1998; **Med School:** Tulane Univ 1982; **Resid:** Surgery, Univ Wash Med Ctr 1987; **Fellow:** Surgical Oncology, Univ Tex-MD Anderson Cancer Ctr 1992; **Fac Appt:** Assoc Prof S, Univ Wash

Chang, Helena MD [S] - **Spec Exp:** Breast Cancer; Cancer Surgery; **Hospital:** UCLA Med Ctr (page 83); **Address:** 200 UCLA Medical Plaza, Ste B265-1, Revlon Breast Clinic, Los Angeles, CA 90095-8344; **Phone:** 310-825-2144; **Board Cert:** Surgery 1997; **Med School:** Temple Univ 1981; **Resid:** Surgery, Episcopal Hosp 1986; **Fellow:** Cellular Molecular Biology, Temple Univ 1977; Surgical Oncology, Meml Sloan-Kettering Cancer Ctr 1988; **Fac Appt:** Prof S, UCLA

Clark, Orlo H MD [S] - **Spec Exp:** Thyroid Cancer & Surgery; Neuroendocrine Tumors; Parathyroid Cancer; **Hospital:** UCSF - Mt Zion Med Ctr, UCSF Med Ctr; **Address:** UCSF Mt Zion Med Ctr, 1600 Divisadero St Fl 3, Box 1674, San Francisco, CA 94115-1926; **Phone:** 415-353-7687; **Board Cert:** Surgery 1974; **Med School:** Cornell Univ-Weill Med Coll 1967; **Resid:** Surgery, UCSF Med Ctr 1970; Surgery, UCSF Med Ctr 1973; **Fellow:** Surgery, Royal Med Sch London 1971; **Fac Appt:** Prof S, UCSF

Eilber, Frederick R MD [S] - **Spec Exp:** Tumor Surgery; Sarcoma; **Hospital:** UCLA Med Ctr (page 83); **Address:** 200 UCLA Medical Plaza, Ste 120, Los Angeles, CA 90095-1718; **Phone:** 310-825-7086; **Board Cert:** Surgery 1973; **Med School:** Univ Mich Med Sch 1965; **Resid:** Surgery, Univ Maryland Hosp 1972; **Fellow:** Surgery, Univ Tex-MD Anderson Hosp 1973; **Fac Appt:** Prof S, UCLA

Ellenhorn, Joshua MD [S] - **Spec Exp:** Gastrointestinal Cancer; Head & Neck Cancer; Cancer Surgery; **Hospital:** City of Hope Natl Med Ctr & Beckman Rsch (page 69); **Address:** City of Hope Med Ctr, 1500 E Duarte Rd, Duarte, CA 91010; **Phone:** 626-359-8111 x65342; **Board Cert:** Surgery 2000; **Med School:** Boston Univ 1984; **Resid:** Surgery, Univ Cincinnati Hosp 1991; **Fellow:** Surgical Oncology, Meml Sloan-Kettering Cancer Ctr 1993

Esserman, Laura J MD [S] - **Spec Exp:** Breast Cancer; **Hospital:** UCSF - Mt Zion Med Ctr, UCSF Med Ctr; **Address:** UCSF-Mt Zion Hosp, Clin Cancer Ctr, 1600 Divisadero St Fl 2, San Francisco, CA 94115; **Phone:** 415-353-7070; **Board Cert:** Surgery 2001; **Med School:** Stanford Univ 1983; **Resid:** Surgery, Stanford Univ Med Ctr 1991; **Fellow:** Oncology, Stanford Univ Med Ctr 1988; **Fac Appt:** Assoc Prof S, UCSF

Essner, Richard MD [S] - **Spec Exp:** Sentinel Node Surgery; Melanoma; Gastrointestinal Surgery; **Hospital:** St John's Hlth Ctr, Santa Monica, Century City Hosp; **Address:** John Wayne Cancer Inst, 2200 Santa Monica Blvd, Santa Monica, CA 90404-2302; **Phone:** 310-998-3906; **Board Cert:** Surgery 1994; **Med School:** Emory Univ 1985; **Resid:** Surgery, Univ NC Hosps 1992; **Fac Appt:** Asst Clin Prof S, USC Sch Med

Giuliano, Armando E MD [S] - **Spec Exp:** Breast Cancer; Thyroid & Parathyroid Surgery; **Hospital:** St John's Hlth Ctr, Santa Monica, UCLA Med Ctr (page 83); **Address:** John Wayne Cancer Inst, 2200 Santa Monica Blvd, Santa Monica, CA 90404; **Phone:** 310-829-8089; **Board Cert:** Surgery 1999; **Med School:** Univ Chicago-Pritzker Sch Med 1973; **Resid:** Surgery, UCSF Med Ctr 1980; **Fellow:** Surgical Oncology, UCLA Med Ctr 1978; **Fac Appt:** Prof S, UCLA

Goodnight, James E MD [S] - **Spec Exp:** Melanoma; Breast Cancer; Bone & Soft Tissue Tumors; **Hospital:** UC Davis Med Ctr; **Address:** UC Davis Med Ctr, Dept Surgery, 2221 Stockton Blvd, rm 3112, Sacramento, CA 95817; **Phone:** 916-734-3190; **Board Cert:** Surgery 1997; **Med School:** Baylor Coll Med 1968; **Resid:** Surgery, Univ Utah Hosp 1976; **Fellow:** Surgical Oncology, UCLA Med Ctr 1978; **Fac Appt:** Prof S, UC Davis

Goodson III, William H MD [S] - **Spec Exp:** Breast Cancer & Surgery; Breast Disease; **Hospital:** CA Pacific Med Ctr - Pacific Campus, UCSF - Mt Zion Med Ctr; **Address:** 2100 Webster St, Ste 401, San Francisco, CA 94115; **Phone:** 415-923-3925; **Board Cert:** Surgery 1996; **Med School:** Harvard Med Sch 1971; **Resid:** Surgery, Univ Hosps 1976; Surgery, Children's Hosp 1977

Hoque, Laura W MD [S] - Spec Exp: Breast Cancer; Breast Disease; **Hospital:** Kapiolani Med Ctr for Women & Chldn, Queen's Med Ctr - Honolulu; **Address:** Kapi'olani Womens Ctr, 1907 S Beretania St, Ste 501, Honolulu, HI 96826; **Phone:** 808-949-3444; **Board Cert:** Surgery 1999; **Med School:** Boston Univ 1993; **Resid:** Surgery, St Vincents Hosp 1998; **Fellow:** Breast Surgery, Meml Sloan Kettering Cancer Ctr 1999; **Fac Appt:** Assoc Clin Prof S, Univ Hawaii JA Burns Sch Med

Johnson, Denise L MD [S] - Spec Exp: Melanoma; Breast Cancer; **Hospital:** Stanford Univ Med Ctr; **Address:** Stanford Univ Med Ctr-Dept Surgery, 300 Pasteur Drive, Ste H3680, MC 5655, Stanford, CA 94305; **Phone:** 650-723-5672; **Board Cert:** Surgery 2001; **Med School:** Washington Univ, St Louis 1978; **Resid:** Surgery, Univ Illinois Med Ctr 1986; Immunology, Univ Texas SW Med Ctr 1982; **Fellow:** Surgical Oncology, City of Hope Med Ctr 1989; **Fac Appt:** Assoc Prof S, Stanford Univ

Kaufman, Cary S MD [S] - Spec Exp: Breast Cancer; Breast Disease; **Hospital:** St Joseph Hosp - Bellingham; **Address:** 2940 Squalicom Pkwy, Ste 101, Bellingham, WA 98225; **Phone:** 360-671-9877; **Board Cert:** Surgery 2000; **Med School:** UCLA 1973; **Resid:** Surgery, Univ Wash Med Ctr 1975; Surgery, Harbor-UCLA Med Ctr 1979; **Fac Appt:** Asst Clin Prof S, Univ Wash

Klein, Andrew S MD [S] - Spec Exp: Transplant-Liver; Liver Cancer; **Hospital:** Cedars-Sinai Med Ctr; **Address:** Cedars-Sinai Medical Center, 8635 W Third St, Ste 590W, Los Angeles, CA 90048; **Phone:** 310-423-2641; **Board Cert:** Surgery 1996; **Med School:** Johns Hopkins Univ 1979; **Resid:** Surgery, Johns Hopkins Hosp 1982; Surgery, Johns Hopkins Hosp 1986; **Fellow:** Transplant Surgery, UCLA-CHS 1988; **Fac Appt:** Clin Prof S, UCLA

Knudson, Mary Margaret MD [S] - Spec Exp: Breast Cancer; **Hospital:** UCSF Med Ctr, San Francisco Genl Hosp; **Address:** 1001 Potrero Ave, Ste 3A, San Francisco, CA 94110; **Phone:** 415-206-8814; **Board Cert:** Surgery 1992; Surgical Critical Care 1998; **Med School:** Univ Mich Med Sch 1976; **Resid:** Surgery, Beth Israel Hosp 1979; Surgery, Univ Mich Med Ctr 1982; **Fellow:** Pediatric Surgery, Stanford Univ Hosps; **Fac Appt:** Assoc Prof S, UCSF

Moossa, AR MD [S] - Spec Exp: Pancreatic Cancer; Gastrointestinal Cancer; Hepatobiliary Surgery; **Hospital:** UCSD Med Ctr; **Address:** 9300 Campus Point Drive, MC 7212, La Jolla, CA 92037; **Phone:** 858-657-6113; **Med School:** England 1965; **Resid:** Surgery, Liverpool Univ Hosps 1970; **Fellow:** Surgical Oncology, Johns Hopkins Hosp 1972; **Fac Appt:** Prof S, UCSD

Norton, Jeffrey A MD [S] - Spec Exp: Pancreatic Cancer; Gastrointestinal Cancer & Surgery; Endocrine Surgery; **Hospital:** Stanford Univ Med Ctr; **Address:** 875 Blake Wilbur Drive, Clinic F, Stanford, CA 94305; **Phone:** 650-723-5461; **Board Cert:** Surgery 2001; **Med School:** SUNY Upstate Med Univ 1973; **Resid:** Surgery, Duke Univ Med Ctr 1978; **Fellow:** Research, Natl Cancer Inst 1982; **Fac Appt:** Prof S, Stanford Univ

Pellegrini, Carlos MD [S] - Spec Exp: Esophageal Cancer; Esophageal Surgery; Gastrointestinal Cancer & Surgery; **Hospital:** Univ Wash Med Ctr; **Address:** Univ Washington Medical Ctr, Dept Surgery, 1959 NE Pacific St, Box 356410, Seattle, WA 98195; **Phone:** 206-543-3106; **Board Cert:** Surgery 1998; **Med School:** Argentina 1971; **Resid:** Surgery, Granadero Hosp 1975; Surgery, Univ Chicago Hosps 1979; **Fac Appt:** Prof S, Univ Wash

Reber, Howard A MD [S] - **Spec Exp:** Pancreatic Cancer; Gastrointestinal Cancer; **Hospital:** UCLA Med Ctr (page 83); **Address:** UCLA Medical Ctr, Dept Surgery, 10833 Le Conte Ave, Los Angeles, CA 90095-6904; **Phone:** 310-825-4976; **Board Cert:** Surgery 1971; **Med School:** Univ Pennsylvania 1964; **Resid:** Surgery, Hosp Univ Penn 1970; **Fac Appt:** Prof S, UCLA

Schneider, Philip D MD/PhD [S] - **Spec Exp:** Cancer Surgery; Minimally Invasive Surgery; **Hospital:** UC Davis Med Ctr; **Address:** UC Davis, Div Surg Oncology, 4501 X St, Ste 3010, Sacramento, CA 95817; **Phone:** 916-734-7280; **Board Cert:** Surgery 2002; **Med School:** St Louis Univ 1972; **Resid:** Surgery, Univ Minn Hosps 1981; Surgical Oncology, Meml Hosp 1976; **Fac Appt:** Prof S, UC Davis

Silverstein, Melvin J MD [S] - **Spec Exp:** Breast Cancer; **Hospital:** USC Norris Comp Cancer Ctr; **Address:** USC Norris Cancer Center, 1441 Eastlake Ave, rm 7415, Los Angeles, CA 90033; **Phone:** 323-865-3535; **Board Cert:** Surgery 1971; **Med School:** Albany Med Coll 1965; **Resid:** Surgery, Boston City Hosp-Tufts Univ 1970; **Fellow:** Surgical Oncology, UCLA Med Ctr 1975; **Fac Appt:** Prof S, USC Sch Med

Sinanan, Mika N MD [S] - **Spec Exp:** Gastrointestinal Surgery; Gastrointestinal Cancer; Liver & Biliary Cancer; Laparoscopic Surgery; **Hospital:** Univ Wash Med Ctr; **Address:** Univ Washington, Dept Surgery, 1959 NE Pacific St, Box 356410, Seattle, WA 98195-6410; **Phone:** 206-543-5511; **Board Cert:** Surgery 1998; **Med School:** Johns Hopkins Univ 1980; **Resid:** Surgery, Univ Washington Hosp 1988; **Fellow:** Gastrointestinal Surgery, Univ Brit Columbia Med Ctr 1986; **Fac Appt:** Prof S, Univ Wash

Traverso, L William MD [S] - **Spec Exp:** Pancreatic Cancer; Laparoscopic Surgery; **Hospital:** Virginia Mason Med Ctr; **Address:** Virginia Mason Med Ctr, Dept Surg, 1100 9th Ave, Seattle, WA 98101; **Phone:** 206-223-8855; **Board Cert:** Surgery 1998; **Med School:** UCLA 1973; **Resid:** Surgery, UCLA Med Ctr 1978; **Fac Appt:** Clin Prof S, Univ Wash

Wagman, Lawrence D MD [S] - **Spec Exp:** Liver Cancer; Gastrointestinal Cancer; Breast Cancer; **Hospital:** City of Hope Natl Med Ctr & Beckman Rsch (page 69), San Dimas Comm Hosp; **Address:** City of Hope Natl Cancer Ctr, Dept Surgery, 1500 Duarte Rd, Duarte, CA 91010; **Phone:** 626-250-4673 x67100; **Board Cert:** Surgery 2005; **Med School:** Columbia P&S 1978; **Resid:** Surgery, Med Coll Virginia Hosp 1985; **Fellow:** Surgical Oncology, NIH/NCI 1982; **Fac Appt:** Assoc Clin Prof S, UCSD

Warren, Robert S MD [S] - **Spec Exp:** Liver Cancer; **Hospital:** UCSF Med Ctr; **Address:** UCSF Comprehensive Cancer Center, 1600 Divisadero St, rm A710, San Francisco, CA 94143-1932; **Phone:** 415-353-9846; **Board Cert:** Surgery 1998; **Med School:** Univ Minn 1980; **Resid:** Surgery, Univ Minn Hosps 1988; **Fellow:** Surgical Oncology, Meml Sloan-Kettering Cancer Ctr 1986; **Fac Appt:** Prof S, UCSF

Cleveland Clinic

Recognized Leader in Breast Health

Cleveland Clinic specialists are leaders in innovative therapies for breast cancer, including treatment that may reduce the risk of onset or progression of the disease. Each year, thousands of women seek help for breast cancer or other breast disorders at Cleveland Clinic's Taussig Cancer Center and Breast Center. For newly diagnosed and second-opinion patients, the Breast Center's team of professionals offers evaluations on the same day, whenever possible.

Early Detection is Vital

Detecting breast cancer early is crucial to survival. Cleveland Clinic radiologists perform more than 4,500 mammograms monthly, providing the latest breast imaging capabilities, including digital mammography; expert interpretation by dedicated breast imaging physicians; and special care if high-risk factors are present.

Breast MRI

Breast Center specialists use breast magnetic resonance imaging to complement existing screening, diagnostic and surgical strategies. Currently, breast MRI is used to stage newly diagnosed patients, particularly those with dense breast tissue; to evaluate women with a history of breast cancer, especially those who have had breast conservation surgery; and to assess patients when diagnostic results are inconclusive.

Treatment and Reconstruction

The Breast Center offers patients the latest treatments for breast cancer, including minimally invasive techniques and reconstructive surgery performed alone or together with therapeutic cancer surgery; radiation therapy, during which the patient's opposite breast is shielded from scatter radiation with a unique device developed at Cleveland Clinic; partial-breast irradiation; neo-adjuvant chemotherapy, given prior to surgery; and access to clinical trials.

For patients with more advanced breast cancer, the physicians and scientists of Cleveland Clinic's Taussig Cancer Center and Lerner Research Institute are at the forefront of clinical trials and anti-cancer drug development, blending standard treatments with innovations in chemotherapy, radiotherapy and biological treatment.

To schedule an appointment or for more information about the Cleveland Clinic Breast Center, call 800.890.2467 or visit www.clevelandclinic.org/breasttopdocs

Cleveland Clinic Breast Center | 9500 Euclid Ave. / W14 | Cleveland, OH 44195

Nipple-Sparing Mastectomy

Cleveland Clinic physicians developed a mastectomy technique that leaves the nipple intact, allowing for a more natural-looking breast reconstruction.

"The response that we are getting from patients to this surgery is the most overwhelming I have seen in 25 years," says Clinic breast surgeon Joseph Crowe, M.D., who developed the technique. "The nipple-sparing procedure is not for every woman with breast cancer," Dr. Crowe is careful to qualify. "The cancer must be a small tumor, confined to one location and at least 3 to 4 centimeters away from the nipple," he explains. To date, Cleveland Clinic's Breast Center has the world's largest experience using nipple-sparing mastectomy, and patient satisfaction has been extraordinary.

FOX CHASE
CANCER CENTER

333 Cottman Avenue
Philadelphia, PA 19111-2497
Phone: 1-888-FOX CHASE • Fax: 215-728-2702
www.fccc.edu

SURGICAL ONCOLOGY

The most experienced surgical oncologists have the best treatment outcomes. Fox Chase surgeons are highly specialized and focus solely on cancer. The comprehensive surgical oncology program at Fox Chase encompasses subspecialties in breast, gastrointestinal, gynecologic, head and neck, orthopedic, thoracic and urologic surgical oncology and plastic surgery and reconstruction.

Breast Cancer Diagnostic techniques include stereotactic breast biopsy and, at the time of surgery, sentinel lymph-node biopsy. Treatment options include breast-preserving surgery (lumpectomy) with radiation therapy as well as mastectomy with reconstructive surgery. Women who choose mastectomy have several options for breast reconstruction. Fox Chase surgeons can perform a skin-sparing mastectomy to ease this process.

Gastrointestinal Cancers Our gastrointestinal surgeons have extensive experience with pancreatic cancer, advanced and recurrent cancer in the gastrointestinal tract and rare tumors such as sarcomas. Laparoscopic surgery for colon and other gastrointestinal cancers is also available.

Genitourinary Cancers Our urologic surgical oncologists have broad expertise in the care of patients with cancers of the prostate, bladder, kidney, ureter, adrenal gland, testes and penis. Fox Chase urologists annually perform hundreds of complex open and laparoscopic surgeries for cancer. These services include minimally invasive robotic surgery, organ-sparing resections, urinary diversions and cryosurgical ablation. They have extensive experience with laparoscopic partial nephrectomy.

Gynecologic Cancers Fox Chase experts in gynecologic cancer offer the most advanced treatments for women with cancers of the uterus, ovary and cervix. Robotic surgery is done when appropriate. We also have a comprehensive research program to develop new treatments for ovarian cancer.

Head and Neck Cancers The head and neck cancer center at Fox Chase provides patients with one-stop consultations with surgical, radiation and medical oncologists. Expertise includes otolaryngology, plastic surgery and microvascular reconstruction. Transoral laser surgery is available for oral cancers, tongue, larynx, and pharynx to aid in organ preservation.

Minimally Invasive Surgery

The highly skilled surgeons at Fox Chase Cancer Center treat many patients with minimally invasive procedures, which usually provide faster recovery time and less discomfort for patients.

Technology includes the most advanced robotic da Vinci S Surgical System, available for prostate cancer and some gynecologic cancers. Minimally invasive laparascopic surgery is available for abdominal surgeries, including surgery for colon and kidney cancers.

Fox Chase patients with small lung cancers may benefit from video-assisted thoracic surgery (VATS), uses smaller chest incisions than conventional surgery. Fox Chase is one of only a few institutions in the country offering VATS for lung cancer.

Organ Preservation

A major focus of surgical oncology at Fox Chase is preserving organs and their function, including breast-conserving surgery and removal of colon or rectal tumors while preserving the bowel and anal sphincter. Minimally invasive procedures, such as transoral laser surgery for head and neck cancers, permit organ preservation and shorten recovery time.

For more about Fox Chase physicians and services, visit our web site, www.fccc.edu, or call 1-888-FOX CHASE.

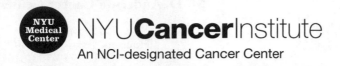

NYU**Cancer**Institute
An NCI-designated Cancer Center

A Collaborative Approach
The NYU Cancer Institute, an NCI designated center, is a "matrix cancer center" without walls operating within the larger NYU Medical Center. With over 200 members and a research funding base of over $81 million, this structure strengthens our capabilities to forge collaborations across medical and scientific disciplines, which translates to comprehensive care for our patients and discoveries that will influence the future of this disease.

Renowned Expertise
Our highly skilled Magnet™ nursing team not only plays a pivotal role in coordinating direct patient care, but is also a source of invaluable patient education. Team members' compassion and expertise help patients better manage the symptoms of their disease as well as their special needs.

A Patient-Focused Setting
The NYU Clinical Cancer Center, with over 70 faculty members from various disciplines at the New York University School of Medicine, is the principal outpatient facility of the Cancer Institute and serves as home for our patients and their caregivers. The center and its multidisciplinary team of experts provide access to the latest treatment options and clinical trials along with a variety of programs in cancer prevention, screening, diagnostics, genetic counseling, and supportive services. When it comes to kids and cancer, the Stephen D. Hassenfeld Children's Center for Cancer and Blood Disorders offers not just innovation but insight. As a leading member of the NCI-sponsored Children's Oncology Group, our physicians are known for developing new ways to treat childhood cancer. Our affiliation with Bellevue Hospital, the oldest public hospital in the country, affords clinically distinctive opportunities to learn and care for patients with cancer by observing its presentation and behavior in a variety of patient groups.

SURGICAL ONCOLOGY PROGRAM

UCLA Health System

1-800-UCLA-MD1 (825-2631)
www.uclahealth.org

Using the latest in surgical technologies — including minimally invasive surgery and robotics — UCLA's surgical oncology program offers a multidisciplinary approach to modern cancer therapy for solid tumors of the breast, lung, colon, liver and pancreas; soft-tissue and bone sarcomas; and melanoma.

Sophisticated diagnostic and therapeutic services, some only available at select medical centers, offer adults and children the accurate staging of cancers and the latest cancer surgery approaches. Post-operative treatments may include the latest the field has to offer in chemotherapy, radiation, biological therapy and gene therapy.

The Center for Advanced Surgical and Interventional Technology (CASIT), a UCLA-based collaboration among surgery, engineering, and industry, is taking surgery to the next step by exploring innovative surgical approaches for the future, including robotics to perform minimally invasive procedures.

UCLA's Jonsson Cancer Center

Designated by the National Cancer Institute as one of only 39 comprehensive cancer centers in the United States, UCLA's Jonsson Cancer Center has earned an international reputation for developing new cancer therapies, providing the best in experimental and traditional treatments, and expertly guiding and training the next generation of medical researchers. The center's 250 physicians and scientists treat upwards of 20,000 patient visits per year and offer hundreds of clinical trials that provide the latest in experimental cancer treatments (www.cancer.mednet.ucla.edu). The center also offers patients and families complete psychological and support services.

UCLA's Jonsson Cancer Center has been ranked the best cancer center in California by *U.S.News & World Report*'s Annual Best Hospitals survey for the seventh year. UCLA Medical Center, of which the Cancer Center is a part, has ranked best in the West for the past 17 years.

UCLA'S SURGICAL ONCOLOGY PROGRAM OFFERS SOPHISTICATED SURGICAL TREATMENTS FOR CANCERS OF THE:

- Breast
- Lung
- Colon
- Liver
- Pancreas
- Bone
- Skin (melanoma)

Call 1-800-UCLA-MD1 (825-2631)
for a referral to a UCLA doctor.

Thoracic Surgery

A thoracic surgeon provides the operative, perioperative care and critical care of patients with pathologic conditions within the chest. Included is the surgical care of coronary artery disease, cancers of the lung, esophagus and chest wall, abnormalities of the trachea, abnormalities of the great vessels and heart valves, congenital anomalies, tumors of the mediastinum and diseases of the diaphragm. The management of the airway and injuries of the chest is within the scope of the specialty.

Thoracic surgeons have the knowledge, experience and technical skills to accurately diagnose, operate upon safely and effectively manage patients with thoracic diseases of the chest. This requires substantial knowledge of cardiorespiratory physiology and oncology, as well as capability in the use of heart assist devices, management of abnormal heart rhythms and drainage of the chest cavity, respiratory support systems, endoscopy and invasive and noninvasive diagnostic techniques.

Training Required: Seven to eight years

Thoracic Surgery

New England

Bueno, Raphael MD [TS] - **Spec Exp:** Lung Cancer; **Hospital:** Brigham & Women's Hosp; **Address:** Brigham and Women's Hospital, 75 Francis St, Boston, MA 02115; **Phone:** 617-732-6824; **Board Cert:** Thoracic Surgery 1997; Surgery 2002; Surgical Critical Care 2003; **Med School:** Harvard Med Sch 1985; **Resid:** Surgery, Brigham & Women's Hosp 1992; **Fellow:** Surgical Critical Care, Brigham & Women's Hosp 1993; Cardiothoracic Surgery, Mass Genl Hosp 1997; **Fac Appt:** Assoc Prof S, Harvard Med Sch

Gaissert, Henning A MD [TS] - **Spec Exp:** Esophageal Cancer; Tracheal Surgery; Lung Cancer; **Hospital:** Mass Genl Hosp; **Address:** Division of Thoracic Surgery, 55 Fruit St, BLK 1570, Boston, MA 02114; **Phone:** 617-726-5341; **Board Cert:** Surgery 2001; Thoracic Surgery 2004; **Med School:** Germany 1984; **Resid:** Surgery, Mass Genl Hosp 1989; Surgery, Barnes Jewish Hosp 1991; **Fellow:** Research, Harvard Med Sch 1993; Cardiothoracic Surgery, Barnes Jewish Hosp 1996; **Fac Appt:** Assoc Prof S, Harvard Med Sch

Mathisen, Douglas MD [TS] - **Spec Exp:** Tracheal Surgery; Lung Cancer; Esophageal Cancer; **Hospital:** Mass Genl Hosp, Newton - Wellesley Hosp; **Address:** Mass Genl Hosp, Dept Thor Surg, 55 Fruit St, Blake 1570, Boston, MA 02114; **Phone:** 617-726-6826; **Board Cert:** Thoracic Surgery 2002; **Med School:** Univ IL Coll Med 1974; **Resid:** Surgery, Mass Genl Hosp 1981; Thoracic Surgery, Mass Genl Hosp 1982; **Fellow:** Surgical Oncology, Natl Cancer Inst 1979; **Fac Appt:** Prof S, Harvard Med Sch

Nugent, William MD [TS] - **Spec Exp:** Thoracic Cancers; **Hospital:** Dartmouth - Hitchcock Med Ctr; **Address:** Dept Cardiothoracic Surgery, 1 Medical Center Drive, Lebanon, NH 03756-1000; **Phone:** 603-650-8572; **Board Cert:** Thoracic Surgery 2002; **Med School:** Albany Med Coll 1975; **Resid:** Surgery, Beth Israel Hosp 1980; Thoracic Surgery, Univ Michigan 1983; **Fellow:** Cardiothoracic Surgery, Mass Genl Hosp 1981; **Fac Appt:** Prof S, Dartmouth Med Sch

Sugarbaker, David J MD [TS] - **Spec Exp:** Mesothelioma; Transplant-Lung; Esophageal Cancer; **Hospital:** Brigham & Women's Hosp, Dana-Farber Cancer Inst; **Address:** Brigham & Women's Hosp, Div Thoracic Surg, 75 Francis St, Boston, MA 02115-6110; **Phone:** 617-732-6824; **Board Cert:** Surgery 1987; Thoracic Surgery 1999; **Med School:** Cornell Univ-Weill Med Coll 1979; **Resid:** Surgery, Brigham & Women's Hosp 1982; Surgery, Brigham & Women's Hosp 1986; **Fellow:** Thoracic Surgery, Toronto Genl Hosp 1988; **Fac Appt:** Prof S, Harvard Med Sch

Wain, John MD [TS] - **Spec Exp:** Lung Cancer; Esophageal Cancer; **Hospital:** Mass Genl Hosp; **Address:** Mass Genl Hosp, Dept Thoracic Surg, 55 Fruit St, Blake 1570, Boston, MA 02114; **Phone:** 617-726-5200; **Board Cert:** Thoracic Surgery 2000; **Med School:** Jefferson Med Coll 1980; **Resid:** Surgery, Mass Genl Hosp 1985; **Fellow:** Cardiothoracic Surgery, Mass Genl Hosp 1988; **Fac Appt:** Asst Prof TS, Harvard Med Sch

Wright, Cameron D MD [TS] - **Spec Exp:** Lung Cancer; Esophageal Cancer; Tracheal Surgery; **Hospital:** Mass Genl Hosp; **Address:** Division of Surgery, 55 Fruit St, Blake 1570, Boston, MA 02114-2696; **Phone:** 617-726-5801; **Board Cert:** Surgery 1995; Thoracic Surgery 1997; **Med School:** Univ Mich Med Sch 1980; **Resid:** Surgery, Mass Genl Hosp 1986; Thoracic Surgery, Mass Genl Hosp 1988; **Fac Appt:** Assoc Prof S, Harvard Med Sch

Mid Atlantic

Altorki, Nasser MD [TS] - **Spec Exp:** Esophageal Cancer; Lung Cancer; Thoracic Cancers; Vaccine Therapy; **Hospital:** NY-Presby Hosp (page 79); **Address:** 525 E 68th St, New York, NY 10021-4870; **Phone:** 212-746-5156; **Board Cert:** Surgery 1996; Thoracic Surgery 1998; **Med School:** Egypt 1978; **Resid:** Surgery, Univ Chicago Hosps 1985; **Fellow:** Cardiothoracic Surgery, Univ Chicago Hosps 1987; **Fac Appt:** Prof S, Cornell Univ-Weill Med Coll

Bains, Manjit MD [TS] - **Spec Exp:** Esophageal Cancer; Lung Cancer; **Hospital:** Meml Sloan Kettering Cancer Ctr (page 76); **Address:** 1275 York Ave, rm C-861, New York, NY 10021; **Phone:** 212-639-7450; **Board Cert:** Surgery 1971; Thoracic Surgery 1972; **Med School:** India 1963; **Resid:** Surgery, Rochester Genl Hosp 1970; **Fellow:** Thoracic Surgery, Sloan Kettering Cancer Ctr 1972; **Fac Appt:** Clin Prof S, Cornell Univ-Weill Med Coll

Demmy, Todd L MD [TS] - **Spec Exp:** Lung Cancer; Thoracic Cancers; Esophageal Cancer; **Hospital:** Roswell Park Cancer Inst, Buffalo General Hosp; **Address:** Roswell Park Cancer Inst, Carlton Bldg, Elm & Carlton Sts, rm 243, Buffalo, NY 14263; **Phone:** 716-845-5873; **Board Cert:** Surgical Critical Care 1992; Surgery 1997; Thoracic Surgery 2000; **Med School:** Jefferson Med Coll 1983; **Resid:** Surgery, Baylor Univ Medical Ctr 1988; Thoracic Surgery, Allegheny Genl Hosp 1991; **Fac Appt:** Assoc Prof S, SUNY Buffalo

Friedberg, Joseph MD [TS] - **Spec Exp:** Lung Cancer; Mesothelioma; Photodynamic Therapy; **Hospital:** Penn Presby Med Ctr - UPHS (page 84), Hosp Univ Penn - UPHS (page 84); **Address:** Penn-Presbyterian Medical Ctr, 51 N 39th St, rm W250, Philadelphia, PA 19104; **Phone:** 215-662-9195; **Board Cert:** Surgery 1996; Thoracic Surgery 1997; **Med School:** Harvard Med Sch 1986; **Resid:** Surgery, Mass General Hosp 1994; **Fellow:** Cardiothoracic Surgery, Brigham & Womens Hosp 1996

Gharagozloo, Farid MD [TS] - **Spec Exp:** Video Assisted Thoracic Surgery (VATS); Lung Cancer; **Hospital:** G Washington Univ Hosp, Harbor Hosp Ctr; **Address:** 2175 K St NW, Ste 300, Washington, DC 20037; **Phone:** 202-775-8600; **Board Cert:** Surgery 1990; Thoracic Surgery 1993; **Med School:** Johns Hopkins Univ 1983; **Resid:** Surgery, Mayo Clinic 1989; Research, Harvard Med Sch 1986; **Fellow:** Cardiothoracic Surgery, Mayo Clinic 1992; **Fac Appt:** Prof S

Goldberg, Melvyn MD [TS] - **Spec Exp:** Lung Cancer; Esophageal Cancer; Barrett's Esophagus; **Hospital:** Fox Chase Cancer Ctr (page 73); **Address:** Fox Chase Cancer Center, 7701 Burholme Ave, Philadelphia, PA 19111; **Phone:** 215-728-2654; **Board Cert:** Surgery 1971; Thoracic Surgery 1977; **Med School:** Canada 1965; **Resid:** Surgery, Toronto General Hosp 1971; **Fellow:** Cardiothoracic Surgery, The London Chest Hosp 1973; **Fac Appt:** Prof S, Temple Univ

Heitmiller, Richard F MD [TS] - **Spec Exp:** Esophageal Surgery; Esophageal Cancer; Lung Cancer; **Hospital:** Union Meml Hosp - Baltimore; **Address:** 3333 N Calvert St, Ste 610, Baltimore, MD 21218; **Phone:** 410-554-2063; **Board Cert:** Surgery 1997; Thoracic Surgery 1999; **Med School:** Johns Hopkins Univ 1979; **Resid:** Surgery, Mass Genl Hosp 1985; **Fellow:** Thoracic Surgery, Mass Genl Hosp 1987; **Fac Appt:** Assoc Prof Surg & Onc, Johns Hopkins Univ

Kaiser, Larry R MD [TS] - **Spec Exp:** Lung Cancer; Esophageal Cancer; Mediastinal Tumors; **Hospital:** Hosp Univ Penn - UPHS (page 84), Pennsylvania Hosp (page 84); **Address:** Hosp Univ Pennsylvania, Dept Surgery, 3400 Spruce St, 4 Silverstein, Philadelphia, PA 19104-4219; **Phone:** 215-662-7538; **Board Cert:** Surgery 2005; Thoracic Surgery 1996; **Med School:** Tulane Univ 1977; **Resid:** Surgery, UCLA Med Ctr 1983; Cardiothoracic Surgery, Univ Toronto Hosps 1985; **Fellow:** Surgical Oncology, UCLA Med Ctr 1981; **Fac Appt:** Prof S, Univ Pennsylvania

Keenan, Robert J MD [TS] - **Spec Exp:** Lung Cancer; Esophageal Cancer; Mediastinal Tumors; **Hospital:** Allegheny General Hosp, Westmoreland Regl Hosp; **Address:** Allegheny Genl Hosp, 14th Fl, 320 E North Ave, Pittsburgh, PA 15212; **Phone:** 412-359-6137; **Board Cert:** Surgery 2000; **Med School:** Canada 1984; **Resid:** Surgery, Univ Toronto Med Ctr 1989; **Fellow:** Thoracic Surgery, Univ Pittsburgh Med Ctr 1990; Thoracic Surgery, Univ Toronto Med Ctr 1991; **Fac Appt:** Prof TS, Drexel Univ Coll Med

Keller, Steven M MD [TS] - **Spec Exp:** Lung Cancer; Esophageal Cancer; **Hospital:** Montefiore Med Ctr; **Address:** Greene Medical Arts Pavilion, 3400 Bainbridge Ave, Ste 5B, Bronx, NY 10467-2404; **Phone:** 718-920-7580; **Board Cert:** Surgery 1996; Thoracic Surgery 1996; **Med School:** Albany Med Coll 1977; **Resid:** Surgery, Mount Sinai Hosp 1985; Thoracic Surgery, Mem Sloan Kettering Cancer Ctr 1987; **Fellow:** Surgical Oncology, NIH/National Cancer Inst 1983; **Fac Appt:** Prof TS, Albert Einstein Coll Med

Krasna, Mark MD [TS] - **Spec Exp:** Esophageal Cancer; Lung Cancer; Mesothelioma; **Hospital:** St Joseph Med Ctr, Univ of MD Med Sys; **Address:** 7505 Osler Drive Odea Bldg - Ste 303, Towson, MD 21204; **Phone:** 410-427-2220; **Board Cert:** Thoracic Surgery 2000; **Med School:** Israel 1982; **Resid:** Surgery, CMDNJ-Rutgers Med Sch 1988; **Fellow:** Cardiothoracic Surgery, New England Deaconess-Harvard 1990; **Fac Appt:** Prof S, Univ MD Sch Med

Krellenstein, Daniel J MD [TS] - **Spec Exp:** Lung Cancer; Minimally Invasive Thoracic Surgery; **Hospital:** Mount Sinai Med Ctr (page 77), Lenox Hill Hosp; **Address:** 16 E 98th St, Ste 1F, New York, NY 10029-6545; **Phone:** 212-423-9311; **Board Cert:** Surgery 1974; Thoracic Surgery 1977; **Med School:** SUNY Buffalo 1964; **Resid:** Surgery, SUNY Downstate Med Ctr 1972; **Fac Appt:** Assoc Clin Prof TS, Mount Sinai Sch Med

Pass, Harvey MD [TS] - **Spec Exp:** Lung Cancer; Mesothelioma; Clinical Trials; **Hospital:** NYU Med Ctr (page 80); **Address:** NYU Cancer Ctr, 160 E 34th St Fl 8, New York, NY 10016; **Phone:** 212-731-5414; **Board Cert:** Thoracic Surgery 2001; **Med School:** Duke Univ 1973; **Resid:** Surgery, Duke Univ Med Ctr 1975; Surgery, Univ Miss Med Ctr 1980; **Fellow:** Cardiothoracic Surgery, MUSC Med Ctr 1982; **Fac Appt:** Prof S, NYU Sch Med

Pierson III, Richard N MD [TS] - **Spec Exp:** Transplant-Lung; Lung Cancer; **Hospital:** Univ of MD Med Sys; **Address:** Univ MD Med Ctr, Dept Cardiothoracic Surg, 22 S Greene St, rm N4W94, Baltimore, MD 21201; **Phone:** 410-328-5842; **Board Cert:** Surgery 2000; Thoracic Surgery 2002; **Med School:** Columbia P&S 1983; **Resid:** Surgery, Univ Mich Med Ctr 1990; **Fellow:** Cardiothoracic Surgery, Mass General Hosp 1992; **Fac Appt:** Assoc Prof TS, Univ MD Sch Med

Shrager, Joseph B MD [TS] - **Spec Exp:** Lung Cancer; **Hospital:** Hosp Univ Penn - UPHS (page 84), Pennsylvania Hosp (page 84); **Address:** Hosp Univ Penn, Div Thoracic Surg, 3400 Spruce St, 4 Silverstein Bldg, Philadelphia, PA 19104; **Phone:** 215-662-4767; **Board Cert:** Thoracic Surgery 1999; Surgery 1996; **Med School:** Harvard Med Sch 1988; **Resid:** Surgery, Hosp U Penn 1995; Cardiothoracic Surgery, Mass General Hosp 1997; **Fac Appt:** Assoc Prof S, Univ Pennsylvania

Sonett, Joshua R MD [TS] - **Spec Exp:** Minimally Invasive Thoracic Surgery; Transplant-Lung; Thoracic Cancers; **Hospital:** NY-Presby Hosp (page 79); **Address:** 161 Fort Washington Ave, New York, NY 10032; **Phone:** 212-305-8086; **Board Cert:** Surgery 1994; Thoracic Surgery 1997; **Med School:** E Carolina Univ 1988; **Resid:** Surgery, Univ Mass Med Ctr 1993; **Fellow:** Cardiothoracic Surgery, Univ Pittsburgh Med Ctr 1994; Thoracic Surgery, Meml Sloan Kettering Cancer Ctr; **Fac Appt:** Assoc Prof S, Columbia P&S

Swanson, Scott J MD [TS] - **Spec Exp:** Lung Cancer; Video Assisted Thoracic Surgery (VATS); Esophageal Cancer; **Hospital:** Mount Sinai Med Ctr (page 77); **Address:** 1190 5th Ave, Box 1028, New York, NY 10029; **Phone:** 212-659-6815; **Board Cert:** Surgery 1991; Thoracic Surgery 1996; **Med School:** Harvard Med Sch 1985; **Resid:** Surgery, Brigham & Womens Hosp 1990; **Fellow:** Cardiothoracic Surgery, Brigham & Womens Hosp 1994

Watson, Thomas J MD [TS] - **Spec Exp:** Esophageal Cancer; Lung Cancer; Thoracic Surgery; **Hospital:** Univ of Rochester Strong Meml Hosp, Highland Hosp - Rochester; **Address:** 601 Elmwood Ave, Box Surg, Rochester, NY 14642; **Phone:** 585-275-1509; **Board Cert:** Thoracic Surgery 1997; Surgery 2003; **Med School:** Univ SC Sch Med 1988; **Resid:** Surgery, LAC-USC Med Ctr 1993; Cardiothoracic Surgery, LAC-USC Med Ctr 1996; **Fellow:** Esophageal Surgery, LAC-USC Med Ctr 1994; **Fac Appt:** Assoc Prof S, Univ Rochester

Yang, Stephen C MD [TS] - **Spec Exp:** Mesothelioma; Lung Cancer; Esophageal Cancer; **Hospital:** Johns Hopkins Hosp - Baltimore, Johns Hopkins Bayview Med Ctr; **Address:** Johns Hopkins Hosp, 600 N Wolfe St Blalock Bldg - rm 240, Baltimore, MD 21287-5674; **Phone:** 410-614-3891; **Board Cert:** Surgery 2004; Thoracic Surgery 2006; **Med School:** Med Coll VA 1984; **Resid:** Surgery, Univ Tex Hlth Sci Ctr 1990; **Fellow:** Thoracic Surgery, MD Anderson Cancer Ctr 1992; Cardiothoracic Surgery, Med Coll Virginia 1994; **Fac Appt:** Assoc Prof TS, Johns Hopkins Univ

Southeast

Cerfolio, Robert J MD [TS] - **Spec Exp:** Lung Cancer; Tracheal Surgery; Chest Wall Tumors; Esophageal Cancer; **Hospital:** Univ of Ala Hosp at Birmingham; **Address:** 703 S 19th St, Ste 739, Birmingham, AL 35294; **Phone:** 205-934-5937; **Board Cert:** Thoracic Surgery 1997; Surgery 2003; **Med School:** Univ Rochester 1988; **Resid:** Surgery, Cornell-NY Hosp 1990; Surgery, Mayo Clinic 1993; **Fellow:** Cardiothoracic Surgery, Mayo Clinic 1996; **Fac Appt:** Prof TS, Univ Ala

D'Amico, Thomas MD [TS] - **Spec Exp:** Lung Cancer; Esophageal Cancer; **Hospital:** Duke Univ Med Ctr; **Address:** Duke Univ Med Ctr, Dept Thoracic Surg, Box 3496, Durham, NC 27710; **Phone:** 919-684-4891; **Board Cert:** Surgery 1995; Thoracic Surgery 1998; **Med School:** Columbia P&S 1987; **Resid:** Surgery, Duke Univ Med Ctr 1989; Cardiothoracic Surgery, Duke Univ Med Ctr 1996; **Fellow:** Thoracic Oncology, Meml Sloan Kettering Cancer Ctr; **Fac Appt:** Assoc Prof S, Duke Univ

Egan, Thomas MD [TS] - **Spec Exp:** Transplant-Lung; Thoracic Cancers; **Hospital:** Univ NC Hosps; **Address:** Univ N Carolina Hosps, 3040 Burnett, CB7065, Womack Bldg, Chapel Hill, NC 27599-7065; **Phone:** 919-966-3381; **Board Cert:** Thoracic Surgery 1999; **Med School:** Univ Toronto 1976; **Resid:** Surgery, Univ Toronto 1986; Thoracic Surgery, Univ Toronto 1988; **Fellow:** Transplant Surgery, Washington Univ 1989; **Fac Appt:** Prof S, Univ NC Sch Med

Harpole Jr, David H MD [TS] - **Spec Exp:** Lung Cancer; Mesothelioma; Esophageal Cancer; **Hospital:** Duke Univ Med Ctr; **Address:** Duke Univ Med Ctr-Thoracic Surgery, 2424 Erwin Rd, Ste 403 - rm 4071, Durham, NC 27705; **Phone:** 919-668-8413; **Board Cert:** Surgery 2002; Thoracic Surgery 2003; **Med School:** Univ VA Sch Med 1984; **Resid:** Surgery, Duke Univ Med Ctr 1991; **Fellow:** Thoracic Surgery, Duke Univ Med Ctr 1993; **Fac Appt:** Prof S, Duke Univ

Jones, David R MD [TS] - **Spec Exp:** Lung Cancer; Esophageal Cancer; Minimally Invasive Thoracic Surgery; **Hospital:** Univ Virginia Med Ctr; **Address:** Department of Surgery, Box 800679, Charlottesville, VA 22901; **Phone:** 434-243-6443; **Board Cert:** Surgery 1996; Thoracic Surgery 1999; **Med School:** W VA Univ 1989; **Resid:** Surgery, West Va Univ 1995; **Fellow:** Thoracic Surgery, Univ North Carolina 1998; **Fac Appt:** Assoc Prof S, Univ VA Sch Med

Kiernan, Paul D MD [TS] - **Spec Exp:** Lung Cancer; Esophageal Cancer; Mediastinal Tumors; **Hospital:** Inova Fairfax Hosp, Inova Alexandria Hosp; **Address:** 2921 Telestar Court, Falls Church, VA 22042; **Phone:** 703-280-5858; **Board Cert:** Thoracic Surgery 2002; **Med School:** Georgetown Univ 1974; **Resid:** Surgery, Mayo Clinic 1979; Cardiothoracic Surgery, Mayo Clinic 1981; **Fellow:** Vascular Surgery, Mayo Clinic 1982; **Fac Appt:** Assoc Clin Prof S, Georgetown Univ

Kiev, Jonathan MD [TS] - **Spec Exp:** Chest Wall Tumors; **Hospital:** Med Coll of VA Hosp; **Address:** 1250 E Marshall St, PO Box 980068, Richmond, VA 23298; **Phone:** 804-828-2775; **Board Cert:** Surgery 1996; Thoracic Surgery 2002; **Med School:** Tulane Univ 1989; **Resid:** Surgery, Hahnemann Univ 1994; **Fellow:** Thoracic Surgery, Univ Pittsburgh 2001; Thoracic Surgery, Mayo Clinic 2001; **Fac Appt:** Prof S, Va Commonwealth Univ

Miller, Daniel L MD [TS] - **Spec Exp:** Esophageal Cancer; Lung Cancer; Mesothelioma; **Hospital:** Emory Univ Hosp; **Address:** Emory Clinic, 1365 Clifton Rd NE, Atlanta, GA 30322; **Phone:** 404-778-3755; **Board Cert:** Thoracic Surgery 2005; Surgery 2001; **Med School:** Univ KY Coll Med 1985; **Resid:** Surgery, Georgetown Univ Hosp 1991; **Fellow:** Cardiothoracic Surgery, Mayo Clinic 1994; **Fac Appt:** Assoc Prof S, Emory Univ

Miller, Joseph MD [TS] - **Spec Exp:** Lung Cancer; **Hospital:** Emory Univ Hosp, Crawford Long Hosp of Emory Univ; **Address:** 550 Peachtree St NE, MOT-6th Fl, Atlanta, GA 30308; **Phone:** 404-686-2515; **Board Cert:** Surgery 1973; Thoracic Surgery 1975; **Med School:** Emory Univ 1965; **Resid:** Surgery, Mayo Clin 1972; Thoracic Surgery, Emory Univ Hosp 1974; **Fac Appt:** Prof S, Emory Univ

Mullett, Timothy W MD [TS] - **Spec Exp:** Lung Cancer; Esophageal Surgery; **Hospital:** Univ of Kentucky Chandler Hosp; **Address:** 900 S Limestone St, Lexington, KY 40536; **Phone:** 859-323-6494; **Board Cert:** Thoracic Surgery 1997; Surgery 2005; **Med School:** Univ Fla Coll Med 1987; **Resid:** Surgery, Shands/Univ of FL 1993; **Fellow:** Pediatric Surgery, Shands/Univ of FL 1994; Cardiothoracic Surgery, Shands/Univ of FL 1995; **Fac Appt:** Assoc Prof S, Univ KY Coll Med

Nesbitt, Jonathan C MD [TS] - **Spec Exp:** Lung Cancer; Esophageal Cancer; **Hospital:** Saint Thomas Hosp - Nashville; **Address:** The Surgical Clinic, St Thomas Med Bldg, 4230 Harding Rd, Ste 525, Nashville, TN 37205; **Phone:** 615-385-1547; **Board Cert:** Surgery 1998; Thoracic Surgery 1998; **Med School:** Georgetown Univ 1981; **Resid:** Surgery, Vanderbilt Univ Medical Ctr 1987; Thoracic Surgery, Albany Medical Ctr 1989; **Fac Appt:** Asst Clin Prof S, Vanderbilt Univ

Ninan, Mathew MD [TS] - **Spec Exp:** Lung Cancer; Transplant-Lung; Esophageal Cancer; **Hospital:** Baptist Memorial Hospital - Memphis, Methodist LeBonheur Germantown Hosp; **Address:** Cardiovascular Surgery Clinic, LLC, 6029 Walnut Grove Rd, Ste 401, East Office, Memphis, TN 38120; **Phone:** 901-747-3066; **Med School:** India 1988; **Resid:** Surgery, University of London 1994; **Fellow:** Cardiothoracic Surgery, Univ Pittsburgh 1998; **Fac Appt:** Asst Prof TS, Vanderbilt Univ

Putnam Jr, Joe B MD [TS] - **Spec Exp:** Lung Cancer; Esophageal Cancer; Sarcoma-Soft Tissue; **Hospital:** Vanderbilt Univ Med Ctr, VA Med Ctr - Nashville; **Address:** Vanderbilt Univ Med Ctr - Thoracic Surgery, 1301 Medical Center Drive, 2971 TVC, Nashville, TN 37232-5734; **Phone:** 615-343-9202; **Board Cert:** Thoracic Surgery 1997; **Med School:** Univ NC Sch Med 1979; **Resid:** Surgery, Univ Rochester 1986; Thoracic Surgery, Univ Mich Med Ctr 1988; **Fellow:** Surgical Oncology, NCI/NIH-Surg Branch 1984; **Fac Appt:** Prof TS, Vanderbilt Univ

Reed, Carolyn E MD [TS] - **Spec Exp:** Esophageal Cancer; Lung Cancer; **Hospital:** MUSC Med Ctr; **Address:** Med Univ S Carolina, Hollings Cancer Ctr, 96 Jonathan Lucas St, Ste 418, Charleston, SC 29425; **Phone:** 843-792-3362; **Board Cert:** Thoracic Surgery 2006; **Med School:** Univ Rochester 1977; **Resid:** Surgery, New York Hosp 1982; Thoracic Surgery, New York Hosp 1985; **Fellow:** Surgical Oncology, Meml Sloan Kettering Cancer Ctr 1983; **Fac Appt:** Prof S, Med Univ SC

Robinson, Lary A MD [TS] - **Spec Exp:** Lung Cancer; Mesothelioma; **Hospital:** H Lee Moffitt Cancer Ctr & Research Inst, Tampa Genl Hosp; **Address:** 12902 Magnolia Drive, Tampa, FL 33612-9497; **Phone:** 813-979-3050; **Board Cert:** Thoracic Surgery 2003; Surgery 2002; Surgical Critical Care 2000; **Med School:** Washington Univ, St Louis 1972; **Resid:** Surgery, Duke Univ Med Ctr 1974; Thoracic Surgery, Duke Univ Med Ctr 1981; **Fellow:** Cardiothoracic Surgery, St Thomas Hosp 1982; Cardiothoracic Surgery, Duke Univ Med Ctr 1983; **Fac Appt:** Prof S, Univ S Fla Coll Med

Midwest

Deschamps, Claude MD [TS] - **Spec Exp:** Esophageal Cancer; Lung Cancer; **Hospital:** St Mary's Hosp - Rochester; **Address:** Mayo Clinic, Div Thoracic Surgery, 200 First St SW, Rochester, MN 55905; **Phone:** 507-284-8462; **Board Cert:** Surgery 1994; **Med School:** Univ Montreal 1979; **Resid:** Surgery, Univ Montreal Hosps 1984; Thoracic Surgery, Univ Montreal Hosp 1985; **Fellow:** Thoracic Surgery, Mayo Clinic 1987; **Fac Appt:** Prof S, Mayo Med Sch

Faber, L Penfield MD [TS] - **Spec Exp:** Lung Cancer; Esophageal Cancer; Thoracic Cancers; **Hospital:** Rush Univ Med Ctr; **Address:** 1725 W Harrison St, Ste 774, Chicago, IL 60612-3817; **Phone:** 312-738-3732; **Board Cert:** Surgery 1962; Thoracic Surgery 1963; **Med School:** Northwestern Univ 1956; **Resid:** Surgery, Presby-St Luke's Hosp 1961; Thoracic Surgery, Hines VA Hosp 1963; **Fac Appt:** Prof TS, Rush Med Coll

Ferguson, Mark MD [TS] - **Spec Exp:** Barrett's Esophagus; Esophageal Cancer; Lung Cancer; **Hospital:** Univ of Chicago Hosps; **Address:** 5841 S Maryland Ave, MC 5035, Univ of Chicago Hospitals, Chicago, IL 60637-1470; **Phone:** 773-702-3551; **Board Cert:** Surgery 1993; Thoracic Surgery 2003; **Med School:** Univ Chicago-Pritzker Sch Med 1977; **Resid:** Surgery, Univ Chicago Hosps 1982; **Fellow:** Cardiothoracic Surgery, Univ Chicago Hosps 1984; **Fac Appt:** Prof S, Univ Chicago-Pritzker Sch Med

Iannettoni, Mark D MD [TS] - **Spec Exp:** Transplant-Lung; Lung Cancer; Esophageal Disorders; **Hospital:** Univ Iowa Hosp & Clinics; **Address:** Univ Iowa Hosp & Clinics, 200 Hawkins Drive, rm SE514GH, Iowa City, IA 52242; **Phone:** 319-356-1133; **Board Cert:** Surgery 2002; Thoracic Surgery 2002; **Med School:** SUNY Upstate Med Univ 1985; **Resid:** Surgery, SUNY Upstate Med Ctr 1991; Thoracic Surgery, Univ Mich Med Ctr 1993; **Fellow:** Thoracic Surgery, Univ Mich Med Sch 1994

Maddaus, Michael A MD [TS] - **Spec Exp:** Esophageal Cancer; Lung Cancer; Minimally Invasive Thoracic Surgery; **Hospital:** Univ Minn Med Ctr, Fairview - Univ Campus, Abbott - Northwestern Hosp; **Address:** Univ Minn Hosps, 420 Delaware St, Box 207 UMHC, Minneapolis, MN 55455; **Phone:** 612-624-9461; **Board Cert:** Surgery 2000; Thoracic Surgery 1993; **Med School:** Univ Minn 1982; **Resid:** Surgery, Univ Minn 1990; Thoracic Surgery, Univ Toronto 1991; **Fellow:** Cardiac Surgery, St Michael's Hosp/Hosp Sick Chldn 1992; Thoracic Oncology, Meml Sloan Kettering Cancer Ctr 1992; **Fac Appt:** Prof S, Univ Minn

Meyers, Bryan MD [TS] - **Spec Exp:** Lung Cancer; Esophageal Cancer; Transplant-Lung; **Hospital:** Barnes-Jewish Hosp, Barnes-Jewish West County Hosp; **Address:** 4921 Parkview Pl, Ste 8B, St Louis, MO 63110; **Phone:** 314-362-8598; **Board Cert:** Surgery 1998; Thoracic Surgery 1999; **Med School:** Univ Chicago-Pritzker Sch Med 1986; **Resid:** Surgery, Mass Genl Hosp 1996; **Fellow:** Cardiothoracic Surgery, Barnes Hosp-Wash Univ 1998; **Fac Appt:** Assoc Prof S, Washington Univ, St Louis

Naunheim, Keith S MD [TS] - **Spec Exp:** Lung Cancer; Esophageal Cancer; Chest Wall Tumors; Video Assisted Thoracic Surgery (VATS); **Hospital:** St Louis Univ Hosp; **Address:** St Lous Univ Med Ctr, Dept Surgery, 3635 Vista Ave, St Louis, MO 63110-0250; **Phone:** 314-577-8360; **Board Cert:** Thoracic Surgery 2004; **Med School:** Univ Chicago-Pritzker Sch Med 1978; **Resid:** Surgery, Univ Chicago Hosp 1983; **Fellow:** Cardiothoracic Surgery, Univ Chicago Hosp 1985; **Fac Appt:** Prof S, St Louis Univ

Orringer, Mark B MD [TS] - **Spec Exp:** Esophageal Cancer; Lung Cancer; Mediastinal Tumors; Lung Cancer; **Hospital:** Univ Michigan Hlth Sys; **Address:** Univ Mich, Taubman Ctr, 1500 E Med Ctr Drive, rm TC 2120, Box 0344, Ann Arbor, MI 48109-0344; **Phone:** 734-936-4975; **Board Cert:** Surgery 1973; Thoracic Surgery 1974; **Med School:** Univ Pittsburgh 1967; **Resid:** Thoracic Surgery, Johns Hopkins Hosp 1973; **Fac Appt:** Prof S, Univ Mich Med Sch

Patterson, G Alexander MD [TS] - **Spec Exp:** Lung Cancer; Esophageal Cancer; Transplant-Lung; **Hospital:** Barnes-Jewish Hosp; **Address:** 660 S Euclid Ave, Box 8234, St Louis, MO 63110; **Phone:** 314-362-6025; **Board Cert:** Surgery 1978; Thoracic Surgery 1981; Vascular Surgery 1982; **Med School:** Canada 1974; **Resid:** Surgery, Queens Univ Med Ctr 1978; Vascular Surgery, Univ Toronto Med Ctr 1979; **Fellow:** Research, Toronto Genl Hosp 1981; Surgical Critical Care, Johns Hopkins Hosp 1982; **Fac Appt:** Prof S, Washington Univ, St Louis

Great Plains and Mountains

Bull, David A MD [TS] - **Spec Exp:** Esophageal Cancer; **Hospital:** Univ Utah Hosps and Clins; **Address:** Univ Utah, Dept Cardiothoracic Surgery, 30 N 1900 East, rm 3C127, Salt Lake City, UT 84132; **Phone:** 801-581-5311; **Board Cert:** Thoracic Surgery 2004; Vascular Surgery 2003; Surgery 1999; Surgical Critical Care 1999; **Med School:** UCSF 1985; **Resid:** Surgery, UCSF Medical Ctr 1987; Surgery, Univ Arizona Hosps 1990; **Fellow:** Vascular Surgery, Univ Arizona Hosps 1992; Cardiothoracic Surgery, Univ Arizona Hosps 1994; **Fac Appt:** Assoc Prof TS, Univ Utah

Karwande, Shreekanth V MD [TS] - **Spec Exp:** Thoracic Cancers; Lung Cancer; **Hospital:** Univ Utah Hosps and Clins; **Address:** Univ Utah Med Ctr, Cardiothoracic Surg, 30 N 1900 E, Ste 3C127, Salt Lake City, UT 84132; **Phone:** 801-581-5311; **Board Cert:** Thoracic Surgery 2003; **Med School:** India 1973; **Resid:** Surgery, Erie Co Med Ctr 1981; Cardiothoracic Surgery, New York Hosp 1985; **Fellow:** Cardiothoracic Surgery, Meml Sloan Kettering Cancer Ctr; **Fac Appt:** Prof S, Univ Utah

Southwest

Lanza, Louis MD [TS] - **Spec Exp:** Lung Cancer; **Hospital:** Mayo Clin Hosp - Scottsdale; **Address:** Mayo Clinic Hosp, 5779 E Mayo Blvd MCSB Bldg Fl 1, Phoenix, AZ 85054; **Phone:** 480-342-2270; **Board Cert:** Thoracic Surgery 2002; **Med School:** Loyola Univ-Stritch Sch Med 1981; **Resid:** Surgery, Univ Michigan Med Ctr 1988; Cardiovascular Surgery, Texas Heart Inst 1991; **Fellow:** Surgical Oncology, Natl Cancer Inst 1986; Thoracic Oncology, MD Anderson Cancer Ctr 1989

Reardon, Michael J MD [TS] - **Spec Exp:** Cardiac Tumors/Cancer; **Hospital:** Methodist Hosp - Houston, UT MD Anderson Cancer Ctr (page 81); **Address:** 6560 Fannin St, Ste 1002, Houston, TX 77030; **Phone:** 713-793-7409; **Board Cert:** Thoracic Surgery 2006; **Med School:** Baylor Coll Med 1978; **Resid:** Surgery, Baylor Affil Hosps 1983; Thoracic Surgery, Texas Heart Inst 1985; **Fac Appt:** Clin Prof S, Baylor Coll Med

Roth, Jack MD [TS] - **Spec Exp:** Esophageal Cancer; Lung Cancer; Gene Therapy; **Hospital:** UT MD Anderson Cancer Ctr (page 81); **Address:** Dept Thoracic & Cardiovasc Surg Unit 445, 1515 Holcombe Blvd, Houston, TX 77030-1402; **Phone:** 713-792-7664; **Board Cert:** Thoracic Surgery 2002; **Med School:** Johns Hopkins Univ 1971; **Resid:** Surgery, Johns Hopkins Hosp 1973; Thoracic Surgery, UCLA Ctr Hlth Sci 1979; **Fellow:** Surgical Oncology, UCLA 1975; **Fac Appt:** Prof TS, Univ Tex, Houston

Swisher, Stephen G MD [TS] - **Spec Exp:** Esophageal Cancer; Lung Cancer; Mesothelioma; Thoracic Cancers; **Hospital:** UT MD Anderson Cancer Ctr (page 81); **Address:** Dept of Thoracic & Cardiovasc Surg, 1515 Holcombe Blvd, Unit 445, Houston, TX 77030; **Phone:** 713-792-8659; **Board Cert:** Surgery 2002; Thoracic Surgery 1997; **Med School:** UCSD 1986; **Resid:** Surgery, UCLA Med Ctr 1993; **Fellow:** Surgical Oncology, UCLA Med Ctr 1990; Cardiothoracic Surgery, MD Anderson Canc Ctr 1996; **Fac Appt:** Prof TS, Univ Tex, Houston

West Coast and Pacific

Cannon, Walter Bradford MD [TS] - **Spec Exp:** Chest Wall Tumors; **Hospital:** Stanford Univ Med Ctr, VA Hlth Care Sys - Palo Alto; **Address:** Stanford Univ Med Ctr, Dept Cardiothoracic Surgery, 300 Pasteur Dr, Falk Bldg CVRB, Stanford, CA 94305-5407; **Phone:** 650-736-7191; **Board Cert:** Thoracic Surgery 1996; Surgery 1996; **Med School:** Harvard Med Sch 1969; **Resid:** Thoracic Surgery, Stanford Univ Hosp 1975; **Fac Appt:** Clin Prof S, Stanford Univ

Thoracic Surgery

De Meester, Tom R MD [TS] - Spec Exp: Stomach Cancer; Esophageal Cancer; Lung Cancer; Tracheal Surgery; **Hospital:** USC Univ Hosp - R K Eamer Med Plz; **Address:** 1510 San Pablo St, Ste 514, Los Angeles, CA 90033; **Phone:** 323-442-5925; **Board Cert:** Surgery 1971; Thoracic Surgery 1971; **Med School:** Univ Mich Med Sch 1963; **Resid:** Surgery, Johns Hopkins Hosp 1966; **Fellow:** Thoracic Surgery, Johns Hopkins Hosp 1968; **Fac Appt:** Prof S, USC Sch Med

Handy Jr, John R MD [TS] - Spec Exp: Lung Cancer; Esophageal Cancer; Mesothelioma; Chest Wall Tumors; **Hospital:** Providence Portland Med Ctr; **Address:** Oregon Clinic-Cardiothoracic Surgery, 1111 NE 99th Ave, Ste 201, Portland, OR 97213; **Phone:** 503-215-2300; **Board Cert:** Thoracic Surgery 2001; Surgery 1999; **Med School:** Duke Univ 1983; **Resid:** Surgery, Brown Univ Hosp 1990; **Fellow:** Cardiothoracic Surgery, MUSC Med Ctr 1993

Jablons, David M MD [TS] - Spec Exp: Lung Cancer; Mesothelioma; Esophageal Surgery; **Hospital:** UCSF - Mt Zion Med Ctr; **Address:** UCSF Thoracic Surg, 1600 Divisadero St Fl 4, San Francisco, CA 94115; **Phone:** 415-885-3882; **Board Cert:** Thoracic Surgery 2002; **Med School:** Albany Med Coll 1984; **Resid:** Surgery, New Eng Med Ctr-Tufts Univ 1986; Surgery, New Eng Med Ctr-Tufts Univ 1991; **Fellow:** Surgical Oncology, Natl Cancer Inst-NIH 1989; Cardiothoracic Surgery, New York Hosp-Cornell 1993; **Fac Appt:** Prof S, UCSF

Kernstine, Kemp H MD/PhD [TS] - Spec Exp: Lung Cancer; Esophageal Cancer; Tracheal Surgery; Esophageal Surgery; **Hospital:** City of Hope Natl Med Ctr & Beckman Rsch (page 69); **Address:** City of Hope Comprehensive Cancer Ctr, 1500 E Duarte Rd, Duarte, CA 91010; **Phone:** 626-359-8111 x68845; **Board Cert:** Thoracic Surgery 1996; Surgery 2001; **Med School:** Duke Univ 1982; **Resid:** Surgery, Univ Minn Med Ctr 1988; **Fellow:** Cardiothoracic Surgery, Brigham & Women's Hosp 1994; **Fac Appt:** Assoc Prof S, Univ Iowa Coll Med

McKenna Jr, Robert J MD [TS] - Spec Exp: Lung Cancer; Video Assisted Thoracic Surgery (VATS); **Hospital:** Cedars-Sinai Med Ctr; **Address:** 8635 W 3rd St, Ste 975 West Twr, Los Angeles, CA 90048-6101; **Phone:** 310-652-0530; **Board Cert:** Thoracic Surgery 1997; **Med School:** USC Sch Med 1977; **Resid:** Surgery, Stanford Univ Hosp 1982; Cardiothoracic Surgery, Good Samaritan Hosp 1987; **Fellow:** Thoracic Surgery, MD Anderson Tumor Inst 1983; **Fac Appt:** Clin Prof TS, UCLA

Vallieres, Eric MD [TS] - Spec Exp: Lung Cancer; Mesothelioma; Mediastinal Tumors; Thoracic Cancers; **Hospital:** Swedish Med Ctr - Seattle; **Address:** 1221 Madison St, Ste 400, Seattle, WA 98104; **Phone:** 206-215-6800; **Med School:** Canada 1982; **Resid:** Surgery, Univ of Toronto 1988; Thoracic Surgery, Univ of Toronto 1989; **Fellow:** Cardiovascular Surgery, Univ of Montreal 1990

Whyte, Richard MD [TS] - Spec Exp: Lung Cancer; Esophageal Cancer; **Hospital:** Stanford Univ Med Ctr; **Address:** Stanford Univ Sch Med, Div Thor Surg, 300 Pasteur Dr, Bldg CVRB - rm 205, Stanford, CA 94305-5407; **Phone:** 650-723-6649; **Board Cert:** Surgery 1991; Thoracic Surgery 1993; **Med School:** Univ Pittsburgh 1983; **Resid:** Surgery, Mass Genl Hosp 1990; Thoracic Surgery, Univ Michigan Hosp 1992; **Fac Appt:** Assoc Prof TS, Stanford Univ

Wood, Douglas E MD [TS] - Spec Exp: Lung Cancer; Esophageal Cancer; Mesothelioma; **Hospital:** Univ Wash Med Ctr, Northwest Hosp; **Address:** Univ Washington, Div Cardiothoracic Surg, 1959 NE Pacific St, AA Bldg - rm 115, Box 356310, Seattle, WA 98195-6310; **Phone:** 206-685-3228; **Board Cert:** Surgery 1999; Thoracic Surgery 2001; Surgical Critical Care 1993; **Med School:** Harvard Med Sch 1983; **Resid:** Surgery, Mass Genl Hosp 1989; Thoracic Surgery, Mass Genl Hosp 1991; **Fellow:** Surgical Critical Care, Mass Genl Hosp 1991; **Fac Appt:** Prof S, Univ Wash

Colon
and
lung
canswers.

At City of Hope, we're one of the few U.S. hospitals to offer robotic-assisted surgery for colon and lung cancers. With this minimally invasive procedure, our patients can experience less discomfort and a faster recovery. For an appointment, call 800-826-HOPE. Or ask your doctor for a referral. Most insurance accepted. At City of Hope, we have answers to cancer.

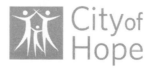

City of
Hope

Science saving lives.
cityofhope.org/topdoctors

Cleveland Clinic

Taussig Cancer Center

At Cleveland Clinic Taussig Cancer Center, we offer expanded services for people with lung cancer. Our goal in the Lung Cancer Clinic is to provide comprehensive assessment, management recommendations and support for people with lung cancer. Our thoracic surgeons, medical oncologists, radiation oncologists, pulmonologists, palliative medicine physicians, pain management physicians, pathologists, radiologists and clinical nurse specialists team up to offer the latest therapies, to reduce treatment complications and to improve overall quality of life.

The colorimetric sensor array system uses a novel optical chemical sensor to detect and identify odor-producing chemicals or patterns, such as those generated by lung cancer. A color fingerprint demonstrates changes in color due to exposure to exhaled breath generated from a colorimetric sensor array.

The use of implantable intrathecal pumps for the long-term delivery of medications such as narcotics can provide superior pain relief with fewer side effects than oral medications.

Combined PET-CT imaging for lung cancer staging offers major clinical advantages. It provides more accurate tumor detection and localization, and can even influence the course of treatment. This PET-CT image shows small-cell lung carcinoma invading the pulmonary vein.

Video-assisted thoracoscopy is of particular benefit to lung cancer patients who develop dangerous fluid levels in the sac surrounding the lung. For patients with early-stage lung cancer, surgical resection offers the best chance of survival. In addition to advanced surgical and palliative procedures, Taussig Cancer Center patients may benefit from treatment with targeted drug therapy or novel technologies such as stereotactic radiotherapy.

Gamma Knife radiosurgery may improve quality of life when lung cancer metastasizes to the brain. The Gamma Knife may also provide extended control of multiple metastatic tumors and even increase survival in some patients. In 2005, Cleveland Clinic upgraded its Gamma Knife equipment to the latest version (4C).

Novel experimental drugs and radiation protocols are also available to Taussig Cancer Center lung cancer patients through the many clinical trials in which we participate.

Second Opinion Clinic
• Offers lung cancer patients a second or confirmatory opinion
• Assessment includes pathology and radiology review
• Treatment plan is discussed with referring physician

Following a consult, patients can return to their primary care physician or oncologist for further recommendations.

Supportive Care Services

• Pain management	• Nutrition	• Imaging review
• Palliative medicine	• Social work services	• Pathology review
• Pulmonary rehabilitation	• Psychology/psychiatry services	• Same-day evaluations

To schedule an appointment or for more information about the Cleveland Clinic Taussig Cancer Center, call 800.890.2467 or visit www.clevelandclinic.org/lungtopdocs.

Taussig Cancer Center | 9500 Euclid Avenue / W14 | Cleveland OH 44195

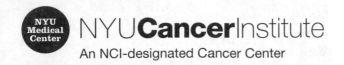

NYU**Cancer**Institute
An NCI-designated Cancer Center

NYU Clinical Cancer Center
160 East 34th Street
New York, New York 10016
www.nyuci.org/atcd

NYU Medical Center
550 First Avenue
(at 31st Street)
New York, New York 10016
www.nyumc.org/atcd

Stephen D. Hassenfeld
Children's Center
for Cancer and Blood
Disorders
160 East 32nd Street
New York, New York 10016
www.nyumc.org/hassenfeld

A Collaborative Approach
The NYU Cancer Institute, an NCI designated center, is a "matrix cancer center" without walls operating within the larger NYU Medical Center. With over 200 members and a research funding base of over $81 million, this structure strengthens our capabilities to forge collaborations across medical and scientific disciplines, which translates to comprehensive care for our patients and discoveries that will influence the future of this disease.

Renowned Expertise
Our highly skilled Magnet™ nursing team not only plays a pivotal role in coordinating direct patient care, but is also a source of invaluable patient education. Team members' compassion and expertise help patients better manage the symptoms of their disease as well as their special needs.

A Patient-Focused Setting
The NYU Clinical Cancer Center, with over 70 faculty members from various disciplines at the New York University School of Medicine, is the principal outpatient facility of the Cancer Institute and serves as home for our patients and their caregivers. The center and its multidisciplinary team of experts provide access to the latest treatment options and clinical trials along with a variety of programs in cancer prevention, screening, diagnostics, genetic counseling, and supportive services. When it comes to kids and cancer, the Stephen D. Hassenfeld Children's Center for Cancer and Blood Disorders offers not just innovation but insight. As a leading member of the NCI-sponsored Children's Oncology Group, our physicians are known for developing new ways to treat childhood cancer. Our affiliation with Bellevue Hospital, the oldest public hospital in the country, affords clinically distinctive opportunities to learn and care for patients with cancer by observing its presentation and behavior in a variety of patient groups.

THORACIC ONCOLOGY PROGRAM

UCLA Health System

1-800-UCLA-MD1 (825-2631)
www.uclahealth.org

UCLA's Thoracic Oncology Program provides highly integrated medical, surgical and radiation oncology services to patients with benign and malignant tumors of the lung, esophagus, pleura, mediastinum, chest wall, and all other areas of the thoracic cavity.

UCLA's program partners scientists specializing in cell signaling, angiogenesis inhibition, immunotherapy and gene therapy with experts in molecular imaging, epidemiology, pathology, biostatistics and patient care.

The Lung Cancer Program at UCLA's Jonsson Cancer Center has been designated a Specialized Program of Research Excellence (SPORE) by the National Cancer Institute, making it one of a handful of programs nationwide to receive national recognition and substantial research funding to improve prevention, detection and treatment of lung cancer. The goal is to translate basic research from the laboratories into patient care much more quickly and effectively.

UCLA's Jonsson Cancer Center

Designated by the National Cancer Institute as one of only 39 comprehensive cancer centers in the United States, UCLA's Jonsson Cancer Center has earned an international reputation for developing new cancer therapies, providing the best in experimental and traditional treatments, and expertly guiding and training the next generation of medical researchers. The center's 250 physicians and scientists treat upwards of 20,000 patient visits per year and offer hundreds of clinical trials that provide the latest in experimental cancer treatments (www.cancer.mednet.ucla.edu). The center also offers patients and families complete psychological and support services.

UCLA's Jonsson Cancer Center has been ranked the best cancer center in California by *U.S.News & World Report*'s Annual Best Hospitals survey for the seventh year. UCLA Medical Center of which the Cancer Center is a part, has ranked best in the West for the past 17 years.

UCLA'S THORACIC ONCOLOGY PROGRAM OFFERS TREATMENTS FOR TUMORS OF THE:

- Lung
- Esophagus
- Pleura
- Mediastinum
- Chest Wall
- All other areas of the thoracic cavity

Call 1-800-UCLA-MD1 (825-2631)
for a referral to a UCLA doctor.

Urology

A urologist manages benign and malignant medical and surgical disorders of the genitourinary system and the adrenal gland. This specialist has comprehensive knowledge of, and skills in, endoscopic, percutaneous and open surgery of congenital and acquired conditions of the urinary and reproductive systems and their contiguous structures.

Training Required: Five years

Urology

New England

Heney, Niall M MD [U] - **Spec Exp:** Urologic Cancer; **Hospital:** Mass Genl Hosp; **Address:** Mass Genl Hosp, Dept Urol, 55 Fruit St, GRB 1102, Boston, MA 02114; **Phone:** 617-726-3011; **Board Cert:** Urology 1977; **Med School:** Ireland 1965; **Resid:** Urology, Regional Hosp 1972; Urology, Mass Genl Hosp 1976; **Fac Appt:** Prof Med, Harvard Med Sch

Janeiro Jr, John J MD [U] - **Spec Exp:** Urologic Cancer; Prostate Disease; **Hospital:** Southern NH Med Ctr, St Joseph Hosp; **Address:** Urology Center Southern New Hampshire, 17 Riverside St, Ste 201, Nashua, NH 03062; **Phone:** 603-883-1550; **Board Cert:** Urology 1999; **Med School:** Univ Mass Sch Med 1982; **Resid:** Urology, Lahey Clinic 1987; **Fellow:** Pediatric Urology, Childrens Hosp 1989

Libertino, John A MD [U] - **Spec Exp:** Kidney Cancer; Prostate Cancer; Adrenal Tumors; **Hospital:** Lahey Clin; **Address:** Lahey Clinic, Dept Urology, 41 Mall Rd, Burlington, MA 01805; **Phone:** 781-744-2511; **Board Cert:** Urology 1973; **Med School:** Georgetown Univ 1965; **Resid:** Urology, Univ Rochester-Strong Meml Hosp 1967; Urology, Yale-New Haven Hosp 1970; **Fellow:** Surgery, Yale-New Haven Hosp 1968; **Fac Appt:** Assoc Clin Prof S, Harvard Med Sch

Loughlin, Kevin R MD [U] - **Spec Exp:** Prostate Cancer; Genitourinary Cancer; **Hospital:** Brigham & Women's Hosp, Dana-Farber Cancer Inst; **Address:** Brigham & Women's Hosp, Div Urology, 45 Francis St, ASBII-3, Boston, MA 02115; **Phone:** 617-732-6325; **Board Cert:** Urology 2004; **Med School:** NY Med Coll 1975; **Resid:** Pediatrics, New York Hosp-Cornell 1978; Surgery, Bellevue Hosp Ctr-NYU 1979; **Fellow:** Urology, Brigham & Women's Hosp 1983; Urologic Oncology, Meml Sloan Kettering Cancer Ctr; **Fac Appt:** Prof S, Harvard Med Sch

McDougal, W Scott MD [U] - **Spec Exp:** Penile Cancer; Prostate Cancer; Urologic Cancer; **Hospital:** Mass Genl Hosp; **Address:** Mass Genl Hosp, 55 Fruit St, Bldg GRB - rm 1102, Boston, MA 02114; **Phone:** 617-726-3010; **Board Cert:** Surgery 1975; Urology 2004; **Med School:** Cornell Univ-Weill Med Coll 1968; **Resid:** Surgery, Univ Hosps Cleveland 1975; Urology, Univ Hosps Cleveland 1975; **Fellow:** Physiology, Yale Med Sch 1972; **Fac Appt:** Prof U, Harvard Med Sch

McGovern, Francis MD [U] - **Spec Exp:** Prostate Cancer; **Hospital:** Mass Genl Hosp; **Address:** One Hawthorne Pl, Ste 109, Boston, MA 02114; **Phone:** 617-726-3574; **Board Cert:** Urology 1999; **Med School:** Case West Res Univ 1983; **Resid:** Urology, Mass Genl Hosp 1989

Richie, Jerome MD [U] - **Spec Exp:** Prostate Cancer; Testicular Cancer; Kidney Cancer; **Hospital:** Brigham & Women's Hosp, Dana-Farber Cancer Inst; **Address:** Brigham & Womens Hosp, 75 Francis St, Ste ASB2, Boston, MA 02115; **Phone:** 617-732-6325; **Board Cert:** Urology 1992; **Med School:** Univ Tex Med Br, Galveston 1969; **Resid:** Surgery, UCLA Med Ctr 1971; Urology, UCLA Med Ctr 1975; **Fac Appt:** Prof U, Harvard Med Sch

Mid Atlantic

Bagley Jr, Demetrius H MD [U] - **Spec Exp:** Kidney Cancer; **Hospital:** Thomas Jefferson Univ Hosp (page 82); **Address:** 833 Chestnut St E, Ste 703, Philadelphia, PA 19107; **Phone:** 215-955-1000; **Board Cert:** Urology 1981; **Med School:** Johns Hopkins Univ 1970; **Resid:** Surgery, Yale-New Haven Hosp 1972; Urology, Yale-New Haven Hosp 1979; **Fellow:** Surgery, NCI-USPHS 1975; **Fac Appt:** Prof U, Thomas Jefferson Univ

Benson, Mitchell C MD [U] - **Spec Exp:** Prostate Cancer/Robotic Surgery; Bladder Cancer; Kidney Cancer; Continent Urinary Diversions; **Hospital:** NY-Presby Hosp (page 79); **Address:** NY Presby Hosp-Columbia, Dept Urology, 161 Ft Washington Ave Fl 11 - rm 1102, New York, NY 10032-3713; **Phone:** 212-305-5201; **Board Cert:** Urology 1984; **Med School:** Columbia P&S 1977; **Resid:** Surgery, Mount Sinai Med Ctr 1979; Urology, Columbia-Presby Hosp 1982; **Fellow:** Oncology, Johns Hopkins Hosp 1984; **Fac Appt:** Prof U, Columbia P&S

Burnett II, Arthur L MD [U] - **Spec Exp:** Prostate Cancer; Erectile Dysfunction; **Hospital:** Johns Hopkins Hosp - Baltimore; **Address:** 600 N Wolfe St, Marburg Bldg, Ste 407, Baltimore, MD 21287; **Phone:** 410-614-3986; **Board Cert:** Urology 1998; **Med School:** Johns Hopkins Univ 1988; **Resid:** Urology, Johns Hopkins Hosp 1994; Surgery, Johns Hopkins Hosp 1990; **Fac Appt:** Prof U, Johns Hopkins Univ

Carter, H Ballentine MD [U] - **Spec Exp:** Prostate Cancer; **Hospital:** Johns Hopkins Hosp - Baltimore; **Address:** Brady Urological Inst, Johns Hopkins Hosp, 600 N Wolfe St Marburg Bldg - rm 145, Baltimore, MD 21287-2101; **Phone:** 410-955-6100; **Board Cert:** Urology 1999; **Med School:** Med Univ SC 1981; **Resid:** Surgery, New York Hosp 1983; Urology, New York Hosp 1987; **Fellow:** Research, Johns Hopkins Hosp 1989; **Fac Appt:** Prof U, Johns Hopkins Univ

Droller, Michael J MD [U] - **Spec Exp:** Urologic Cancer; Bladder Cancer; Prostate Cancer; Kidney Cancer; **Hospital:** Mount Sinai Med Ctr (page 77); **Address:** 5 E 98th St Fl 6th, Box 1272, New York, NY 10029-6501; **Phone:** 212-241-3868; **Board Cert:** Urology 2001; **Med School:** Harvard Med Sch 1968; **Resid:** Surgery, Peter Bent Brigham Hosp 1970; Urology, Stanford Univ Med Ctr 1976; **Fellow:** Immunology, Univ Stockholm 1977; **Fac Appt:** Prof U, Mount Sinai Sch Med

Gomella, Leonard G MD [U] - **Spec Exp:** Prostate Cancer; Laparoscopic Surgery; Urologic Cancer; **Hospital:** Thomas Jefferson Univ Hosp (page 82); **Address:** Thomas Jefferson Univ, 1015 Walnut St Fl 11 - Ste 1112, Philadelphia, PA 19107-5001; **Phone:** 215-955-1000; **Board Cert:** Urology 1998; **Med School:** Univ KY Coll Med 1980; **Resid:** Surgery, Univ Kentucky Med Ctr 1982; Urology, Univ Kentucky Med Ctr 1986; **Fellow:** Urologic Oncology, Natl Cancer Inst 1988; **Fac Appt:** Prof U, Jefferson Med Coll

Grasso, Michael MD [U] - **Spec Exp:** Urologic Cancer; Laparoscopic Surgery; **Hospital:** St Vincent Cath Med Ctrs - Manhattan; **Address:** 170 W 12th St, Ste 205, Dept Urology - Cronin 205, New York, NY 10011; **Phone:** 212-604-1270; **Board Cert:** Urology 2002; **Med School:** Jefferson Med Coll 1986; **Resid:** Surgery, Jefferson Univ Hosp 1988; Urology, Jefferson Univ Hosp 1992; **Fac Appt:** Prof U, NY Med Coll

Greenberg, Richard E MD [U] - **Spec Exp:** Prostate Cancer; Bladder Cancer; Kidney Cancer; **Hospital:** Fox Chase Cancer Ctr (page 73), Abington Mem Hosp; **Address:** Fox Chase Cancer Ctr, Div Urol Dept Surg, 333 Cottman Ave, Ste H3 - rm H3-116, Philadelphia, PA 19111; **Phone:** 215-728-5341; **Board Cert:** Urology 2005; **Med School:** Cornell Univ-Weill Med Coll 1976; **Resid:** Surgery, New York Hosp 1979; Urology, New York Hosp 1983; **Fac Appt:** Prof U, Temple Univ

Urology

Herr, Harry W MD [U] - **Spec Exp:** Bladder Cancer; Prostate Cancer; Testicular Cancer; **Hospital:** Meml Sloan Kettering Cancer Ctr (page 76), NY-Presby Hosp (page 79); **Address:** Meml Sloan Kettering Canc Ctr, Dept Urol, 1275 York Ave, New York, NY 10021; **Phone:** 646-422-4411; **Board Cert:** Urology 1976; **Med School:** UCSF 1969; **Resid:** Urology, UC Irvine Med Ctr 1974; **Fellow:** Urology, Meml Sloan Kettering Cancer Ctr 1976; **Fac Appt:** Assoc Prof S, Cornell Univ-Weill Med Coll

Huben, Robert P MD [U] - **Spec Exp:** Prostate Cancer; Kidney Cancer; Urologic Cancer; **Hospital:** Roswell Park Cancer Inst; **Address:** Roswell Park Cancer Inst, Elm & Carlton Sts, Buffalo, NY 14263-0001; **Phone:** 716-845-3389; **Board Cert:** Urology 1983; **Med School:** Cornell Univ-Weill Med Coll 1976; **Resid:** Urology, East Virginia Med Ctr 1981; **Fellow:** Urologic Oncology, Roswell Park Meml Inst 1982

Jarow, Jonathan P MD [U] - **Spec Exp:** Prostate Cancer; Erectile Dysfunction; Incontinence after Prostate Cancer; **Hospital:** Johns Hopkins Hosp - Baltimore; **Address:** Johns Hopkins Outpatient Ctr-Urology, 601 N Caroline St, Fl 4, Baltimore, MD 21287; **Phone:** 410-955-3617; **Board Cert:** Urology 1999; **Med School:** Northwestern Univ 1980; **Resid:** Surgery, Johns Hopkins Hosp 1982; Urology, Johns Hopkins Hosp 1986; **Fellow:** Andrology, Baylor Univ 1989; **Fac Appt:** Assoc Prof U, Johns Hopkins Univ

Kaplan, Steven A MD [U] - **Spec Exp:** Incontinence after Prostate Cancer; **Hospital:** NY-Presby Hosp (page 79); **Address:** NY Presbyterian-Weill Cornell Medical Ctr, 525 E 68th St, rm F9West, New York, NY 10021; **Phone:** 212-746-4811; **Board Cert:** Urology 2001; **Med School:** Mount Sinai Sch Med 1982; **Resid:** Surgery, Mount Sinai Hosp 1984; Urology, Columbia Presby Med Ctr 1988; **Fellow:** Urology, Columbia Presby Med Ctr 1990; **Fac Appt:** Prof U, Cornell Univ-Weill Med Coll

Katz, Aaron E MD [U] - **Spec Exp:** Prostate Cancer-Cryosurgery; Kidney Cancer-Cryosurgery; Complementary Medicine; **Hospital:** NY-Presby Hosp (page 79); **Address:** NY Presby Med Ctr, Herbert Irving Pav, 161 Ft Washington Ave Fl 11, New York, NY 10032; **Phone:** 212-305-6408; **Board Cert:** Urology 2006; **Med School:** NY Med Coll 1986; **Resid:** Urology, Maimonides Med Ctr 1992; **Fellow:** Urologic Oncology, Columbia Presby Med Ctr 1993; **Fac Appt:** Assoc Clin Prof U, Columbia P&S

Kirschenbaum, Alexander M MD [U] - **Spec Exp:** Prostate Cancer; Bladder Cancer; Kidney Cancer; **Hospital:** Mount Sinai Med Ctr (page 77); **Address:** 58A E 79th St, New York, NY 10021; **Phone:** 646-422-0926; **Board Cert:** Urology 2005; **Med School:** Mount Sinai Sch Med 1980; **Resid:** Surgery, Mount Sinai Hosp 1982; Urology, Mount Sinai Hosp 1985; **Fellow:** Urologic Oncology, Mount Sinai Hosp 1987; **Fac Appt:** Assoc Prof U, Mount Sinai Sch Med

Lanteri, Vincent J MD [U] - **Spec Exp:** Prostate Cancer/Robotic Surgery; Urologic Cancer; Minimally Invasive Urologic Surgery; **Hospital:** Hackensack Univ Med Ctr (page 74), Valley Hosp; **Address:** 5 Summit Ave Fl 2, Hackensack, NJ 07601; **Phone:** 201-487-8866; **Board Cert:** Urology 1982; **Med School:** Mexico 1974; **Resid:** Surgery, UMDNJ Med Ctr 1977; Urology, UMDNJ Med Ctr 1980; **Fellow:** Urologic Oncology, Roswell Park Cancer Inst 1981

Lepor, Herbert MD [U] - **Spec Exp:** Prostate Cancer; **Hospital:** NYU Med Ctr (page 80); **Address:** 150 E 32nd St Fl 2, New York, NY 10016; **Phone:** 646-825-6327; **Board Cert:** Urology 2005; **Med School:** Johns Hopkins Univ 1975; **Resid:** Urology, Johns Hopkins Hosp 1986; **Fac Appt:** Prof U, NYU Sch Med

Lowe, Franklin MD [U] - Spec Exp: Complementary Medicine; Prostate Cancer; **Hospital:** St Luke's - Roosevelt Hosp Ctr - Roosevelt Div (page 72), NY-Presby Hosp (page 79); **Address:** 425 W 59th St, Ste 3A, New York, NY 10019; **Phone:** 212-523-7790; **Board Cert:** Urology 2006; **Med School:** Columbia P&S 1979; **Resid:** Surgery, Johns Hopkins Hosp 1981; Urology, Johns Hopkins Hosp 1984; **Fac Appt:** Clin Prof U, Columbia P&S

Macchia, Richard MD [U] - Spec Exp: Prostate Disease; Prostate Cancer; Voiding Dysfunction; **Hospital:** SUNY Downstate Med Ctr, Kings County Hosp Ctr; **Address:** SUNY Downstate Med School, Dept Urology, 445 Lenox Rd, Box 79, Brooklyn, NY 11203-2098; **Phone:** 718-270-2554; **Board Cert:** Urology 1977; **Med School:** NY Med Coll 1969; **Resid:** Surgery, St Vincent's Hosp 1971; Urology, SUNY Downstate Med Ctr 1974; **Fellow:** Urologic Oncology, Meml Sloan Kettering Cancer Ctr 1976; **Fac Appt:** Prof U, SUNY Downstate

Malkowicz, S Bruce MD [U] - Spec Exp: Urologic Cancer; **Hospital:** Hosp Univ Penn - UPHS (page 84); **Address:** Hosp Univ Penn, Dept Urology, 3400 Spruce St, 9 Penn Tower, Philadelphia, PA 19104; **Phone:** 215-662-2891; **Board Cert:** Urology 2000; **Med School:** Univ Pennsylvania 1981; **Resid:** Surgery, Hosp Univ Penn 1983; Urology, Hosp Univ Penn 1987; **Fellow:** Urologic Oncology, USC Med Ctr 1998; Urologic Oncology, Hosp Univ Penn/Wistar Inst 1990; **Fac Appt:** Assoc Prof U, Univ Pennsylvania

Mostwin, Jacek L MD/PhD [U] - Spec Exp: Prostate Cancer; **Hospital:** Johns Hopkins Hosp - Baltimore; **Address:** Johns Hopkins Hosp, 600 N Wolfe St, Marburg-401C, Baltimore, MD 21287; **Phone:** 410-955-4461; **Board Cert:** Urology 1997; **Med School:** Univ MD Sch Med 1975; **Resid:** Surgery, Univ Michigan Med Ctr 1978; Urology, Johns Hopkins Hosp 1983; **Fac Appt:** Prof U, Johns Hopkins Univ

Naslund, Michael MD [U] - Spec Exp: Prostate Cancer; Prostate Disease; **Hospital:** Univ of MD Med Sys; **Address:** Maryland Prostate Ctr, 419 W Redwood St, Ste 320, Baltimore, MD 21201; **Phone:** 410-328-0800; **Board Cert:** Urology 2000; **Med School:** Johns Hopkins Univ 1981; **Resid:** Surgery, Johns Hopkins Hosp 1983; Urology, Johns Hopkins Hosp 1987; **Fac Appt:** Prof U, Univ MD Sch Med

Nelson, Joel B MD [U] - Spec Exp: Prostate Cancer; **Hospital:** UPMC Shadyside; **Address:** UPMC Shadyside Med Ctr, 5200 Centre Ave, Ste 209, Pittsburgh, PA 15232; **Phone:** 412-605-3013; **Board Cert:** Urology 1998; **Med School:** Northwestern Univ 1988; **Resid:** Surgery, Northwestern Meml Hosp 1990; Urology, Northwestern Meml Hosp 1994; **Fellow:** Urology, Johns Hopkins Hosp; **Fac Appt:** Prof U, Univ Pittsburgh

Partin, Alan W MD/PhD [U] - Spec Exp: Prostate Cancer; Prostate Disease; **Hospital:** Johns Hopkins Hosp - Baltimore; **Address:** Johns Hopkins Hosp, 600 N Wolfe St Marburg Bldg - rm 134, Baltimore, MD 21287; **Phone:** 410-614-4876; **Board Cert:** Urology 1998; **Med School:** Johns Hopkins Univ 1989; **Resid:** Surgery, Johns Hopkins Hosp 1991; Urology, Johns Hopkins Hosp 1994; **Fac Appt:** Prof U, Johns Hopkins Univ

Sawczuk, Ihor S MD [U] - Spec Exp: Kidney Cancer; Bladder Cancer; Prostate Cancer/Robotic Surgery; **Hospital:** Hackensack Univ Med Ctr (page 74), NY-Presby Hosp (page 79); **Address:** Hackensack Univ Med Ctr, 360 Essex St, Hackensack, NJ 07601; **Phone:** 201-336-8090; **Board Cert:** Urology 1996; **Med School:** Med Coll PA Hahnemann 1979; **Resid:** Surgery, St Vincent's Hosp & Med Ctr 1981; Urology, Columbia-Presby Med Ctr 1984; **Fellow:** Urologic Oncology, Columbia-Presby Med Ctr 1986; **Fac Appt:** Prof U, Columbia P&S

Scardino, Peter T MD [U] - **Spec Exp:** Prostate Cancer; **Hospital:** Meml Sloan Kettering Cancer Ctr (page 76); **Address:** 1275 York Ave, Box 27, New York, NY 10021; **Phone:** 646-422-4329; **Board Cert:** Urology 1981; **Med School:** Duke Univ 1971; **Resid:** Surgery, Mass Genl Hosp 1973; Urology, UCLA Med Ctr 1979; **Fellow:** Urology, Natl Cancer Inst 1976; **Fac Appt:** Prof U, Cornell Univ-Weill Med Coll

Schlegel, Peter MD [U] - **Spec Exp:** Prostate Cancer; Fertility Preservation in Cancer; Erectile Dysfunction; **Hospital:** NY-Presby Hosp (page 79); **Address:** 525 E 68th St, Starr 900, New York, NY 10021-4870; **Phone:** 212-746-5491; **Board Cert:** Urology 2007; **Med School:** Univ Mass Sch Med 1983; **Resid:** Surgery, Johns Hopkins Hosp 1985; Urology, Johns Hopkins Hosp 1989; **Fellow:** Medical Oncology, Johns Hopkins Hosp 1987; Male Reproduction, NY Hosp-Cornell Med Ctr 1991; **Fac Appt:** Prof U, Cornell Univ-Weill Med Coll

Sheinfeld, Joel MD [U] - **Spec Exp:** Testicular Cancer; Bladder Cancer; Fertility Preservation in Cancer; **Hospital:** Meml Sloan Kettering Cancer Ctr (page 76); **Address:** Meml Sloan Kettering Canc Ctr-Kimmel Ctr, 353 E 68th St, New York, NY 10021; **Phone:** 646-422-4311; **Board Cert:** Urology 2000; **Med School:** Univ Fla Coll Med 1981; **Resid:** Urology, Strong Meml Hosp 1986; **Fellow:** Urologic Oncology, Meml Sloan Kettering Cancer Ctr 1989; **Fac Appt:** Assoc Prof U, Cornell Univ-Weill Med Coll

Taneja, Samir S MD [U] - **Spec Exp:** Kidney Cancer; Prostate Cancer; Urologic Cancer; Laparoscopic Surgery; **Hospital:** NYU Med Ctr (page 80); **Address:** 150 E 32nd St, Ste 200, New York, NY 10016; **Phone:** 646-825-6321; **Board Cert:** Urology 1999; **Med School:** Northwestern Univ 1990; **Resid:** Urology, UCLA Med Ctr 1996; **Fac Appt:** Assoc Prof U, NYU Sch Med

Tewari, Ashutosh MD [U] - **Spec Exp:** Prostate Cancer/Robotic Surgery; **Hospital:** NY-Presby Hosp (page 79); **Address:** Weill Cornell Brady Urologic Health Ct, 525 E 68th St, Starr 916, New York, NY 10021; **Phone:** 212-746-5638; **Med School:** India 1983; **Resid:** Surgery, GSVM Medical College 1990; Urology, Henry Ford Hosp 2003; **Fellow:** Transplant Surgery, Liverpool 1993; Urologic Oncology, Shands Healthcare 1995; **Fac Appt:** Assoc Prof U, Cornell Univ-Weill Med Coll

Uzzo, Robert MD [U] - **Spec Exp:** Kidney Cancer; Bladder Cancer; Prostate Cancer; Testicular Cancer; **Hospital:** Fox Chase Cancer Ctr (page 73); **Address:** 333 Cottman Ave, rm H3116, Philadelphia, PA 19111; **Phone:** 215-728-3501; **Board Cert:** Urology 2001; **Med School:** Cornell Univ-Weill Med Coll 1991; **Resid:** Surgery, New York Hosp-Cornell Med Ctr 1993; Urology, New York Hosp-Cornell Med Ctr 1997; **Fellow:** Urologic Oncology, Cleveland Clinic 1999; Renal Transplant, Cleveland Clinic 2000; **Fac Appt:** Assoc Prof S, Temple Univ

Van Arsdalen, Keith N MD [U] - **Spec Exp:** Urologic Cancer; **Hospital:** Hosp Univ Penn - UPHS (page 84), Chldns Hosp of Philadelphia, The; **Address:** Hosp Univ Penn, Div Urol, 3400 Spruce St, 9 Penn Tower, Philadelphia, PA 19104-4283; **Phone:** 215-662-2891; **Board Cert:** Urology 1984; **Med School:** Med Coll VA 1977; **Resid:** Surgery, Univ Maryland Hosp 1979; Urology, Med Coll Virginia 1982; **Fellow:** Urodynamics, Hosp Univ Penn 1983; **Fac Appt:** Prof U, Univ Pennsylvania

Vaughan, Edwin D MD [U] - **Spec Exp:** Urologic Cancer; Adrenal Tumors; Prostate Disease; **Hospital:** NY-Presby Hosp (page 79), Meml Sloan Kettering Cancer Ctr (page 76); **Address:** New York Presby Hosp, Dept Urology, 525 E 68th St, Starr 900, Box 94, New York, NY 10021-4870; **Phone:** 212-746-5480; **Board Cert:** Urology 1986; **Med School:** Univ VA Sch Med 1965; **Resid:** Surgery, Vanderbilt Univ Med Ctr 1967; Urology, Univ Virginia Hosp 1971; **Fellow:** Internal Medicine, Columbia Univ 1973; **Fac Appt:** Prof U, Cornell Univ-Weill Med Coll

von Eschenbach, Andrew C MD [U] - **Spec Exp:** Prostate Cancer; Urologic Cancer; **Hospital:** Natl Inst of Hlth - Clin Ctr; **Address:** Natl Cancer Inst, 5600 Fischers Ln, rm 1471, MC 259, Park Lawn, Rockville, MD 20857; **Phone:** 301-496-5615; **Board Cert:** Urology 1978; **Med School:** Georgetown Univ 1967; **Resid:** Surgery, Penn Hosp 1972; Penn Hosp 1975; **Fellow:** Urologic Oncology, Univ Texas-MD Anderson Hosp 1977

Waldbaum, Robert MD [U] - **Spec Exp:** Prostate Cancer; Prostate Disease; Urologic Cancer; **Hospital:** N Shore Univ Hosp at Manhasset, St Francis Hosp - The Heart Ctr; **Address:** 535 Plandome Rd, Ste 3, Manhasset, NY 11030-1961; **Phone:** 516-627-6188; **Board Cert:** Urology 1973; **Med School:** Columbia P&S 1962; **Resid:** Surgery, Columbia Presby Med Ctr 1966; Urology, New York Hosp-Cornell 1970; **Fac Appt:** Clin Prof U, Cornell Univ-Weill Med Coll

Walsh, Patrick MD [U] - **Spec Exp:** Prostate Cancer; Urologic Cancer; **Hospital:** Johns Hopkins Hosp - Baltimore; **Address:** Brady Urological Inst, 600 N Wolfe St, Phipps 554A, Baltimore, MD 21287-2101; **Phone:** 410-955-6100; **Board Cert:** Urology 1975; **Med School:** Case West Res Univ 1964; **Resid:** Surgery, Peter Bent Brigham Hosp/Childrens Hosp 1967; Urology, UCLA Med Ctr 1971; **Fellow:** Endocrinology, Harbor Genl Hosp 1970; **Fac Appt:** Prof U, Johns Hopkins Univ

Wein, Alan J MD [U] - **Spec Exp:** Prostate Cancer; Testicular Cancer; Urologic Cancer; **Hospital:** Hosp Univ Penn - UPHS (page 84), Pennsylvania Hosp (page 84); **Address:** Univ Penn Hlth System, Div Urology, 3400 Spruce St, 9 Penn Tower, Philadelphia, PA 19104-4283; **Phone:** 215-662-2891; **Board Cert:** Urology 1995; **Med School:** Univ Pennsylvania 1966; **Resid:** Surgery, Hosp Univ Penn 1968; Urology, Hosp Univ Penn 1972; **Fellow:** Urology, Hosp Univ Penn 1969; **Fac Appt:** Prof U, Univ Pennsylvania

Weiss, Robert E MD [U] - **Spec Exp:** Bladder Cancer; Kidney Cancer; Testicular Cancer; **Hospital:** Robert Wood Johnson Univ Hosp - New Brunswick, Univ Med Ctr - Princeton; **Address:** 1 Robert Wood Johnson Pl Ste MB588, New Brunswick, NJ 08901-1928; **Phone:** 732-235-7775; **Board Cert:** Urology 2003; **Med School:** NYU Sch Med 1985; **Resid:** Surgery, Mount Sinai Med Ctr 1987; Urology, Mount Sinai Med Ctr 1991; **Fellow:** Urologic Oncology, Meml Sloan Kettering Cancer Ctr 1994; **Fac Appt:** Assoc Prof U, UMDNJ-RW Johnson Med Sch

Yu, George W MD [U] - **Spec Exp:** Urologic Cancer; Nutrition & Disease Prevention/Control; Nutrition & Cancer Prevention/Control; **Hospital:** G Washington Univ Hosp, Anne Arundel Med Ctr; **Address:** 116 Defense Hwy, Ste 200, Annapolis, MD 21401; **Phone:** 410-897-0540, **Board Cert:** Urology 1983; **Med School:** Tufts Univ 1973; **Resid:** Surgery, Brigham & Women's Hosp 1976; Urology, Johns Hopkins Hosp 1981; **Fac Appt:** Prof U, Geo Wash Univ

Southeast

Amling, Christopher L MD [U] - **Spec Exp:** Urologic Cancer; Prostate Cancer/Robotic Surgery; Kidney Cancer; Bladder Cancer; **Hospital:** Univ of Ala Hosp at Birmingham; **Address:** 1530 3rd Ave S, Ste FOT-1105, Birmingham, AL 35294; **Phone:** 205-975-0088; **Board Cert:** Urology 1999; **Med School:** Oregon Hlth Sci Univ 1985; **Resid:** Urology, Duke Univ Med Ctr 1996; **Fellow:** Urologic Oncology, Mayo Clinic 1997; **Fac Appt:** Prof U, Univ Ala

Beall, Michael E MD [U] - **Spec Exp:** Prostate Cancer; Testicular Cancer; **Hospital:** Inova Fairfax Hosp, Reston Hosp Ctr; **Address:** 8503 Arlington Blvd, Ste 310, Fairfax, VA 22030; **Phone:** 703-208-4200; **Board Cert:** Urology 1979; **Med School:** Geo Wash Univ 1972; **Resid:** Surgery, Geo Wash Univ Hosp 1974; Urology, Geo Wash Univ Hosp 1977; **Fac Appt:** Assoc Clin Prof U, Geo Wash Univ

Cookson, Michael MD [U] - **Spec Exp:** Bladder Cancer; Testicular Cancer; Prostate Cancer; **Hospital:** Vanderbilt Univ Med Ctr, Saint Thomas Hosp - Nashville; **Address:** Vanderbilt Univ Med Ctr, Urol Surg A1302 MCN, Nashville, TN 37232; **Phone:** 615-322-2880; **Board Cert:** Urology 1998; **Med School:** Univ Okla Coll Med 1988; **Resid:** Urology, Univ Tex San Antonio-Univ Hosp 1994; **Fellow:** Urologic Oncology, Meml Sloan-Kettering Cancer Ctr 1996; **Fac Appt:** Assoc Prof U, Vanderbilt Univ

El-Galley, Rizk MD [U] - **Spec Exp:** Urologic Cancer; Laparoscopic Surgery; Bladder Cancer; **Hospital:** Univ of Ala Hosp at Birmingham; **Address:** UAB Hosp FOT-1105, 1530 3rd Ave S, Birmingham, AL 35294-3411; **Phone:** 205-996-8765; **Board Cert:** Urology 2003; **Med School:** Egypt 1983; **Resid:** Urology, Emory Univ Hosp 1999; **Fac Appt:** Asst Prof U, Univ Ala

Fraser, Lionel B MD [U] - **Spec Exp:** Prostate Cancer; Incontinence after Prostate Cancer; Erectile Dysfunction; **Hospital:** Baptist Hosp - Jackson; **Address:** Metropolitan Urology-St Dominic East Med Tower, 971 Lakeland Drive, Ste 315, Jackson, MS 39216; **Phone:** 601-982-0982; **Board Cert:** Urology 2005; **Med School:** Univ Mich Med Sch 1977; **Resid:** Surgery, New England Deaconness Hosp 1979; **Fellow:** Urology, Brigham & Womens Hosp 1983

Harty, James MD [U] - **Spec Exp:** Urologic Cancer; **Hospital:** Norton Hosp, Jewish Hosp HlthCre Svcs Inc; **Address:** 210 E Gray St, Ste 1000, Louisville, KY 40202; **Phone:** 502-629-5904; **Board Cert:** Urology 1979; **Med School:** Ireland 1969; **Resid:** Surgery, Johns Hopkins Hosp 1973; Urology, Johns Hopkins Hosp 1977; **Fac Appt:** Prof S, Univ Louisville Sch Med

Jordan, Gerald H MD [U] - **Spec Exp:** Urinary Reconstruction; Prostate Cancer; **Hospital:** Sentara Norfolk Genl Hosp; **Address:** 400 W Brambleton Ave, Ste 100, Norfolk, VA 23510; **Phone:** 757-457-5100; **Board Cert:** Urology 1984; **Med School:** Univ Tex, San Antonio 1977; **Resid:** Urology, Naval Reg Med Ctr 1978; **Fellow:** Reconstructive Surgery, Eastern Va Med Sch 1984; **Fac Appt:** Prof U, Eastern VA Med Sch

Keane, Thomas E MD [U] - **Spec Exp:** Urologic Cancer; Genitourinary Cancer; Prostate Cancer; Clinical Trials; **Hospital:** MUSC Med Ctr; **Address:** MUSC-Urology Dept, 96 Jonathan Lucas St, Ste CSB644, Charleston, SC 29425; **Phone:** 843-792-1666; **Board Cert:** Urology 2003; **Med School:** Ireland 1981; **Resid:** Urology, St Vincents Hosp 1986; Urology, N Tees Gen Hosp 1988; **Fellow:** Urology, Duke Univ Med Ctr 1993; **Fac Appt:** Prof U, Univ SC Sch Med

Kim, Edward D MD [U] - **Spec Exp:** Prostate Cancer; Bladder Cancer; **Hospital:** Univ of Tennesee Mem Hosp; **Address:** 1928 Alcoa Hwy, Med Office Bldg B, Ste 127, Knoxville, TN 37920; **Phone:** 865-544-9254; **Board Cert:** Urology 1998; **Med School:** Northwestern Univ 1989; **Resid:** Urology, Northwestern Meml Hosp 1995; **Fellow:** Baylor Coll Med 1996; **Fac Appt:** Assoc Prof U, Univ Tenn Coll Med, Memphis

Lockhart, Jorge L MD [U] - **Spec Exp:** Urologic Cancer; **Hospital:** H Lee Moffitt Cancer Ctr & Research Inst, Tampa Genl Hosp; **Address:** H Lee Moffitt Cancer Ctr, Dept Urology, 12902 Magnolia Drive, Tampa, FL 33612; **Phone:** 813-745-6033; **Board Cert:** Urology 1980; **Med School:** Uruguay 1973; **Resid:** Urology, Duke Univ Med Ctr 1977; **Fellow:** Urodynamics, Duke Univ Med Ctr 1978; **Fac Appt:** Prof S, Univ S Fla Coll Med

Marshall, Fray F MD [U] - **Spec Exp:** Urologic Cancer; Prostate Cancer; Kidney Cancer; **Hospital:** Emory Univ Hosp; **Address:** Emory Clinic, Dept Urology, 1365 Clifton Rd NE B Bldg - Ste 1400, Atlanta, GA 30322; **Phone:** 404-778-4898; **Board Cert:** Urology 1977; **Med School:** Univ VA Sch Med 1969; **Resid:** Surgery, Univ Mich Hosps 1972; Urology, Mass Genl Hosp 1975; **Fac Appt:** Prof U, Emory Univ

Moul, Judd W MD [U] - **Spec Exp:** Prostate Cancer; Testicular Cancer; **Hospital:** Duke Univ Med Ctr, Durham Regional Hosp; **Address:** Duke Univ Med Ctr, Div Urologic Surgery, Box 3707, Durham, NC 27710; **Phone:** 919-684-2446; **Board Cert:** Urology 1999; **Med School:** Jefferson Med Coll 1982; **Resid:** Urology, Walter Reed Army Med Ctr 1987; **Fellow:** Urologic Oncology, Duke Univ Med Ctr 1989; **Fac Appt:** Prof S, Duke Univ

Pow-Sang, Julio MD [U] - **Spec Exp:** Prostate Cancer; **Hospital:** H Lee Moffitt Cancer Ctr & Research Inst; **Address:** H Lee Moffitt Cancer Ctr, GU Clinic, 12902 Magnolia Drive, Tampa, FL 33612-9416; **Phone:** 813-972-8418; **Board Cert:** Urology 1999; **Med School:** Mexico 1978; **Resid:** Surgery, Univ Miami Sch Med 1983; Urology, Univ Miami Sch Med 1986; **Fellow:** Urologic Oncology, Univ Fla Coll Med 1987; **Fac Appt:** Prof S, Univ S Fla Coll Med

Robertson, Cary N MD [U] - **Spec Exp:** Prostate Cancer; Kidney Cancer; Testicular Cancer; **Hospital:** Duke Univ Med Ctr; **Address:** Duke Univ Med Ctr, Trent Drive, Box 3833, Durham, NC 27710; **Phone:** 919-681-6768; **Board Cert:** Urology 2005; **Med School:** Tulane Univ 1977; **Resid:** Urology, Duke Univ Med Ctr 1985; **Fellow:** Urologic Oncology, Natl Inst Hlth 1987; **Fac Appt:** Assoc Prof U, Duke Univ

Rowland, Randall MD [U] - **Spec Exp:** Urologic Cancer; **Hospital:** Univ of Kentucky Chandler Hosp; **Address:** Univ Kentucky Med Ctr, Div Urology, 800 Rose St, rm MS283, Lexington, KY 40536-0298; **Phone:** 859-323-6677; **Board Cert:** Urology 1980; **Med School:** Northwestern Univ 1972; **Resid:** Urology, Northwestern Meml Hosp 1978; **Fac Appt:** Prof U, Univ KY Coll Med

Sanders, William H MD [U] - **Spec Exp:** Prostate Cancer; Kidney Cancer; Bladder Cancer; **Hospital:** St Joseph's Hosp - Atlanta, Northside Hosp; **Address:** 5673 Peachtree Dunwoody Rd, Ste 910, Atlanta, GA 30342-1767; **Phone:** 404-255-3822; **Board Cert:** Urology 2006; **Med School:** Emory Univ 1988; **Resid:** Urology, Yale-New Haven Hosp 1993

Schellhammer, Paul MD [U] - **Spec Exp:** Prostate Cancer; Urologic Cancer; **Hospital:** Sentara Norfolk Genl Hosp; **Address:** 6333 Center Drive Bldg 16, Norfolk, VA 23502; **Phone:** 757-457-5100; **Board Cert:** Urology 1999; **Med School:** Cornell Univ-Weill Med Coll 1966; **Resid:** Surgery, Univ Hosps 1968; Urology, Med Coll Va Hosp 1973; **Fellow:** Urology, Memorial Hosp 1974; **Fac Appt:** Prof U, Eastern VA Med Sch

Smith, Joseph A MD [U] - **Spec Exp:** Prostate Cancer/Robotic Surgery; Bladder Cancer; Kidney Cancer; **Hospital:** Vanderbilt Univ Med Ctr; **Address:** Vanderbilt Univ Med Ctr, Dept Urology, A-1302 MCN, Nashville, TN 37232-2765; **Phone:** 615-343-0234; **Board Cert:** Urology 2000; **Med School:** Univ Tenn Coll Med, Memphis 1974; **Resid:** Surgery, Parkland Meml Hosp 1976; Urology, Univ Utah 1979; **Fellow:** Urologic Oncology, Meml Sloan Kettering Cancer Ctr 1980; **Fac Appt:** Prof U, Vanderbilt Univ

Soloway, Mark S MD [U] - **Spec Exp:** Bladder Cancer; Kidney Cancer; Prostate Cancer; **Hospital:** Jackson Meml Hosp, Cedars Med Ctr - Miami; **Address:** 1150 NW 14th St, Ste 309, Miami, FL 33136; **Phone:** 305-243-6596; **Board Cert:** Urology 1977; **Med School:** Case West Res Univ 1968; **Resid:** Surgery, Univ Hosps 1970; Urology, Univ Hosps 1975; **Fellow:** Surgery, Natl Cancer Inst 1972; **Fac Appt:** Prof U, Univ Miami Sch Med

Urology

Teigland, Chris M MD [U] - **Spec Exp:** Prostate Cancer/Robotic Surgery; Kidney Cancer; **Hospital:** Carolinas Med Ctr; **Address:** Mckay Urology, 1023 Edgehill Rd S, Charlotte, NC 28207; **Phone:** 704-355-8686; **Board Cert:** Urology 1999; **Med School:** Duke Univ 1980; **Resid:** Surgery, Univ Utah Affil Hosps 1982; Urology, Univ Texas SW Med Ctr 1987; **Fac Appt:** Clin Prof S, Univ NC Sch Med

Terris, Martha K MD [U] - **Spec Exp:** Prostate Cancer; Brachytherapy; Urologic Cancer; Bladder Cancer; **Hospital:** VA Medical Ctr - Augusta, Med Coll of GA Hosp and Clin; **Address:** Augusta VA Administration Hosp, 1 Freedom Way, Augusta, GA 30904; **Phone:** 706-733-0188; **Board Cert:** Urology 1998; **Med School:** Univ Miss 1986; **Resid:** Surgery, Duke Univ Med Ctr 1988; Urology, Stanford Univ Med Ctr 1995; **Fellow:** Ultrasound, Stanford Univ Med Ctr 1991; **Fac Appt:** Prof S, Med Coll GA

Theodorescu, Dan MD/PhD [U] - **Spec Exp:** Prostate Cancer; Clinical Trials; Bladder Cancer; Kidney Cancer; **Hospital:** Univ Virginia Med Ctr; **Address:** UVA Health System, Dept Urology, PO Box 800422, Charlottesville, VA 22908; **Phone:** 434-924-0042; **Board Cert:** Urology 1999; **Med School:** Canada 1986; **Resid:** Urology, Univ Toronto Med Ctr 1993; **Fellow:** Urologic Oncology, Meml Sloan Kettering Cancer Ctr 1995; **Fac Appt:** Prof U, Univ VA Sch Med

Wajsman, Zev Lew MD [U] - **Spec Exp:** Urologic Cancer; **Hospital:** North Florida Regl Med Ctr; **Address:** Urology Assocs, 1179 NW 64th Terrace, Gainesville, FL 32607; **Phone:** 352-333-5400; **Med School:** Israel 1965; **Resid:** Surgery, Central Emek Hosp 1970; Urology, Central Emek Hosp 1973; **Fellow:** Urology, Rosewell Park Meml Inst 1975

Midwest

Andriole, Gerald L MD [U] - **Spec Exp:** Urologic Cancer; Prostate Cancer; Laparoscopic Surgery; **Hospital:** Barnes-Jewish Hosp; **Address:** 4960 Children's Place, Campus Box 8242, St Louis, MO 63110; **Phone:** 314-362-8212; **Board Cert:** Urology 2003; **Med School:** Jefferson Med Coll 1978; **Resid:** Surgery, Strong Meml Hosp 1980; Urology, Brigham & Womens Hosp 1983; **Fellow:** Urologic Oncology, NCI/NIH 1985; **Fac Appt:** Prof U, Washington Univ, St Louis

Bahnson, Robert MD [U] - **Spec Exp:** Prostate Cancer; Bladder Cancer; Continent Urinary Diversions; **Hospital:** Ohio St Univ Med Ctr, Arthur G James Cancer Hosp & Research Inst; **Address:** 456 West 10th Avenue, Dept of Urology, 4980 Cramblett Med Ctr, Columbus, OH 43210-1240; **Phone:** 614-293-8155; **Board Cert:** Urology 2006; **Med School:** Tufts Univ 1979; **Resid:** Surgery, Northwestern Univ 1981; Urology, Northwestern Univ 1985; **Fellow:** Urology, Northwestern Univ 1984; Research, Univ Pittsburgh 1991; **Fac Appt:** Prof U, Ohio State Univ

Brendler, Charles B MD [U] - **Spec Exp:** Prostate Cancer; **Hospital:** Evanston NW Hlthcare; **Address:** Evanston Northwestern Hosp, 2650 Ridge Ave Walgreen Bldg - Ste 2507, Evanston, IL 60201; **Phone:** 847-547-1090; **Board Cert:** Urology 1981; **Med School:** Univ VA Sch Med 1974; **Resid:** Surgery, Duke Univ Med Ctr 1976; Urology, Duke Univ Med Ctr 1979; **Fellow:** Urologic Oncology, Univ Hosp Wales 1980; Urologic Oncology, Johns Hopkins Hosp 1982; **Fac Appt:** Prof U, Univ Chicago-Pritzker Sch Med

Bruskewitz, Reginald C MD [U] - **Spec Exp:** Urologic Cancer; Prostate Disease; **Hospital:** Univ WI Hosp & Clins; **Address:** Univ Wisconsin Hosp, Urology, 600 Highland Ave, C-52, Madison, WI 53792; **Phone:** 608-263-4757; **Board Cert:** Urology 1981; **Med School:** Univ Wisc 1973; **Resid:** Urology, Univ Wisconsin Hosp 1978; **Fellow:** Urodynamics, UCLA Med Ctr 1979; **Fac Appt:** Assoc Prof S, Univ Wisc

Castle Connolly America's Top Doctors® for Cancer 3rd Edition

Campbell, Steven C MD/PhD [U] - **Spec Exp:** Kidney Cancer; Prostate Cancer; Bladder Cancer; **Hospital:** Cleveland Clin Fdn (page 71); **Address:** Cleveland Clinic/Glickman Urological Inst, 9500 Euclid Ave, Desk A100, Cleveland, OH 44195; **Phone:** 216-444-5595; **Board Cert:** Urology 1999; **Med School:** Univ Chicago-Pritzker Sch Med 1989; **Resid:** Urology, Cleveland Clinic 1995; **Fellow:** Urology, Meml Sloan Kettering Cancer Ctr 1996; **Fac Appt:** Prof S, Cleveland Cl Coll Med/Case West Res

Catalona, William J MD [U] - **Spec Exp:** Urologic Cancer; Prostate Cancer; Prostate Disease; **Hospital:** Northwestern Meml Hosp; **Address:** Northwestern Med Faculty Foundation, 675 N St Clair St, Ste 20-150, Chicago, IL 60611; **Phone:** 312-695-6126; **Board Cert:** Urology 1978; **Med School:** Yale Univ 1968; **Resid:** Surgery, UCSF Med Ctr 1970; Urology, Johns Hopkins Hosp 1976; **Fellow:** Surgical Oncology, Natl Cancer Inst 1972; **Fac Appt:** Prof U, Northwestern Univ

Chodak, Gerald MD [U] - **Spec Exp:** Prostate Cancer; Prostate Disease; **Hospital:** Weiss Meml Hosp; **Address:** 4646 N Marine Drive, Ste A5500, Chicago, IL 60640-5759; **Phone:** 773-564-5006; **Board Cert:** Urology 1984; **Med School:** SUNY Buffalo 1975; **Resid:** Surgery, UCLA Med Ctr 1977; Urology, Brigham & Womens Hosp 1979; **Fellow:** Research, Univ Chicago 1981; Research, Harvard/Chldns Hosp 1982

Coplen, Douglas E MD [U] - **Spec Exp:** Pediatric Urology; Urologic Cancer-Pediatric; Testicular Cancer-Pediatric; **Hospital:** St Louis Chldns Hosp; **Address:** St. Louis Children's Hosp, 4990 Children's Pl, Ste 1120, St Louis, MO 63110; **Phone:** 314-454-6034; **Board Cert:** Urology 1996; **Med School:** Indiana Univ 1985; **Resid:** Urology, Barnes Jewish Hosp 1992; **Fellow:** Pediatric Urology, Children's Hosp 1994; **Fac Appt:** Asst Prof S, Washington Univ, St Louis

Donovan Jr, James F MD [U] - **Spec Exp:** Prostate Cancer/Robotic Surgery; Kidney Cancer; Adrenal Tumors; Laparoscopic Surgery; **Hospital:** Univ Hosp - Cincinnati, Christ Hospital; **Address:** Univ Cincinnati Med Ctr, Medical Arts Bldg, 222 Piedmont Ave, Ste 7000, Cincinnati, OH 45219; **Phone:** 513-475-8787; **Board Cert:** Surgery 1997; Urology 1999; **Med School:** Northwestern Univ 1978; **Resid:** Surgery, Northwestern Meml Hosp 1982; Urology, Northwestern Meml Hosp 1986; **Fellow:** Male Infertility, Baylor Coll Med 1986; **Fac Appt:** Prof U, Univ Cincinnati

Flanigan, Robert C MD [U] - **Spec Exp:** Prostate Cancer; Bladder Cancer; Kidney Cancer; **Hospital:** Loyola Univ Med Ctr, Hines VA Hosp; **Address:** Loyola Univ Med-Fahey Bldg 54, 2160 S First Ave, rm 267, Maywood, IL 60153; **Phone:** 708-216-5100; **Board Cert:** Surgery 1998; Urology 2001; **Med School:** Case West Res Univ 1972; **Resid:** Surgery, Case West Univ Med Ctr 1978; Urology, Case West Univ Med Ctr 1978; **Fac Appt:** Prof U, Loyola Univ-Stritch Sch Med

Foster, Richard S MD [U] - **Spec Exp:** Testicular Cancer; **Hospital:** Indiana Univ Hosp (page 70); **Address:** 535 N Barnhill Drive, Ste 420, Indianapolis, IN 46202; **Phone:** 317-274-3458; **Board Cert:** Urology 1998; **Med School:** Indiana Univ 1980; **Resid:** Urology, Indiana Univ Hosp 1986; **Fac Appt:** Prof U, Indiana Univ

Gill, Inderbir Singh MD [U] - **Spec Exp:** Prostate Cancer; Kidney Cancer; Urologic Cancer; Laparoscopic Surgery; **Hospital:** Cleveland Clin Fdn (page 71); **Address:** Cleveland Clinic Urological Inst, 9500 Euclid Ave, Ste A100, Cleveland, OH 44195; **Phone:** 216-445-1530; **Board Cert:** Urology 1997; **Med School:** India 1980; **Resid:** Surgery, Dayanand Med Coll & Hosp; Urology, Univ Kentucky Hosp 1993; **Fellow:** Cleveland Clinic

Gluckman, Gordon MD [U] - **Spec Exp:** Prostate Cancer; Kidney Cancer; Minimally Invasive Urologic Surgery; **Hospital:** Adv Luth Genl Hosp, Resurrection Med Ctr; **Address:** Parkside Center, 1875 Dempster St, Ste 506, Park Ridge, IL 60068; **Phone:** 847-823-4700; **Board Cert:** Urology 2005; **Med School:** Northwestern Univ 1989; **Resid:** Surgery, UCSF Med Ctr 1991; Urology, UCSF Med Ctr 1995

Kibel, Adam S MD [U] - **Spec Exp:** Prostate Cancer; Bladder Cancer; Kidney Cancer; **Hospital:** Barnes-Jewish Hosp; **Address:** Washington Univ Sch Med, Urologic Surgery, 660 S Euclid Ave, Box 8242, St Louis, MO 63110; **Phone:** 314-362-8295; **Board Cert:** Urology 2001; **Med School:** Cornell Univ-Weill Med Coll 1991; **Resid:** Urology, Brigham & Women's Hosp 1996; **Fellow:** Urologic Oncology, Johns Hopkins Med Ctr 1999; **Fac Appt:** Assoc Prof U, Washington Univ, St Louis

Klein, Eric A MD [U] - **Spec Exp:** Prostate Cancer; Testicular Cancer; Urologic Cancer; **Hospital:** Cleveland Clin Fdn (page 71); **Address:** Cleveland Clinic Fdn, Dept Urol, Sect Urol-Onc, 9500 Euclid Ave, Fl A100, Cleveland, OH 44195-0001; **Phone:** 216-444-5591; **Board Cert:** Urology 1999; **Med School:** Univ Pittsburgh 1981; **Resid:** Urology, Cleveland Clinic Fdn 1986; **Fellow:** Urologic Oncology, Meml Sloan Kettering Canc Ctr 1989; **Fac Appt:** Prof S, Cleveland Cl Coll Med/Case West Res

Koeneman, Kenneth MD [U] - **Spec Exp:** Prostate Cancer/Robotic Surgery; Urologic Cancer; **Hospital:** Univ Minn Med Ctr, Fairview - Univ Campus; **Address:** MN Hosp Dept of Urology, 420 Delaware St SE Mayo Bldg - Ste B-435, Minneapolis, MN 55455; **Phone:** 612-625-6401; **Board Cert:** Urology 2002; **Med School:** Univ IL Coll Med 1992; **Resid:** Urology, Loyola Univ Med Ctr 1998; **Fellow:** Urologic Oncology, Univ VA 2000; **Fac Appt:** Assoc Prof U, Univ Minn

Kozlowski, James M MD [U] - **Spec Exp:** Prostate Cancer; Continent Urinary Diversions; Laparoscopic Surgery; **Hospital:** Northwestern Meml Hosp, Jesse A Brown VA Med Ctr; **Address:** 675 N St Clair St, Galter Bldg Fl 20 - Ste 150, Chicago, IL 60611; **Phone:** 312-695-8146; **Board Cert:** Surgery 1993; Urology 1983; **Med School:** Northwestern Univ 1975; **Resid:** Surgery, Northwestern Univ-McGaw 1979; Urology, Northwestern Univ-McGaw 1981; **Fellow:** Research, NCI-Frederick Cancer Rsch 1984; **Fac Appt:** Assoc Prof U, Northwestern Univ

McVary, Kevin MD [U] - **Spec Exp:** Prostate Cancer; Erectile Dysfunction; **Hospital:** Northwestern Meml Hosp; **Address:** 675 N St Clair St, Galter Bldg Fl 20 - Ste 150, Chicago, IL 60611-4813; **Phone:** 312-695-8146; **Board Cert:** Urology 2000; **Med School:** Northwestern Univ 1983; **Resid:** Surgery, Northwestern Meml Hosp 1985; Urology, Northwestern Meml Hosp 1988; **Fellow:** Research, Northwestern Meml Hosp; **Fac Appt:** Prof U, Northwestern Univ

Menon, Mani MD [U] - **Spec Exp:** Prostate Cancer/Robotic Surgery; Transplant-Kidney; Urologic Cancer; **Hospital:** Henry Ford Hosp; **Address:** Henry Ford Hosp - Vattikuti Urology Inst, 2799 W Grand Bvd, Clinic Bldg - #K-9, Detroit, MI 48202; **Phone:** 313-916-2062; **Board Cert:** Urology 1982; **Med School:** India 1969; **Resid:** Urology, Bryn Mawr Hosp 1974; Urology, Johns Hopkins Hosp 1980; **Fellow:** Transplant Surgery, Johns Hopkins Univ 1977; **Fac Appt:** Prof S, Univ Mass Sch Med

Montie, James MD [U] - **Spec Exp:** Bladder Cancer; Prostate Cancer; Genitourinary Cancer; **Hospital:** Univ Michigan Hlth Sys; **Address:** 1500 E Medical Ctr Dr, Dept Urology, Taubman Hlth Care Ctr, rm 3876, Box 0330, Ann Arbor, MI 48109-0330; **Phone:** 734-647-8903; **Board Cert:** Urology 1978; **Med School:** Univ Mich Med Sch 1971; **Resid:** Urology, Cleveland Clinic Fdn 1976; **Fellow:** Urologic Oncology, Meml Sloan-Kettering Cancer Ctr 1979; **Fac Appt:** Prof U, Univ Mich Med Sch

Myers, Robert P MD [U] - Spec Exp: Prostate Cancer; **Hospital:** Mayo Med Ctr & Clin - Rochester, Rochester Meth Hosp; **Address:** Mayo Clinic, Dept Urology, 200 First St SW, Rochester, MN 55905; **Phone:** 507-284-3077; **Board Cert:** Urology 1976; **Med School:** Columbia P&S 1967; **Resid:** Urology, Mayo Clinic 1972; **Fac Appt:** Prof U, Mayo Med Sch

Novick, Andrew MD [U] - Spec Exp: Transplant-Kidney; Kidney Cancer; Urologic Cancer; **Hospital:** Cleveland Clin Fdn (page 71); **Address:** Cleveland Clinic-Urological Inst, 9500 Euclid Ave, Desk A100, Cleveland, OH 44195; **Phone:** 216-444-5600; **Board Cert:** Urology 1996; **Med School:** McGill Univ 1972; **Resid:** Surgery, Royal Victoria Hosp 1974; Urology, Cleveland Clinic 1977; **Fac Appt:** Prof S, Cleveland Cl Coll Med/Case West Res

O'Donnell, Michael A MD [U] - Spec Exp: Bladder Cancer; Immunotherapy; Urologic Cancer; **Hospital:** Univ Iowa Hosp & Clinics; **Address:** Univ Iowa Hosp & Clins, Dept Urology, 200 Hawkins Drive, 3RCP, Iowa City, IA 52242-1089; **Phone:** 319-384-6040; **Board Cert:** Urology 2005; **Med School:** Duke Univ 1984; **Resid:** Surgery, Brigham & Womens Hosp 1987; Urology, Brigham & Womens Hosp 1991; **Fellow:** Urology, Brigham & Womens Hosp 1993; **Fac Appt:** Prof U, Univ Iowa Coll Med

Patel, Vipul R MD [U] - Spec Exp: Prostate Cancer/Robotic Surgery; Kidney Cancer; **Hospital:** Ohio St Univ Med Ctr; **Address:** 538 Doan Hall, 410 W 10th Ave, Columbus, OH 43210; **Phone:** 614-293-0981; **Board Cert:** Urology 2004; **Med School:** Baylor Coll Med 1995; **Resid:** Urology, Univ Miami; **Fellow:** Urologic Laparoscopic Surgery-Endourology, Univ Miami; **Fac Appt:** Assoc Clin Prof U, Ohio State Univ

Resnick, Martin MD [U] - Spec Exp: Prostate Cancer; Urologic Cancer; **Hospital:** Univ Hosps Case Med Ctr, MetroHealth Med Ctr; **Address:** Univ Hosp, Dept Urology, 11100 Euclid Ave, Cleveland, OH 44106-5046; **Phone:** 216-844-3011; **Board Cert:** Urology 1998; **Med School:** Wake Forest Univ 1969; **Resid:** Surgery, Univ Hosps 1971; Urology, Northwestern Univ Med Ctr 1975; **Fac Appt:** Prof U, Case West Res Univ

Schaeffer, Anthony MD [U] - Spec Exp: Incontinence after Prostate Cancer; **Hospital:** Northwestern Meml Hosp; **Address:** 675 N St Clair, Galter Bldg Fl 20 - Ste 150, Chicago, IL 60611; **Phone:** 312-695-8146; **Board Cert:** Urology 1978; **Med School:** Northwestern Univ 1968; **Resid:** Surgery, Northwestern Meml Hosp 1970; Urology, Stanford Med Ctr 1976; **Fac Appt:** Prof U, Northwestern Univ

See, William MD [U] - Spec Exp: Prostate Cancer; Bladder Cancer; Testicular Cancer; **Hospital:** Froedtert Meml Lutheran Hosp; **Address:** Med Coll Wisconsin, Dept Urology, 9200 W Wisconsin Ave, Milwaukee, WI 53226; **Phone:** 414-456-6950; **Board Cert:** Urology 2000; **Med School:** Univ Chicago-Pritzker Sch Med 1982; **Resid:** Urology, Univ Washington 1988; **Fellow:** Research, Natl Kidney Fdn/Univ Wash 1986; Research, Amer Fdn for Urol Dis/Univ Iowa 1990; **Fac Appt:** Prof U, Med Coll Wisc

Steinberg, Gary D MD [U] - Spec Exp: Bladder Cancer; Kidney Cancer; Prostate Cancer; **Hospital:** Univ of Chicago Hosps; **Address:** 5841 S Maryland Ave, rm J653, MC 6038, Chicago, IL 60637; **Phone:** 773-702-3080; **Board Cert:** Urology 2003; **Med School:** Univ Chicago-Pritzker Sch Med 1985; **Resid:** Surgery, Johns Hopkins Hosp 1987; Urology, Brady Urol Inst/Johns Hopkins 1991; **Fellow:** Oncology, Johns Hopkins Hosp 1989; **Fac Appt:** Assoc Prof U, Univ Chicago-Pritzker Sch Med

Thomas Jr, Anthony J MD [U] - **Spec Exp:** Fertility Preservation in Cancer; **Hospital:** Cleveland Clin Fdn (page 71); **Address:** Cleveland Clinic-Urological Inst, 9500 Euclid Ave, Desk A100, Cleveland, OH 44195; **Phone:** 216-444-5600; **Board Cert:** Urology 1978; **Med School:** Univ Cincinnati 1969; **Resid:** Surgery, Wayne State Univ Affil Hosp 1971; Urology, Wayne State Univ Affil Hosp 1976

Williams, Richard D MD [U] - **Spec Exp:** Kidney Cancer; Bladder Cancer; Prostate Cancer; **Hospital:** Univ Iowa Hosp & Clinics; **Address:** Univ Iowa Hosp, Dept Urology, 200 Hawkins Dr, rm 3251 RCP, Iowa City, IA 52242-1089; **Phone:** 319-356-0760; **Board Cert:** Urology 1979; **Med School:** Univ Kans 1970; **Resid:** Surgery, Univ Minn Hosp 1972; Urology, Univ Minn Hosp 1976; **Fellow:** Urologic Oncology, Univ Minn Hosp 1979; **Fac Appt:** Prof U, Univ Iowa Coll Med

Wood, David P MD [U] - **Spec Exp:** Genitourinary Cancer; Bladder Cancer; Prostate Cancer; **Hospital:** Univ Michigan Hlth Sys; **Address:** Univ Mich, Dept Urology, 3875 Taubman Cancer Ctr, 1500 E Medical Center Drive, Ann Arbor, MI 48109-0999; **Phone:** 734-763-9269; **Board Cert:** Urology 2002; **Med School:** Univ Mich Med Sch 1983; **Resid:** Urology, Cleveland Clinic 1988; **Fellow:** Urologic Oncology, Meml Sloan-Kettering Cancer Ctr 1991; **Fac Appt:** Prof U, Univ Mich Med Sch

Zippe, Craig D MD [U] - **Spec Exp:** Prostate Cancer; Bladder Cancer; Incontinence after Prostate Cancer; **Hospital:** Cleveland Clin Fdn (page 71); **Address:** 12000 McCracken Rd, Ste 451, Garfield Heights, OH 44125; **Phone:** 216-587-4370; **Board Cert:** Urology 1997; **Med School:** Rush Med Coll 1980; **Resid:** Urology, Columbia Presby Med Ctr 1989; **Fellow:** Urologic Oncology, Meml Sloan Kettering Cancer Ctr 1992

Great Plains and Mountains

Childs, Stacy J MD [U] - **Spec Exp:** Prostate Cancer; Bladder Cancer; **Hospital:** Yampa Valley Med Ctr, Memorial Hosp - Craig; **Address:** 501 Anglers Drive, Ste 202, Steamboat Springs, CO 80487-8841; **Phone:** 970-871-9710; **Board Cert:** Urology 1979; **Med School:** Louisiana State Univ 1972; **Resid:** Urology, Carraway Meth Med Ctr 1977; **Fac Appt:** Clin Prof U, Univ Colorado

Crawford, E David MD [U] - **Spec Exp:** Prostate Cancer; Testicular Cancer; Bladder Cancer; **Hospital:** Univ Colorado Hosp; **Address:** Urologic Oncology, MS F710, 1665 N Ursula St, rm 1004, Box 6510, Aurora, CO 80045; **Phone:** 720-848-0170; **Board Cert:** Urology 1980; **Med School:** Univ Cincinnati 1973; **Resid:** Urology, Good Samaritan Hosp 1977; **Fellow:** Genitourinary Surgery, UCLA Med Ctr 1978; **Fac Appt:** Prof U, Univ Colorado

Davis, Bradley E MD [U] - **Spec Exp:** Urologic Cancer; Bladder Cancer; Reconstructive Surgery; Prostate Cancer; **Hospital:** Overland Pk Regl Med Ctr, St Luke's Hosp of Kansas City; **Address:** Urologic Surgical Associates, 10550 Quivira Rd, Ste 105, Overland Park, KS 66215; **Phone:** 913-438-3833; **Board Cert:** Urology 2004; **Med School:** Univ Kans 1986; **Resid:** Surgery, St Lukes Hosp 1991; Urology, Univ Kansas Med Ctr 1991; **Fellow:** Urologic Oncology, Meml Sloan-Kettering Cancer Ctr 1993; **Fac Appt:** Asst Clin Prof U, Univ Kans

Lugg, James A MD [U] - **Spec Exp:** Prostate Cancer; Laparoscopic Surgery; Incontinence after Prostate Cancer; **Hospital:** Cheyenne Regl Med Ctr, Univ Colorado Hosp; **Address:** 2301 House Ave, Ste 502, Cheyenne, WY 82001; **Phone:** 307-635-4131; **Board Cert:** Urology 1998; **Med School:** Northwestern Univ 1990; **Resid:** Urology, UCLA Med Ctr 1995; **Fac Appt:** Asst Prof U, Univ Colorado

Middleton, Richard MD [U] - **Spec Exp:** Urologic Cancer; **Hospital:** Univ Utah Hosps and Clins, VA Medical Center - Salt Lake City; **Address:** University of Utah Medical Ctr, 50 N Medical Drive, Salt Lake City, UT 84132; **Phone:** 801-587-4888; **Board Cert:** Urology 1970; **Med School:** Cornell Univ-Weill Med Coll 1958; **Resid:** Surgery, New York Hosp-Cornell Med Ctr 1961; Urology, New York Hosp-Cornell Med Ctr 1967; **Fac Appt:** Prof U, Univ Utah

Southwest

Babaian, Richard MD [U] - **Spec Exp:** Prostate Cancer; **Hospital:** UT MD Anderson Cancer Ctr (page 81); **Address:** MD Anderson Cancer Ctr, 1515 Holcombe Blvd, Unit 1373, Houston, TX 77030; **Phone:** 713-792-3250; **Board Cert:** Urology 1980; **Med School:** Georgetown Univ 1972; **Resid:** Surgery, Univ Wisconsin 1974; Urology, Univ NC Hosp 1977; **Fellow:** Urologic Oncology, MD Anderson Cancer Ctr 1979; Immunology, Univ NC Hosps 1978; **Fac Appt:** Prof U, Univ Tex, Houston

Bans, Larry L MD [U] - **Spec Exp:** Prostate Cancer; Prostate Disease; **Hospital:** Banner Good Samaritan Regl Med Ctr - Phoenix; **Address:** Prostate Solutions of Arizona, 2525 E Arizona Biltmore Cir, Ste C236, Phoenix, AZ 85016; **Phone:** 602-426-9772; **Board Cert:** Urology 2004; **Med School:** Cornell Univ-Weill Med Coll 1978; **Resid:** Urology, Ind Univ Med Ctr 1983

Bardot, Stephen F MD [U] - **Spec Exp:** Urologic Cancer; Prostate Cancer; **Hospital:** Ochsner Fdn Hosp, Summit Hosp-Baton Rouge; **Address:** Ochsner Clinic, 1514 Jefferson Hwy Fl 4, Atrium 4 West, Dept of Urology, New Orleans, LA 70121-2483; **Phone:** 504-842-4083; **Board Cert:** Urology 1993; **Med School:** Univ Kans 1985; **Resid:** Surgery, St Luke's Hosp 1987; Urology, Kansas City Univ Med Ctr 1990; **Fellow:** Urologic Oncology, Cleveland Clinic 1991

Basler, Joseph W MD [U] - **Spec Exp:** Prostate Cancer; Urologic Cancer; **Hospital:** Audie L Murphy Meml Vets Hosp, Santa Rosa Hlth care Corp; **Address:** 7703 Floyd Curl Dr, MC-7845, San Antonio, TX 78229-3900; **Phone:** 210-567-5640; **Board Cert:** Urology 1992; **Med School:** Univ MO-Columbia Sch Med 1984; **Resid:** Surgery, Univ Missouri 1986; Urology, Barnes Hosp/Wash Univ 1990; **Fac Appt:** Prof U, Univ Tex, San Antonio

Greene, Graham MD [U] - **Spec Exp:** Urologic Cancer; **Hospital:** UAMS Med Ctr, Arkansas Chldns Hosp; **Address:** 4301 W Markham, Slot 774, Little Rock, AR 72205; **Phone:** 501-296-1545, **Board Cert:** Urology 1999; **Med School:** Dalhousie Univ 1989; **Resid:** Urology, Victoria Genl 1994; **Fellow:** Urologic Oncology, M.D. Anderson Cancer Ctr 1997; **Fac Appt:** Assoc Prof U, Univ Ark

Kadmon, Dov MD [U] - **Spec Exp:** Prostate Cancer; **Hospital:** St Luke's Episcopal Hosp - Houston, Methodist Hosp - Houston; **Address:** Baylor College of Medicine, 6560 Fannin St, Ste 2100, Houston, TX 77030; **Phone:** 713-798-7893; **Board Cert:** Urology 1984; **Med School:** Israel 1970; **Resid:** Surgery, Barnes Jewish Hosp 1977; Urology, Barnes Jewish Hosp 1980; **Fellow:** Urology, Barnes Jewish Hosp 1982; **Fac Appt:** Prof U, Baylor Coll Med

Lerner, Seth P MD [U] - **Spec Exp:** Bladder Cancer; Testicular Cancer; Urinary Reconstruction; **Hospital:** St Luke's Episcopal Hosp - Houston, Methodist Hosp - Houston; **Address:** 6560 Fannin St, Ste 2100, Houston, TX 77030; **Phone:** 713-798-6841; **Board Cert:** Urology 1994; **Med School:** Baylor Coll Med 1984; **Resid:** Surgery, Virginia Mason Hosp 1986; Urology, Baylor Coll Med 1990; **Fellow:** Urologic Oncology, LAC-USC Med Ctr 1992; **Fac Appt:** Prof U, Baylor Coll Med

Urology

McConnell, John D MD [U] - **Spec Exp:** Prostate Cancer; **Hospital:** UT Southwestern Med Ctr - Dallas, Chldns Med Ctr of Dallas; **Address:** Univ Texas SW Med Ctr, 5323 Harry Hines Blvd, Dallas, TX 75390-9131; **Phone:** 214-648-5630; **Board Cert:** Urology 2004; **Med School:** Loyola Univ-Stritch Sch Med 1978; **Resid:** Surgery, Univ Tex Hlth Sci Ctr-Parkland 1980; Urology, Univ Tex Hlth Sci Ctr-Parkland 1984; **Fac Appt:** Prof U, Univ Tex SW, Dallas

Miles, Brian J MD [U] - **Spec Exp:** Prostate Cancer; Urologic Cancer; Gene Therapy; **Hospital:** Methodist Hosp - Houston, St Luke's Episcopal Hosp - Houston; **Address:** Dept Urology, Scurlock Tower, 6560 Fannin St, Ste 2100, Houston, TX 77030-2769; **Phone:** 713-798-4001; **Board Cert:** Urology 1984; **Med School:** Univ Mich Med Sch 1974; **Resid:** Urology, Walter Reed Army Med Ctr 1982; **Fac Appt:** Prof U, Baylor Coll Med

Pisters, Louis L MD [U] - **Spec Exp:** Prostate Cancer; Bladder Cancer; Genitourinary Cancer; Prostate Cancer/Robotic Surgery; **Hospital:** UT MD Anderson Cancer Ctr (page 81); **Address:** MD Anderson Cancer Ctr, 1515 Holcombe Blvd, Unit 1373, Houston, TX 77030; **Phone:** 713-792-3250; **Board Cert:** Urology 2003; **Med School:** Univ Western Ontario 1986; **Resid:** Urology, Shands Hosp/UNIV Florida 1991; **Fellow:** Urologic Oncology, MD Anderson Cancer Ctr 1993; **Fac Appt:** Assoc Prof U, Univ Tex, Houston

Sagalowsky, Arthur I MD [U] - **Spec Exp:** Urologic Cancer; Transplant-Kidney; Testicular Cancer; **Hospital:** UT Southwestern Med Ctr - Dallas; **Address:** UT SW Med Ctr, Dept Urology, 5323 Harry Hines Blvd, J8.114, Dallas, TX 75390-9110; **Phone:** 214-648-3976; **Board Cert:** Urology 1980; **Med School:** Indiana Univ 1973; **Resid:** Surgery, Indiana Univ Hosps 1975; Urology, Indiana Univ Hosps 1978; **Fellow:** Clinical Pharmacology, Univ Tex SW Med Ctr 1980; **Fac Appt:** Prof U, Univ Tex SW, Dallas

Slawin, Kevin Mark MD [U] - **Spec Exp:** Prostate Cancer; Prostate Cancer/Robotic Surgery; Prostate Disease; **Hospital:** Methodist Hosp - Houston, St Luke's Episcopal Hosp - Houston; **Address:** 6560 Fannin St, Ste 2100, Houston, TX 77030; **Phone:** 713-798-8670; **Board Cert:** Urology 2005; **Med School:** Columbia P&S 1986; **Resid:** Surgery, Mt Sinai Med Ctr 1988; Urology, Columbia-Presby Hosp 1992; **Fellow:** Urologic Oncology, Am Fdn Urol Dis/Baylor Coll Med 1994; **Fac Appt:** Prof U, Baylor Coll Med

Swanson, David A MD [U] - **Spec Exp:** Kidney Cancer; Prostate Cancer; Testicular Cancer; **Hospital:** UT MD Anderson Cancer Ctr (page 81); **Address:** UT MD Anderson Canc Ctr, Dept Urol, 1515 Holcombe Blvd, Unit 1373, Houston, TX 77030-4009; **Phone:** 713-792-3250; **Board Cert:** Urology 1977; **Med School:** Univ Pennsylvania 1967; **Resid:** Surgery, Harbor Genl Hosp 1969; Urology, UC Davis Med Ctr 1975; **Fellow:** Urologic Oncology, Univ Tex-MD Anderson Hosp 1978

Thompson Jr, Ian M MD [U] - **Spec Exp:** Prostate Cancer; Prostate Disease; **Hospital:** Univ Hlth Sys - Univ Hosp; **Address:** Univ Tex Hlth Scis Ctr, Dept Urol, 7703 Floyd Curl Drive, rm 216L, MC 7845, San Antonio, TX 78229-3900; **Phone:** 210-567-5643; **Board Cert:** Urology 2005; **Med School:** Tulane Univ 1980; **Resid:** Urology, Brooke Army Med Ctr 1985; **Fellow:** Medical Oncology, Meml Sloan-Kettering Canc Ctr 1988; **Fac Appt:** Prof S, Univ Tex, San Antonio

West Coast and Pacific

Belldegrun, Arie S MD [U] - **Spec Exp:** Urologic Cancer; Gene Therapy; **Hospital:** UCLA Med Ctr (page 83); **Address:** UCLA-Geffen Sch Med, Dep Urology, 108-33 Leconte Ave, rm 66-118, Los Angeles, CA 90095; **Phone:** 310-206-1434; **Board Cert:** Urology 1999; **Med School:** Israel 1974; **Resid:** Urology, Brigham and Women's Hosp 1985; **Fellow:** Urologic Oncology, Natl Cancer Inst, NIH 1988; **Fac Appt:** Prof U, UCLA

Boyd, Stuart D MD [U] - Spec Exp: Urologic Cancer; **Hospital:** USC Norris Comp Cancer Ctr, USC Univ Hosp - R K Eamer Med Plz; **Address:** 1441 Eastlake Ave, Ste 7416, Los Angeles, CA 90089-9178; **Phone:** 323-865-3704; **Board Cert:** Urology 1984; **Med School:** UCLA 1975; **Resid:** Urology, UCLA Med Ctr 1982; **Fac Appt:** Prof U, USC Sch Med

Carroll, Peter R MD [U] - Spec Exp: Testicular Cancer; Prostate Cancer; Bladder Cancer; Bladder Reconstruction; **Hospital:** UCSF - Mt Zion Med Ctr; **Address:** UCSF Urologic Oncology Practice, Box 1711, San Francisco, CA 94143-1711; **Phone:** 415-353-7171; **Board Cert:** Urology 1998; **Med School:** Georgetown Univ 1979; **Resid:** Surgery, UCSF Med Ctr 1984; **Fellow:** Urology, Meml Sloan Kettering Cancer Ctr 1986; **Fac Appt:** Prof U, UCSF

Danoff, Dudley S MD [U] - Spec Exp: Prostate Cancer; Bladder Cancer; **Hospital:** Cedars-Sinai Med Ctr; **Address:** 8635 W 3rd St, Ste 1 West, Los Angeles, CA 90048; **Phone:** 310-854-9898; **Board Cert:** Urology 1974; **Med School:** Yale Univ 1963; **Resid:** Urology, Yale-New Haven Hosp 1965; Urology, Columbia-Presby Med Ctr 1969

de Kernion, Jean B MD [U] - Spec Exp: Urologic Cancer; Kidney Cancer; Prostate Cancer; Prostate Disease; **Hospital:** UCLA Med Ctr (page 83); **Address:** UCLA-Geffen Sch Med, Dept Urology, rm 66-133CHS, Box 951738, Los Angeles, CA 90095-1738; **Phone:** 310-206-6453; **Board Cert:** Surgery 1973; Urology 1975; **Med School:** Louisiana State Univ 1965; **Resid:** Surgery, Univ Hosps-Case West Res 1967; Urology, Univ Hosps-Case West Res 1973; **Fellow:** Urologic Oncology, Natl Cancer Inst 1969; **Fac Appt:** Prof U, UCLA

Ellis, William J MD [U] - Spec Exp: Prostate Cancer; Kidney Cancer; Prostate Disease; **Hospital:** Univ Wash Med Ctr; **Address:** Univ Wash Med Ctr, Dept Urology, Box 356158, Seattle, WA 98195; **Phone:** 206-598-4294; **Board Cert:** Urology 2001; **Med School:** Johns Hopkins Univ 1985; **Resid:** Surgery, Northwestern Meml Hosp 1987; Urology, Northwestern Meml Hosp 1991; **Fac Appt:** Assoc Prof U, Univ Wash

Gill, Harcharan Singh MD [U] - Spec Exp: Urologic Cancer; Prostate Cancer; **Hospital:** Stanford Univ Med Ctr; **Address:** 875 Blake Wilbur Drive, Stanford, CA 94305-5826; **Phone:** 650-725-5544; **Board Cert:** Urology 1995; **Med School:** Kenya 1977; **Resid:** Urology, Inst of Urol; Urology, Univ Penn 1991; **Fellow:** Urology, Univ Penn 1986; **Fac Appt:** Prof U, Stanford Univ

Holden, Stuart MD [U]   Spec Exp: Kidney Cancer; **Hospital:** Cedars-Sinai Med Ctr; **Address:** 8635 W 3rd St, Ste 1 West, Los Angeles, CA 90048; **Phone:** 310-854-9898; **Board Cert:** Urology 1977; **Med School:** Cornell Univ-Weill Med Coll 1968; **Resid:** Surgery, NY Hosp-Cornell 1970; Urology, Emory Univ Hosp 1975; **Fellow:** Urology, Meml Sloan Kettering Cancer Ctr 1978

Huffman, Jeffry L MD [U] - Spec Exp: Kidney Cancer; Bladder Cancer; Prostate Cancer; **Hospital:** USC Univ Hosp - R K Eamer Med Plz, USC Norris Comp Cancer Ctr; **Address:** 1975 Zonal Ave, rm 512, Los Angeles, CA 90033; **Phone:** 323-442-6284; **Board Cert:** Urology 2005; **Med School:** Loyola Univ-Stritch Sch Med 1978; **Resid:** Surgery, St Francis Hosp 1980; Urology, Univ Chicago Hosps 1983; **Fellow:** Urologic Oncology, Meml Sloan Kettering Cancer Ctr 1985; **Fac Appt:** Prof U, USC-Keck School of Medicine

Kawachi, Mark H MD [U] - Spec Exp: Prostate Cancer/Robotic Surgery; Minimally Invasive Urologic Surgery; **Hospital:** City of Hope Natl Med Ctr & Beckman Rsch (page 69); **Address:** City of Hope Natl Med Ctr, Div Urologic Onc, 1500 E Duarte Rd, Duarte, CA 91010-3012; **Phone:** 626-359-8111 x62655; **Board Cert:** Urology 2004; **Med School:** USC Sch Med 1979; **Resid:** Urology, USC Med Ctr 1984

Lange, Paul MD [U] - **Spec Exp:** Prostate Cancer; **Hospital:** Univ Wash Med Ctr; **Address:** Univ Wash Med Ctr, Dept Urology, Box 356158, Seattle, WA 98195; **Phone:** 206-598-4294; **Board Cert:** Urology 1978; **Med School:** Washington Univ, St Louis 1967; **Resid:** Surgery, Duke Univ Med Ctr 1972; Urology, Univ Minn Med Ctr 1975; **Fellow:** Immunology, Univ Minn 1973; Research, Natl Inst Hlth 1970; **Fac Appt:** Prof U, Univ Wash

Lieskovsky, Gary MD [U] - **Spec Exp:** Prostate Cancer; **Hospital:** USC Norris Comp Cancer Ctr, USC Univ Hosp - R K Eamer Med Plz; **Address:** 1441 Eastlake Ave, Ste 7416, Los Angeles, CA 90089-0112; **Phone:** 323-865-3702; **Board Cert:** Urology 1980; **Med School:** Canada 1973; **Resid:** Urology, Univ Alberta Hosp 1978; **Fellow:** Urology, UCLA Med Ctr 1980; **Fac Appt:** Prof U, USC Sch Med

Presti Jr, Joseph C MD [U] - **Spec Exp:** Prostate Cancer; Bladder Cancer; Kidney Cancer; **Hospital:** Stanford Univ Med Ctr; **Address:** Stanford Univ Sch Med-Dept Urology, 875 Blake Wilbur Dr MC 5826, Stanford, CA 94305; **Phone:** 650-725-5544; **Board Cert:** Urology 2002; **Med School:** UC Irvine 1984; **Resid:** Surgery, UCSF Med Ctr 1986; Urology, UCSF Med Ctr 1989; **Fellow:** Urologic Oncology, Meml Sloan-Kettering Cancer Ctr 1992; **Fac Appt:** Prof U, Stanford Univ

Schmidt, Joseph MD [U] - **Spec Exp:** Prostate Cancer; Clinical Trials; **Hospital:** UCSD Med Ctr; **Address:** 200 W Arbor Drive, San Diego, CA 92103-8897; **Phone:** 619-543-5904; **Board Cert:** Urology 1971; **Med School:** Univ IL Coll Med 1961; **Resid:** Surgery, Rush-Presby-St Lukes Hosp 1963; Urology, Johns Hopkins Hosp 1967; **Fellow:** Urology, Johns Hopkins Sch Med 1967; **Fac Appt:** Prof U, UCSD

Skinner, Donald G MD [U] - **Spec Exp:** Bladder Cancer; Testicular Cancer; Prostate Cancer; **Hospital:** USC Norris Comp Cancer Ctr, USC Univ Hosp - R K Eamer Med Plz; **Address:** 1441 Eastlake Ave, Ste 7416, Los Angeles, CA 90089-9178; **Phone:** 323-865-3707; **Board Cert:** Urology 1974; **Med School:** Yale Univ 1964; **Resid:** Surgery, Mass Genl Hosp 1966; Urology, Mass Genl Hosp 1971; **Fac Appt:** Prof U, USC Sch Med

Skinner, Eila C MD [U] - **Spec Exp:** Urologic Cancer; Urinary Reconstruction; **Hospital:** USC Norris Comp Cancer Ctr, USC Univ Hosp - R K Eamer Med Plz; **Address:** USC-Keck Sch Med, Dept Urology, 1441 Eastlake Ave, Ste 7416, Los Angeles, CA 90089; **Phone:** 323-865-3700; **Board Cert:** Urology 2001; **Med School:** USC Sch Med 1983; **Resid:** Urology, LAC-USC Med Ctr 1988; **Fellow:** Urologic Oncology, LAC-USC Med Ctr 1990; **Fac Appt:** Assoc Prof U, USC Sch Med

Smith, Robert B MD [U] - **Spec Exp:** Urologic Cancer; **Hospital:** UCLA Med Ctr (page 83); **Address:** UCLA-Geffen Sch Med, Dept Urology, Box 951738, Los Angeles, CA 90095-1738; **Phone:** 310-825-9273; **Board Cert:** Urology 1972; **Med School:** UCLA 1963; **Resid:** Surgery, UCLA Med Ctr 1965; Urology, UCLA Med Ctr 1969; **Fac Appt:** Prof S, UCLA

Stein, John P MD [U] - Spec Exp: Bladder Cancer; Prostate Cancer; Testicular Cancer; **Hospital:** USC Norris Comp Cancer Ctr; **Address:** 1441 Eastlake Ave, Ste 7416, Los Angeles, CA 90089; **Phone:** 323-865-3709; **Board Cert:** Urology 1999; **Med School:** Loyola Univ-Stritch Sch Med 1989; **Resid:** Surgery, LAC-USC Med Ctr 1991; Urology, LAC-USC Med Ctr 1993; **Fellow:** Urologic Oncology, LAC-USC Med Ctr 1997; **Fac Appt:** Assoc Prof U, USC Sch Med

Tomera, Kevin M MD [U] - Spec Exp: Urologic Cancer; Voiding Dysfunction; **Hospital:** Alaska Regl Hosp, Providence Alaska Med Ctr; **Address:** 1200 Airport Heights Drive, Ste 101, Anchorage, AK 99508-2944; **Phone:** 907-276-2803; **Board Cert:** Urology 1995; **Med School:** Northwestern Univ 1978; **Resid:** Urology, Mayo Clinic 1983

Wilson, Timothy G MD [U] - Spec Exp: Prostate Cancer/Robotic Surgery; Minimally Invasive Urologic Surgery; Urinary Reconstruction; **Hospital:** City of Hope Natl Med Ctr & Beckman Rsch (page 69); **Address:** City of Hope Natl Med Ctr, Div Urologic Onc, 1500 E Duarte Rd, Duarte, CA 91010; **Phone:** 626-359-8111 x62655; **Board Cert:** Urology 2001; **Med School:** Oregon Hlth Sci Univ 1984; **Resid:** Urology, USC Med Ctr 1990; **Fellow:** Urologic Oncology, City Hosp Natl Med Ctr 1991; **Fac Appt:** Assoc Clin Prof U, USC Sch Med

Breast
and
prostate
canswers.

At City of Hope, we use state-of-the-art surgical techniques for our treatment of breast and prostate cancers. Many of these are less invasive, so our patients can have fewer side effects and a faster recovery. For an appointment, call 800-826-HOPE. Or ask your doctor for a referral. Most insurance accepted. At City of Hope, we have answers to cancer.

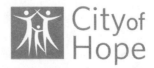

Science saving lives.
cityofhope.org/topdoctors

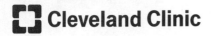

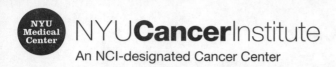

NYU**Cancer**Institute
An NCI-designated Cancer Center

A Collaborative Approach

The NYU Cancer Institute, an NCI designated center, is a "matrix cancer center" without walls operating within the larger NYU Medical Center. With over 200 members and a research funding base of over $81 million, this structure strengthens our capabilities to forge collaborations across medical and scientific disciplines, which translates to comprehensive care for our patients and discoveries that will influence the future of this disease.

Renowned Expertise

Our highly skilled Magnet™ nursing team not only plays a pivotal role in coordinating direct patient care, but is also a source of invaluable patient education. Team members' compassion and expertise help patients better manage the symptoms of their disease as well as their special needs.

A Patient-Focused Setting

The NYU Clinical Cancer Center, with over 70 faculty members from various disciplines at the New York University School of Medicine, is the principal outpatient facility of the Cancer Institute and serves as home for our patients and their caregivers. The center and its multidisciplinary team of experts provide access to the latest treatment options and clinical trials along with a variety of programs in cancer prevention, screening, diagnostics, genetic counseling, and supportive services. When it comes to kids and cancer, the Stephen D. Hassenfeld Children's Center for Cancer and Blood Disorders offers not just innovation but insight. As a leading member of the NCI-sponsored Children's Oncology Group, our physicians are known for developing new ways to treat childhood cancer. Our affiliation with Bellevue Hospital, the oldest public hospital in the country, affords clinically distinctive opportunities to learn and care for patients with cancer by observing its presentation and behavior in a variety of patient groups.

GENITOURINARY ONCOLOGY PROGRAM

UCLA Health System

1-800-UCLA-MD1 (825-2631)
www.uclahealth.org

UCLA's Genitourinary Oncology Program specializes in the management of localized and advanced urologic cancers of the:

Prostate • Kidney • Bladder

UCLA's Prostate Cancer Program brings together a multidisciplinary team to treat benign prostate hyperplasia (BPH) and prostate cancer. At UCLA, more than 100 prostatectomies are performed for prostate cancer annually, and potency-sparing surgery is performed in appropriate cases with good results. Other options include external beam radiation therapy, radioactive seed implantation for localized disease, cryosurgery for localized or minimally invasive disease, hormonal and chemotherapeutic treatment of advanced disease, and clinical trials of new drugs for hormone-refractory metastatic prostate cancer.

The UCLA Kidney Cancer Program provides expertise in developing individualized treatment plans, using both standard and innovative experimental therapies, including immunotherapy, gene therapy, chemotherapy and tumor vaccines. The program has achieved a more than 35 percent response rate with a combination of surgery and immunotherapy, while the average in the country remains between 12 and 15 percent.

UCLA's Jonsson Cancer Center

Designated by the National Cancer Institute as one of only 39 comprehensive cancer centers in the United States, UCLA's Jonsson Cancer Center has earned an international reputation for developing new cancer therapies, providing the best in experimental and traditional treatments, and expertly guiding and training the next generation of medical researchers. The center's 250 physicians and scientists treat upwards of 20,000 patient visits per year and offer hundreds of clinical trials that provide the latest in experimental cancer treatments (www.cancer. mednet.ucla.edu). The center also offers patients and families complete psychological and support services.

UCLA's Jonsson Cancer Center has been ranked the best cancer center in California by *U.S.News & World Report*'s Annual Best Hospitals survey for the seventh year. UCLA Medical Center, of which the Cancer Center is a part, has ranked best in the West for the past 17 years.

Call 1-800-UCLA-MD1 (825-2631)
for a referral to a UCLA doctor.

THE END OF CANCER BEGINS WITH RESEARCH

In 2002, the Prostate Cancer Program at UCLA's Jonsson Cancer Center was designated by the National Cancer Institute as a site of research excellence, making it one of the few institutions nationwide tapped to improve prevention, detection and treatment of prostate cancer.

The designation as a Specialized Program of Research (SPORE) comes with a five-year $11.5 million grant to further expand UCLA's renowned prostate cancer program. Researchers are focusing on two major areas: new molecular targets for therapies, and investigating nutritional strategies to prevent the disease and impede tumor growth.

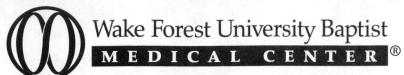

Wake Forest University Baptist
MEDICAL CENTER ®

Comprehensive Cancer Center
Prostate Cancer Center of Excellence

Medical Center Boulevard • Winston-Salem, NC 27157
PAL® (Physician-to-physician calls) 1-800-277-7654
Health On-Call® (Patient access) 1-800-446-2255
www.wfubmc.edu/cancer/

OVERVIEW

The Prostate Cancer Center of Excellence was established in 1999 as a center for innovative research and treatment of this common but complex cancer. The Prostate Cancer Center of Excellence has three broad areas of emphasis: chemoprevention, molecular epidemiology and novel therapies.

RESEARCH

Because the optimal treatment for many prostate cancers is still uncertain, the greatest impact on reducing mortality and morbidity from prostate cancer can be achieved by research focused on chemoprevention, on identifying men at high risk for the disease or its recurrence, and on the development of new therapies for men with existing prostate cancer.

In chemoprevention, studies are being conducted on soy protein with isoflavones and vitamin D as preventive agents. Risk factor research is examining aberrations at the cellular and molecular level that contribute to increased risk for the disease. Among the new therapies being explored are the use of dendritic (immune) cells and vitamin D to fight off prostate cancer.

MULTIDISCIPLINARY CARE

In clinical treatment, Wake Forest Baptist has brought together experts in genitourinary medical oncology, radiation oncology, urologic oncology, pathology and radiology in a unique and comprehensive multidisciplinary clinic. Through a weekly clinic, the Genitourinary Oncology Group provides assessment of all new patients to determine the most effective treatment program including initial treatment, long-term follow-up and quality of life issues. The clinic sees patients with prostate, bladder, testicular, adrenal and other related cancers.

Genetic screening is available for those who are concerned about hereditary risk factors. Patients who are at high risk may elect to participate in breast cancer prevention trials.

THE LATEST TREATMENT MODALITIES

3D Conformal and Intensity Modulated Radiation Therapy — Among the newer treatment options for cancer of the prostate, brain, lung, and head and neck are two methods of focusing radiation on the tumor and surrounding at-risk tissues while optimally sparing nearby normal tissues, 3-dimensional (3D) conformal radiation therapy, and intensity modulated radiation therapy (IMRT). This approach uses anatomic computed tomographic and/or magnetic resonance images of the patient, computer-generated radiation dose calculations, and a computer-controlled linear accelerator to conform or "paint" the radiation dose very precisely to match the shape of the tumor to be treated, avoiding critical structures that may be only millimeters away.

The linear accelerator radiation beam intensity is varied, or modulated, over space and time during the patient's treatment, hence the term "Intensity Modulated" radiation therapy. In combination with advanced imaging techniques like magnetic resonance spectroscopy and positron emission tomography that image both tumor anatomy and biology, IMRT holds great promise for improving local tumor control and survival, even in the most resistant and aggressive human cancers.

Brachytherapy — involves the implantation of radioactive sources in or near a tumor. A full range of brachytherapy treatment options are available for treating cancers of the prostate, breast, cervix, uterus, vagina, head and neck, soft tissues, brain, and eye. With the availability of both high dose rate (HDR) and low dose rate (LDR) brachytherapy technology and expertise, virtually any area of the body can be implanted if appropriate.

**To make an appointment or find a specialist at Wake Forest University Baptist Medical Center,
call Health On-Call® 1-800-446-2255**

KNOWLEDGE MAKES ALL THE DIFFERENCE.

Other Specialists

Cardiology
(a subspecialty of INTERNAL MEDICINE)

Cardiovascular Disease: A cardiologist specializes in diseases of the heart, lungs and blood vessels and manages complex cardiac conditions such a heart attacks and life-threatening, abnormal heartbeat rhythms.

Cardiac Electrophysiology: A field of special interest within the subspecialty of cardiovascular disease which involves intricate technical procedures to evaluate heart rhythms and determine appropriate treatment for them.

Interventional Cardiology: An area of medicine within the subspecialty of cardiology which uses specialized imaging and other diagnostic techniques to evaluate blood flow and pressure in the coronary arteries and chambers of the heart, and uses technical procedures and medications to treat abnormalities that impair the function of the heart.

Training Required: Three years in internal medicine plus additional training and examination for certification in cardiovascular disease, clinical electrophysiology or interventional cardiology.

Clinical Genetics: A specialist trained in diagnostic and therapeutic procedures for patients with genetically linked diseases.

This specialist uses modern cytogenetics, radiologic and biochemical testing to assist in specialized genetic counseling, implements needed therapeutic interventions and provides prevention through prenatal diagnosis. A clinical geneticist demonstrates competence in providing comprehensive diagnostic, management and counseling services for genetic disorders. A medical geneticist plans and coordinates large scale screening programs for inborn errors of metabolism, hemoglobinopathies, chromosome abnormalities and neural tube defects.

Training Required: Two or four years

Infectious Disease:
(a subspecialty of INTERNAL MEDICINE)

An internist who deals with infectious diseases of all types and in all organs. Conditions requiring selective use of antibodies call for this special skill. This physician often diagnoses and treats AIDS patients and patients with fevers which have not been explained. Infectious disease specialists may also have expertise in preventive medicine and conditions associated with travel.

Training Required: Three years in internal medicine plus additional training and examination for certification in infectious disease.

Internal Medicine: An internist is a personal physician who provides long-term, comprehensive care in the office and the hospital, managing both common and complex illness of adolescents, adults and the elderly. Internists are trained in the diagnosis and treatment of cancer, infections and diseases affecting the heart, blood, kidneys, joints and digestive, respiratory and vascular systems. They are also trained in the essentials of primary care internal medicine, which incorporates an understanding of disease prevention, wellness, substance abuse, mental health and effective treatment of common problems of the eyes, ears, skin, nervous system and reproductive organs.

Note: Internal Medicine normally includes many primary care physicians. However; for the purpose of this directory, no primary care physicians are included.

Training Required: Three years

Physical Medicine & Rehabilitation:

Physical medicine and rehabilitation, also referred to as rehabilitation medicine, is the medical specialty concerned with diagnosing, evaluations and treating patients with physical disabilities. these disabilities may arise from conditions affecting the musculoskeletal system such as neck and back pain, sports injuries, or other painful conditions affecting the limbs, for example carpal tunnel syndrome. Alternatively, the disabilities may result from neurological trauma or disease such as spinal cord injury, head injury or stroke.

A physician certified in physical medicine and rehabilitation is often called a physiatrist. The primary goal of the physiatrist is to achieve maximal comprehensive rehabilitation. Pain management is often an important part of the role of the physiatrist. for diagnosis and evaluation, a physiatrist may include the techniques of electromyography to supplement the standard history, physical, X-ray and laboratory examinations. the physiatrist has expertise in orthotics and mechanical and electrical devices.

Training Required: Four years plus one year clinical practice.

Preventive Medicine: A preventative medicine specialist

focuses on the health of individuals and defined populations in order to protect, promote and maintain health and well-bing and prevent disease, disability and premature death. a preventive medicine physician may be a specialist in general preventive medicine, public health, occupational medicine, or aerospace medicine. this specialist works with large population groups as well as with individual patients to promote health and understand the resks of disease, injury, disability and death, seeking to modify and eliminate these risks.

Training Required: Three years

Cardiovascular Disease

Mid Atlantic

Steingart, Richard MD [Cv] - **Spec Exp:** Heart Disease in Cancer Patients; **Hospital:** Meml Sloan Kettering Cancer Ctr (page 76); **Address:** Meml Sloan-Kettering Cancer Ctr, Dept Cardiology, 1275 York Ave, New York, NY 10021; **Phone:** 212-639-8488; **Board Cert:** Internal Medicine 1977; Cardiovascular Disease 1979; **Med School:** Mount Sinai Sch Med 1974; **Resid:** Internal Medicine, Yale-New Haven Hosp 1977; **Fellow:** Cardiovascular Disease, Mt Sinai Med Ctr 1979; **Fac Appt:** Prof Med, Cornell Univ-Weill Med Coll

Clinical Genetics

Mid Atlantic

Ostrer, Harry MD [CG] - **Spec Exp:** Genetic Disorders; Hereditary Cancer; **Hospital:** NYU Med Ctr (page 80); **Address:** NYU Medical Ctr, 550 1st Ave, rm MSB136, New York, NY 10016; **Phone:** 212-263-5746; **Board Cert:** Clinical Genetics 1984; Pediatrics 1985; Clinical Cytogenetics 1990; Clinical Molecular Genetics 2004; **Med School:** Columbia P&S 1976; **Resid:** Pediatrics, Johns Hopkins Hosp 1978; Clinical Genetics, Natl Inst Health 1981; **Fellow:** Molecular Genetics, Johns Hopkins Hosp 1983; **Fac Appt:** Prof Ped, NYU Sch Med

Shapiro, Lawrence R MD [CG] - **Spec Exp:** Hereditary Cancer; **Hospital:** Westchester Med Ctr; **Address:** Regional Med Genetics Ctr, 19 Bradhurst Ave, Ste 1600, Hawthorne, NY 10532-2140; **Phone:** 914-593-8900; **Board Cert:** Pediatrics 1967; Clinical Genetics 1982; Clinical Cytogenetics 1982; **Med School:** NYU Sch Med 1962; **Resid:** Pediatrics, Chldns Hosp 1964; Pediatrics, Bellevue Hosp 1965; **Fellow:** Clinical Genetics, Mount Sinai Med Ctr 1968; **Fac Appt:** Prof Ped, NY Med Coll

Southeast

Sutphen, Rebecca MD [CG] - **Spec Exp:** Genetic Disorders; Hereditary Cancer; Cancer Risk Assessment; **Hospital:** H Lee Moffitt Cancer Ctr & Research Inst; **Address:** H Lee Moffitt Cancer Ctr & Rsch Inst, 12902 Magnolia Drive, Tampa, FL 33612; **Phone:** 813-903-4990; **Board Cert:** Pediatrics 2001; Clinical Cytogenetics 2006; Clinical Molecular Genetics 1996; Clinical Genetics 2006; **Med School:** Temple Univ 1990; **Resid:** Pediatrics, All Children's Hosp 1993; **Fellow:** Clinical Genetics, Univ S Fla Coll Med 1995; **Fac Appt:** Assoc Prof CG, Univ S Fla Coll Med

Midwest

Rubinstein, Wendy S MD/PhD [CG] - **Spec Exp:** Breast Cancer; Colon Cancer; Pancreatic Cancer; **Hospital:** Evanston Hosp; **Address:** Ctr for Medical Genetics, 1000 Central St, Ste 620, Evanston, IL 60201; **Phone:** 847-570-1029; **Board Cert:** Internal Medicine 2003; Clinical Genetics 2007; Clinical Molecular Genetics 2007; **Med School:** Mount Sinai Sch Med 1989; **Resid:** Internal Medicine, Strong Meml Hosp 1992; **Fellow:** Clinical Genetics, Univ Pittsburgh 1996; Clinical Molecular Genetics, Univ Pittsburgh 1996; **Fac Appt:** Asst Prof Med, Northwestern Univ

Whelan, Alison MD [CG] - **Spec Exp:** Gynecologic Cancer Risk Assessment; Colon & Rectal Cancer Risk Assessment; Hereditary Cancer; **Hospital:** Barnes-Jewish Hosp, St Louis Chldns Hosp; **Address:** Washington Univ Sch Med, 660 S Euclid Ave, Campus Box 8073, St Louis, MO 63110; **Phone:** 314-454-6093; **Board Cert:** Clinical Genetics 1996; **Med School:** Washington Univ, St Louis 1986; **Resid:** Internal Medicine, Barnes Hosp 1989; Pediatrics, Wash Univ Sch Med 1994; **Fellow:** Research, Wash Univ Sch Med 1991; Clinical Genetics, Wash Univ Sch Med 1994; **Fac Appt:** Prof Med, Washington Univ, St Louis

Southwest

Mulvihill, John J MD [CG] - **Spec Exp:** Genetic Disorders; Fertility in Cancer Survivors; **Hospital:** Chldns Hosp OU Med Ctr; **Address:** Childrens Hosp, 940 NE 13th St, rm 2B2418, Oklahoma City, OK 73104; **Phone:** 405-271-8685; **Board Cert:** Pediatrics 1975; Clinical Genetics 1982; **Med School:** Univ Wash 1969; **Resid:** Pediatrics, Johns Hopkins Hosp 1974; **Fellow:** Research, NCI-Natl Inst Hlth 1972; **Fac Appt:** Prof CG, Univ Okla Coll Med

West Coast and Pacific

Grody, Wayne W MD/PhD [CG] - **Spec Exp:** Genetic Disorders; Hereditary Cancer; **Hospital:** UCLA Med Ctr (page 83); **Address:** UCLA School Medicine, Division of Genetic Molecular Pathology, 10833 Le Conte Ave, #37-121CHS Ave, Los Angeles, CA 90095-1732; **Phone:** 310-825-5648; **Board Cert:** Clinical Genetics 1990; Anatomic & Clinical Pathology 1987; Clinical Biochemical Genetics 1990; Molecular Genetic Pathology 2001; **Med School:** Baylor Coll Med 1977; **Resid:** Pathology, UCLA Med Ctr 1986; **Fellow:** Clinical Genetics, UCLA Med Ctr 1987; **Fac Appt:** Prof CG, UCLA

Weitzel, Jeffrey N MD [CG] - **Spec Exp:** Breast Cancer; Ovarian Cancer; Hereditary Cancer; **Hospital:** City of Hope Natl Med Ctr & Beckman Rsch (page 69); **Address:** City of Hope Cancer Ctr, 1500 E Duarte Rd, Duarte, CA 91010; **Phone:** 626-256-8662; **Board Cert:** Internal Medicine 1986; Medical Oncology 1989; Clinical Genetics 1996; **Med School:** Univ Minn 1983; **Resid:** Internal Medicine, Univ Minn Hosps 1986; Hematology, Hammersmith Hosp 1987; **Fellow:** Hematology & Oncology, Tufts -New England Med Ctr 1992; Clinical Genetics, Tufts-New England Med Ctr 1996; **Fac Appt:** Assoc Clin Prof Med, USC Sch Med

Infectious Disease

Mid Atlantic

Polsky, Bruce MD [Inf] - **Spec Exp:** Infections in Cancer Patients; AIDS Related Cancers; **Hospital:** St Luke's - Roosevelt Hosp Ctr - Roosevelt Div (page 72); **Address:** 1111 Amsterdam Ave, New York, NY 10025; **Phone:** 212-523-2525; **Board Cert:** Internal Medicine 1983; Infectious Disease 1986; **Med School:** Wayne State Univ 1980; **Resid:** Internal Medicine, Montefiore Hosp 1983; **Fellow:** Infectious Disease, Meml Sloan Kettering Cancer Ctr 1986; **Fac Appt:** Prof Med, Columbia P&S

Sepkowitz, Kent MD [Inf] - **Spec Exp:** Infections in Cancer Patients; **Hospital:** Meml Sloan Kettering Cancer Ctr (page 76); **Address:** 1275 York Ave, New York, NY 10021-0033; **Phone:** 212-639-2441; **Board Cert:** Internal Medicine 1983; Infectious Disease 2000; **Med School:** Univ Okla Coll Med 1980; **Resid:** Internal Medicine, Roosevelt Hosp 1984; **Fellow:** Infectious Disease, Meml Sloan Kettering Cancer Ctr 1991; **Fac Appt:** Prof Med, Cornell Univ-Weill Med Coll

Great Plains and Mountains

Freifeld, Alison D MD [Inf] - **Spec Exp:** Infectious Disease during Chemotherapy; Infections in Cancer Patients; **Hospital:** Nebraska Med Ctr; **Address:** University of Nebraska, 985400 Nebraska Medical Center, Omaha, NE 68198-5400; **Phone:** 402-559-8650; **Board Cert:** Internal Medicine 1985; Infectious Disease 1988; **Med School:** Johns Hopkins Univ 1982; **Resid:** Internal Medicine, Johns Hopkins Univ Med Ctr 1985

West Coast and Pacific

Palefsky, Joel M MD [Inf] - **Spec Exp:** AIDS Related Cancers; **Hospital:** UCSF - Mt Zion Med Ctr; **Address:** UCSF Med Ctr, Infectious Disease, 505 Parnassus Ave, rm M1203, San Francisco, CA 94143-0126; **Phone:** 415-353-2626; **Board Cert:** Internal Medicine 1984; Infectious Disease 1988; **Med School:** McGill Univ 1980; **Resid:** Internal Medicine, Royal Victoria Hosp 1984; **Fellow:** Infectious Disease, Stanford Univ 1989

Internal Medicine

New England

Billings, J Andrew MD [IM] - **Spec Exp:** Palliative Care; Pain Management; **Hospital:** Mass Genl Hosp; **Address:** 55 Fruit St, FND 600, Boston, MA 02114; **Phone:** 617-724-9197; **Board Cert:** Internal Medicine 1975; **Med School:** Harvard Med Sch 1972; **Resid:** Internal Medicine, Univ California Hosps 1975; **Fellow:** Internal Medicine, Mass Genl Hosp 1977; **Fac Appt:** Assoc Prof Med, Harvard Med Sch

Mid Atlantic

Rivlin, Richard S MD [IM] - **Spec Exp:** Cancer Prevention; Nutrition & Cancer Prevention; **Hospital:** NY-Presby Hosp (page 79); **Address:** Anne Fisher Nutrition Ctr, Strang Cancer Prevention Ctr, 480 E 72nd St, Ste 600, New York, NY 10021; **Phone:** 212-794-4900 x152; **Board Cert:** Internal Medicine 1969; **Med School:** Harvard Med Sch 1959; **Resid:** Internal Medicine, Bellevue Hosp 1960; Internal Medicine, Johns Hopkins Hosp 1961; **Fellow:** Endocrinology, Diabetes & Metabolism, Natl Inst Hlth 1963; Biochemistry, Johns Hopkins Hosp 1966; **Fac Appt:** Prof Med, Cornell Univ-Weill Med Coll

Southeast

Heimburger, Douglas C MD [IM] - **Spec Exp:** Nutrition & Disease Prevention/Control; Nutrition & Cancer Prevention; **Hospital:** Univ of Ala Hosp at Birmingham, VA Med Ctr; **Address:** Univ Alabama, Dept Nutrition Sci & Med, 1675 University Blvd, Webb 439, Birmingham, AL 35294-3360; **Phone:** 205-934-7058; **Board Cert:** Internal Medicine 1981; **Med School:** Vanderbilt Univ 1978; **Resid:** Internal Medicine, Washington Univ Hosps 1981; **Fellow:** Nutrition, Univ Alabama Med Ctr 1982

Southwest

Witte, Marlys H MD [IM] - **Spec Exp:** Lymphedema; **Hospital:** Univ Med Ctr - Tucson; **Address:** Univ Arizona Hlth Scis Ctr, 1501 N Campbell Ave, rm 4406, Box 245200, Tucson, AZ 85724-5063; **Phone:** 520-626-6118; **Board Cert:** Internal Medicine 1967; **Med School:** NYU Sch Med 1960; **Resid:** Internal Medicine, Bellevue Hosp 1963; **Fellow:** Internal Medicine, NYU Med Ctr 1966; **Fac Appt:** Prof S, Univ Ariz Coll Med

Wolff, Robert A MD [IM] - **Spec Exp:** Gastrointestinal Cancer; Pancreatic Cancer; Colon & Rectal Cancer; Clinical Trials; **Hospital:** UT MD Anderson Cancer Ctr (page 81); **Address:** MD Anderson Cancer Ctr, Faculty Center Unit 426, Box 301402, Houston, TX 77230; **Phone:** 713-745-5476; **Board Cert:** Internal Medicine 1989; **Med School:** Albany Med Coll 1986; **Resid:** Internal Medicine, Duke Univ Med Ctr 1989; **Fellow:** Hematology & Oncology, Duke Univ Med Ctr 1992; **Fac Appt:** Assoc Prof Med, Univ Tenn Coll Med, Memphis

Physical Medicine & Rehabilitation

Mid Atlantic

Cheville, Andrea MD [PMR] - **Spec Exp:** Lymphedema; Cancer Rehabilitation; Pain-Cancer; **Hospital:** Hosp Univ Penn - UPHS (page 84); **Address:** Hosp Univ Penn, 3400 Spruce St, 5 W Gates, Philadelphia, PA 19104; **Phone:** 215-349-8769; **Board Cert:** Physical Medicine & Rehabilitation 1998; **Med School:** Harvard Med Sch 1993; **Resid:** Physical Medicine & Rehabilitation, UMDNJ Med Ctr 1997; **Fellow:** Pain & Palliative Care, Meml Sloan Kettering Cancer Ctr 1999; **Fac Appt:** Asst Prof PMR, Univ Pennsylvania

Francis, Kathleen MD [PMR] - **Spec Exp:** Lymphedema; **Address:** 200 S Orange Ave, Livingston, NJ 07039; **Phone:** 973-322-7366; **Board Cert:** Physical Medicine & Rehabilitation 2004; **Med School:** UMDNJ-NJ Med Sch, Newark 1989; **Resid:** Physical Medicine & Rehabilitation, UMDNJ-Kessler Inst Rehab 1993; **Fac Appt:** Asst Clin Prof PMR, UMDNJ-NJ Med Sch, Newark

Schwartz, L Matthew MD [PMR] - **Spec Exp:** Lymphedema; Head & Neck Cancer; Pain-Cancer; Cancer Rehabilitation; **Hospital:** Hosp Univ Penn - UPHS (page 84), Chestnut Hill Rehab Hosp; **Address:** Hosp Univ Penn, Dept Phys Med & Rehab, 3400 Spruce St, 5 West Gates, Philadelphia, PA 19104; **Phone:** 215-662-3259; **Board Cert:** Physical Medicine & Rehabilitation 1992; Pain Medicine 2003; **Med School:** UMDNJ-NJ Med Sch, Newark 1987; **Resid:** Physical Medicine & Rehabilitation, Hosp Univ Penn 1989; Physical Medicine & Rehabilitation, Thomas Jefferson Univ Hosp 1991; **Fac Appt:** Clin Prof PMR, Univ Pennsylvania

Stubblefield, Michael MD [PMR] - **Spec Exp:** Cancer Rehabilitation; Pain-Cancer; **Hospital:** Meml Sloan Kettering Cancer Ctr (page 76); **Address:** Meml Sloan Kettering Cancer Ctr, 1275 York Ave, Box 349, New York, NY 10021; **Phone:** 212-639-7834; **Board Cert:** Internal Medicine 2001; Physical Medicine & Rehabilitation 2002; **Med School:** Columbia P&S 1996; **Resid:** Internal Medicine, Columbia Presby Med Ctr 2001; Physical Medicine & Rehabilitation, Columbia Presby Med Ctr 2001

Southeast

King Jr, Richard W MD [PMR] - **Spec Exp:** Cancer Rehabilitation; Lymphedema; Soft Tissue Radiation Necrosis; **Hospital:** WellStar Windy Hill Hosp; **Address:** HyOx Medical Treatment Ctr, 2550 Windy Hill Rd, Ste 110, Marietta, GA 30067; **Phone:** 678-303-3200; **Board Cert:** Physical Medicine & Rehabilitation 1988; Undersea & Hyperbaric Medicine 2002; **Med School:** Emory Univ 1979; **Resid:** Physical Medicine & Rehabilitation, Emory Univ Hosp 1987; **Fac Appt:** Asst Clin Prof PMR, Emory Univ

Stewart, Paula JB MD [PMR] - **Spec Exp:** Lymphedema; Brain Tumors; Spinal Cord Tumors; Cancer Rehabilitation; **Hospital:** Healthsouth Lakeshore Rehab Hosp; **Address:** Healthsouth Lakeshore Rehab Hosp, 3800 Ridgeway Drive, Birmingham, AL 35209; **Phone:** 205-868-2347; **Board Cert:** Physical Medicine & Rehabilitation 1996; Spinal Cord Injury Medicine 2000; **Med School:** Univ Minn 1987; **Resid:** Physical Medicine & Rehabilitation, Mayo Clinic 1991

Midwest

DePompolo, Robert W MD [PMR] - **Spec Exp:** Cancer Rehabilitation; Lymphedema; **Hospital:** St Mary's Hosp - Rochester, Mayo Med Ctr & Clin - Rochester; **Address:** Mayo Clinic, Dept Phys Med & Rehab, 200 1st St SW, Rochester, MN 55905; **Phone:** 507-255-8972; **Board Cert:** Physical Medicine & Rehabilitation 1981; **Med School:** Wayne State Univ 1977; **Resid:** Physical Medicine & Rehabilitation, Univ Minnesota 1980

Feldman, Joseph MD [PMR] - **Spec Exp:** Lymphedema; Pain-Back; **Hospital:** Evanston Hosp; **Address:** Evantston Hospital, 2650 Ridge Rd, rm 2204, Evanston, IL 60201-1718; **Phone:** 847-570-2066; **Board Cert:** Physical Medicine & Rehabilitation 1971; **Med School:** Univ IL Coll Med 1965; **Resid:** Physical Medicine & Rehabilitation, Univ of Ilinois 1969; **Fac Appt:** Asst Prof PMR, Northwestern Univ

Gamble, Gail L MD [PMR] - **Spec Exp:** Lymphedema; Head & Neck Cancer; Bone Tumors-Metastatic; **Hospital:** Mayo Med Ctr & Clin - Rochester; **Address:** Mayo Clinic, Dept Phys Med & Rehab, 200 1st St SW, Rochester, MN 55905; **Phone:** 507-284-2608; **Board Cert:** Physical Medicine & Rehabilitation 1985; **Med School:** Mayo Med Sch 1979; **Resid:** Physical Medicine & Rehabilitation, Mayo Clinic 1983

Preventive Medicine

Mid Atlantic

Lane, Dorothy S MD [PrM] - **Spec Exp:** Cancer Prevention; Health Promotion & Disease Prevention; **Hospital:** Stony Brook Univ Med Ctr; **Address:** Stony Brook Univ Sch Med, HSC L2, rm 142, Stony Brook, NY 11794-8437; **Phone:** 631-444-2094; **Board Cert:** Public Health & Genl Preventive Med 1970; Family Medicine 2000; **Med School:** Columbia P&S 1965; **Resid:** Public Health & Genl Preventive Med, NY Health Dept 1968; **Fac Appt:** Prof PrM, SUNY Stony Brook

Weiss, Stanley H MD [PrM] - **Spec Exp:** Cancer Epidemiology & Control; Infections in Cancer Patients; **Hospital:** UMDNJ-Univ Hosp-Newark; **Address:** NJ Medical School, 30 Bergen St, ADMC, Ste 1614, Newark, NJ 07107-3000; **Phone:** 973-972-7716; **Board Cert:** Internal Medicine 1981; Medical Oncology 1985; **Med School:** Harvard Med Sch 1978; **Resid:** Internal Medicine, Montefiore Med Ctr 1981; **Fellow:** Medical Oncology, National Cancer Inst 1985; Epidemiology, National Cancer Inst 1987; **Fac Appt:** Prof PrM, UMDNJ-NJ Med Sch, Newark

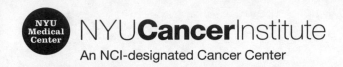

NYU**Cancer**Institute

An NCI-designated Cancer Center

NYU Clinical Cancer Center
160 East 34th Street
New York, New York 10016
www.nyuci.org/atcd

NYU Medical Center
550 First Avenue
(at 31st Street)
New York, New York 10016
www.nyumc.org/atcd

Stephen D. Hassenfeld
Children's Center
for Cancer and Blood
Disorders
160 East 32nd Street
New York, New York 10016
www.nyumc.org/hassenfeld

A Collaborative Approach

The NYU Cancer Institute, an NCI designated center, is a "matrix cancer center" without walls operating within the larger NYU Medical Center. With over 200 members and a research funding base of over $81 million, this structure strengthens our capabilities to forge collaborations across medical and scientific disciplines, which translates to comprehensive care for our patients and discoveries that will influence the future of this disease.

Renowned Expertise

Our highly skilled Magnet™ nursing team not only plays a pivotal role in coordinating direct patient care, but is also a source of invaluable patient education. Team members' compassion and expertise help patients better manage the symptoms of their disease as well as their special needs.

A Patient-Focused Setting

The NYU Clinical Cancer Center, with over 70 faculty members from various disciplines at the New York University School of Medicine, is the principal outpatient facility of the Cancer Institute and serves as home for our patients and their caregivers. The center and its multidisciplinary team of experts provide access to the latest treatment options and clinical trials along with a variety of programs in cancer prevention, screening, diagnostics, genetic counseling, and supportive services. When it comes to kids and cancer, the Stephen D. Hassenfeld Children's Center for Cancer and Blood Disorders offers not just innovation but insight. As a leading member of the NCI-sponsored Children's Oncology Group, our physicians are known for developing new ways to treat childhood cancer. Our affiliation with Bellevue Hospital, the oldest public hospital in the country, affords clinically distinctive opportunities to learn and care for patients with cancer by observing its presentation and behavior in a variety of patient groups.

Section IV
Appendices

Appendix A:
Medical Boards

Intro to ABMS and Osteopathic Specialties

The following pages contain descriptions of the "official" medical specialties, approved by the American Board of Medical Specialists (for M.D.s) or by the American Osteopathic Association (for D.O.s). These are important because they are the only specialties recognized by the official governing boards. There may be physicians who call themselves one kind of specialist or another, but they may not be certified by the "official" boards. There are, in fact, over 100 such "self-designated" boards, some simply groups of physicians interested in a given area of medicine with no qualifications for membership to other groups with very specific qualifications for membership.

It is important for the medical consumer to seek out physicians certified by the ABMS or AOA to assure their doctor has had the appropriate training and passed the board certification exam.

ABMS

The ABMS is an organization of ABMS approved medical specialty boards. The mission of the ABMS is to maintain and improve the quality of medical care by assisting the Member Boards in their efforts to develop and utilize professional and educational standards for the evaluation and certification of physician specialists. The intent of certification of physicians is to provide assurance to the public that a physician specialist certified by a Member Board of the ABMS has successfully completed an approved educational program and evaluation process which includes an examination designed to assess the knowledge, skills, and experience required to provide quality patient care in that specialty. The ABMS serves to coordinate the activities of its Member Boards and to provide information to the public, the government, the profession and its Members concerning issues involving specialization and certification in medicine.

Following is a list of the addresses of the various medical specialty boards approved by the ABMS. Note that there are 24 board organizations for 25 medical specialties. Psychiatry and Neurology share the same board.

To find out if a physician is certified, consumers can call the individual boards which may charge a fee for the information, or they can contact the ABMS at 866-275-2267 (no fee) or www.abms.org.

American Board of Allergy and Immunology
111 S. Independence Mall E. Suite 701
Philadelphia, PA 19106-3699
(215) 592-9466, (866) 264-5568

General Certification in Allergy and Immunology. Certifications awarded since 1989 are valid for 10 years. For those certified prior to 1989 there is no recertification requirement.

American Board of Anesthesiology
4101 Lake Boone Trail, Suite 510
Raleigh, NC 27607-7506
(919) 881-2570

General Certification in Anesthesiology; with Special and Added Qualifications in Critical Care Medicine and Pain Management. Certifications awarded since 2000 are valid for 10 years.

American Board of Colon and Rectal Surgery
20600 Eureka Road, Suite 600
Taylor, MI 48180
(734) 282-9400

General Certification in Colon and Rectal Surgery. Certifications awarded since 1990 are valid for 10 years.

American Board of Dermatology
Henry Ford Health System
One Ford Place
Detriot, MI 48202-3450
(313) 874-1088

General Certification in Dermatology; with Special Qualifications in Dermatopathology, and Pediatric Dermatology. Certifications awarded since 1991 are valid for 10 years with no recertification required.

American Board of Emergency Medicine
3000 Coolidge Road
East Lansing, MI 48823-6319
(517) 332-4800

General Certification in Emergency Medicine; with Special and Added Qualifications in
Medical Toxicology, Pediatric Emergency Medicine, Sports Medicine and Undersea and
Hyperbaric Medicine. Certifications awarded since 1980 are valid for 10 years.

American Board of Family Practice
2228 Young Drive
Lexington, KY 40505-4294
(859) 269-5626, (888) 995-5700

General Certification in Family Practice; with Added Qualifications in Adolescent
Medicine, Geriatric Medicine and Sports Medicine. Certifications awarded since 1970
are valid for 7 years.

American Board of Internal Medicine
510 Walnut Street, Suite 1700
Philadelphia, PA 19106-3699
(215) 446-3500, (800) 441-2246

General Certification in Internal Medicine; with Special Qualifications in Cardiovascular
Disease, Endocrinology, Diabetes and Metabolism, Gastroenterology, Hematology,
Infectious Disease, Medical Oncology, Nephrology, Pulmonary Disease, and
Rheumatology; and Added Qualifications in Adolescent Medicine, Clinical Cardiac
Electrophysiology, Critical Care Medicine, Geriatric Medicine, Interventional Cardiology,
Sleep Medicine, Sports Medicine and Transplant Hepatology. Certifications awarded
since 1990 are valid for 10 years.

American Board of Medical Genetics
9650 Rockville Pike
Bethesda, MD 20814-3998
(301) 634-7315

General Certification in Clinical Genetics (MD), PhD Medical Genetics, Clinical
Biochemical Genetics, Clinical Cytogenetics and Clinical Molecular Genetics; with
Added Qualifications in Molecular Genetic Pathology. Certifications awarded since 2002
are valid for 2 years.

Appendix A: Medical Boards

American Board of Neurological Surgery
6550 Fannin Street, Suite 2139
Houston, TX 77030-2701
(713) 441-6015

General Certification in Neurological Surgery. Certifications awarded since 1999 are valid for 10 years.

American Board of Nuclear Medicine
4555 Forest Park Boulevard, Suite 119
St. Louis, MO 63108
(314) 367-2225

General Certification in Nuclear Medicine. Certifications awarded since 1992 are valid for 10 years.

American Board of Obstetrics and Gynecology
2915 Vine Street, Suite 300
Dallas, TX 75204
(214) 871-1619

General Certification in Obstetrics and Gynecology; with Special Qualifications in Gynecologic Oncology, Maternal and Fetal Medicine, Reproductive Endocrinology; and Added Qualifications in Critical Care Medicine. Certifications awarded since 1986 are valid for 6 years.

American Board of Ophthalmology
111 Presidential Boulevard, Suite 241
Bala Cynwyd, PA 19004-1075
(610) 664-1175

General Certification in Ophthalmology - Certifications awarded since 1992 are valid for 10 years. For those certified prior to 1992, there is no recertification requirement.

American Board of Orthopaedic Surgery
400 Silver Cedar Court
Chapel Hill, NC 27514
(919) 929-7103

General Certification in Orthopaedic Surgery; with Added Qualification in Hand Surgery and Orthopaedics Sports Medicine. Certificates awared since 1996 are valid for 10 years.

American Board of Otolaryngology
5615 Kirby Drive, Suite 600
Houston, TX 77005
(713) 850-0399

General Certification in Otolaryngology; with Added Qualifications in Neurotology, Pediatric Otolaryngology and Plastic Surgery within the Head and Neck. Certifications awarded since 2002 are valid for 10 years.

American Board of Pathology
P.O. Box 25915
Tampa, FL 33622-5915
(813) 286-2444

General Certification in Anatomic and Clinical Pathology, Anatomic Pathology and Clinical Pathology; with Special Qualifications in Blood Banking/Transfusion Medicine, Chemical Pathology, Dermatopathology, Forensic Pathology, Hematology, Medical Microbiology, Molecular Genetic Pathology, Neuropathology and Pediatric Pathology; and Added Qualifications in Cytopathology. Certifications awarded since 1997 are valid for 10 years.

American Board of Pediatrics
111 Silver Cedar Court
Chapel Hill, NC 27514-1651
(919) 929-0461

General Certification in Pediatrics; with Special Qualifications in Adolescent Medicine, Developmental-Behavioral Pediatrics, Neonatal-Perinatal Medicine, Pediatric Cardiology, Pediatric Critical Care Medicine, Pediatric Emergency Medicine, Pediatric Endocrinology, Pediatric Gastroenterology, Pediatric Hematology-Oncology, Pediatric Infectious Diseases, Pediatric Nephrology, Pediatric Pulmonology, and Pediatric Rheumatology; and Added Qualifications in Medical Toxicology, Neurodevelopmental Disabilities, Pediatric Transplant Hepatology and Sports Medicine. Certifications awarded since 1988 are valid for 7 years.

American Board of Physical Medicine and Rehabilitation
3015 Allegro Park Lane, S.W.
Rochester, MN 55902-4139
(507) 282-1776

General Certification in Physical Medicine and Rehabilitation; with Special Qualifications in Pain Medicine, Pediatric Rehabilitation Medicine, and Spinal Cord Injury Medicine. Certifications awarded since 1993 are valid for 10 years.

Appendix A: Medical Boards

American Board of Plastic Surgery
  Seven Penn Center, Suite 400
  1635 Market Street
  Philadelphia, PA 19103-2204
  (215) 587-9322

General Certification in Plastic Surgery; with Added Qualifications in Hand Surgery.
Certifications awarded since 1995 are valid for 10 years.

American Board of Preventive Medicine
  330 South Wells Street, Suite 1018
  Chicago, IL 60606-7106
  (312) 939-ABPM [2276]

General Certification in Aerospace Medicine, Occupational Medicine and Public Health
and General Preventive Medicine; with Added Qualifications in Undersea and
Hyperbaric Medicine and Medical Toxicology. Certifications awarded since 1997 are
valid for 10 years.

American Board of Psychiatry and Neurology
  500 Lake Cook Road, Suite 335
  Deerfield, IL 60015-5349
  (847) 945-7900

General Certification in Psychiatry, Neurology and Neurology with Special Qualification
in Child Neurology; with Special Qualifications in Child and Adolescent Psychiatry, Pain
Medicine and Sleep Medicine; and Added Qualifications in Addiction Psychiatry,
Clinical Neurophysiology, Forensic Psychiatry, Geriatric Psychiatry, Neurodevelopmental
Disabilities, Psychosomatic Medicine and Vascular Neurology . Certifications awarded
since 1994 are valid for 10 years.

American Board of Radiology
  5441 E. Williams Boulevard, Suite 200
  Tucson, AZ 85711
  (520) 790-2900

General Certification in Diagnostic Radiology or Radiation Oncology; with Special
Competency in Nuclear Radiology; and Added Qualifications in Neuroradiology,
Pediatric Radiology and Vascular and Interventional Radiology. Radiological Physics is a
non-clinical certification. Certificates are valid for 10 years.

American Board of Surgery
1617 John F. Kennedy Boulevard, Suite 860
Philadelphia, PA 19103-1847
(215) 568-4000

General Certification in Surgery and Vascular Surgery; with Special Qualifications in
Pediatric Surgery and Surgery of the Hand; and Added Qualifications in Surgical Critical
Care. Certifications awarded since 1976 are valid for 10 years.

American Board of Thoracic Surgery
633 North St. Clair Street, Suite 2320
Chicago, IL 60611
(312) 202-5900

General Certification in Thoracic Surgery. Certifications awarded since 1976 are valid
for 10 years.

American Board of Urology
2216 Ivy Road, Suite 210
Charlottesville, VA 22903
(434) 979-0059

General Certification in Urology. Certifications awarded as of 1985 are valid for 10 years.

Osteopathic

The American Osteopathic Association (AOA) is a member association
representing more than 56,000 osteopathic physicians (D.O.s). The AOA serves as
the primary certifying body for D.O.s, and is the accrediting agency for all
osetopathic medical colleges and healthcare facilities. The AOA's mission is to
advance the philosophy and practice of osteopathic medicine by promoting
excellence in education, research, and the delivery of quality, cost-effective
healthcare within a distinct, unified profession.

American Osteopathic Association
142 E Ontario Street
Chicago, IL 60611

Consumers may call the American Osteopathic Association at (800) 621-1773 or
visit the website, www.osteopathic.org, for general certification information.

Appendix A: Medical Boards

American Osteopathic Board of Anesthesiology

General certification in Anesthesiology; with Added Qualifications in Addiction Medicine, Critical Care Medicine, and Pain Management. Certifications awarded since 2002 are valid for 10 years. For those certified prior to 2002 there is no recertification requirement.

American Osteopathic Board of Dermatology

General certification in Dermatology; with Added Qualifications in Dermatopathology and Mohs'-Micrographic Surgery. Certifications awarded since 2004 are valid for 10 years.

American Osteopathic Board of Emergency Medicine

General certification in Emergency Medicine; with Added Qualifications in Emergency Medical Services, Medical Toxicology, and Sports Medicine. Certifications awarded since 1994 are valid for 10 years.

American Osteopathic Board of Family Physicians

General certification in Family Practice and Osteopathic Manipulative Treatment (OMT); with Added Qualifications in Geriatric Medicine and Sports Medicine. Certifications awarded since March 1,1997 are valid for 8 years.

American Osteopathic Board of Internal Medicine

General certification in Internal Medicine; with Special Qualifications in Allergy/Immunology, Cardiology, Endocrinology, Gastroenterology, Hematology, Infectious Disease, Nephrology, Oncology, Pulmonary Disease, Rheumatology; with Added Qualifications in Addiction Medicine, Critical Care Medicine, Clinical Cardiac Electrophysiology, Geriatric Medicine, Interventional Cardiology and Sports Medicine. Certifications awarded since 1993 are valid for 10 years.

American Osteopathic Board of Neurology and Psychiatry

General certification in Neurology and Psychiatry; with Special Qualifications in Child/Adolescent Psychiatry and Child/Adolescent Neurology; with Added Qualifications in Addiction Medicine, Neurophysiology, and Sports Medicine. Certifications awarded since 1995 are valid for 10 years.

American Osteopathic Board of Neuromusculoskeletal Medicine

(Formerly American Osteopathic Board of Special Proficiency in Osteopathic Manipulative Medicine). Additional Certification in sports medicine. Certification awarded since 1995 are valid for 10 years.

American Osteopathic Board of Nuclear Medicine

General certification in Nuclear Medicine. Certifications awarded since 1995 are valid for 10 years.

American Osteopathic Board of Obstetrics and Gynecology

General certification in Obstetrics and Gynecology; with Special Qualifications in Gynecologic Oncology; Maternal and Fetal Medicine and Reproductive Endocrinology. Certifications awarded since June 2002 are valid for 6 years.

American Osteopathic Board of Ophthalmology and Otolaryngology/Head and Neck Surgery

General certification in Ophthalmology, Otolaryngology, Facial Plastic Surgery and Otolaryngology/Facial Plastic Surgery; with Added Qualifications in Otolaryngic Allergy. Certifications awarded in Ophthalmology since 2000 are valid for 10 years. For those certified prior to 2000 there is no recertification requirement. Certifications awarded in Otolaryngology and/or Otolaryngology/Facial Plastic Surgery since 2002 are valid for 10 years.

American Osteopathic Board of Orthopaedic Surgery

General certification in Orthopaedic Surgery; with Added Qualifications in Hand Surgery. Certifications awarded since 1994 are valid for 10 years.

American Osteopathic Board of Pathology

General certification in Laboratory Medicine, Anatomic Pathology and Anatomic Pathology and Laboratory Medicine; with Special Qualifications in Forensic Pathology; and with Added Qualifications in Dermatopathology. Certifications awarded since 1995 are valid for 10 years.

American Osteopathic Board of Pediatrics

General certification in Pediatrics with Special Qualifications in Adolescent and Young Adult Medicine, Neonatology, Pediatric Allergy/Immunology and Pediatric Endocrinology; with Added Qualifications in Sports Medicine. Certifications awarded since 1995 are valid for 7 years.

American Osteopathic Board of Physical Medicine and Rehabilitation Medicine

General certification in Physical Medicine and Rehabilitation; with Added Qualifications in Sports Medicine. Certifications awarded since 2004 are valid for 10 years.

Appendix A: Medical Boards

American Osteopathic Board of Preventive Medicine

General certification in Preventive Medicine/Aerospace Medicine, Preventive Medicine/Occupational-Environmental Medicine and Preventive Medicine/Public Health; with Added Qualifications in Occupational Medicine and Sports Medicine. Certifications awarded since 1994 are valid for 10 years.

American Osteopathic Board of Proctology

General certification in Proctology. Certifications awarded since 2004 are valid for 10 years.

American Osteopathic Board of Radiology

General certification in Diagnostic Radiology and Radiation Oncology; with Added Qualifications in Body Imaging, Diagnostic Ultrasound, Neuroradiology, Pediatric Radiology and Vascular and Interventional Radiology. Certifications awarded since 2002 are valid for 10 years.

American Osteopathic Board of Surgery

General certification in Surgery, Neurological Surgery, Plastic and Reconstructive Surgery, Cardiothoracic Surgery, Urological Surgery and General Vascular Surgery; with Added Qualifications in Surgical Critical Care. Certifications awarded since 1997 are valid for 10 years.

APPENDIX B:
Hospital Listings

Following is an alphabetical listing of hospitals noted in doctors' entries. Institutions listed in **Bold** are profiled in this guide. The abbreviations as they appear in the listings are in *italics* below. Due to the many mergers taking place in the hospital industry the names on this list may have changed subsequent to publication of this guide.

Abbott - Northwestern Hospital		(612) 863-4000
Abbott - Northwestern Hosp		
800 E 28th St	Minneapolis, MN 55407	MIDWEST
Advocate Christ Medical Center		(708) 684-8000
Adv Christ Med Ctr		
4440 W 95th St	Oak Lawn, IL 60453	MIDWEST
Advocate Illinois Masonic Medical Center		(773) 975-1600
Adv Illinois Masonic Med Ctr		
836 W Wellington Ave	Chicago, IL 60657-5147	MIDWEST
Advocate Lutheran General Hospital		(847) 723-2210
Adv Luth Genl Hosp		
1775 West Dempster St	Park Ridge, IL 60068	MIDWEST
Alaska Regional Hospital		(907) 276-1131
Alaska Regl Hosp		
2801 DeBarr Rd	Anchorage, AK 99508	WEST COAST AND PACIFIC
Albany Medical Center		(518) 262-3125
Albany Med Ctr		
43 New Scotland Ave	Albany, NY 12208	MID ATLANTIC
Alfred I duPont Hospital for Children		(302) 651-4000
Alfred I duPont Hosp for Children		
1600 Rockland Rd	Wilmington, DE 19803	MID ATLANTIC
All Children's Hospital		(727) 767-7451
All Children's Hosp		
801 Sixth Street South	St. Petersburg, FL 33701	SOUTHEAST
Allegheny General Hospital		(412) 359-3131
Allegheny General Hosp		
320 E. North Avenue	Pittsburgh, PA 15212	MID ATLANTIC

Alta Bates Summit Medical Center		(510) 204-4444
Alta Bates Summit Med Ctr		
2450 Ashby Avenue	Berkeley, CA 94705	WEST COAST AND PACIFIC
Anne Arundel Medical Center		(443) 481-1000
Anne Arundel Med Ctr		
64 Franklin Street	Annapolis, MD 21401	MID ATLANTIC
Arkansas Children's Hospital		(501) 364-1100
Arkansas Chldns Hosp		
800 Marshall St	Little Rock, AR 72202	SOUTHWEST
Arthur G. James Cancer Hospital & Research Institute		(614) 293-3300
Arthur G James Cancer Hosp & Research Inst		
300 West 10th Avenue	Columbus, OH 43210	MIDWEST
Audie L Murphy Memorial Veterans Hospital		(210) 617-5300
Audie L Murphy Meml Vets Hosp		
7400 Merton Minter Blvd	San Antonio, TX 78229	SOUTHWEST
Aultman Hospital		(330) 452-9911
Aultman Hosp		
2600 6th St SW	Canton, OH 44710-1799	MIDWEST
Banner Desert Medical Center		(480) 512-3000
Banner Desert Med Ctr		
1400 S Dobson Rd	Mesa, AZ 85202	SOUTHWEST
Banner Good Samaritan Regional Medical Center - Phoenix		(602) 239-2000
Banner Good Samaritan Regl Med Ctr - Phoenix		
1111 E McDowell Rd	Phoenix, AZ 85060	SOUTHWEST
Baptist Hospital - Jackson		(601) 968-1000
Baptist Hosp - Jackson		
1225 N State St	Jackson, MS 39202	SOUTHEAST
Baptist Hospital - Nashville		(615) 284-5555
Baptist Hosp - Nashville		
2000 Church St	Nashville, TN 37236	SOUTHEAST
Baptist Hospital of Miami		(786) 596-1960
Baptist Hosp of Miami		
8900 N Kendall Dr	Miami, FL 33176	SOUTHEAST
Baptist Medical Center - Jacksonville		(904) 202-2000
Baptist Medical Center - Jacksonville		
800 Prudential Drive	Jacksonville, FL 32207	SOUTHEAST
Baptist Memorial Hospital - Memphis		(901) 226-5000
Baptist Memorial Hospital - Memphis		
6019 Walnut Grove Rd	Memphis, TN 38120	SOUTHEAST

Barnes-Jewish Hospital   (314) 362-5000
Barnes-Jewish Hosp
One Barnes-Jewish Hospital Plaza   St. Louis, MO 63110   MIDWEST

Bascom Palmer Eye Institute   (305) 326-6000
Bascom Palmer Eye Inst.
900 NW 17 St   Miami, FL 33136   SOUTHEAST

Baylor University Medical Center   (214) 820-0111
Baylor Univ Medical Ctr
3500 Gaston Avenue   Dallas, TX 75246   SOUTHWEST

Ben Taub General Hospital   (713) 873-2000
Ben Taub General Hosp
1504 Taub Loop   Houston, TX 77001   SOUTHWEST

Beth Israel Deaconess Medical Center - Boston   (617) 667-7000
Beth Israel Deaconess Med Ctr - Boston
330 Brookline Ave   Boston, MA 02215   NEW ENGLAND

Beth Israel Medical Center - Milton & Caroll Petrie Division   (212) 420-2000
Beth Israel Med Ctr - Petrie Division
First Avenue @ 16th Street   New York, NY 10003   MID ATLANTIC

Boston Medical Center   (617) 638-8000
Boston Med Ctr
1 Boston Medical Center Pl   Boston, MA 02118   NEW ENGLAND

Brigham & Women's Hospital   (617) 732-5500
Brigham & Women's Hosp
75 Francis St   Boston, MA 02115   NEW ENGLAND

Bryn Mawr Hospital   (610) 526-3000
Bryn Mawr Hosp
130 S Bryn Mawr Ave   Bryn Mawr, PA 19010-3143   MID ATLANTIC

California Pacific Medical Center - Pacific Campus   (415) 600-6000
CA Pacific Med Ctr - Pacific Campus
2333 Buchanan St   San Francisco, CA 94115   WEST COAST AND PACIFIC

Cancer Treatment Centers of America-Midwestern Regional Medical Center   (847) 872-4561
Cancer Treatment Ctrs of Amer-Midwest Reg Med Ctr
2520 Elisha Ave   Zion, IL 60099   MIDWEST

Carolinas Medical Center   (704) 355-2000
Carolinas Med Ctr
1000 Blythe Blvd   Charlotte, NC 28203-5871   SOUTHEAST

Cedars Medical Center - Miami   (305) 325-5511
Cedars Med Ctr - Miami
1400 NW 12 Ave   Miami, FL 33136   SOUTHEAST

Cedars-Sinai Medical Center		(310) 423-3277
Cedars-Sinai Med Ctr		
8700 Beverly Boulevard	Los Angeles, CA 90048	WEST COAST AND PACIFIC
Centennial Medical Center		(615) 342-1000
Centennial Med Ctr		
2300 Patterson Street	Nashville, TN 37203	SOUTHEAST
Cheyenne Regional Medical Center		(307) 634-2273
Cheyenne Regl Med Ctr		
214 E 23rd St	Cheyenne, WY 82001	GREAT PLAINS AND MOUNTAINS
Children's Healthcare of Atlanta - Egleston		(404) 325-6000
Chldns Hlthcare Atlanta - Egleston		
1405 Clifton Rd NE	Atlanta, GA 30322	SOUTHEAST
Children's Hospital - Boston		(617) 355-6000
Children's Hospital - Boston		
300 Longwood Avenue	Boston, MA 02115	NEW ENGLAND
Children's Hospital - Denver, The		(303) 861-8888
Chldn's Hosp - Denver, The		
1056 E 19th Ave	Denver, CO 80218-1088	GREAT PLAINS AND MOUNTAINS
Children's Hospital - Los Angeles		(323) 660-2450
Chldns Hosp - Los Angeles		
4650 Sunset Blvd	Los Angeles, CA 90027	WEST COAST AND PACIFIC
Children's Hospital - Omaha		(402) 955-5400
Children's Hosp - Omaha		
8200 Dodge St	Omaha, NE 68114	GREAT PLAINS AND MOUNTAINS
Children's Hospital and Clinics - Minneapolis		(612) 813-6111
Chldns Hosp and Clinics - Minneapolis		
2525 Chicago Ave S	Minneapolis, MN 55404	MIDWEST
Children's Hospital and Regional Medical Center - Seattle		(206) 987-2000
Chldns Hosp and Regl Med Ctr - Seattle		
4800 Sand Point Way NE	Seattle, WA 98145	WEST COAST AND PACIFIC
Children's Hospital at OU Medical Center		(405) 271-5437
Chldns Hosp OU Med Ctr		
940 Northeast 13th St	Oklahoma City, OK 73104	SOUTHWEST
Children's Hospital Medical Center - Akron		(330) 379-8200
Children's Hosp & Med Ctr- Akron		
One Perkins Square	Akron, OH 44308	MIDWEST
Children's Hospital of Alabama - Birmingham		(205) 939-9100
Children's Hospital - Birmingham		
1600 7th Ave South	Birmingham, AL 35233	SOUTHEAST

Children's Hospital of Michigan   (313) 745-5437
Chldns Hosp of Michigan
3901 Beaubian Blvd   Detroit, MI 48201   MIDWEST

Children's Hospital of Philadelphia, The   (215) 590-1000
Chldns Hosp of Philadelphia, The
34th St & Civic Center Blvd   Philadelphia, PA 19104   MID ATLANTIC

Children's Hospital of Pittsburgh - UPMC   (412) 692-8583
Chldns Hosp of Pittsburgh - UPMC
3705 Fifth Avenue   Pittsburgh, PA 15213   MID ATLANTIC

Children's Hospital of Wisconsin   (414) 266-2000
Chldns Hosp - Wisconsin
9000 W Wisconsin Ave   Milwaukee, WI 53201   MIDWEST

Children's Medical Center of Dallas   (214) 456-7000
Chldns Med Ctr of Dallas
1935 Motor St   Dallas, TX 75235   SOUTHWEST

Children's Memorial Hospital   (773) 880-4000
Children's Mem Hosp
2300 Children's Plaza   Chicago, IL 60614   MIDWEST

Children's Mercy Hospitals & Clinics   (816) 234-3000
Chldns Mercy Hosps & Clinics
2401 Gilham Rd   Kansas City, MO 64108   MIDWEST

Children's National Medical Center - DC   (202) 884-5000
Chldns Natl Med Ctr
111 Michigan Ave NW   Washington, DC 20010   MID ATLANTIC

Christiana Care Health Services   (302) 428-2229
Christiana Care Hlth Svs
501 W 14th St   Wilmington, DE 19899-1038   MID ATLANTIC

Christiana Hospital   (302) 733-1000
Christiana Hospital
4755 Ogletown-Stanton Rd   Newark, DE 19718-0001   MID ATLANTIC

Cincinnati Children's Hospital Medical Center   (800) 344-2462
Cincinnati Chldns Hosp Med Ctr
3333 Burnet Ave   Cincinnati, OH 45229-3039   MIDWEST

City of Hope National Medical Center & Beckman Research   (626) 359-8111
City of Hope Natl Med Ctr & Beckman Rsch
1500 E Duarte Rd   Duarte, CA 91010   WEST COAST AND PACIFIC

Cleveland Clinic Florida - Weston   (954) 659-5000
Cleveland Clin - Weston
2950 Cleveland Clinic Blvd   Weston, FL 33331   SOUTHEAST

Cleveland Clinic Foundation   (800) 223-2273
Cleveland Clin Fdn
9500 Euclid Avenue   Cleveland, OH 44195   MIDWEST

Community Medical Center - Toms River   (908) 240-8000
Comm Med Ctr - Toms River
99 Highway 37 W   Toms River, NJ 08755   MID ATLANTIC

Concord Hospital   (603) 225-2711
Concord Hospital
250 Pleasant St   Concord, NH 03301-2598   NEW ENGLAND

Connecticut Children's Medical Center   (860) 545-9000
CT Chldns Med Ctr
282 Washington St   Hartford, CT 06106   NEW ENGLAND

Cooper University Hospital   (856) 342-2000
Cooper Univ Hosp
1 Cooper Plaza   Camden, NJ 08103-1489   MID ATLANTIC

Dana-Farber Cancer Institute   (617) 632-3000
Dana-Farber Cancer Inst
44 Binney St   Boston, MA 02115   NEW ENGLAND

Dartmouth - Hitchcock Medical Center   (603) 650-5000
Dartmouth - Hitchcock Med Ctr
1 Medical Center Dr   Lebanon, NH 03756-0002   NEW ENGLAND

Delnor - Community Hospital   (630) 208-3000
Delnor - Comm Hosp
300 Randall Road   Geneva, IL 60134   MIDWEST

Doctors' Hospital   (305) 666-2111
Doctors' Hosp
5000 University Dr   Coral Gables, FL 33146   SOUTHEAST

Doernbecher Children's Hospital/Oregon Health Science University   (503) 494-8811
Doernbecher Chldns Hosp/OHSU
3181 SW Sam Jackson Park Rd   Portland, OR 97201-3098   WEST COAST AND PACIFIC

Duke University Medical Center   (919) 684-8111
Duke Univ Med Ctr
DUMC, Box 3708   Durham, NC 27710   SOUTHEAST

East Cooper Regional Medical Center   (843) 881-0100
E Cooper Reg Med Ctr
1200 Johnnie Dodds Blvd   Mount Pleasant, SC 29464-3231   SOUTHEAST

Elliot Hospital   (603) 669-5300
Elliot Hosp
1 Elliot Way   Manchester, NH 03103   NEW ENGLAND

Emory University Hospital		(404) 712-2000
Emory Univ Hosp		
1364 Clifton Rd NE	Atlanta, GA 30322	SOUTHEAST

Englewood Hospital & Medical Center		(201) 894-3000
Englewood Hosp & Med Ctr		
350 Engle Street	Englewood, NJ 07631	MID ATLANTIC

Evanston Hospital		(847) 570-2000
Evanston Hosp		
2650 Ridge Ave	Evanston, IL 60201	MIDWEST

Evanston Northwestern Healthcare		(847) 570-2000
Evanston NW Hlthcare		
1301 Central Ave	Evanston, IL 60201	MIDWEST

Fletcher Allen Health Care - Medical Center Campus		(802) 847-0000
FAHC - Med Ctr Campus		
111 Colchester Ave (Burgess 1)	Burlington, VT 05401	NEW ENGLAND

Fletcher Allen Health Care - UHC Campus		(802) 847-0000
FAHC - UHC Campus		
1 S Prospect St	Burlington, VT 05401	NEW ENGLAND

Forsyth Medical Center		(336) 718-5000
Forsyth Med Ctr		
3333 Silas Creek Pkwy	Winston-Salem, NC 27103	SOUTHEAST

Four Winds Hospital		(914) 763-8151
Four Winds Hosp		
800 Cross River Road	Katonah, NY 10536	MID ATLANTIC

Fox Chase Cancer Center		(215) 728-6900
Fox Chase Cancer Ctr		
333 Cottman Avenue	Philadelphia, PA 19111	MID ATLANTIC

Franklin Square Hospital		(410) 682-7000
Franklin Square Hosp		
9000 Franklin Square Drive	Baltimore, MD 21237	MID ATLANTIC

Froedtert Memorial Lutheran Hospital		(414) 805-6644
Froedtert Meml Lutheran Hosp		
9200 W Wisconsin Ave	Milwaukee, WI 53226	MIDWEST

George Washington University Hospital		(202) 715-4000
G Washington Univ Hosp		
900 23rd St NW	Washington, DC 20037	MID ATLANTIC

Georgetown University Hospital		(202) 444-2000
Georgetown Univ Hosp		
3800 Reservoir Rd NW	Washington, DC 20007	MID ATLANTIC

Goshen General Hospital		(574) 533-2141
Goshen Genl Hosp		
200 High Park Ave	Goshen, IN 46526	MIDWEST

Greater Baltimore Medical Center		(443) 849-2000
Greater Baltimore Med Ctr		
6701 N Charles St	Baltimore, MD 21204	MID ATLANTIC

Greenwich Hospital		(203) 863-3000
Greenwich Hosp		
Five Perryridge Road	Greenwich, CT 06830	NEW ENGLAND

H Lee Moffitt Cancer Center & Research Institute		(813) 972-4673
H Lee Moffitt Cancer Ctr & Research Inst		
12902 Magnolia Drive	Tampa, FL 33612-9497	SOUTHEAST

Hackensack University Medical Center		(201) 996-2000
Hackensack Univ Med Ctr		
30 Prospect Avenue	Hackensack, NJ 07601	MID ATLANTIC

Hahnemann University Hospital		(215) 762-7000
Hahnemann Univ Hosp		
Broad & Vine St	Philadelphia, PA 19102	MID ATLANTIC

Harborview Medical Center		(206) 731-3000
Harborview Med Ctr		
325 9th Ave, Box 359717	Seattle, WA 98104	WEST COAST AND PACIFIC

Harper University Hospital		(313) 745-8040
Harper Univ Hosp		
3990 John R St	Detroit, MI 48201-2097	MIDWEST

Harrison Memorial Hospital		(360) 377-3911
Harrison Meml Hosp		
2520 Cherry Ave	Bremerton, WA 98310-4270	WEST COAST AND PACIFIC

Hartford Hospital		(860) 545-5000
Hartford Hosp		
80 Seymour St, Box 5037	Hartford, CT 06102-5037	NEW ENGLAND

Healthsouth Lakeshore Rehabilitation Hospital		(205) 868-2000
Healthsouth Lakeshore Rehab Hosp		
3800 Ridgeway	Birmingham, AL 35209	SOUTHEAST

Henry Ford Hospital		(313) 916-2600
Henry Ford Hosp		
2799 W Grand Blvd	Detroit, MI 48202	MIDWEST

Hospital for Joint Diseases		(212) 598-6000
Hosp For Joint Diseases		
301 East 17th Street	New York, NY 10003	MID ATLANTIC

Hospital for Special Surgery		(212) 606-1000
Hosp For Special Surgery		
535 East 70th Street	New York, NY 10021	MID ATLANTIC

Hospital of the University of Pennsylvania - UPHS		(215) 662-4000
Hosp Univ Penn - UPHS		
3400 Spruce Street	Philadelphia, PA 19104	MID ATLANTIC

Indiana University Hospital		(317) 274-5000
Indiana Univ Hosp		
550 N University Blvd	Indianapolis, IN 46202	MIDWEST

Inova Fairfax Hospital		(703) 698-1110
Inova Fairfax Hosp		
3300 Gallows Road	Falls Church, VA 22042	SOUTHEAST

Jackson Memorial Hospital		(305) 585-1111
Jackson Meml Hosp		
1611 NW 12th Ave	Miami, FL 33136	SOUTHEAST

Johns Hopkins Hospital - Baltimore, The		(410) 955-5000
Johns Hopkins Hosp - Baltimore		
600 N Wolfe St	Baltimore, MD 21287	MID ATLANTIC

Kaiser Permanente Santa Clara Medical Center		(408) 236-6400
Kaiser Permanente Santa Clara Med Ctr		
900 Kiley Blvd	Santa Clara, CA 95051	WEST COAST AND PACIFIC

Kapiolani Medical Center for Women & Children		(808) 983-6000
Kapiolani Med Ctr for Women & Chldn		
1319 Punahou St	Honolulu, HI 96826	WEST COAST AND PACIFIC

Karmanos Cancer Institute		(800) 527-6266
Karmanos Cancer Inst		
4100 John R	Detroit, MI 48201	MIDWEST

Kootenai Medical Center		(208) 666-2000
Kootenai Med Ctr		
2003 Lincoln Way	Coeur d'Alene, ID 83814-2677	GREAT PLAINS AND MOUNTAINS

Kosair Children's Hospital		(502) 629-6000
Kosair Chldn's Hosp		
231 E Chestnut St	Louisville, KY 40202	SOUTHEAST

LAC & USC Medical Center		(323) 226-2622
LAC & USC Med Ctr		
1200 N State St	Los Angeles, CA 90033-4525	WEST COAST AND PACIFIC

LAC - Harbor - UCLA Medical Center		(310) 222-2345
LAC - Harbor - UCLA Med Ctr		
1000 W Carson St	Torrance, CA 90509-2059	WEST COAST AND PACIFIC

Lahey Clinic
Lahey Clin
41 Mall Road Burlington, MA 01805 (781) 744-5100
NEW ENGLAND

Lakeland Regional Medical Center
Lakeland Regl Med Ctr
1324 Lakeland Hills Blvd Lakeland, FL 33805 (863) 687-1100
SOUTHEAST

Lankenau Hospital
Lankenau Hosp
100 Lancaster Ave Wynnewood, PA 19096-3498 (610) 645-2000
MID ATLANTIC

LDS Hospital
LDS Hosp
8th Ave & C St Salt Lake City, UT 84143 (801) 408-1100
GREAT PLAINS AND MOUNTAINS

Le Bonheur Children's Medical Center
Le Bonheur Chldns Med Ctr
50 N Dunlap Memphis, TN 38103-2893 (901) 572-3000
SOUTHEAST

Lenox Hill Hospital
Lenox Hill Hosp
100 East 77th Street New York, NY 10021 (212) 434-2000
MID ATLANTIC

Loma Linda University Medical Center
Loma Linda Univ Med Ctr
11234 Anderson St Loma Linda, CA 92354 (909) 558-4000
WEST COAST AND PACIFIC

Long Beach Memorial Medical Center
Long Beach Meml Med Ctr
2801 Atlantic Ave Long Beach, CA 90801 (562) 933-2000
WEST COAST AND PACIFIC

Long Island College Hospital
Long Island Coll Hosp
339 Hicks Street Brooklyn, NY 11201 (718) 780-1000
MID ATLANTIC

Long Island Jewish Medical Center
Long Island Jewish Med Ctr
270-05 76th Avenue New Hyde Park, NY 11040 (516) 470-7000
MID ATLANTIC

Louis A Weiss Memorial Hospital
Weiss Meml Hosp
4646 N Marine Dr Chicago, IL 60640 (773) 878-8700
MIDWEST

Louisiana State University Hospital
Louisiana State Univ Hosp
1501 Kings Highway P.O. Box 33932 Shreveport, LA 71130 (318) 675-4239
SOUTHWEST

Loyola University Medical Center
Loyola Univ Med Ctr
2160 S 1st Ave Maywood, IL 60153 (708) 216-9000
MIDWEST

Lucile Packard Children's Hospital/Stanford University Medical Center   (650) 497-8000
Lucile Packard Chldns Hosp/Stanford Univ Med Ctr
725 Welch Rd   Palo Alto, CA 94304   WEST COAST AND PACIFIC

Magee-Womens Hospital - UPMC   (412) 641-1000
Magee-Womens Hosp - UPMC
300 Halket Street   Pittsburgh, PA 15213   MID ATLANTIC

Maimonides Medical Center   (718) 283-6000
Maimonides Med Ctr
4802 Tenth Avenue   Brooklyn, NY 11219   MID ATLANTIC

Maine Medical Center   (207) 871-0111
Maine Med Ctr
22 Bramhall St   Portland, ME 04102   NEW ENGLAND

Marin General Hospital   (415) 925-7000
Marin Genl Hosp
250 Bon Air Rd   Greenbrae, CA 94904   WEST COAST AND PACIFIC

Massachusetts Eye and Ear Infirmary   (617) 523-7900
Mass Eye & Ear Infirmary
243 Charles Street   Boston, MA 02114   NEW ENGLAND

Massachusetts General Hospital   (617) 726-2000
Mass Genl Hosp
55 Fruit St   Boston, MA 02114   NEW ENGLAND

Mayo Clinic - Jacksonville, FL   (904) 953-2000
Mayo - Jacksonville
4500 San Pablo Road   Jacksonville, FL 32224   SOUTHEAST

Mayo Clinic - Rochester, MN   (507) 284-2511
Mayo Med Ctr & Clin - Rochester
200 First St SW   Rochester, MN 55905   MIDWEST

Mayo Clinic - Scottsdale   (480) 301-8000
Mayo Clin Hosp - Scottsdale
13400 E Shea Blvd   Scottsdale, AZ 85259   SOUTHWEST

Mayo Clinic Hospital - Phoenix   (480) 515-6296
Mayo - Phoenix
5777 E Mayo Blvd   Phoenix, AZ 85054   SOUTHWEST

McLaren Regional Medical Center   (810) 342-2000
McLaren Reg Med Ctr
401 S. Ballenger Highway   Flint, MI 48532   MIDWEST

Medical Center of Louisiana @ New Orleans (University Hospital)   (504) 903-3000
Med Ctr LA @ New Orleans (Univ Hosp)
2021 Perdido St   New Orleans, LA 70112   SOUTHWEST

Medical City Dallas Hospital		(972) 566-7000
Med City Dallas Hosp		
7777 Forest Ln	Dallas, TX 75230-2594	SOUTHWEST

Medical College of Georgia Hospital and Clinic		(706) 721-6569
Med Coll of GA Hosp and Clin		
1120 15th Street	Augusta, GA 30912	SOUTHEAST

Medical College of Virginia Hospitals		(804) 828-9000
Med Coll of VA Hosp		
1250 E Marshall St, Box 980510	Richmond, VA 23219	SOUTHEAST

Medical University of South Carolina Medical Center		(843) 792-2300
MUSC Med Ctr		
169 Ashley Ave	Charleston, SC 29425	SOUTHEAST

Memorial Health University Medical Center - Savannah		(912) 350-8000
Meml Hlth Univ Med Ctr - Savannah		
4700 Waters Ave	Savannah, GA 31404	SOUTHEAST

Memorial Regional Hospital - Hollywood		(954) 987-2000
Meml Regl Hosp - Hollywood		
3501 Johnson Street	Hollywood, FL 33021	SOUTHEAST

Memorial Sloan-Kettering Cancer Center		(212) 639-2000
Meml Sloan Kettering Cancer Ctr		
1275 York Avenue	New York, NY 10021	MID ATLANTIC

Mercy Hospital - Miami, FL		(305) 854-4400
Mercy Hosp - Miami		
3663 S Miami Ave	Miami, FL 33133	SOUTHEAST

Methodist Children's Hospital of South Texas		(210) 575-7105
Methodist Chldns Hosp of South Texas		
7700 Floyd Curl Dr	San Antonio, TX 78229-3311	SOUTHWEST

Methodist Hospital - Houston		(713) 790-3311
Methodist Hosp - Houston		
6565 Fannin St, D200	Houston, TX 77030	SOUTHWEST

Methodist University Hospital		(901) 516-7000
Methodist Univ Hosp - Memphis		
1265 Union Ave	Memphis, TN 38104	SOUTHEAST

MetroHealth Medical Center		(216) 778-7800
MetroHealth Med Ctr		
2500 MetroHealth Drive	Cleveland, OH 44109-1998	MIDWEST

Metropolitan Hospital Center - NY		(212) 423-6262
Metropolitan Hosp Ctr - NY		
1901 First Avenue	New York, NY 10029	MID ATLANTIC

Metropolitan Methodist Hospital		(210) 208-2200
Metro Methodist Hosp		
1310 McCullough Ave	San Antonio, TX 78212	SOUTHWEST
Miami Children's Hospital		(305) 666-6511
Miami Children's Hosp		
3100 SW 62nd Ave	Miami, FL 33155	SOUTHEAST
Michigan State University-Sparrow Hospital		(517) 364-1000
Mich State Univ-Sparrow Hos		
1215 E Michigan Ave, MS 0	Lansing, MI 48912	MIDWEST
Mobile Infirmary Medical Center		(334) 431-2400
Mobile Infirmary Med Ctr		
5 Mobile Infirmary Circle	Mobile, AL 36607-3513	SOUTHEAST
Montefiore Medical Center		(718) 920-4321
Montefiore Med Ctr		
111 East 210 Street	Bronx, NY 10467	MID ATLANTIC
Mott Children's Hospital		(734) 936-4000
Mott Chldns Hosp		
1500 E Medical Center Dr	Ann Arbor, MI 48109	MIDWEST
Mount Sinai Medical Center		(212) 241-6500
Mount Sinai Med Ctr		
One Gustave L. Levy Pl	New York, NY 10029	MID ATLANTIC
Mount Sinai Medical Center - Miami		(305) 674-2121
Mount Sinai Med Ctr - Miami		
4300 Alton Rd	Miami Beach, FL 33140	SOUTHEAST
National Institutes of Health - Clinical Center		(301) 496-4000
Natl Inst of Hlth - Clin Ctr		
6100 Executive Blvd, rm 3C01, MS 7511	Bethesda, MD 20892-7511	MID ATLANTIC
Nebraska Medical Center		(402) 552-2000
Nebraska Med Ctr		
987400 Nebraska Med Ctr	Omaha, NE 68198-7400	GREAT PLAINS AND MOUNTAINS
Nebraska Methodist Hospital		(402) 354-4000
Nebraska Meth Hosp		
8303 Dodge St	Omaha, NE 68114	GREAT PLAINS AND MOUNTAINS
New York Eye & Ear Infirmary		(212) 979-4000
New York Eye & Ear Infirm		
310 East 14th Street	New York, NY 10003	MID ATLANTIC
NewYork-Presbyterian Hospital		(212) 305-2500
NY-Presby Hosp		
161 Fort Washington Ave	New York, NY 10032	MID ATLANTIC

North Florida Regional Medical Center   (352) 333-4000
North Florida Regl Med Ctr
6500 Newberry Rd   Gainesville, FL 32605   SOUTHEAST

North Shore University Hospital at Manhasset   (516) 562-0100
N Shore Univ Hosp at Manhasset
300 Community Dr   Manhasset, NY 11030   MID ATLANTIC

Northern Westchester Hospital   (914) 666-1200
Northern Westchester Hosp
400 East Main Street   Mount Kisco, NY 10549   MID ATLANTIC

Northwestern Memorial Hospital   (312) 926-2000
Northwestern Meml Hosp
251 E Huron St   Chicago, IL 60611   MIDWEST

Norton Hospital   (502) 629-8000
Norton Hosp
200 E Chestnut St   Louisville, KY 40202   SOUTHEAST

NYU Medical Center   (212) 263-7300
NYU Med Ctr
550 First Avenue   New York, NY 10016   MID ATLANTIC

Ochsner Baptist Medical Center   (504) 899-9311
Ochsner Baptist Med Ctr
2700 Napoleon Ave   New Orleans, LA 70115   SOUTHWEST

Ochsner Foundation Hospital   (504) 842-3000
Ochsner Fdn Hosp
1516 Jefferson Hwy   New Orleans, LA 70121   SOUTHWEST

Ohio State University Medical Center   (614) 293-8000
Ohio St Univ Med Ctr
410 W 10th Avenue   Columbus, OH 43210   MIDWEST

Olathe Medical Center   (913) 791-4200
Olathe Med Ctr
20333 W 151st St   Olathe, KS 66061-5352   GREAT PLAINS AND MOUNTAINS

Oregon Health & Science University   (503) 494-8311
OR Hlth & Sci Univ
3181 SW Sam Jackson Park Rd   Portland, OR 97239-3098   WEST COAST AND PACIFIC

OU Medical Center   (405) 271-4700
OU Med Ctr
1200 Everett Dr   Oklahoma City, OK 73104-5098   SOUTHWEST

Our Lady of Mercy Medical Center   (718) 920-9000
Our Lady of Mercy Med Ctr
600 E 233rd St   Bronx, NY 10466   MID ATLANTIC

Our Lady of the Lake Regional Medical Center		(225) 765-6565
Our Lady of the Lake Regl Med Ctr		
5000 Hennessy Blvd	Baton Rouge, LA 70808-4398	SOUTHWEST

Overlake Hospital Medical Center		(425) 688-5000
Overlake Hosp Med Ctr		
1035 116th Ave NE	Bellevue, WA 98004-4687	WEST COAST AND PACIFIC

Overland Park Regional Medical Center		(913) 541-5000
Overland Pk Regl Med Ctr		
10500 Quivira Rd	Overland Park, KS 66215	GREAT PLAINS AND MOUNTAINS

Palmetto Richland Memorial Hospital		(803) 434-7000
Palmetto Richland Mem Hosp		
5 Richland Medical Park Drive	Columbia, SC 29203	SOUTHEAST

Penn Presbyterian Medical Center - UPHS		(215) 662-8000
Penn Presby Med Ctr - UPHS		
51 N 39th St	Philadelphia, PA 19104	MID ATLANTIC

Pennsylvania Hospital		(215) 829-3000
Pennsylvania Hosp		
3600 Market St, Ste 240	Philadelphia, PA 19104	MID ATLANTIC

Phoenix Baptist Hospital & Medical Center		(602) 249-0212
Phoenix Baptist Hosp & Med Ctr		
2000 West Bethany Home Rd	Phoenix, AZ 85015-2184	SOUTHWEST

Phoenix Children's Hospital		(602) 546-1000
Phoenix Children's Hosp		
1919 E Thomas Rd	Phoenix, AZ 85106	SOUTHWEST

Physicians Regional Medical Center		(239) 348-4000
Physicians Regl Med Ctr		
6101 Pine Ridge Rd	Naples, FL 34119	SOUTHEAST

Pitt County Memorial Hospital - Univ Health System East Carolina		(252) 847-4100
Pitt Cty Mem Hosp - Univ Med Ctr East Carolina		
2100 Stantonsburg Rd	Greenville, NC 27835-6028	SOUTHEAST

Presbyterian - St Luke's Medical Center		(303) 839-6000
Presby - St Luke's Med Ctr		
1719 E 19th Ave	Denver, CO 80218	GREAT PLAINS AND MOUNTAINS

Presbyterian Hospital - Albuquerque		(505) 841-1234
Presbyterian Hospital - Albuquerque		
1100 Central Ave SE	Albuquerque, NM 87106	SOUTHWEST

Presbyterian Hospital of Dallas		(214) 345-6789
Presby Hosp of Dallas		
8200 Walnut Hill Ln	Dallas, TX 75231	SOUTHWEST

Primary Children's Medical Center   (801) 588-2000
Primary Children's Med Ctr
100 N Medical Drive   Salt Lake City, UT 84113-1100   GREAT PLAINS AND MOUNTAINS

Providence Hospital - Southfield   (248) 424-3000
Providence Hosp - Southfield
16001 W Nine Mile Rd   Southfield, MI 48075   MIDWEST

Providence Portland Medical Center   (503) 215-1111
Providence Portland Med Ctr
4805 NE Glisan   Portland, OR 97213-2967   WEST COAST AND PACIFIC

Providence St Vincent Medical Center   (503) 216-1234
Providence St Vincent Med Ctr
9205 SW Barnes Rd   Portland, OR 97225-6622   WEST COAST AND PACIFIC

Queen's Medical Center - Honolulu   (808) 538-9011
Queen's Med Ctr - Honolulu
1301 Punchbowl Street   Honolulu, HI 96813   WEST COAST AND PACIFIC

Rady Children's Hospital - San Diego   (858) 576-1700
Rady Children's Hosp - San Diego
3020 Children's Way   San Diego, CA 92123   WEST COAST AND PACIFIC

Rainbow Babies & Children's Hospital   (216) 844-1000
Rainbow Babies & Chldns Hosp
11100 Euclid Ave   Cleveland, OH 44106   MIDWEST

Rapid City Regional Hospital   (605) 719-1000
Rapid City Reg Hosp
353 Fairmount Blvd   Rapid City, SD 57701   GREAT PLAINS AND MOUNTAINS

Regional Medical Center - Memphis   (901) 545-7100
Regional Med Ctr - Memphis
877 Jefferson Avenue   Memphis, TN 38103   SOUTHEAST

Rhode Island Hospital   (401) 444-4000
Rhode Island Hosp
593 Eddy Street   Providence, RI 02903   NEW ENGLAND

Riley Hospital for Children   (317) 274-5000
Riley Hosp for Children
702 Barnhill Drive   Indianapolis, IN 46202   MIDWEST

Riverview Medical Center   (732) 741-2700
Riverview Med Ctr
1 Riverview Plaza   Red Bank, NJ 07701   MID ATLANTIC

Robert Wood Johnson University Hospital - New Brunswick   (732) 828-3000
Robert Wood Johnson Univ Hosp - New Brunswick
1 Robert Wood Johnson Pl   New Brunswick, NJ 08901   MID ATLANTIC

Rochester Methodist Hospital (507) 284-2511
Rochester Meth Hosp
201 W Center St Rochester, MN 55905-3003 MIDWEST

Roswell Park Cancer Institute (716) 845-5770
Roswell Park Cancer Inst
Elm and Carlton Streets Buffalo, NY 14263 MID ATLANTIC

Rush University Medical Center (312) 942-5000
Rush Univ Med Ctr
1653 W Congress Pkwy Chicago, IL 60612-3833 MIDWEST

Sacred Heart Medical Center (541) 686-7300
Sacred Heart Med Ctr
1255 Hilyard St Eugene, OR 97440-3700 WEST COAST AND PACIFIC

Saint Francis Hospital - Memphis (901) 765-1000
St Francis Hosp - Memphis
5959 Park Ave Memphis, TN 38119 SOUTHEAST

Saint John's Health Center (310) 829-5511
St John's Hlth Ctr, Santa Monica
1328 22nd St Santa Monica, CA 90404 WEST COAST AND PACIFIC

Saint Thomas Hospital - Nashville (615) 222-2111
Saint Thomas Hosp - Nashville
4220 Harding Road Nashville, TN 37205 SOUTHEAST

Saint Vincent Catholic Medical Centers - St Vincent's Manhattan (212) 604-7000
St Vincent Cath Med Ctrs - Manhattan
170 West 12th Street New York, NY 10011 MID ATLANTIC

Salt Lake Regional Medical Center (801) 350-4111
Salt Lake Regional Med Ctr
1050 E South Temple Salt Lake City, UT 84102 GREAT PLAINS AND MOUNTAINS

San Francisco General Hospital (415) 206-8000
San Francisco Genl Hosp
1001 Potrero Avenue San Francisco, CA 94110 WEST COAST AND PACIFIC

Santa Clara Valley Medical Center (408) 885-5000
Santa Clara Vly Med Ctr
751 S Bascom Ave San Jose, CA 95128 WEST COAST AND PACIFIC

Santa Monica - UCLA Medical Center (310) 319-4000
Santa Monica - UCLA Med Ctr
1250 16th St Santa Monica, CA 90404 WEST COAST AND PACIFIC

Sarasota Memorial Hospital (941) 917-9000
Sarasota Meml Hosp
1700 S Tamiami Trail Sarasota, FL 34239 SOUTHEAST

Schneider Children's Hospital   (718) 470-3000
Schneider Chldn's Hosp
269-01 76th Ave   New Hyde Park, NY 11040   MID ATLANTIC

Scott & White Memorial Hospital   (254) 724-2111
Scott & White Mem Hosp
2401 South 31st Street   Temple, TX 76508-0001   SOUTHWEST

Scottsdale Healthcare - Shea   (480) 860-3000
Scottsdale Hlthcare - Shea
9000 E Shea Blvd   Scottsdale, AZ 85258-4514   SOUTHWEST

Scripps Green Hospital   (858) 455-9100
Scripps Green Hosp
10666 N Torrey Pines Rd   La Jolla, CA 92037   WEST COAST AND PACIFIC

Scripps Memorial Hospital - La Jolla   (858) 457-4123
Scripps Meml Hosp - La Jolla
9888 Genesee Ave   La Jolla, CA 92037   WEST COAST AND PACIFIC

Sentara Norfolk General Hospital   (757) 668-3000
Sentara Norfolk Genl Hosp
600 Gresham Dr   Norfolk, VA 23507   SOUTHEAST

Shands Healthcare at University of Florida   (352) 265-0111
Shands Hlthcre at Univ of FL
1600 SW Archer Rd   Gainesville, FL 32610   SOUTHEAST

Shands Jacksonville   (904) 244-0411
Shands Jacksonville
655 W 8th St   Jacksonville, FL 32209   SOUTHEAST

Sibley Memorial Hospital   (202) 537-4000
Sibley Mem Hosp
5255 Loughboro Road NW   Washington, DC 20016   MID ATLANTIC

Sioux Valley Hospital USD Medical Center   (605) 333-1000
Sioux Valley Hosp
1100 S Euclid Ave, PO Box 5039   Sioux Falls, SD 57717   GREAT PLAINS AND MOUNTAINS

Southern New Hampshire Medical Center   (603) 577-2000
Southern NH Med Ctr
8 Prospect St   Nashua, NH 03061   NEW ENGLAND

Southwest Texas Methodist Hospital   (210) 575-4000
SW TX Meth Hosp
7700 Floyd Curl Dr   San Antonio, TX 78229   SOUTHWEST

Spectrum Health - Blodgett Campus   (616) 774-7444
Spectrum Hlth Blodgett Campus
1840 Wealthy St SE   Grand Rapids, MI 49506   MIDWEST

St Anthony Hospital *St Anthony Hosp* 1000 N Lee St	Oklahoma City, OK 73102	(405) 272-7000 SOUTHWEST
St Anthony's Hospital - St Petersburg *St Anthony's Hosp - St Petersburg* 1200 7th Avenue North	St Petersburg, FL 33705	(727) 893-6814 SOUTHEAST
St Barnabas Medical Center *St Barnabas Med Ctr* 94 Old Short Hills Rd	Livingston, NJ 07039-5672	(973) 322-5000 MID ATLANTIC
St Francis Hospital and Health Center *St Francis Hosp* 8111 S Emerson Ave	Indianapolis, IN 46143	(317) 865-5000 MIDWEST
St John's Hospital - Springfield *St John's Hosp - Springfield* 800 E Carpenter St	Springfield, IL 62769	(217) 544-6464 MIDWEST
St John's Regional Medical Center *St John's Regional Med Ctr* 1600 N Rose Ave	Oxnard, CA 93030	(805) 988-2500 WEST COAST AND PACIFIC
St Joseph Hospital *St Joseph Hosp* 172 Kinsley St	Nashua, NH 03060	(603) 882-3000 NEW ENGLAND
St Joseph Hospital *St Joseph Hosp - Bellingham* 2901 Squalicum Pkwy	Bellingham, WA 98225-1898	(360) 734-5400 WEST COAST AND PACIFIC
St Joseph Medical Center *St Joseph Med Ctr* 7601 Osler Drive	Baltimore, MD 21208	(410) 337-1000 MID ATLANTIC
St Joseph's Children's Hospital *St Josephs Chldns Hosp* 3001 W Dr Martin Luther King Jr Blvd	Tampa, FL 33607	(813) 554-8500 SOUTHEAST
St Joseph's Hospital & Medical Center - Phoenix *St Joseph's Hosp & Med Ctr - Phoenix* 350 W Thomas Rd	Phoenix, AZ 85013-4496	(602) 406-3000 SOUTHWEST
St Joseph's Hospital - Atlanta *St Joseph's Hosp - Atlanta* 5665 Peachtree Dunwoody Rd NE	Atlanta, GA 30342	(404) 851-7001 SOUTHEAST
St Joseph's Hospital - Tucson *St Joseph's Hosp - Tucson* 350 N Wilmot Rd	Tucson, AZ 85711	(520) 296-3211 SOUTHWEST

St Jude Children's Research Hospital   (901) 495-3300
St Jude Children's Research Hosp
332 N Lauderdale St   Memphis, TN 38105   SOUTHEAST

St Louis Children's Hospital   (314) 454-6000
St Louis Chldns Hosp
One Children's Pl   St Louis, MO 63110   MIDWEST

St Louis University Hospital   (314) 577-8000
St Louis Univ Hosp
3635 Vista at Grand Blvd   St Louis, MO 63110   MIDWEST

St Luke's - Roosevelt Hospital Center - Roosevelt Division   (212) 523-4000
St Luke's - Roosevelt Hosp Ctr - Roosevelt Div
1000 Tenth Avenue   New York, NY 10019   MID ATLANTIC

St Luke's Episcopal Hospital - Houston   (832) 355-1000
St Luke's Episcopal Hosp - Houston
6720 Bertner Avenue   Houston, TX 77030   SOUTHWEST

St Luke's Hospital - Bethlehem   (610) 954-4000
St Luke's Hosp - Bethlehem
801 Ostrum Street   Bethlehem, PA 18015   MID ATLANTIC

St Luke's Hospital - Chesterfield, MO   (314) 434-1500
St Luke's Hosp - Chesterfield, MO
232 S Woods Mill Rd   Chesterfield, MO 63017   MIDWEST

St Luke's Hospital - Jacksonville   (904) 296-3700
St Luke's Hosp - Jacksonville
4201 Belfort Rd   Jacksonville, FL 32216   SOUTHEAST

St Luke's Hospital of Kansas City   (816) 932-2000
St Luke's Hosp of Kansas City
4401 Wornall Rd   Kansas City, MO 64111   MIDWEST

St Mary's Hospital - Rochester, MN (Mayo Clinic)   (507) 255-5123
St Mary's Hosp - Rochester
1216 2nd St SW   Rochester, MN 55902   MIDWEST

St Mary's Medical Center - Huntington   (304) 526-1234
St Mary's Med Ctr - Huntington
2900 First Ave   Huntington, WV 25702-1272   MID ATLANTIC

St Mary's Medical Center - West Palm Beach   (561) 844-6300
St Mary's Med Ctr - W Palm Bch
901 45th St   West Palm Beach, FL 33407   SOUTHEAST

St Patrick Hospital & Health Sciences Center   (406) 543-7271
St Patrick Hospital - Missoula
500 W Broadway   Missoula, MT 59802   GREAT PLAINS AND MOUNTAINS

St Peter's University Hospital   (732) 745-8600
St Peter's Univ Hosp
254 Easton Ave   New Brunswick, NJ 08901-1780   MID ATLANTIC

St Vincent Carmel Hospital   (317) 573-7000
St Vincent Carmel Hosp
13500 N Meridian St   Carmel, IN 46032-1496   MIDWEST

St Vincent Hospital - Santa Fe   (505) 983-3361
St Vincent Hosp - Santa Fe
455 St Michaels Dr   Santa Fe, NM 87504-2107   SOUTHWEST

St Vincent's Medical Center - Jacksonville   (904) 308-7300
St Vincent's Med Ctr - Jacksonville
1800 Barrs St   Jacksonville, FL 32204   SOUTHEAST

St. Luke's Regional Medical Center   (208) 381-2222
St. Luke's Reg Med Ctr - Boise
190 E Bannock St   Boise, ID 83712   GREAT PLAINS AND MOUNTAINS

Stanford University Medical Center   (650) 723-4000
Stanford Univ Med Ctr
300 Pasteur Dr   Stanford, CA 94305   WEST COAST AND PACIFIC

Stony Brook University Medical Center   (631) 689-8333
Stony Brook Univ Med Ctr
Nicolls Rd   Stony Brook, NY 11794-8410   MID ATLANTIC

Suburban Hospital Healthcare Systems   (301) 896-3100
Suburban Hosp - Bethesda
8600 Old Georgetown Road   Bethesda, MD 20814   MID ATLANTIC

SUNY Downstate Medical Center   (718) 270-1000
SUNY Downstate Med Ctr
450 Clarkson Ave   Brooklyn, NY 11203   MID ATLANTIC

Swedish Medical Center - Seattle   (206) 386-6000
Swedish Med Ctr - Seattle
747 Broadway   Seattle, WA 98122   WEST COAST AND PACIFIC

Tacoma General Hospital   (253) 403-1000
Tacoma Genl Hosp
315 Martin Luther King Jr Way   Tacoma, WA 98405   WEST COAST AND PACIFIC

Tampa General Hospital   (813) 844-7000
Tampa Genl Hosp
PO BOX 1289   Tampa, FL 33601   SOUTHEAST

Temple University Hospital   (215) 707-2000
Temple Univ Hosp
3401 N Broad St   Philadelphia, PA 19140-5189   MID ATLANTIC

Texas Children's Hospital - Houston *Texas Chldns Hosp - Houston* 6621 Fannin St	Houston, TX 77030	(832) 824-1000 SOUTHWEST
Thomas Jefferson University Hospital *Thomas Jefferson Univ Hosp* 111 S 11th St	Philadelphia, PA 19107	(215) 955-6000 MID ATLANTIC
Tucson Medical Center *Tucson Med Ctr* 5301 E Grant Rd	Tucson, AZ 85712-2874	(520) 327-5461 SOUTHWEST
Tufts - New England Medical Center *Tufts-New England Med Ctr* 750 Washington Street	Boston, MA 02111	(617) 636-5000 NEW ENGLAND
Tulane University Hospital & Clinic *Tulane Univ Hosp & Clin* 1415 Tulane Ave	New Orleans, LA 70112	(504) 588-5263 SOUTHWEST
UCLA Medical Center *UCLA Med Ctr* 10833 Le Conte Avenue	Los Angeles, CA 90095	(310) 825-9111 WEST COAST AND PACIFIC
UCSD Medical Center *UCSD Med Ctr* 200 W Arbor Dr	San Diego, CA 92103	(619) 543-6222 WEST COAST AND PACIFIC
UCSF - Mount Zion Medical Center *UCSF - Mt Zion Med Ctr* 1600 Divisadero St	San Francisco, CA 94115	(415) 567-6600 WEST COAST AND PACIFIC
UCSF Medical Center *UCSF Med Ctr* 500 Parnassus Ave	San Francisco, CA 94143	(415) 476-1000 WEST COAST AND PACIFIC
UMass Memorial Medical Center *UMass Memorial Med Ctr* 55 Lake Ave N	Worcester, MA 01655	(508) 334-1000 NEW ENGLAND
UMDNJ-University Hospital-Newark *UMDNJ-Univ Hosp-Newark* 150 Bergen St	Newark, NJ 07103-2406	(973) 972-4300 MID ATLANTIC
Uniformed Services University of the Health Sciences *Unif Serv Univ of the Hlth Sci* 4301 Jones Bridge Rd	Bethesda, MD 20814-4799	(301) 295-9390 MID ATLANTIC
Union Memorial Hospital - Baltimore *Union Meml Hosp - Baltimore* 201 E University Pkwy	Baltimore, MD 21218	(410) 554-2000 MID ATLANTIC

University Health System - University Hospital   (210) 358-4000
Univ Hlth Sys - Univ Hosp
4502 Medical Dr   San Antonio, TX 78229   SOUTHWEST

University Hospital & Clinics- Mississippi   (601) 984-1000
Univ Hosps & Clins - Jackson
2500 N State St   Jackson, MS 39216   SOUTHEAST

University Hospital - Cincinnati   (513) 584-1000
Univ Hosp - Cincinnati
234 Goodman St   Cincinnati, OH 45219   MIDWEST

University Hospital - SUNY Upstate Medical University   (315) 464-5540
Univ. Hosp.- SUNY Upstate
750 E Adams Street   Syracuse, NY 13210   MID ATLANTIC

University Hospitals Case Medical Center   (216) 844-1000
Univ Hosps Case Med Ctr
11100 Euclid Ave   Cleveland, OH 44106   MIDWEST

University Medical Center Health System   (806) 775-8200
Univ Med Ctr - Lubbock
PO Box 5980   Lubbock, TX 79408   SOUTHWEST

University Medical Center of Southern Nevada - Las Vegas   (702) 383-2000
Univ Med Ctr - Las Vegas
1800 W Charleston Blvd   Las Vegas, NV 89102   WEST COAST AND PACIFIC

University Medical Center- Tucson   (520) 694-0111
Univ Med Ctr - Tucson
1501 N Campbell Ave   Tucson, AZ 85724-5128   SOUTHWEST

University New Mexico Health & Science Center   (505) 272-2111
Univ NM Hlth & Sci Ctr
2211 Lomas Blvd NE   Albuquerque, NM 87106   SOUTHWEST

University of Alabama Hospital at Birmingham   (205) 934-4011
Univ of Ala Hosp at Birmingham
619 South 19th Street   Birmingham, AL 35249-6544   SOUTHEAST

University of Arkansas for Medical Sciences Medical Center   (501) 686-7000
UAMS Med Ctr
4301 W Markham St   Little Rock, AR 72205   SOUTHWEST

University of California - Davis Medical Center   (916) 734-2011
UC Davis Med Ctr
2315 Stockton Blvd   Sacramento, CA 95817   WEST COAST AND PACIFIC

University of California - Irvine Medical Center   (714) 456-6011
UC Irvine Med Ctr
101 The City Dr   Orange, CA 92868   WEST COAST AND PACIFIC

University of Chicago Hospitals   (773) 702-1000
Univ of Chicago Hosps
5841 S Maryland Ave   Chicago, IL 60637   MIDWEST

University of Colorado Hospital   (303) 372-0000
Univ Colorado Hosp
4200 E 9th Ave   Denver, CO 80262   GREAT PLAINS AND MOUNTAINS

University of Connecticut Health Center, John Dempsey Hospital   (860) 679-2100
Univ of Conn Hlth Ctr, John Dempsey Hosp
263 Farmington Ave   Farmington, CT 06030   NEW ENGLAND

University of Illinois Medical Center at Chicago   (312) 996-7000
Univ of IL Med Ctr at Chicago
1740 W Taylor St   Chicago, IL 60612   MIDWEST

University of Iowa Hospitals and Clinics   (319) 356-1616
Univ Iowa Hosp & Clinics
200 Hawkins Drive   Iowa City, IA 52242   MIDWEST

University of Kansas Hospital   (913) 588-5000
Univ of Kansas Hosp
3901 Rainbow Blvd   Kansas City, KS 66160   GREAT PLAINS AND MOUNTAINS

University of Kentucky Chandler Hospital   (800) 333-8874
Univ of Kentucky Chandler Hosp
800 Rose Street   Lexington, KY 40536   SOUTHEAST

University of Louisville Hospital   (502) 562-3000
Univ of Louisville Hosp
530 S Jackson St   Louisville, KY 40202   SOUTHEAST

University of Maryland Medical System   (410) 328-8667
Univ of MD Med Sys
22 S Greene St   Baltimore, MD 21201   MID ATLANTIC

University of Miami Hosp & Clinics/Sylvester Comprehensive Cancer Cntr   (305) 243-1000
Univ of Miami Hosp & Clins/Sylvester Comp Canc Ctr
1475 NW 12th Ave   Miami, FL 33136   SOUTHEAST

University of Michigan Health System   (734) 936-4000
Univ Michigan Hlth Sys
1500 E Medical Center Dr   Ann Arbor, MI 48109   MIDWEST

University of Minnesota Medical Center, Fairview - University Campus   (612) 273-3000
Univ Minn Med Ctr, Fairview - Univ Campus
420 Delaware St SE   Minneapolis, MN 55455   MIDWEST

University of Missouri Hospitals & Clinics   (573) 882-4141
Univ of Missouri Hosp & Clins
1 Hospital Dr   Columbia, MO 65212   MIDWEST

University of North Carolina Hospitals		(919) 966-4131
Univ NC Hosps		
101 Manning Drive, Box 7600	Chapel Hill, NC 27514	SOUTHEAST

University of Rochester Strong Memorial Hospital		(585) 275-2121
Univ of Rochester Strong Meml Hosp		
601 Elmwood Ave	Rochester, NY 14642	MID ATLANTIC

University of South Florida - Tampa		(813) 974-2011
Univ of S FL - Tampa		
4202 E Fowler Ave	Tampa, FL 33620	SOUTHEAST

University of Tennessee Memorial Hospital		(865) 544-9000
Univ of Tennessee Mem Hosp		
1924 Alcoa Hwy	Knoxville, TN 37920	SOUTHEAST

University of Texas MD Anderson Cancer Center		(713) 792-2121
UT MD Anderson Cancer Ctr		
1515 Holcombe Blvd	Houston, TX 77030-4095	SOUTHWEST

University of Texas Southwestern Medical Center at Dallas, The		(214) 648-3111
UT Southwestern Med Ctr - Dallas		
5323 Harry Hines Blvd	Dallas, TX 75390	SOUTHWEST

University of Toledo Medical Center		(419) 383-4000
Univ of Toledo Med Ctr		
3000 Arlington Ave	Toledo, OH 43614	MIDWEST

University of Utah Hospitals and Clinics		(801) 581-2121
Univ Utah Hosps and Clins		
50 N Medical Dr	Salt Lake City, UT 84132	GREAT PLAINS AND MOUNTAINS

University of Virginia Medical Center		(434) 924-0211
Univ Virginia Med Ctr		
1215 Lee Street	Charlottesville, VA 22908-0001	SOUTHEAST

University of Washington Medical Center		(206) 598-3300
Univ Wash Med Ctr		
1959 NE Pacific St, Box 356355	Seattle, WA 98195	WEST COAST AND PACIFIC

University of Wisconsin Hospital & Clinics		(608) 263-6400
Univ WI Hosp & Clins		
600 Highland Avenue	Madison, WI 53792	MIDWEST

UPMC Montefiore		(412) 647-2345
UPMC Montefiore		
200 Lothrop St	Pittsburgh, PA 15213	MID ATLANTIC

UPMC Presbyterian		(412) 647-2345
UPMC Presby, Pittsburgh		
200 Lothrop St	Pittsburgh, PA 15213	MID ATLANTIC

UPMC Shadyside   (412) 623-2121
UPMC Shadyside
5230 Centre Ave   Pittsburgh, PA 15232   MID ATLANTIC

USC Norris Comprehensive Cancer Center and Hospital   (323) 865-3000
USC Norris Comp Cancer Ctr
1441 Eastlake Ave   Los Angeles, CA 90033   WEST COAST AND PACIFIC

USC University Hospital - Richard K. Eamer Medical Plaza   (323) 442-8444
USC Univ Hosp - R K Eamer Med Plz
1500 San Pablo St   Los Angeles, CA 90033   WEST COAST AND PACIFIC

VA Health Care System - Palo Alto   (650) 493-5000
VA Hlth Care Sys - Palo Alto
3801 Miranda Ave   Palo Alto, CA 94304   WEST COAST AND PACIFIC

VA Medical Center - Ann Arbor   (734) 769-7100
VA Med Ctr - Ann Arbor
2215 Fuller Rd   Ann Arbor, MI 48105   MIDWEST

VA Medical Center - Atlanta   (404) 321-6111
VA Med Ctr - Atlanta
1670 Clairmont Rd   Decatur, GA 30033   SOUTHEAST

VA Medical Center - Portland   (503) 220-8262
VA Medical Center - Portland
3710 SW US Veteran Hospital Rd   Portland, OR 97239   WEST COAST AND PACIFIC

VA Medical Center - West Los Angeles   (310) 478-3711
VA Med Ctr - W Los Angeles
11301 Wilshire Blvd   Los Angeles, CA 90073   WEST COAST AND PACIFIC

Vanderbilt Children's Hospital   (615) 936-1000
Vanderbilt Children's Hosp
2200 Children's Way   Nashville, TN 37232   SOUTHEAST

Vanderbilt University Medical Center   (615) 322-5000
Vanderbilt Univ Med Ctr
1313 21st Avenue South   Nashville, TN 37232   SOUTHEAST

Veterans Affairs Medical Center - Augusta   (706) 733-0188
VA Medical Ctr - Augusta
One Freedom Way   Augusta, GA 30904   SOUTHEAST

Veterans Affairs Medical Center - Tucson   (520) 792-1450
VA Medical Center - Tucson
3601 S 6th Avenue   Tucson, AZ 85723   SOUTHWEST

Virginia Hospital Center - Arlington   (703) 558-5000
Virginia Hosp Ctr - Arlington
1701 N George Mason Dr   Arlington, VA 22205-3698   SOUTHEAST

Virginia Mason Medical Center   (206) 223-6600
Virginia Mason Med Ctr
1100 Ninth Ave, Box 900   Seattle, WA 98111   WEST COAST AND PACIFIC

Wake Forest University Baptist Medical Center   (336) 716-2011
Wake Forest Univ Baptist Med Ctr
Medical Center Blvd   Winston-Salem, NC 27157-1015   SOUTHEAST

WakeMed Cary Hospital   (919) 350-2300
WakeMed Cary
1900 Kildaire Farm Rd   Cary, NC 27511-6616   SOUTHEAST

Washington Hospital Center   (202) 877-7000
Washington Hosp Ctr
110 Irving St NW   Washington, DC 20010   MID ATLANTIC

Washington University Medical Center   (314) 362-6828
Washington Univ Med Ctr
4444 Forest Park Ave   St Louis, MO 63108   MIDWEST

WellStar Kennestone Hospital   (770) 793-5000
WellStar Kennestone Hosp
677 Church Street   Marietta, GA 30060   SOUTHEAST

WellStar Windy Hill Hospital   (770) 644-1000
WellStar Windy Hill Hosp
2540 Windy Hill Road   Marietta, GA 30067   SOUTHEAST

West Virginia University Hospital - Ruby Memorial   (304) 598-4000
WV Univ Hosp - Ruby Memorial
1 Medical Center Drive   Morgantown, WV 26506   MID ATLANTIC

Westchester Medical Center   (914) 493-7000
Westchester Med Ctr
95 Grasslands Road   Valhalla, NY 10595   MID ATLANTIC

Western Pennsylvania Hospital   (412) 578-5120
Western Penn Hosp
4800 Friendship Avenue   Pittsburgh, PA 15224   MID ATLANTIC

William Beaumont Hospital   (248) 551-5000
William Beaumont Hosp
3601 W 13 Mile Rd   Royal Oak, MI 48073   MIDWEST

Wills Eye Hospital   (215) 928-3000
Wills Eye Hosp
840 Walnut St   Philadelphia, PA 19107-5598   MID ATLANTIC

Winthrop - University Hospital   (516) 663-0333
Winthrop - Univ Hosp
259 1st St   Mineola, NY 11501   MID ATLANTIC

Wolfson Children's Hospital   (904) 202-8000
Wolfson Chldns Hosp
800 Prudential Dr   Jacksonville, FL 32207   SOUTHEAST

Women's and Children's Hospital of Buffalo, The   (716) 878-7000
Women's & Chldn's Hosp of Buffalo, The
219 Bryant St   Buffalo, NY 14222   MID ATLANTIC

Yakima Valley Memorial Hospital   (509) 575-8000
Yakima Valley Mem Hosp
2811 Tieton Dr   Yakima, WA 98902-3799   WEST COAST AND PACIFIC

Yale - New Haven Hospital   (203) 688-4242
Yale - New Haven Hosp
20 York St   New Haven, CT 06510   NEW ENGLAND

Yampa Valley Medical Center   (970) 879-1322
Yampa Valley Med Ctr
1024 Central Park Dr   Steamboat Springs, CO 80487   GREAT PLAINS AND MOUNTAINS

Appendix C:
Selected Cancer Resources

GENERAL RESOURCES

AMERICAN CANCER SOCIETY
A site with many resources on types of cancer, treatments, coping, support, clinical research data, volunteering and current news articles. It also has a database which allows one to search by zip code to locate local resources, activities and news.

National Office
1599 Clifton Road, NE
Atlanta, GA 30329

800-ACS-2345
www.cancer.org

AMERICAN INSTITUTE FOR CANCER RESEARCH
Discusses current research findings on diet, nutrition and cancer prevention and provides an online Cancer Resource Book.

1759 R Street, NW
Washington, DC 20009-2552

800-843-8114
www.aicr.org

ANNIE APPLESEED PROJECT
Provides information, education, advocacy and awareness those interested in complementary and alternative medical treatments.

7319 Serrano Terrace
Delray Beach, FL 33446-2215

www.annieappleseedproject.org
annfonfa@aol.com

ASSOCIATION OF CANCER ONLINE RESOURCES (ACOR)
Maintains many support groups and cancer-specific information, treatment options, clinical trial findings and a large collection of cancer-related online communities.

173 Duane Street
Suite 3A
New York, NY 10013-3334

212-226-5525
www.acor.org

CANCER CARE
Provides free resources and support to cancer patients, caregivers and families with all cancers through counseling, education, information, referrals and direct financial assistance.

National Office
275 7th Ave, Fl 22
New York, NY 10001

800-813-HOPE or 212-302-2400
www.cancercare.org

CANCER NEWS
News and information on cancer diagnosis, treatment and prevention.

www.cancernews.com

CANCER RESEARCH & PREVENTION FOUNDATION OF AMERICA
Scientific research and cancer education with a focus on cancers that can be prevented through lifestyle changes or early detection followed by prompt treatment. Includes breast, cervical, colorectal, lung, prostate, skin, oral and testicular cancers.

1600 Duke Street
Suite 500
Alexandria, VA 22314

800-227-2732
www.preventcancer.org

CANCER TRACK

Comprehensive source for links to news, research, medications, treatments, support groups, regulatory agencies and online references.

www.cancertrack.com

CANCERBACKUP

Europe-based organization with over 4,500 pages of online cancer information, practical advice and support for cancer patients and their families.

www.cancerbackup.org.uk

CANCEREDUCATION.COM

Provides cancer-specific information and educational programming for patients, their families and physicians.

750 Lexington Avenue	212-531-5960
26th Floor	www.cancereducation.com
New York, NY 10022	webmaster@cancereducation.com
NexCura, Inc.	206-270-0225
1215 Fourth Ave	www.cancerfacts.com
Suite 1925	answers@support.nextura.com
Seattle, WA 98161	

CANCERNETWORK.COM

Provides research findings and information on cancers, complications, therapies and insurance and payment issues.

CMP Heathcare Media	516-562-5000
Oncology Publishing Group	www.cancernetwork.com
600 Community Drive	info@cancernetwork.com
Manhasset, NY	

CANCERSOURCE.COM

Information, articles, advice, interactive tools and community resources for patients, physicians, children, women and nurses.

280 Summer Street, 9th Fl	866-234-5025
Boston, MA 02210	www.cancersource.com

HEALTH FINDER

A service of the Department of Health and Human Services, Health Finder has many resources ranging from topics specifically related to cancer to broader health topics such as locating public clinics, nursing homes, health fraud advice, medical privacy and links to universities, medical dictionaries and journals. It also has a guide that presents information and resources to help patients and families get better quality healthcare.

www.healthfinder.gov

NATIONAL CANCER INSTITUTE (NCI)

A branch of the US National Institutes of Health, NCI provides information about cancer, clinical trials, statistics, and research.

www.cancer.gov

The National Cancer Institute's (NCI's) Cancer Information Service (CIS) is a national information and education network. The CIS is a free public service of the NCI, the Nation's primary agency for cancer research. The CIS provides current cancer information to patients, their families, the public, and health professionals. The CIS provides personalized, confidential responses to specific questions about cancer.

NCI-Designated Cancer Centers

Cancer centers listed by state.

www3.cancer.gov/cancercenters

NCI Dictionary of Cancer Terms

www.cancer.gov/dictionary

Cancer Information Service (CIS)
Building 31
Room 20892
Bethesda, MD

800-422-6237 or 800-4-CANCER
cis.nci.nih.gov

NATIONAL COMPREHENSIVE CANCER NETWORK (NCCN)

Outlines cancer treatment guidelines and offers cancer patients and their families information to help work with their physicians to make more informed decisions about care and treatments.

Treatment Guidelines for Patients

National Comprehensive Cancer Network
500 Old York Road
Suite 250
Jenkintown, PA 19046

215-690-0300 or 888-909-NCCN (6226)
www.nccn.org

ONCOLINK

Informaton on specific types of cancer, updates on cancer treatments and news about research advances

OncoLink
Abramson Cancer Center of the University of Pennsylvania
3400 Spruce Street - 2 Donner
Philadelphia, PA 19104

www.oncolink.com

ONCOLOGY NURSING SOCIETY (ONS)

Resources on prevention, detection, diagnosis, treatment and survivorship.

Oncology Nursing Society
125 Enterprise Drive
Pittsburgh, PA 15275

866-257-4ONS
www.ons.org/patientEd
customer.service@ons.org

ONCOLOGY TOOLS

Information related to cancers and approved cancer drug therapies organized by disease category.

www.fda.gov/cder/cancer

Appendix C

PEOPLE LIVING WITH CANCER

A website by the American Society of Clinical Oncology for patients that provides oncologist-approved information on more than 50 types of cancer and their treatments, side effects, coping, and clinical trials. It includes a "Find an Oncologist" database, live chats, message boards, a drug database and links to patient support organizations.

American Society of Clinical Oncology
1900 Duke Street
Suite 200
Alexandria, VA 22314

703-519-2927 or 800-651-3038
www.peoplelivingwithcancer.org
contactus@plwc.org

SPECIAL POPULATIONS NETWORKS FOR CANCER AWARENESS, RESEARCH AND TRAINING

Resources and programs for minority communities.
http://www.cancer.gov/newscenter/special-populations-network-QA

YOUR DISEASE RISK

Provides education on cancers and focuses on prevention as the primary approach to controlling cancer and other chronic diseases.

Harvard Center for Cancer Prevention
677 Huntington Ave, Landmark 3 East
Boston, MA 02115

617-998-1034
www.yourdiseaserisk.harvard.edu

CHILDREN AND YOUNG ADULTS

BRAVE KIDS

Provides online resources for children with chronic, life-threatening illnesses and disabilities and their families. Local resources searchable by zip code.

Brave Kids: West Coast
1223 Wilshire Boulevard
#1411
Santa Monica, CA

800-568-1008
www.bravekids.org
info@bravekids.org

Brave Kids: East Coast
1208 Lake Cove Court
Ponte Verde Beach, FL 32082

904-827-9571
www.bravekids.org
info@bravekids.org

CANDLELIGHTERS CHILDHOOD CANCER FOUNDATION

Offers support, education and advocacy for families of children with cancer, survivors of childhood cancer and the professionals who care for them.

National Office
P.O. Box 498
Kensington, MD 20895-0498

800-366-CCCF or 301-962-3520
www.candlelighters.org
staff@candlelighters.org

CHILDREN'S ONCOLOGY GROUP

The Children's Oncology Group, in partnership with the National Childhood Cancer Foundation. Offers education and support resources.

Rush Operation Ctr
440 E. Huntington Dr., Ste 400
Arcadia, CA 91006

626-447-0064

www.childrensoncologygroup.org

CureSearch
Provides educational resources about cancer diagnoses, the different phases of treatment and support resources

CureSearch Headquarters
4600 East West Highway
Suite 600
Bethesda, MD

800-458-6223
www.curesearch.org

KidsHealth.org
Site designed for parents, kids and teens that discusses many health topics including cancer.

The Nemours Foundation, 1600 Rockland Rd.
Wilmington, DE 19803

302-651-4046
www.kidshealth.org

LIVESTRONG™ Young Adult Alliance (The Lance Armstrong Foundation).
The mission of the LIVESTRONG™ Young Adult Alliance is to improve survival rates and quality of life for young adults living with cancer by promoting relevant research and the delivery of patient care, generating awareness of the issue, being a voice for young adults with cancer and advancing helpful community-based programs and services.

PO Box 161150
Austin TX, 78716

512-236-8820
www.livestrong.org/yaa

National Childhood Cancer Foundation
National Childhood Cancer Foundation
440 E Huntington Drive
Suite 300
Arcadia, CA 91066-0012

800.458.NCCF
www.curesearch.org

Pediatric Oncology Resource Center
A site with resources, Internet links, and references for parents, friends and families of children who have or had childhood cancer.

www.acor.org/ped-onc

Planet Cancer
A website for young adults with cancer that provides support and other resources, including an online forum.

www.planetcancer.org

Teens Living with Cancer
A website for teenagers with cancer with information on treatments, combating fear, testimonials from other teens who have or had cancer and support chat rooms.

Melissa's Living Legacy Foundation
245 Citation Drive
Henrietta, NY 14467

585-334-0858
teenslivingwithcancer.org
info@teenslivingwithcancer.org

CLINICAL TRIALS

American Cancer Society
Free clinical trial matching and referral service.

http://clinicaltrials.cancer.org

Association of Clinical Research Professionals (ACRP)
Provides information regarding participating in a clinical trial, including important questions to ask, resources and a glossary of common terms associated with clinical trials.

http://www.acrpnet.org/resources/trial/questions.html

CENTERWATCH

Provides information and resources used by patients, pharmaceutical, biotechnology and medical device companies, CROs and research centers involved in clinical research around the world. The web site provides an extensive list of IRB approved clinical trials being conducted internationally and also lists promising therapies newly approved by the Food and Drug Administration. CenterWatch also offers reports on specific illnesses, clinical trial information and therapies that patients and advocates can buy.

Thomson CenterWatch   617-856-5900
22 Thompson Place   www.centerwatch.com
47F1
Boston, MA 02110

COALITION OF NATIONAL CANCER COOPERATIVE GROUPS (CNCC)

A network of cancer clinical trials specialists including cooperative groups, cancer centers, academic medical centers, community hospitals, physician practices, and patient advocate groups, CNCC aims at improving the clinical trials experience for patients and physicians, and providing professional support services, regulatory requirements, and providing professional support services. It offers a variety of programs and information for physicians, patient advocate groups, and patients designed to increase awareness of, and participation in cancer clinical trials.

1818 Market Street   877-520-4457
#1100   www.cancertrialshelp.org
Philadelphia, PA 19103

INTERNATIONAL FEDERATION OF PHARMACEUTICAL MANUFACTURERS & ASSOCIATIONS (IFPMA)

Provides a portal that allows one to search for comprehensive information on on-going clinical trials or results of completed trials conducted by the pharmaceutical industry.

www.ifpma.org/clinicaltrials

NATIONAL CANCER INSTITUTE (NCI)

A branch of the US National Institutes of Health, NCI provides information about cancer, clinical trials, statistics, and research.

www.cancer.gov/clinicaltrials

NATIONAL COMPREHENSIVE CANCER NETWORK (NCCN)

An alliance of 19 of the world's leading cancer centers, NCCN is a source of information to help patients and health professionals make informed decisions about cancer care. Through the collective expertise of its member institutions, the NCCN develops, updates, and disseminates a complete library of clinical practice guidelines.

Treatment Guidelines for Patients: 215-690-0300 or 888-909-NCCN

National Comprehensive Cancer Network   Fax: 215-690-0280
500 Old York Road   www.nccn.org
Suite 250
Jenkintown, PA

SPECIFIC CANCERS

RARE CANCER ALLIANCE
Provides support and other resources for adults and children with rare cancers.

Note: You are encouraged to explore the other websites listed in this appendix, as many also include information on rare cancers.

www.rare-cancer.org

SUPPORT

FERTILE HOPE
Provides reproductive information and support to cancer patients whose medical treatments present the risk of infertility.

Note: You are encouraged to explore the other websites listed in this appendix, as many also include resources for support including education materials, chat rooms, community groups and clinical advice.

www.fertilehope.org

SURVIVORS

CANCER SURVIVORS NETWORK
(American Cancer Soceity) Provides a forum for cancer survivors to share their stories, join chats, post messages on discussion boards and create their own webpage about their stories.

www.acscsn.org

CANCERVIVE
Provides support, public education and advocacy to those who have had cancer.

11636 Chayote Street
Los Angeles, CA 90049

800-4TO-CURE or 310-203-9232
www.cancervive.org
cancervivr@aol.com

LANCE ARMSTRONG FOUNDATION (LAF)
LAF provides advocacy, education, support and research for both cancer survivors and people who currently have cancer.

PO Box 161150
Austin, TX 78716-1150

512-236-8820
www.livestrong.org

NATIONAL COALITION FOR CANCER SURVIVORSHIP (NCCS)
Provides education, advocacy and support to those affected by cancer and cancer survivors. Specifically addresses quality of care and minority issues.

1010 Wayne Avenue
Suite 770
Silver Spring, MD 20910

877-622-7937
www.canceradvocacy.org
info@canceradvocacy.org

OUTLOOK - LIFE BEYOND CHILDHOOD CANCER
Addresses the needs and provides information to help give survivors and their families the tools to help them become their own advocate and is a forum for support.

www.outlook-life.org

TRAVEL ASSISTANCE

NATIONAL PATIENT AIR TRANSPORT HELPLINE (NPATH)
Provides information about and referrals to charitable medical air transportation programs that provide long-distance travel for medical, low income, and financially vulnerable patients. The information is provided at no cost and the HELPLINE is available 24 hours a day.

1-800-296-1217
www.npath.org or www.patienttravel.org

TREATMENT

AMERICAN SOCIETY FOR THERAPEUTIC RADIOLOGY AND ONCOLOGY
Provides downloadable brochures and publications on treatment options for several specific cancers.

ASTRO Headquarters
8280 Willow Oaks Corporate Drive
Suite 500
Fairfax, VA 22031

800-962-7876 or 703-502-1550
Fax 703-502-7852
www.astro.org

BLOOD AND MARROW TRANSPLANT INFORMATION NETWORK
Provides information about blood and marrow transplants, support groups, a list of transplant centers and testimonials from survivors.

www.bmtinfonet.org

CANCERSYMPTOMS.ORG
(Oncology Nursing Soceity) Provides information and resources for learning about and managing symptoms often associated with cancer treatment.

www.cancersymptoms.org

WOMEN

BREASTCANCER.ORG
Offers information on breast cancer prevention, symptoms, treatment, research, recovery and support.

www.breastcancer.org

ENTRE MUJERES
Un guia sobre la recuperación física y emocional después de la mastectomía.

www.cancerlinks.com/Mujeres/mujeres_index.html

LOOK GOOD. . . FEEL BETTER
Provides resources and links for women who are undergoing cancer treatment including cosmetic advice and support.

www.lookgoodfeelbetter.org

NATIONAL WOMEN'S HEALTH RESOURCE CENTER
Women's health site that includes information on various cancers.

NWHRC
157 Broad Street
Suite 315
Red Bank, NJ

www.healthywomen.org (Note: Click on "Health Center" and select the appropriate topic.)

NCI WOMEN OF COLOR
Provides basic data on how cancer affects women in minority populations.

http://cancercontrol.cancer.gov/womenofcolor

WOMEN'S CANCER CENTER
Many resources for women with various kinds of cancer.

www.womenscancercenter.com

YWCA
"ENCOREplus", a program available at some YWCA locations that focuses on cancer prevention, nutrition and rehabilitation.

YWCA USA
1015 18th Street, NW
Suite 1100
Washington, DC 20036

800-YWCA-US1 or 202-467-0801
www.ywca.org (Note: click on the "I need help" link.)

Section V
Indices

Subject Index

A

B

C

D

F

J

L

M

N

P

R

S

T

U

V

W

Special Expertise Index

This index lists the areas which the physicians listed in the Guide have identified as their "special expertise." These are not medical specialities. They are specific elements of disease, procedures, techniques and treatments for which these physicians are best known and are referred patients.

Special Expertise Index

Special Expertise Index

Special Expertise Index

Special Expertise Index

Special Expertise Index

Special Expertise Index

Special Expertise Index

Special Expertise Index

Special Expertise Index

Special Expertise Index

P

Special Expertise Index

Spec	Name	St	Pg
Pancreatic Surgery			
PS	Meyers, R	UT	363
S	Cameron, J	MD	427
S	Hoffman, J	PA	429
S	Pappas, T	NC	437
S	Warshaw, A	MA	426
S	Willis, I	FL	438
Pancreatic/Biliary Endoscopy (ERCP)			
Ge	Goldberg, M	IL	125
Ge	Haluszka, O	PA	122
Pap Smear Abnormalities			
GO	Dunton, C	PA	257
GO	Jones, H	TN	260
Parathyroid Cancer			
Oto	Shindo, M	NY	296
Oto	Weber, S	TX	305
S	Clark, O	CA	451
S	Harkema, J	MI	441
S	Leight, G	NC	436
S	Shaha, A	NY	432
S	Udelsman, R	CT	425
Parathyroid Surgery			
S	Roses, D	NY	431
Parent Guidance in Parental Cancer			
Psyc	Rauch, P	MA	378
Parotid Gland Tumors			
Oto	Burkey, B	TN	297
Oto	Fee, W	CA	305
Oto	Myers, E	PA	295
Pediatric Cancers			
Path	Triche, T	CA	331
Ped	Sallan, S	MA	364
PHO	Adamson, P	PA	338
PHO	Carroll, W	NY	339
PHO	Civin, C	MD	340
PHO	Drachtman, R	NJ	340
PHO	Dunkel, I	NY	340
PHO	Garvin, J	NY	340
PHO	Korones, D	NY	342
PHO	Meyers, P	NY	343
PHO	Moscow, J	KY	347
PHO	Neuberg, R	SC	347
PHO	Parker, R	NY	343
PHO	Sencer, S	MN	352
PHO	Sondel, P	WI	352
PHO	Steinherz, P	NY	344
PS	Ehrlich, P	MI	362
PS	Paidas, C	FL	361
PS	Sawin, R	WA	364
PS	Stolar, C	NY	361
RadRO	Constine, L	NY	389
RadRO	Donaldson, S	CA	404
RadRO	Douglas, J	WA	405
RadRO	Kun, L	TN	395
RadRO	Marcus, R	GA	395
RadRO	Mehta, M	WI	399
RadRO	Michalski, J	MO	400
RadRO	Roberts, K	CT	388
RadRO	Sailer, S	NC	396
RadRO	Schomberg, P	MN	400

Spec	Name	St	Pg
RadRO	Stea, B	AZ	404
RadRO	Wharam, M	MD	393
Pediatric Eye Reconstructive Surgery			
Oph	Piest, K	TX	278
Pediatric Neuroradiology			
NRad	Vezina, L	DC	412
Pediatric Neurosurgery			
NS	Albright, A	WI	230
NS	Boggan, J	CA	236
NS	Boop, F	TN	228
NS	Carmel, P	NJ	224
NS	Carson, B	MD	224
NS	Chapman, P	MA	222
NS	Cherny, W	ID	234
NS	Cohen, A	OH	231
NS	Duhaime, A	NH	222
NS	Edwards, M	CA	236
NS	Ellenbogen, R	WA	237
NS	Ewend, M	NC	228
NS	Feldstein, N	NY	225
NS	Frim, D	IL	231
NS	Fuchs, H	NC	228
NS	Goodrich, J	NY	225
NS	Goumnerova, L	MA	223
NS	Greene, C	MO	231
NS	Kaufman, B	WI	232
NS	Mapstone, T	OK	235
NS	Morrison, G	FL	229
NS	Parent, A	MS	229
NS	Park, T	MO	232
NS	Pollack, I	PA	226
NS	Raffel, C	MN	233
NS	Ruge, J	IL	233
NS	Sanford, R	TN	229
NS	Tomita, T	IL	234
NS	Wisoff, J	NY	227
Pediatric Ophthalmology			
Oph	Lueder, G	MO	277
Oph	Murphree, A	CA	278
Oph	Shields, C	PA	275
Oph	Shields, J	PA	275
Pediatric Orthopaedic Cancers			
OrS	O'Donnell, R	CA	287
OrS	Peabody, T	IL	286
OrS	Simon, M	IL	286
Pediatric Orthopaedic Surgery			
OrS	Conrad, E	WA	287
OrS	Malawer, M	DC	283
OrS	Randall, R	UT	286
Pediatric Orthopedic Surgery			
OrS	Dormans, J	PA	283
Pediatric Pathology			
Path	Triche, T	CA	331
Pediatric Plastic Surgery			
PlS	Bartlett, S	PA	370

Spec	Name	St	Pg
Pediatric Urology			
PS	Ginsburg, H	NY	361
U	Coplen, D	MO	485
Pelvic Imaging			
DR	McCarthy, S	CT	407
Pelvic Reconstruction			
GO	Clarke-Pearson, D	NC	259
GO	Currie, J	CT	254
GO	Fowler, J	OH	262
GO	Kohler, M	SC	260
GO	Lentz, S	NC	260
GO	Mutch, D	MO	263
GO	Sevin, B	FL	261
GO	Smith, H	NM	266
Pelvic Tumors			
GO	Barnes, W	DC	255
GO	Cohen, C	NY	256
GO	Penalver, M	FL	260
GO	Podratz, K	MN	263
GO	Sevin, B	FL	261
S	Paty, P	NY	431
Penile Cancer			
U	McDougal, W	MA	476
Peritoneal Carcinomatosis			
GO	Gershenson, D	TX	265
S	Bartlett, D	PA	427
S	Kuhn, J	TX	448
S	Levine, E	NC	436
S	Sugarbaker, P	DC	432
PET Imaging			
DR	Patz, E	NC	410
NuM	Carrasquillo, J	NY	414
NuM	Coleman, R	NC	416
NuM	Dillehay, G	IL	416
NuM	Goldsmith, S	NY	415
NuM	Larson, S	NY	415
NuM	Scheff, A	CA	417
NuM	Siegel, B	MO	416
NuM	Wahl, R	MD	415
PET Imaging-Brain			
NuM	Alavi, A	PA	414
NuM	Waxman, A	CA	417
PET Imaging-Breast			
NuM	Wahl, R	MD	415
Photodynamic Therapy			
D	Hanke, C	IN	108
Pul	Downie, G	NC	383
RadRO	Glatstein, E	PA	390
TS	Friedberg, J	PA	463
Phototherapy in Skin Disease			
D	Elmets, C	AL	106
Pigmented Lesions			
D	Johr, R	FL	107

Special Expertise Index

Special Expertise Index

Special Expertise Index

Spec	Name	St	Pg
Oto	Weber, R	TX	304
Oto	Weisman, R	CA	307
S	Bland, K	AL	434
S	Edney, J	NE	445
S	Grant, C	MN	441
S	Siperstein, A	OH	444

Thyroid & Parathyroid Surgery

Spec	Name	St	Pg
Oto	Har-El, G	NY	293
Oto	Kraus, D	NY	294
S	Chabot, J	NY	427
S	Giuliano, A	CA	451
S	Jackson, G	TX	447

Thyroid Cancer

Spec	Name	St	Pg
EDM	Ain, K	KY	117
EDM	Ball, D	MD	116
EDM	Fitzgerald, P	CA	119
EDM	Gagel, R	TX	118
EDM	Kandeel, F	CA	119
EDM	Kloos, R	OH	117
EDM	Koch, C	MS	117
EDM	Kopp, P	IL	117
EDM	Ladenson, P	MD	116
EDM	Levine, R	NH	116
EDM	Ridgway, E	CO	118
EDM	Robbins, R	TX	118
EDM	Rubenfeld, S	TX	118
EDM	Sherman, S	TX	118
EDM	Tuttle, R	NY	116
EDM	Waguespack, S	TX	118
EDM	Wartofsky, L	DC	116
NuM	Goldsmith, S	NY	415
NuM	Lamonica, D	NY	415
NuM	Larson, S	NY	415
NuM	Silberstein, E	OH	416
NuM	Waxman, A	CA	417
Onc	Jahan, T	CA	198
Onc	Pfister, D	NY	161
Oto	Chalian, A	PA	292
Oto	Couch, M	NC	297
Oto	Eisele, D	CA	305
Oto	Fee, W	CA	305
Oto	Keane, W	PA	294
Oto	Lavertu, P	OH	301
Oto	Lydiatt, W	NE	303
Oto	McCaffrey, T	FL	298
Oto	Persky, M	NY	295
Oto	Petruzzelli, G	IL	301
Oto	Shindo, M	NY	296
Oto	Teknos, T	MI	302
Oto	Valentino, J	KY	299
Oto	Weber, S	TX	305
Path	DeLellis, R	RI	318
Path	Li Volsi, V	PA	321
Path	Sanchez, M	NJ	322
Path	Wheeler, T	TX	329
PEn	Zimmerman, D	IL	359
PIS	Loree, T	NY	371
PS	Ehrlich, P	MI	362
PS	Skinner, M	NC	362
RadRO	Charboneau, J	MN	398
RadRO	Grigsby, P	MO	398
S	Alfonso, A	NY	426
S	Butler, J	CA	450
S	Cady, B	RI	424
S	Evans, D	TX	447

Spec	Name	St	Pg
S	Farrar, W	OH	440
S	Harkema, J	MI	441
S	Leight, G	NC	436
S	Roses, D	NY	431
S	Shah, J	NY	432
S	Shaha, A	NY	432
S	Udelsman, R	CT	425

Thyroid Cancer & Surgery

Spec	Name	St	Pg
Oto	Clayman, G	TX	303
Oto	Schantz, S	NY	296
S	Clark, O	CA	451
S	Hanks, J	VA	435
S	Moley, J	MO	442
S	Ridge, J	PA	431

Thyroid Disorders

Spec	Name	St	Pg
EDM	Ain, K	KY	117
EDM	Ladenson, P	MD	116
EDM	Levine, R	NH	116
EDM	Wartofsky, L	DC	116
NuM	Strauss, H	NY	415
Oto	Davidson, B	DC	293
Oto	Donovan, D	TX	303
Path	Wheeler, T	TX	329
PEn	Zimmerman, D	IL	359

Thyroid Imaging

Spec	Name	St	Pg
NuM	Scheff, A	CA	417

Thyroid Ultrasound

Spec	Name	St	Pg
DR	Hann, L	NY	409

Tongue Cancer

Spec	Name	St	Pg
Oto	Myers, J	TX	304

Tracheal Surgery

Spec	Name	St	Pg
Oto	McCaffrey, T	FL	298
TS	Cerfolio, R	AL	465
TS	De Meester, T	CA	470
TS	Gaissert, H	MA	462
TS	Kernstine, K	CA	470
TS	Mathisen, D	MA	462
TS	Wright, C	MA	462

Transfusion Medicine

Spec	Name	St	Pg
PHO	Wolfe, L	MA	338

Transplant Medicine-Liver

Spec	Name	St	Pg
Ge	Brown, K	MI	125
Ge	Crippin, J	MO	125
Ge	Gish, R	CA	126

Transplant-Kidney

Spec	Name	St	Pg
PS	Colombani, P	MD	360
S	Fung, J	OH	440
U	Menon, M	MI	486
U	Novick, A	OH	487
U	Sagalowsky, A	TX	490

Transplant-Liver

Spec	Name	St	Pg
PS	Colombani, P	MD	360
PS	Meyers, R	UT	363
S	Brems, J	IL	439
S	Chari, R	TN	434
S	Emond, J	NY	428

Spec	Name	St	Pg
S	Fung, J	OH	440
S	Hemming, A	FL	435
S	Jenkins, R	MA	424
S	Klein, A	CA	452
S	Marsh, J	PA	430
S	Pinson, C	TN	437
S	Wood, R	TX	450

Transplant-Liver-Adult & Pediatric

Spec	Name	St	Pg
S	Chapman, W	MO	440
S	Millis, J	IL	442

Transplant-Lung

Spec	Name	St	Pg
TS	Egan, T	NC	466
TS	Iannettoni, M	IA	468
TS	Meyers, B	MO	468
TS	Ninan, M	TN	467
TS	Patterson, G	MO	468
TS	Pierson, R	MD	464
TS	Sonett, J	NY	465
TS	Sugarbaker, D	MA	462

Transplant-Lung (Pathology)

Spec	Name	St	Pg
Path	Yousem, S	PA	323

Transplant-Pancreas

Spec	Name	St	Pg
S	Millis, J	IL	442

Tumor Banking

Spec	Name	St	Pg
Path	Balla, A	IL	325
Path	Melamed, J	NY	321
Path	Orenstein, J	DC	321

Tumor Diagnosis

Spec	Name	St	Pg
Path	Brooks, J	PA	319

Tumor Imaging

Spec	Name	St	Pg
NuM	Coleman, R	NC	416

Tumor Surgery

Spec	Name	St	Pg
PS	Aiken, J	WI	362
PS	Ginsburg, H	NY	361
S	Byrd, D	WA	450
S	Crowe, J	OH	440
S	Eilber, F	CA	451

Tumor Surgery-Pediatric

Spec	Name	St	Pg
OrS	Dormans, J	PA	283
PS	Meyers, R	UT	363
PS	Ziegler, M	CO	363

Tumors-Rare & Multiple

Spec	Name	St	Pg
S	Dooley, W	OK	446

U

Unknown Primary Cancer

Spec	Name	St	Pg
Onc	Greco, F	TN	168
Onc	Jacobs, C	CA	198
Onc	Kelsen, D	NY	157
Onc	Sikic, B	CA	201
Onc	Stewart, F	WA	201
Onc	Stooler, M	NY	163
Onc	Tschetter, L	SD	188

Alphabetical Listing of Doctors

Alphabetical Listing of Doctors

Name	Specialty	Pg	Name	Specialty	Pg
Bains, Manjit (NY)	TS	463	Benson, Mitchell (NY)	U	477
Bakay, Roy (IL)	NS	230	Bentz, Brandon (UT)	Oto	302
Balch, Charles (MD)	S	426	Benz, Edward (MA)	Hem	130
Balducci, Lodovico (FL)	Onc	164	Berchuck, Andrew (NC)	GO	259
Ball, Douglas (MD)	EDM	116	Berek, Jonathan (CA)	GO	266
Ball, Edward D (CA)	Onc	195	Berg, Christine (MD)	RadRO	388
Balla, Andre (IL)	Path	325	Berg, Daniel (WA)	D	110
Ballantyne, Garth (NJ)	S	426	Berg, Stacey (TX)	PHO	354
Banks, Peter (NC)	Path	323	Berg, Wendie A (MD)	DR	408
Bans, Larry (AZ)	U	489	Berger, Mitchel (CA)	NS	236
Barakat, Richard (NY)	GO	255	Berke, Gerald (CA)	Oto	305
Baranko, Paul (AZ)	PHO	354	Berkowitz, Ross (MA)	GO	254
Bardot, Stephen (LA)	U	489	Berlin, Jordan (TN)	Onc	165
Barger, Geoffrey R (MI)	N	245	Berliner, Nancy (CT)	Hem	130
Barkin, Jamie (FL)	Ge	124	Berman, Michael (CA)	GO	266
Barlogie, Bart (AR)	Hem	140	Bernard, Stephen (NC)	Onc	165
Barnes, Willard (DC)	GO	255	Berrey, B (FL)	OrS	284
Barnett, Gene (OH)	NS	230	Berson, Anthony (NY)	RadRO	389
Baron, Joseph (IL)	Hem	136	Bertolone, Salvatore (KY)	PHO	344
Barredo, Julio (FL)	PHO	344	Bhan, Atul (MA)	Path	318
Barter, James (MD)	GO	256	Bierman, Philip (NE)	Onc	186
Bartlett, David (PA)	S	427	Biermann, J Sybil (MI)	OrS	285
Bartlett, Scott (PA)	PlS	370	Bigelow, Carolyn (MS)	Hem	134
Basch, Samuel (NY)	Psyc	378	Bilchik, Anton (CA)	S	450
Bashevkin, Michael (NY)	Onc	150	Billings, J Andrew (MA)	IM	507
Basler, Joseph (TX)	U	489	Bilsky, Mark (NY)	NS	223
Bassett, Lawrence (CA)	DR	411	Bitran, Jacob (IL)	Onc	175
Bastian, Boris C (CA)	Path	329	Black, Keith (CA)	NS	236
Bauer, Jerry (IL)	NS	230	Black, Peter (MA)	NS	222
Beall, Michael (VA)	U	482	Blair, Norman (IL)	Oph	276
Beart, Robert (CA)	CRS	97	Bland, Kirby (AL)	S	434
Beatty, Patrick (MT)	Onc	186	Blaney, Susan (TX)	PHO	354
Beauchamp, Robert (TN)	S	433	Blanke, Charles (OR)	Onc	196
Beck, David E (LA)	CRS	96	Blasko, John C (WA)	RadRO	404
Becker, James (MA)	S	424	Blatt, Julie (NC)	PHO	345
Beer, Tomasz (OR)	Onc	195	Bleday, Ronald (MA)	CRS	90
Behm, Frederick (IL)	Path	325	Block, Susan (MA)	Psyc	378
Behrns, Kevin (FL)	S	434	Blom, Dennis (IN)	S	439
Beitsch, Peter (TX)	S	446	Bockenstedt, Paula (MI)	Hem	136
Belani, Chandra (PA)	Onc	150	Boggan, James (CA)	NS	236
Belinson, Jerome (OH)	GO	262	Bojrab, Dennis (MI)	Oto	300
Bell, Debra (MA)	Path	318	Boland, C Richard (TX)	Ge	126
Belldegrun, Arie (CA)	U	490	Boldt, David (TX)	Hem	140
Ben-Josef, Edgar (MI)	RadRO	397	Bolger, Graeme (AL)	Onc	165
Benedetti, Costantino (OH)	PM	313	Bollen, Andrew (CA)	Path	329
Benedetto, Pasquale (FL)	Onc	164	Bolwell, Brian (OH)	Onc	175
Benevenia, Joseph (NJ)	OrS	282	Bonner, James (AL)	RadRO	394
Benjamin, Robert (TX)	Onc	189	Bonomi, Philip (IL)	Onc	175
Bennett, Richard (CA)	D	110	Boop, Frederick (TN)	NS	228
Bensinger, William (WA)	Onc	196	Borden, Ernest (OH)	Onc	175
Benson, Al (IL)	Onc	175	Borgen, Patrick (NY)	S	427

Name	Specialty	Pg	Name	Specialty	Pg
Borges, Lawrence (MA)	NS	222	Bumpous, Jeffrey (KY)	Oto	297
Boronow, Richard C (MS)	GO	259	Bunn, Paul (CO)	Onc	186
Bos, Gary D (WA)	OrS	287	Burger, Peter (MD)	Path	319
Bosl, George (NY)	Onc	150	Burkey, Brian (TN)	Oto	297
Boston, Barry (TN)	Onc	165	Burnett, Arthur (MD)	U	477
Bostwick, David (VA)	Path	323	Burris, Howard A (TN)	Onc	165
Bowen, Glen (UT)	D	109	Burstein, Harold J (MA)	Onc	144
Boxrud, Cynthia (CA)	Oph	278	Burt, Randall (UT)	Ge	125
Boyce, H Worth (FL)	Ge	124	Burt, Richard (IL)	Onc	176
Boyd, Stuart (CA)	U	491	Burton, Allen (TX)	PM	314
Bradford, Carol (MI)	Oto	300	Bussel, James (NY)	PHO	339
Brandt, Keith (MO)	PlS	373	Butler, David (TX)	D	109
Braun, Martin (DC)	D	103	Butler, John (CA)	S	450
Braverman, Irwin (CT)	D	102	Butler, William (SC)	Onc	166
Brawley, Otis (GA)	Onc	165	Buys, Saundra (UT)	Onc	186
Braylan, Raul (FL)	Path	323	Buzdar, Aman (TX)	Onc	189
Brecher, Martin (NY)	PHO	339	Byrd, David (WA)	S	450
Breitbart, William (NY)	Psyc	378	Byrd, John (OH)	Onc	176
Brem, Henry (MD)	NS	224	Bystryn, Jean (NY)	D	104
Brem, Steven (FL)	NS	228			
Brems, John (IL)	S	439	## C		
Brendler, Charles (IL)	U	484			
Brennan, Murray (NY)	S	427	Cady, Blake (RI)	S	424
Brenner, Malcolm (TX)	Hem	140	Cagle, Philip (TX)	Path	327
Bresalier, Robert (TX)	Ge	126	Cain, Joanna (OR)	GO	266
Brescia, Frank J (SC)	Onc	165	Cairo, Mitchell (NY)	PHO	339
Brewer, Molly (CT)	GO	254	Calvo, Benjamin (NC)	S	434
Bricker, Leslie J (MI)	Onc	176	Cameron, John (MD)	S	427
Bristow, Robert (MD)	GO	256	Camins, Martin (NY)	NS	224
Brizel, David (NC)	RadRO	394	Camitta, Bruce (WI)	PHO	349
Brockstein, Bruce (IL)	Onc	176	Camoriano, John (AZ)	Onc	190
Brodeur, Garrett (PA)	PHO	339	Campbell, Bruce (WI)	Oto	300
Brodland, David (PA)	D	103	Campbell, Steven (OH)	U	485
Brooks, John (PA)	Path	319	Cance, William (FL)	S	434
Brown, Kimberly (MI)	Ge	125	Canellos, George P (MA)	Onc	144
Bruce, Jeffrey (NY)	NS	224	Cannon, Walter (CA)	TS	469
Bruera, Eduardo (TX)	Onc	189	Caputo, Thomas (NY)	GO	256
Brufsky, Adam (PA)	Onc	150	Carbone, David (TN)	Onc	166
Bruggers, Carol (UT)	PHO	353	Carducci, Michael (MD)	Onc	150
Bruner, Janet (TX)	Path	327	Carey, Lisa A (NC)	Onc	166
Brunicardi, F Charles (TX)	S	446	Carlson, John (NJ)	GO	256
Brunt, L Michael (MO)	S	439	Carlson, Robert (CA)	Onc	196
Bruskewitz, Reginald (WI)	U	484	Carmel, Peter (NJ)	NS	224
Buadi, Francis (TN)	Hem	134	Carney, John (AR)	D	109
Buchholz, Thomas (TX)	RadRO	402	Carpenter, John (AL)	Onc	166
Buckner, Jan (MN)	Onc	176	Carrasquillo, Jorge (NY)	NuM	414
Buckwalter, Joseph (IA)	OrS	285	Carrau, Ricardo (PA)	Oto	292
Budd, George (OH)	Onc	176	Carroll, Peter (CA)	U	491
Bueno, Raphael (MA)	TS	462	Carroll, William (NY)	PHO	339
Bukowski, Ronald (OH)	Onc	176	Carson, Benjamin (MD)	NS	224
Bull, David (UT)	TS	469	Carter, H Ballentine (MD)	U	477
			Cascino, Terrence (MN)	N	245

Alphabetical Listing of Doctors

Name	Specialty	Pg	Name	Specialty	Pg
Cassisi, Nicholas (FL)	Oto	297	Clarke-Pearson, Daniel (NC)	GO	259
Castle, Valerie (MI)	PHO	349	Clayman, Gary (TX)	Oto	303
Castleberry, Robert (AL)	PHO	345	Cleary, James (WI)	Onc	177
Catalona, William (IL)	U	485	Clinton, Steven (OH)	Onc	177
Cerfolio, Robert (AL)	TS	465	Clohisy, Denis (MN)	OrS	285
Chabner, Bruce (MA)	Onc	145	Close, Lanny G (NY)	Oto	292
Chabot, John (NY)	S	427	Cloughesy, Timothy (CA)	N	247
Chait, Alan (WA)	EDM	119	Clutter, William E (MO)	EDM	117
Chakravarthy, Anuradha (TN)	RadRO	394	Cobleigh, Melody (IL)	Onc	177
Chalas, Eva (NY)	GO	256	Cobos, Everardo (TX)	Hem	140
Chalian, Ara (PA)	Oto	292	Coccia, Peter (NE)	PHO	353
Chambers, Setsuko (AZ)	GO	265	Cochran, Alistair (CA)	Path	330
Champlin, Richard (TX)	Hem	140	Cockerham, Kimberly (CA)	Oph	278
Chanan-Khan, Asher (NY)	Onc	150	Cohen, Alan (OH)	NS	231
Chandler, William F (MI)	NS	230	Cohen, Bruce (OH)	ChiN	248
Chandrasoma, Parakrama (CA)	Path	329	Cohen, Carmel (NY)	GO	256
Chang, Alfred (MI)	S	440	Cohen, James I (OR)	Oto	305
Chang, Helena (CA)	S	450	Cohen, Michael (IA)	Path	325
Chang, Jenny (TX)	Onc	190	Cohen, Philip (DC)	Onc	151
Chao, Nelson (NC)	Onc	166	Cohen, Roger (PA)	Onc	151
Chap, Linnea (CA)	Onc	196	Cohen, Seymour (NY)	Onc	151
Chapman, Paul (NY)	Onc	150	Cohn, Susan (IL)	PHO	349
Chapman, Paul (MA)	NS	222	Coia, Lawrence (NJ)	RadRO	389
Chapman, Robert A (MI)	Onc	176	Coit, Daniel (NY)	S	427
Chapman, William (MO)	S	440	Coker, Newton (TX)	Oto	303
Char, Devron (CA)	Oph	278	Colby, Thomas (AZ)	Path	327
Charboneau, J William (MN)	RadRO	398	Cole, David (SC)	S	434
Chari, Ravi (TN)	S	434	Coleman, John J (IN)	PlS	373
Chen, Allen (MD)	PHO	339	Coleman, Morton (NY)	Onc	151
Cheng, Edward (MN)	OrS	285	Coleman, Ralph E (NC)	NuM	416
Cherny, W Bruce (ID)	NS	234	Coller, John (MA)	CRS	90
Cheson, Bruce (DC)	Hem	131	Collins, Eva (NH)	PlS	370
Cheville, Andrea (PA)	PMR	508	Colombani, Paul (MD)	PS	360
Childs, Stacy (CO)	U	488	Colon-Otero, Gerardo (FL)	Onc	166
Chingos, James (FL)	Onc	166	Come, Steven (MA)	Onc	145
Chiocca, E Antonio (OH)	NS	231	Comis, Robert (PA)	Onc	151
Chitambar, Christopher (WI)	Onc	177	Conant, Emily (PA)	DR	408
Chlebowski, Rowan (CA)	Onc	196	Conant, Marcus (CA)	D	110
Cho, Kathleen (MI)	Path	325	Connolly, James (MA)	Path	318
Chodak, Gerald (IL)	U	485	Conrad, Ernest (WA)	OrS	287
Choi, Noah (MA)	RadRO	387	Conry, Robert (AL)	Onc	167
Choti, Michael (MD)	S	427	Constine, Louis (NY)	RadRO	389
Chow, Warren (CA)	Onc	196	Cook, Jonathan (NC)	D	106
Chowdhury, Khalid (CO)	Oto	303	Cookson, Michael (TN)	U	482
Choy, Hak (TX)	RadRO	402	Cooper, Barry (TX)	Hem	141
Chu, Edward (CT)	Onc	145	Cooper, Jay (NY)	RadRO	389
Cioffi, William (RI)	S	424	Copeland, Larry J (OH)	GO	262
Civin, Curt (MD)	PHO	340	Copeland III, Edward (FL)	S	434
Clamon, Gerald (IA)	Onc	177	Coplen, Douglas (MO)	U	485
Clark, Joseph (IL)	Onc	177	Cordeiro, Peter (NY)	PlS	371
Clark, Orlo (CA)	S	451	Corey, Seth (TX)	PHO	354

Alphabetical Listing of Doctors

Name	Specialty	Pg	Name	Specialty	Pg
Dottino, Peter (NY)	GO	257	El-Galley, Rizk (AL)	U	482
Douglas, James (WA)	RadRO	405	Ellenbogen, Richard (WA)	NS	237
Downie, Gordon (NC)	Pul	383	Ellenhorn, Joshua (CA)	S	451
Drachtman, Richard (NJ)	PHO	340	Ellis, Georgiana (WA)	Onc	197
Drebin, Jeffrey (PA)	S	427	Ellis, Lee (TX)	S	447
Dreicer, Robert (OH)	Onc	178	Ellis, William (WA)	U	491
Dreyer, ZoAnn (TX)	PHO	354	Ellison, E Christopher (OH)	S	440
Dritschilo, Anatoly (DC)	RadRO	390	Elmets, Craig (AL)	D	106
Driver, Larry (TX)	PM	314	Eloubeidi, Mohamad (AL)	Ge	124
Droller, Michael (NY)	U	477	Emami, Bahman (IL)	RadRO	398
Drucker, David (FL)	PS	361	Emanuel, Peter (AL)	Hem	134
Druker, Brian (OR)	Onc	197	Emerson, Stephen (PA)	Hem	131
Du Pen, Stuart (WA)	PM	314	Emond, Jean (NY)	S	428
Dubeau, Louis (CA)	Path	330	Eng, Charis (OH)	Onc	178
Ducore, Jonathan (CA)	PHO	356	Eng, Kenneth (NY)	S	428
Duffner, Patricia (NY)	ChiN	248	Ennis, Ronald (NY)	RadRO	390
Duhaime, Ann (NH)	NS	222	Ensminger, William (MI)	Onc	178
Dunkel, Ira (NY)	PHO	340	Epstein, Jonathan (MD)	Path	319
Dunphy, Frank (NC)	Onc	167	Erba, Harry (MI)	Hem	136
Dunton, Charles (PA)	GO	257	Erban, John (MA)	Onc	145
Dutcher, Janice (NY)	Onc	152	Esserman, Laura (CA)	S	451
Dutton, Jonathan (NC)	Oph	275	Essner, Richard (CA)	S	451
Duvic, Madeleine (TX)	D	110	Estabrook, Alison (NY)	S	428
Dzubow, Leonard (PA)	D	104	Estey, Elihu (TX)	Onc	190
			Ettinger, David (MD)	Onc	153

E

Name	Specialty	Pg	Name	Specialty	Pg
			Euhus, David (TX)	S	447
Earle, Craig (MA)	Onc	145	Evans, Douglas (TX)	S	447
Earp, H Shelton (NC)	EDM	117	Evers, Kathryn (PA)	DR	408
Ebbert, Larry (SD)	Onc	187	Ewend, Matthew (NC)	NS	228
Eberlein, Timothy (MO)	S	440			

F

Name	Specialty	Pg	Name	Specialty	Pg
Eckardt, Jeffrey (CA)	OrS	287			
Eckhardt, S (CO)	Onc	187	Faber, L Penfield (IL)	TS	467
Edelson, Richard (CT)	D	102	Fabian, Carol J (KS)	Onc	187
Edelstein, Barbara (NY)	DR	408	Falletta, John (NC)	PHO	345
Edge, Stephen (NY)	S	428	Fallon, Robert (IN)	PHO	350
Edington, Howard (PA)	S	428	Fann, Jesse (WA)	Psyc	379
Edney, James (NE)	S	445	Fanucchi, Michael (NY)	Onc	153
Edwards, Michael (AR)	S	446	Farrar, William (OH)	S	440
Edwards, Michael S (CA)	NS	236	Fay, Joseph (TX)	Onc	190
Efron, Jonathan (AZ)	CRS	96	Fee, Willard (CA)	Oto	305
Egan, Thomas (NC)	TS	466	Feig, Barry (TX)	S	447
Ehrlich, Peter (MI)	PS	362	Feinstein, Donald I (CA)	Hem	142
Ehya, Hormoz (PA)	Path	319	Feldman, Joseph (IL)	PMR	509
Eichler, Craig (FL)	D	106	Feldstein, Neil (NY)	NS	225
Eifel, Patricia (TX)	RadRO	403	Felix, Carolyn (PA)	PHO	340
Eilber, Frederick (CA)	S	451	Fenske, Neil A (FL)	D	106
Einhorn, Lawrence (IN)	Onc	178	Fenske, Neil A (FL)	D	106
Eisele, David (CA)	Oto	305	Ferguson, Mark (IL)	TS	468
Eisenberg, Burton (NH)	S	424	Ferrara, James (MI)	PHO	350
Eisenberger, Mario (MD)	Onc	153	Ferraz, Francisco (VA)	NS	228
Eisenstat, Theodore (NJ)	CRS	91	Fewkes, Jessica (MA)	D	102
			Fields, Karen (TX)	Hem	141

Alphabetical Listing of Doctors

Name	Specialty	Pg	Name	Specialty	Pg
Geschwind, Jean (MD)	VIR	413	Goodwin, W Jarrard (FL)	Oto	297
Gewirtz, Alan (PA)	Hem	131	Gordon, Leo I (IL)	Hem	137
Geyer, Charles (PA)	Onc	154	Gorfine, Stephen (NY)	CRS	91
Geyer, J Russell (WA)	PHO	356	Goulet, Robert (IN)	S	441
Gharagozloo, Farid (DC)	TS	463	Goumnerova, Liliana (MA)	NS	223
Giannotta, Steven (CA)	NS	237	Gradishar, William (IL)	Onc	179
Gibbs, John F (NY)	S	429	Grado, Gordon (AZ)	RadRO	403
Gigantelli, James (OK)	Oph	277	Graham, Mark (NC)	Onc	168
Gilbert, Mark (TX)	N	246	Graham, Michael (AZ)	PHO	355
Gilchrest, Barbara (MA)	D	102	Graham-Pole, John (FL)	PHO	346
Gill, Harcharan (CA)	U	491	Gralow, Julie (WA)	Onc	198
Gill, Inderbir (OH)	U	485	Grana, Generosa (NJ)	Onc	155
Ginsburg, Elizabeth (MA)	RE	269	Grandis, Jennifer (PA)	Oto	293
Ginsburg, Howard (NY)	PS	361	Granstein, Richard (NY)	D	104
Gish, Robert (CA)	Ge	126	Grant, Clive S (MN)	S	441
Giuliano, Armando (CA)	S	451	Grant, Michael (TX)	S	447
Glaspy, John (CA)	Onc	198	Grasso, Michael (NY)	U	477
Glass, Jon (PA)	N	244	Greco, F Anthony (TN)	Onc	168
Glassburn, John (PA)	RadRO	390	Green, Daniel (NY)	PHO	340
Glatstein, Eli (PA)	RadRO	390	Green, Howard (FL)	D	107
Glick, John (PA)	Onc	154	Greenberg, Donna (MA)	Psyc	378
Glisson, Bonnie (TX)	Onc	190	Greenberg, Harry (MI)	N	246
Glode, L (CO)	Onc	187	Greenberg, Richard (PA)	U	477
Glogau, Richard (CA)	D	111	Greenberger, Joel (PA)	RadRO	390
Gluckman, Gordon (IL)	U	486	Greene, Clarence (MO)	NS	231
Gluckman, Jack (OH)	Oto	300	Greene, Frederick (NC)	S	435
Gockerman, Jon (NC)	Onc	167	Greene, Graham (AR)	U	489
Godder, Kamar (VA)	PHO	346	Greenson, Joel K (MI)	Path	325
Godwin, John (IL)	Hem	137	Greenwald, Bruce (MD)	Ge	122
Goff, Barbara (WA)	GO	267	Greenway, Hubert T (CA)	D	111
Goggins, Michael (MD)	Ge	122	Greer, Benjamin (WA)	GO	267
Gold, Stuart (NC)	PHO	346	Greer, John P (TN)	Hem	134
Goldberg, Jack (NJ)	Hem	131	Gregory, Stephanie (IL)	Hem	137
Goldberg, Melvyn (PA)	TS	463	Greiner, Carl (NE)	Psyc	379
Goldberg, Michael (IL)	Ge	125	Greipp, Philip R (MN)	Hem	137
Goldberg, Richard (NC)	Onc	168	Grem, Jean L (NE)	Onc	187
Goldblum, John (OH)	Path	325	Grever, Michael (OH)	Hem	137
Goldman, Allan (FL)	Pul	383	Grichnik, James M (NC)	D	107
Goldman, Stanton (TX)	PHO	354	Grier, Holcombe (MA)	PHO	337
Goldman, Stewart (IL)	PHO	350	Grigsby, Perry (MO)	RadRO	398
Goldsmith, Stanley (NY)	NuM	415	Grody, Wayne (CA)	CG	506
Goldstein, Lori (PA)	Onc	154	Grogan, Thomas (AZ)	Path	328
Golomb, Harvey (IL)	Onc	179	Groopman, Jerome E (MA)	Hem	130
Golub, Richard (FL)	CRS	93	Grosfeld, Jay L (IN)	PS	362
Gomella, Leonard (PA)	U	477	Grosh, William (VA)	Onc	168
Goodman, Annekathryn (MA)	GO	254	Grossbard, Michael (NY)	Onc	155
Goodman, Robert (NJ)	RadRO	390	Grossman, Stuart (MD)	Onc	155
Goodnight, James (CA)	S	451	Grossniklaus, Hans (GA)	Oph	275
Goodrich, James (NY)	NS	225	Grubb, Robert (MO)	NS	231
Goodson, William (CA)	S	451	Gruber, Stephen (MI)	Onc	179
Goodwin, Scott (CA)	VIR	414	Grunberg, Steven Marc (VT)	Onc	146

Alphabetical Listing of Doctors

Name	Specialty	Pg	Name	Specialty	Pg
Hong, Waun (TX)	Onc	191	Jaffe, Elaine (MD)	Path	320
Hoppe, Richard (CA)	RadRO	405	Jahan, Thierry (CA)	Onc	198
Hoque, Laura (HI)	S	452	Jahanzeb, Mohammad (TN)	Onc	168
Hord, Jeffrey (OH)	PHO	351	Jain, Subhash (NY)	PM	312
Horn, Biljana N (CA)	PHO	356	Jakacki, Regina (PA)	PHO	341
Horn, Thomas (AR)	D	110	Janeiro, John J (NH)	U	476
Horning, Sandra (CA)	Onc	198	Janjan, Nora (TX)	RadRO	403
Horowitz, Ira (GA)	GO	260	Janss, Anna (GA)	N	245
Hortobagyi, Gabriel (TX)	Onc	191	Jarow, Jonathan (MD)	U	478
Horwitz, Eric (PA)	RadRO	391	Jenkins, Roger (MA)	S	424
Howe, James (IA)	S	441	Jett, James (MN)	Pul	383
Hricak, Hedvig (NY)	DR	409	Jewell, Mark (OR)	PIS	374
Hruban, Ralph (MD)	Path	320	Jhingran, Anuja (TX)	RadRO	403
Hruza, George J (MO)	D	108	Jillella, Anand (GA)	Onc	169
Huben, Robert (NY)	U	478	Johnson, Bruce (MA)	Onc	146
Huber, Philip (TX)	CRS	96	Johnson, David (TN)	Onc	169
Hudes, Gary (PA)	Onc	156	Johnson, Denise (CA)	S	452
Hudis, Clifford (NY)	Onc	156	Johnson, Jonas (PA)	Oto	294
Hudson, Melissa (TN)	PHO	346	Johnson, Ronald (PA)	S	429
Huffman, Jeffry (CA)	U	491	Johnson, Stephen (CO)	NS	234
Hughes, Kevin (MA)	S	424	Johnson, Timothy (MI)	D	108
Hunt, Kelly (TX)	S	447	Johnston, Carolyn Marie (MI)	GO	262
Huntoon, Marc (MN)	PM	314	Johnston, J Martin (ID)	PHO	353
Hurd, David (NC)	Onc	168	Johr, Robert (FL)	D	107
Hurwitz, Craig (ME)	PHO	337	Jones, David (VA)	TS	466
Hussain, Maha (MI)	Onc	180	Jones, Howard (TN)	GO	260
Hutchins, Laura (AR)	Onc	191	Jones, Robert (DC)	Path	320
Hutchinson, Raymond (MI)	PHO	351	Jones, Stephen (TX)	Onc	191
Huynh, Phan Tuong (TX)	DR	411	Jordan, Gerald (VA)	U	482
			Jose, Baby (KY)	RadRO	394
			Joyce, Michael (OH)	OrS	285

I

Name	Specialty	Pg	Name	Specialty	Pg
Iannettoni, Mark (IA)	TS	468	Judy, Kevin (PA)	NS	225
Iglehart, J Dirk (MA)	S	424	Julian, Thomas (PA)	S	429
Iliff, Nicholas Taylor (MD)	Oph	274	Jurcic, Joseph (NY)	Onc	156
Ilson, David (NY)	Onc	156			
Ingle, James (MN)	Onc	180			

K

Name	Specialty	Pg	Name	Specialty	Pg
Irwin, Ronald B (MI)	OrS	285	Kadmon, Dov (TX)	U	489
Isaacs, Claudine (DC)	Onc	156	Kadota, Richard (CA)	PHO	357
Isaacson, Steven (NY)	RadRO	391	Kaelin, William (MA)	Onc	146
Isik, F (WA)	PIS	374	Kaiser, Larry (PA)	TS	464
Israel, Mark (NH)	PHO	338	Kalaycio, Matt (OH)	Onc	180
Israel, Philip (GA)	S	435	Kalemkerian, Gregory (MI)	Onc	180
Itzkowitz, Steven (NY)	Ge	123	Kamani, Naynesh (DC)	PA&I	358
			Kamen, Barton A (NJ)	PHO	341

J

Name	Specialty	Pg	Name	Specialty	Pg
			Kaminski, Mark (MI)	Onc	180
Jablons, David M (CA)	TS	470	Kandeel, Fouad (CA)	EDM	119
Jackler, Robert (CA)	Oto	306	Kane, Javier (TN)	PHO	346
Jackson, Gilchrist (TX)	S	447	Kane, Madeleine (CO)	Onc	188
Jackson, Richard (AR)	PS	363	Kantarjian, Hagop (TX)	Hem	141
Jackson, Valerie P (IN)	DR	410	Kantoff, Philip (MA)	Onc	147
Jacobs, Charlotte (CA)	Onc	198	Kaplan, Lawrence (CA)	Onc	198

Name	Specialty	Pg	Name	Specialty	Pg
Kaplan, Michael J (CA)	Oto	306	Kirschenbaum, Alexander (NY)	U	478
Kaplan, Steven (NY)	U	478	Klagsbrun, Samuel (NY)	Psyc	378
Kapoor, Neena (CA)	PHO	357	Klein, Andrew (CA)	S	452
Karlan, Beth Young (CA)	GO	267	Klein, Eric (OH)	U	486
Karp, Daniel (TX)	Onc	191	Kleinberg, Lawrence (MD)	RadRO	391
Karp, Judith (MD)	Onc	157	Klimberg, Vicki (AR)	S	448
Karpeh, Martin (NY)	S	429	Kloos, Richard (OH)	EDM	117
Karwande, Shreekanth (UT)	TS	469	Kneisl, Jeffrey (NC)	OrS	284
Kassam, Amin (PA)	NS	225	Knisely, Jonathan (CT)	RadRO	387
Katz, Aaron (NY)	U	478	Knowles, Daniel (NY)	Path	320
Katzenstein, Anna-Luise (NY)	Path	320	Knudson, Mary (CA)	S	452
Kaufman, Bruce (WI)	NS	232	Kobrine, Arthur (DC)	NS	225
Kaufman, Cary (WA)	S	452	Koch, Christian (MS)	EDM	117
Kaufman, Howard (NY)	S	429	Koch, Wayne (MD)	Oto	294
Kaufman, Peter (NH)	Onc	147	Koczywas, Marianna (CA)	Onc	198
Kavanah, Maureen (MA)	S	424	Kodner, Ira (MO)	CRS	94
Kawachi, Mark (CA)	U	491	Koeller, Kelly (MN)	NRad	412
Keane, Thomas (SC)	U	482	Koeneman, Kenneth (MN)	U	486
Keane, William (PA)	Oto	294	Koh, Wui-Jin (WA)	RadRO	405
Keating, Michael (TX)	Hem	141	Kohler, Matthew (SC)	GO	260
Keenan, Robert (PA)	TS	464	Komaki, Ritsuko (TX)	RadRO	403
Keller, Frank (GA)	PHO	346	Kondziolka, Douglas (PA)	NS	226
Keller, Steven (NY)	TS	464	Konski, Andre (PA)	RadRO	391
Kelley, Joseph (PA)	GO	257	Kopans, Daniel (MA)	DR	407
Kelley, Mark (TN)	S	436	Kopel, Samuel (NY)	Hem	132
Kelly, Karen (KS)	Onc	188	Kopp, Peter (IL)	EDM	117
Kelly, Patrick (NY)	NS	225	Korones, David (NY)	PHO	342
Kelsen, David (NY)	Onc	157	Kosova, Leonard (IL)	Onc	180
Kemeny, Nancy (NY)	Onc	157	Koss, Michael (CA)	Path	330
Kempin, Sanford (NY)	Hem	132	Koulos, John (NY)	GO	257
Kenan, Samuel (NY)	OrS	283	Kozlowski, James M (IL)	U	486
Kennedy, David (PA)	Oto	294	Kraft, Andrew (SC)	Onc	169
Kern, Robert (IL)	Oto	300	Krag, David (VT)	S	425
Kernstine, Kemp (CA)	TS	470	Kramer, Elissa (NY)	NuM	415
Kessler, Craig (DC)	Hem	132	Kranzler, Leonard (IL)	NS	232
Kibel, Adam S (MO)	U	486	Krasna, Mark (MD)	TS	464
Kiel, Krystyna D (IL)	RadRO	398	Kraus, Dennis (NY)	Oto	294
Kieran, Mark (MA)	PHO	338	Kraut, Eric H (OH)	Hem	137
Kiernan, Paul D (VA)	TS	466	Kraybill, William (MO)	S	441
Kies, Merrill (TX)	Onc	191	Kreissman, Susan (NC)	PHO	346
Kiev, Jonathan (VA)	TS	466	Kreitzer, Joel (NY)	PM	312
Kim, Edward (IN)	U	482	Krellenstein, Daniel (NY)	TS	464
Kim, Jae (MI)	RadRO	399	Krespi, Yosef (NY)	Oto	295
Kim, Julian (OH)	S	441	Kretschmar, Cynthia S (MA)	PHO	338
Kim, Woo Shin (MI)	GO	262	Kriegel, David (NY)	D	104
Kim, Youn-Hee (CA)	D	111	Kris, Mark (NY)	Onc	157
Kindler, Hedy (IL)	Onc	180	Krouse, Robert (AZ)	S	448
King, Richard (GA)	PMR	508	Kuettel, Michael (NY)	RadRO	391
Kinney, Marsha (TX)	Path	328	Kuhn, Joseph (TX)	S	448
Kinsella, Timothy J (OH)	RadRO	399	Kun, Larry (TN)	RadRO	395
Kirkwood, John (PA)	Onc	157	Kung, Faith (CA)	PHO	357

Alphabetical Listing of Doctors

Alphabetical Listing of Doctors

Name	Specialty	Pg	Name	Specialty	Pg
Mauch, Peter (MA)	RadRO	387	Meyers, Paul (NY)	PHO	343
Mauro, Matthew (NC)	VIR	413	Meyers, Rebecka (UT)	PS	363
Maxwell, G Patrick (TN)	PlS	372	Meyskens, Frank (CA)	Onc	199
May, James (MA)	PlS	370	Michalski, Jeff M (MO)	RadRO	400
Mayberg, Marc (WA)	NS	237	Michelassi, Fabrizio (NY)	S	430
Mayer, Robert J (MA)	Onc	147	Mickey, Bruce (TX)	NS	235
Maziarz, Richard (OR)	Hem	143	Middleton, Richard (UT)	U	489
McCaffrey, Thomas (FL)	Oto	298	Mieler, William (IL)	Oph	277
McCarthy, Shirley (CT)	DR	407	Mies, Carolyn (PA)	Path	321
McConnell, John (TX)	U	490	Mihm, Martin (MA)	D	103
McCormick, Beryl (NY)	RadRO	392	Mikkelsen, Tommy (MI)	N	246
McCormick, Paul C (NY)	NS	226	Miles, Brian (TX)	U	490
McCormick, Steven (NY)	Path	321	Millenson, Michael (PA)	Hem	132
McCraw, John (MS)	PlS	372	Miller, Daniel (GA)	TS	466
McCurley, Thomas (TN)	Path	324	Miller, Donald (KY)	Onc	170
McDermott, Michael (CA)	NS	238	Miller, Joseph (GA)	TS	466
McDonald, Charles (RI)	D	103	Miller, Kenneth (MA)	Hem	130
McDonald, Douglas (MO)	OrS	285	Miller, Stanley (MD)	D	105
McDougal, W Scott (MA)	U	476	Miller, Thomas (AZ)	Onc	192
McGahan, John (CA)	VIR	414	Miller, Timothy (CA)	PlS	375
McGill, Trevor (MA)	PO	359	Millikan, Randall (TX)	Onc	193
McGlave, Philip (MN)	Hem	138	Millis, J Michael (IL)	S	442
McGovern, Francis (MA)	U	476	Mills, Stacey (VA)	Path	324
McGrath, Patrick (KY)	S	437	Milsom, Jeffrey (NY)	CRS	91
McGuire, William (MD)	Onc	159	Mintzer, David (PA)	Onc	159
McKenna, Robert J (CA)	TS	470	Mischel, Paul (CA)	Path	331
McLennan, Geoffrey (IA)	Pul	383	Mitchell, Beverly (CA)	Onc	199
McMasters, Kelly (KY)	S	437	Mitnick, Julie (NY)	DR	409
McMenomey, Sean O (OR)	Oto	306	Mittal, Bharat (IL)	RadRO	400
McVary, Kevin (IL)	U	486	Moley, Jeffrey (MO)	S	442
Meacham, Lillian (GA)	PEn	359	Molo, Mary (IL)	RE	270
Meadows, Anna (PA)	PHO	342	Monsees, Barbara (MO)	DR	410
Mears, John (NY)	Hem	132	Montgomery, Elizabeth (MD)	Path	321
Medbery, Clinton (OK)	RadRO	404	Montie, James (MI)	U	486
Medich, David (PA)	CRS	91	Moore, Anne (NY)	Onc	159
Medina, Jesus (OK)	Oto	304	Moore, David (IN)	GO	263
Meehan, Kenneth (NH)	Hem	130	Moore, Joseph (NC)	Onc	170
Meek, Rita (DE)	PHO	343	Moossa, AR (CA)	S	452
Mehta, Minesh (WI)	RadRO	399	Moran, Cesar (TX)	Path	328
Melamed, Jonathan (NY)	Path	321	Morgan, Elaine (IL)	PHO	351
Melmed, Shlomo (CA)	EDM	119	Morgan, Linda (FL)	ObG	268
Melvin, W Scott (OH)	S	442	Morgan, Mark (PA)	GO	258
Mendenhall, Nancy (FL)	RadRO	395	Morgan, Walter (TN)	PS	361
Mendenhall, William (FL)	RadRO	396	Morrison, Glenn (FL)	NS	229
Menick, Frederick (AZ)	PlS	373	Morrow, Monica (PA)	S	430
Menon, Mani (MI)	U	486	Mortimer, Joanne (CA)	Onc	199
Merchant, Thomas (TN)	RadRO	396	Moscow, Jeffrey (KY)	PHO	347
Meredith, Ruby (AL)	RadRO	396	Mostwin, Jacek (MD)	U	479
Meropol, Neal (PA)	Onc	159	Motzer, Robert (NY)	Onc	159
Merrick, Hollis (OH)	S	442	Moul, Judd (NC)	U	483
Meyers, Bryan (MO)	TS	468	Movsas, Benjamin (MI)	RadRO	400

Alphabetical Listing of Doctors

Name	Specialty	Pg	Name	Specialty	Pg
Orringer, Mark B (MI)	TS	468	Persky, Mark (NY)	Oto	295
Osborne, Charles (TX)	Onc	193	Peschel, Richard (CT)	RadRO	387
Osborne, Michael (NY)	S	430	Peters, Glenn (AL)	Oto	298
Osguthorpe, John (SC)	Oto	298	Petersdorf, Stephen (WA)	Onc	200
Oster, Martin (NY)	Onc	160	Peterson, Bruce (MN)	Onc	181
Ostrer, Harry (NY)	CG	505	Petrelli, Nicholas (DE)	S	431
Otley, Clark C (MN)	D	109	Petruzzelli, Guy (IL)	Oto	301
Ott, Kenneth (CA)	NS	238	Petrylak, Daniel (NY)	Onc	161
Otto, Pamela (TX)	DR	411	Pezner, Richard (CA)	RadRO	406
Otto, Randal (TX)	Oto	304	Pfister, David (NY)	Onc	161
Ozols, Robert (PA)	Onc	160	Phillips, Peter (PA)	ChiN	248

P

Name	Specialty	Pg	Name	Specialty	Pg
			Phuphanich, Surasak (GA)	N	245
			Picozzi, Vincent (WA)	Onc	200
Packer, Roger (DC)	ChiN	248	Picus, Joel (MO)	Onc	182
Page, David L (TN)	Path	324	Pienta, Kenneth (MI)	Onc	182
Paidas, Charles (FL)	PS	361	Piepmeier, Joseph (CT)	NS	223
Palefsky, Joel (CA)	Inf	507	Pierce, Lori (MI)	RadRO	400
Panicek, David (NY)	DR	409	Pierson, Richard (MD)	TS	464
Papadopoulos, Nicholas (TX)	Onc	193	Piest, Kenneth (TX)	Oph	278
Papel, Ira (MD)	Oto	295	Pinson, C Wright (TN)	S	437
Pappas, Theodore N (NC)	S	437	Pinto, Harlan (CA)	Onc	200
Parent, Andrew (MS)	NS	229	Pisano, Etta (NC)	DR	410
Park, Tae Sung (MO)	NS	232	Pistenmaa, David (TX)	RadRO	404
Parker, Robert (NY)	PHO	343	Pisters, Katherine (TX)	Onc	194
Partin, Alan (MD)	U	479	Pisters, Louis (TX)	U	490
Partridge, Edward (AL)	GO	260	Pisters, Peter (TX)	S	448
Pasmantier, Mark (NY)	Onc	160	Pitman, Karen (MS)	Oto	298
Pass, Harvey (NY)	TS	464	Pitts, Lawrence (CA)	NS	238
Patchefsky, Arthur (PA)	Path	321	Pochapin, Mark (NY)	Ge	123
Patchell, Roy (KY)	N	245	Pockaj, Barbara (AZ)	S	449
Patel, Vipul (OH)	U	487	Podoloff, Donald (TX)	NuM	417
Patrizio, Pasquale (CT)	RE	269	Podratz, Karl (MN)	GO	263
Patt, Yehuda (NM)	Onc	193	Poliakoff, Steven (FL)	GO	261
Patterson, G Alexander (MO)	TS	468	Polk, Hiram C (KY)	S	437
Paty, Philip (NY)	S	431	Pollack, Alan (PA)	RadRO	392
Patz, Edward (NC)	DR	410	Pollack, Ian (PA)	NS	226
Payne, Richard (NC)	PM	313	Pollack, Jed (NY)	RadRO	392
Peabody, Terrance (IL)	OrS	286	Pollock, Raphael (TX)	S	449
Pearlman, Nathan W (CO)	S	446	Polsky, Bruce (NY)	Inf	506
Pecora, Andrew (NJ)	Onc	161	Pomeroy, Scott (MA)	ChiN	247
Pegram, Mark (CA)	Onc	200	Ponn, Teresa (NH)	S	425
Pellegrini, Carlos (WA)	S	452	Porcu, Pierluigi (OH)	Hem	139
Pelzer, Harold (IL)	Oto	301	Portenoy, Russell (NY)	PM	313
Pemberton, John (MN)	CRS	94	Porter, David (PA)	Hem	132
Penalver, Manuel A (FL)	GO	260	Posey, James (AL)	Onc	171
Penar, Paul (VT)	NS	223	Posner, Jerome (NY)	N	244
Pendergrass, Thomas (WA)	PHO	358	Posner, Marshall (MA)	Onc	148
Pensak, Myles (OH)	Oto	301	Posner, Mitchell (IL)	S	443
Perez, Edith (FL)	Onc	171	Post, Kalmon (NY)	NS	226
Perry, Arie (MO)	Path	326	Postier, Russell (OK)	S	449
Perry, Michael (MO)	Onc	181	Potkul, Ronald (IL)	GO	263

Name	Specialty	Pg
Potsic, William (PA)	PO	359
Pow-Sang, Julio (FL)	U	483
Powell, Bayard (NC)	Hem	135
Powell, Catherine (CA)	GO	267
Prados, Michael (CA)	Onc	200
Press, Oliver W (WA)	Onc	200
Presti, Joseph C (CA)	U	492
Prieto, Victor (TX)	Path	328
Prosnitz, Leonard (NC)	RadRO	396
Provenzale, James (NC)	NRad	412
Puccetti, Diane (WI)	PHO	352
Pui, Ching (TN)	PHO	347
Putnam, Joe (TN)	TS	467

Q

Name	Specialty	Pg
Quinn, David (CA)	Onc	200
Quivey, Jeanne Marie (CA)	RadRO	406

R

Name	Specialty	Pg
Rabinovitch, Rachel (CO)	RadRO	402
Raffel, Corey (MN)	NS	233
Raghavan, Derek (OH)	Onc	182
Rai, Kanti (NY)	Hem	132
Raiford, David (TN)	Ge	124
Ramsay, David (NY)	D	105
Randall, Marcus (KY)	RadRO	396
Randall, R Lor (UT)	OrS	286
Rao, Vijay (PA)	DR	410
Raphael, Bruce (NY)	Hem	133
Rashid, Asif (TX)	Path	329
Rassekh, Christopher (WV)	Oto	295
Ratain, Mark J (IL)	Onc	182
Rauch, Paula (MA)	Psyc	378
Rauck, Richard (NC)	PM	313
Rausen, Aaron (NY)	PHO	343
Read, Thomas (PA)	CRS	92
Ready, John (MA)	OrS	282
Ready, L Brian (WA)	PM	315
Reaman, Gregory (DC)	PHO	343
Reardon, Michael (TX)	TS	469
Reber, Howard (CA)	S	453
Recht, Abram (MA)	RadRO	387
Reed, Carolyn (SC)	TS	467
Regine, William (MD)	RadRO	392
Reintgen, Douglas (FL)	S	437
Remick, Scot C (OH)	Onc	182
Resnick, Martin (OH)	U	487
Reynolds, R Kevin (MI)	GO	263
Rheingold, Susan R (PA)	PHO	343
Riba, Michelle (MI)	Psyc	379
Rice, Dale (CA)	Oto	306

Name	Specialty	Pg
Rice, Henry (NC)	PS	362
Rice, Laurel (VA)	GO	261
Rich, Keith (MO)	NS	233
Rich, Tyvin (VA)	RadRO	396
Richards, Jon (IL)	Onc	182
Richie, Jerome (MA)	U	476
Ricketts, Richard (GA)	PS	362
Ridge, John A (PA)	S	431
Ridgway, E (CO)	EDM	118
Rigel, Darrell (NY)	D	105
Rikkers, Layton (WI)	S	443
Rilling, William (WI)	VIR	414
Ritchey, Arthur (PA)	PHO	344
Rivlin, Richard (NY)	IM	507
Roach, Mack (CA)	RadRO	406
Robb, Geoffrey (TX)	PlS	374
Robbins, Richard (TX)	EDM	118
Robert, Nicholas (VA)	Onc	171
Robert-Vizcarrondo, Francisco (AL)	Onc	171
Roberts, Kenneth (CT)	RadRO	388
Roberts, Patricia L (MA)	CRS	90
Robertson, Cary N (NC)	U	483
Robins, Perry (NY)	D	105
Robinson, Lary A (FL)	TS	467
Rock, Jack (MI)	NS	233
Rodgers, George (UT)	Path	327
Rogers, Lisa (MI)	N	246
Roh, Mark (PA)	S	431
Rohrich, Rod (TX)	PlS	374
Roman-Lopez, Juan J (AR)	GO	266
Rombeau, John (PA)	CRS	92
Romond, Edward H (KY)	Onc	171
Roodman, G David (PA)	Hem	133
Rook, Alain (PA)	D	105
Rosato, Ernest (PA)	S	431
Rose, Christopher (CA)	RadRO	406
Rose, Peter (OH)	GO	263
Rosemurgy, Alexander (FL)	S	437
Rosen, Paul (NY)	Path	321
Rosen, Steven (IL)	Onc	182
Rosenberg, Steven (MD)	S	431
Rosenblatt, Joseph (FL)	Hem	135
Rosenblum, Mark (MI)	NS	233
Rosenblum, Norman (PA)	GO	258
Rosenfeld, Myrna (PA)	N	244
Rosenfeld, Steven (NY)	N	244
Rosenman, Julian (NC)	RadRO	396
Rosenthal, Joseph (CA)	PHO	358
Rosenwaks, Zev (NY)	RE	270
Rosenwasser, Robert (PA)	NS	227
Roses, Daniel (NY)	S	431

Alphabetical Listing of Doctors

Name	Specialty	Pg	Name	Specialty	Pg
Rosner, Howard (CA)	PM	315	Sandler, Eric (FL)	PHO	348
Rosoff, Phillip (NC)	PHO	348	Sandler, Howard (MI)	RadRO	400
Ross, Helen (OR)	Onc	201	Sandlund, John T (TN)	PHO	348
Ross, Jeffrey (NY)	Path	322	Sanford, Robert A (TN)	NS	229
Ross, Merrick (TX)	S	449	Santana, Victor (TN)	PHO	348
Rossi, Carl (CA)	RadRO	406	Saroja, Kurubarahalli (IL)	Onc	183
Roth, Bruce (TN)	Onc	172	Sarr, Michael (MN)	S	443
Roth, Jack (TX)	TS	469	Sasaki, Clarence (CT)	Oto	292
Rothenberg, Mace (TN)	Onc	172	Sasson, Aaron (NE)	S	446
Rothenberger, David (MN)	CRS	94	Savage, David (NY)	Hem	133
Rotman, Marvin (NY)	RadRO	392	Savage, John (MN)	GO	264
Rotmensch, Jacob (IL)	GO	264	Saven, Alan (CA)	Hem	143
Rowland, Randall (KY)	U	483	Sawaya, Raymond (TX)	NS	235
Rubenfeld, Sheldon (TX)	EDM	118	Sawczuk, Ihor (NJ)	U	479
Rubin, Brian (OH)	Path	326	Sawin, Robert (WA)	PS	364
Rubin, Peter (MA)	Oph	274	Scarborough, Mark (FL)	OrS	284
Rubin, Stephen (PA)	GO	258	Scardino, Peter (NY)	U	480
Rubinstein, Wendy (IL)	CG	505	Schaeffer, Anthony (IL)	U	487
Ruckdeschel, John C (MI)	Onc	183	Schantz, Stimson P (NY)	Oto	296
Ruge, John (IL)	NS	233	Schechter, Neil (CT)	Ped	364
Rugo, Hope (CA)	Onc	201	Scheff, Alice M (CA)	NuM	417
Russell, Christy (CA)	Onc	201	Scheinberg, David (NY)	Onc	161
Russell, Kenneth (WA)	RadRO	406	Scheithauer, Bernd (MN)	Path	326
Russo, Carolyn (CA)	PHO	358	Schellhammer, Paul (VA)	U	483
Rutgers, Joanne (CA)	Path	331	Schepps, Barbara (RI)	DR	408
Rutherford, Thomas (CT)	GO	255	Scher, Charles (LA)	PHO	355
Ryken, Timothy (IA)	NS	233	Scher, Howard (NY)	Onc	161
			Schiff, David (VA)	N	245
S			Schiff, Peter (NY)	RadRO	393
			Schiffer, Charles (MI)	Onc	183
Saclarides, Theodore (IL)	CRS	95	Schilder, Russell (PA)	Onc	161
Safai, Bijan (NY)	D	105	Schiller, Alan (NY)	Path	322
Sagalowsky, Arthur (TX)	U	490	Schiller, Gary J (CA)	Hem	144
Sagar, Stephen (OH)	N	246	Schiller, Joan (TX)	Onc	194
Sagel, Stuart (MO)	DR	411	Schilsky, Richard (IL)	Onc	183
Saha, Sukamal (MI)	S	443	Schink, Julian C (IL)	GO	264
Saiki, John (NM)	Onc	194	Schlegel, Peter (NY)	U	480
Sailer, Scott (NC)	RadRO	396	Schmidt, Joseph (CA)	U	492
Salem, Philip (TX)	Onc	194	Schnabel, Freya (NY)	S	431
Salem, Riad (IL)	VIR	414	Schneider, Philip (CA)	S	453
Salem, Ronald R (CT)	S	425	Schnipper, Lowell (MA)	Onc	148
Salgia, Ravi (IL)	Onc	183	Schnitt, Stuart (MA)	Path	319
Sallan, Stephen (MA)	Ped	364	Schoetz, David (MA)	CRS	90
Salo, Jonathan (NC)	S	437	Schold, S Clifford (FL)	N	245
Saltz, Leonard B (NY)	Onc	161	Schomberg, Paula (MN)	RadRO	400
Salvi, Sharad (IL)	PHO	352	Schraut, Wolfgang (PA)	S	432
Samlowski, Wolfram E (UT)	Onc	188	Schuchter, Lynn (PA)	Onc	162
Sampson, John (NC)	NS	229	Schuller, David (OH)	Oto	302
Samuels, Brian L (ID)	Onc	188	Schuster, Michael (NY)	Hem	133
Sanchez, Miguel (NJ)	Path	322	Schusterman, Mark (TX)	PlS	374
Sanders, William (GA)	U	483	Schwartz, Burton (MN)	Onc	183
Sandler, Alan (TN)	Onc	172			

Name	Specialty	Pg	Name	Specialty	Pg
Schwartz, Cindy (RI)	PHO	338	Shochat, Stephen J (TN)	PS	362
Schwartz, Gordon (PA)	S	432	Shrager, Joseph (PA)	TS	464
Schwartz, Herbert (TN)	OrS	284	Shrieve, Dennis (UT)	RadRO	402
Schwartz, L Matthew (PA)	PMR	508	Shulman, Lawrence (MA)	Onc	148
Schwartz, Michael (FL)	Onc	172	Shulman, Lee (IL)	ObG	269
Schwartz, Peter (CT)	GO	255	Sibley, Richard (CA)	Path	331
Schwartzberg, Lee (TN)	Hem	135	Sidransky, David (MD)	Onc	162
Schwartzentruber, Douglas (IN)	S	443	Siegel, Barry (MO)	NuM	416
Scott-Conner, Carol E.H. (IA)	S	443	Siegel, Gordon (IL)	Oto	302
Scully, Sean (FL)	OrS	284	Siegel, Herrick J (AL)	OrS	284
See, William (WI)	U	487	Siegel, Stuart (CA)	PHO	358
Seewaldt, Victoria (NC)	Onc	172	Sielaff, Timothy (MN)	S	444
Seiden, Michael (MA)	Onc	148	Sigurdson, Elin (PA)	S	432
Seiff, Stuart (CA)	Oph	279	Sikic, Branimir I (CA)	Onc	201
Sekhar, Laligam (WA)	NS	238	Silbergeld, Daniel (WA)	NS	238
Sen, Chandranath (NY)	NS	227	Silberstein, Edward (OH)	NuM	416
Senagore, Anthony (MI)	CRS	95	Sills, Allen (TN)	NS	229
Sencer, Susan (MN)	PHO	352	Silva, Elvio (TX)	Path	329
Sener, Stephen (IL)	S	444	Silver, Michael (IL)	Pul	383
Senzer, Neil (TX)	RadRO	404	Silverberg, Steven (MD)	Path	322
Sepkowitz, Kent (NY)	Inf	506	Silverman, Jan F (PA)	Path	322
Serletti, Joseph (PA)	PlS	371	Silverman, Paula (OH)	Onc	184
Serody, Jonathan (NC)	Onc	172	Silverstein, Melvin (CA)	S	453
Sevin, Bernd-Uwe (FL)	GO	261	Sim, Franklin (MN)	OrS	286
Sewell, C Whitaker (GA)	Path	324	Simon, Michael (IL)	OrS	286
Shaffrey, Mark E (VA)	NS	229	Sinanan, Mika (WA)	S	453
Shah, Jatin (NY)	S	432	Singer, Daniel (HI)	OrS	287
Shaha, Ashok (NY)	S	432	Singer, Mark (CA)	Oto	306
Shamberger, Robert (MA)	PS	360	Singer, Samuel (NY)	S	432
Shapiro, Charles (OH)	Onc	183	Singhal, Seema (IL)	Hem	139
Shapiro, Lawrence (NY)	CG	505	Singletary, Sonja (TX)	S	449
Shapiro, Scott (IN)	NS	233	Sinha, Uttam (CA)	Oto	306
Shapiro, William R (AZ)	N	247	Siperstein, Allan (OH)	S	444
Shapshay, Stanley (NY)	Oto	296	Skibber, John (TX)	S	449
Shaw, Edward (NC)	RadRO	397	Skinner, Donald G (CA)	U	492
Shea, Thomas (NC)	Onc	172	Skinner, Eila (CA)	U	492
Shearer, Patricia (FL)	PHO	348	Skinner, Kristin (NY)	S	432
Sheinfeld, Joel (NY)	U	480	Skinner, Michael (NC)	PS	362
Shellito, Paul (MA)	CRS	91	Sklar, Charles (NY)	PEn	359
Shenk, Robert (OH)	S	444	Slatkin, Neal (CA)	PM	315
Sherman, Randolph (CA)	PlS	375	Slawin, Kevin (TX)	U	490
Sherman, Steven (TX)	EDM	118	Sledge, George (IN)	Onc	184
Shibata, Stephen (CA)	Onc	201	Slezak, Sheri (MD)	PlS	371
Shields, Carol (PA)	Oph	275	Slingluff, Craig (VA)	S	438
Shields, Jerry (PA)	Oph	275	Small, Eric (CA)	Onc	201
Shields, Peter (DC)	Onc	162	Small, William (IL)	RadRO	400
Shike, Moshe (NY)	Ge	123	Smalley, Stephen (KS)	RadRO	402
Shin, Dong Moon (GA)	Onc	173	Smith, Barbara (MA)	S	425
Shina, Donald (NM)	RadRO	404	Smith, David (FL)	PlS	372
Shindo, Maisie (NY)	Oto	296	Smith, Donna (IL)	GO	264
Shipley, William U (MA)	RadRO	388	Smith, Harriet (NM)	GO	266

Alphabetical Listing of Doctors

Name	Specialty	Pg	Name	Specialty	Pg
Smith, Joseph A (TN)	U	483	Stern, Jeffrey (CA)	GO	268
Smith, Lee (DC)	CRS	92	Sternberg, Paul (TN)	Oph	275
Smith, Lloyd (CA)	GO	267	Stewart, Forrest (WA)	Onc	201
Smith, Mitchell (PA)	Onc	162	Stewart, Paula (AL)	PMR	509
Smith, Robert (CA)	U	492	Stieg, Philip E (NY)	NS	227
Smith, Thomas (VA)	Onc	173	Stiff, Patrick (IL)	Hem	139
Snyder, David S (CA)	Hem	144	Stock, Richard (NY)	RadRO	393
Snyder, Peter (PA)	EDM	116	Stockdale, Frank (CA)	Onc	201
Snyderman, Carl (PA)	Oto	296	Stolar, Charles (NY)	PS	361
Sobel, Stuart (FL)	D	107	Stolier, Alan (LA)	S	449
Sober, Arthur (MA)	D	103	Stone, Joel (FL)	Onc	173
Socinski, Mark (NC)	Onc	173	Stone, Richard (MA)	Hem	131
Soisson, Andrew (UT)	GO	265	Stoopler, Mark (NY)	Onc	163
Sokoloff, Daniel (FL)	D	107	Stopeck, Alison (AZ)	Onc	194
Solberg, Lawrence (FL)	Hem	135	Stout, John (OR)	Oph	279
Solin, Lawrence (PA)	RadRO	393	Strasberg, Steven M (MO)	S	444
Soloway, Mark (FL)	U	483	Straus, David (NY)	Onc	163
Sondak, Vernon K (FL)	S	438	Strauss, H William (NY)	NuM	415
Sondel, Paul (WI)	PHO	352	Strauss, James (TX)	Hem	141
Sonett, Joshua (NY)	TS	465	Streeter, Oscar (CA)	RadRO	407
Soparkar, Charles (TX)	Oph	278	Stringer, Scott (MS)	Oto	299
Soper, John (NC)	GO	261	Strome, Marshall (OH)	Oto	302
Sosman, Jeffrey (TN)	Onc	173	Strouse, Thomas (CA)	Psyc	379
Sotomayor, Eduardo (FL)	Onc	173	Stryker, Steven (IL)	CRS	95
Soulen, Michael (PA)	VIR	413	Stubblefield, Michael (NY)	PMR	508
Spann, Cyril (GA)	GO	261	Suen, James Y (AR)	Oto	304
Spear, Scott (DC)	PlS	371	Sugarbaker, David (MA)	TS	462
Spence, Alexander (WA)	N	247	Sugarbaker, Paul (DC)	S	432
Spetzler, Robert (AZ)	NS	235	Suh, John (OH)	RadRO	401
Speyer, James (NY)	Onc	162	Sultan, Mark (NY)	PlS	371
Spiegel, David (CA)	Psyc	379	Suster, Saul (OH)	Path	326
Spirtos, Nicola (NV)	GO	267	Sutphen, Rebecca (FL)	CG	505
Spitzer, Thomas (MA)	Hem	130	Sutton, John (NH)	S	425
Spivak, Jerry (MD)	Hem	133	Sutton, Leslie (PA)	NS	227
Spriggs, David (NY)	Onc	162	Sutton, Linda (NC)	Onc	173
Springfield, Dempsey (MA)	OrS	282	Swanson, David (TX)	U	490
Staats, Peter (NJ)	PM	313	Swanson, Neil (OR)	D	111
Stadelmann, Wayne (NH)	PlS	370	Swanson, Scott (NY)	TS	465
Stadler, Walter (IL)	Onc	184	Swarm, Robert (MO)	PM	314
Stadtmauer, Edward (PA)	Onc	162	Swensen, Stephen (MN)	DR	411
Stahl, Richard (CT)	PlS	370	Swerdlow, Steven (PA)	Path	322
Stamos, Michael (CA)	CRS	97	Swetter, Susan (CA)	D	111
Staren, Edgar (IL)	S	444	Swisher, Stephen (TX)	TS	469
Stea, Baldassarre (AZ)	RadRO	404	Swistel, Alexander (NY)	S	433
Stehman, Frederick (IN)	GO	264	Szabo, Robert (CA)	HS	288
Stein, John (CA)	U	493			
Steinberg, Gary (IL)	U	487	**T**		
Steinberg, Harry (NY)	Pul	382			
Steingart, Richard (NY)	Cv	505	Tabak, Brian (CA)	D	111
Steinhagen, Randolph (NY)	CRS	92	Tafra, Lorraine (MD)	S	433
Steinherz, Peter (NY)	PHO	344	Takimoto, Chris (TX)	Onc	194
			Talamonti, Mark (IL)	S	444

Alphabetical Listing of Doctors

Name	Specialty	Pg	Name	Specialty	Pg
von Eschenbach, Andrew (MD)	U	481	Weiner, George J (IA)	Onc	185
Von Hoff, Daniel (AZ)	Onc	195	Weiner, Louis M (PA)	Onc	164
Von Roenn, Jamie H (IL)	Onc	184	Weiner, Michael (NY)	PHO	344
von-Mehren, Margaret (PA)	Onc	163	Weingeist, Thomas (IA)	Oph	277
Vonderheid, Eric (MD)	D	105	Weinreb, Jeffrey (CT)	DR	408
Vose, Julie M (NE)	Hem	140	Weinstein, Gregory (PA)	Oto	296
			Weinstein, Howard J (MA)	PHO	338

W

Name	Specialty	Pg	Name	Specialty	Pg
			Weinstein, James (NH)	OrS	282
Wade, James C (WI)	Onc	185	Weinstein, Sharon (UT)	PM	314
Waggoner, Steven (OH)	GO	264	Weisberg, Tracey (ME)	Onc	148
Wagman, Lawrence D (CA)	S	453	Weisenburger, Dennis (NE)	Path	327
Waguespack, Steven (TX)	EDM	118	Weisman, Robert (CA)	Oto	307
Wahl, Richard (MD)	NuM	415	Weiss, Geoffrey R (VA)	Onc	174
Wain, John (MA)	TS	462	Weiss, Lawrence M (CA)	Path	331
Wajsman, Zev (FL)	U	484	Weiss, Marisa C (PA)	RadRO	393
Waldbaum, Robert (NY)	U	481	Weiss, Martin (CA)	NS	238
Walker, Alonzo (WI)	S	445	Weiss, Robert (NJ)	U	481
Walker, Joan (OK)	GO	266	Weiss, Sharon (GA)	Path	324
Wall, Donna (TX)	PHO	355	Weiss, Stanley H (NJ)	PrM	509
Wallace, Mark (CA)	PM	315	Weissler, Mark (NC)	Oto	299
Wallach, Robert (NY)	GO	258	Weissman, David (WI)	Onc	185
Walling, Arthur (FL)	OrS	284	Weitzel, Jeffrey N (CA)	CG	506
Walsh, Patrick (MD)	U	481	Welton, Mark L (CA)	CRS	97
Walsh, R Matthew (OH)	S	445	Wexler, Leonard (NY)	PHO	344
Walsh, T Declan (OH)	Onc	185	Wexner, Steven (FL)	CRS	93
Walters, Theodore (ID)	Hem	140	Weymuller, Ernest (WA)	Oto	307
Walton, Robert (IL)	PlS	373	Wharam, Moody (MD)	RadRO	393
Ward, Barbara (CT)	S	425	Wharen, Robert E (FL)	NS	230
Ward, John H (UT)	Onc	188	Wheeland, Ronald (MO)	D	110
Ward, William (NC)	OrS	284	Wheeler, Thomas (TX)	Path	329
Warner, Brad (OH)	PS	363	Whelan, Alison (MO)	CG	506
Warnick, Ronald (OH)	NS	234	Whelan, Richard (NY)	CRS	92
Warnke, Roger A (CA)	Path	331	Whitaker, Linton (PA)	PlS	372
Warren, Robert (CA)	S	453	White, Dorothy (NY)	Pul	382
Warshaw, Andrew L (MA)	S	426	White, Richard (NC)	S	438
Wartofsky, Leonard (DC)	EDM	116	Whitlock, James (TN)	PHO	349
Watson, Thomas (NY)	TS	465	Whitworth, Pat (TN)	S	438
Wax, Mark (OR)	Oto	307	Whyte, Richard (CA)	TS	470
Waxman, Alan (CA)	NuM	417	Wicha, Max S (MI)	Onc	185
Waxman, Irving (IL)	Ge	125	Wilczynski, Sharon (CA)	Path	332
Waye, Jerome (NY)	Ge	123	Wilding, George (WI)	Onc	185
Wazen, Jack (FL)	Oto	299	Wilkins, Edwin (MI)	PlS	373
Wazer, David E (RI)	RadRO	388	Wilkins, Ross M (CO)	OrS	286
Weber, Jeffrey S (CA)	Onc	203	Wilkinson, Robert (HI)	PHO	360
Weber, Randal (TX)	Oto	304	Willett, Christopher (NC)	RadRO	397
Weber, Samuel (TX)	Oto	305	Willey, Shawna (DC)	S	433
Weichselbaum, Ralph R (IL)	RadRO	401	Williams, Michael (VA)	Onc	174
Weigel, Ronald (IA)	S	445	Williams, Richard (IA)	U	488
Wein, Alan (PA)	U	481	Williams, Ronald (TX)	OrS	286
Weinberger, Malvin (FL)	PS	362	Williams, Stephen (IN)	Onc	185
Weinberger, Michael (NY)	PM	313	Willis, Irvin (FL)	S	438
Weinblatt, Mark (NY)	PHO	344	Willson, James (TX)	Onc	195
			Wilson, David (OR)	Oph	279

Castle Connolly America's Top Doctors® for Cancer 3rd Edition

Alphabetical Listing of Doctors

Name	Specialty	Pg
Wilson, J Frank (WI)	RadRO	401
Wilson, Keith (OH)	Oto	302
Wilson, Lynn (CT)	RadRO	388
Wilson, Matthew (TN)	Oph	276
Wilson, Timothy (CA)	U	493
Winawer, Sidney (NY)	Ge	124
Winer, Eric (MA)	Onc	149
Wingard, John R (FL)	Onc	174
Winick, Naomi (TX)	PHO	355
Winter, Jane (IL)	Hem	139
Wisch, Nathaniel (NY)	Hem	133
Wiseman, Gregory (MN)	NuM	416
Wisoff, Jeffrey (NY)	NS	227
Witt, Thomas (IL)	S	445
Witte, Marlys (AZ)	IM	507
Wolf, Gregory (MI)	Oto	302
Wolfe, Lawrence (MA)	PHO	338
Wolff, Antonio (MD)	Onc	164
Wolff, Bruce (MN)	CRS	95
Wolff, Robert (TX)	IM	508
Woltering, Eugene (LA)	S	450
Wong, Jeffrey (CA)	RadRO	407
Wong, W Douglas (NY)	CRS	92
Woo, Peak (NY)	Oto	296
Wood, Bradford (MD)	VIR	413
Wood, David (MI)	U	488
Wood, Douglas (WA)	TS	470
Wood, Gary (WI)	D	109
Wood, R Patrick (TX)	S	450
Wood, William (GA)	S	439
Woods, William (GA)	PHO	349
Worden, Francis (MI)	Onc	185
Wright, Cameron (MA)	TS	462

Y

Name	Specialty	Pg
Yaddanapudi, Ravindranath (MI)	PHO	353
Yahalom, Joachim (NY)	RadRO	393
Yang, James (MD)	S	433
Yang, Stephen C (MD)	TS	465
Yarbrough, Wendell (TN)	Oto	299
Yasko, Alan (IL)	OrS	286
Yeager, Andrew (AZ)	Hem	142
Yeatman, Timothy (FL)	S	439
Yee, Douglas (MN)	Onc	186
Yen, Yun (CA)	Onc	203
Yetman, Randall (OH)	PlS	373
Young, A Byron (KY)	NS	230
Young, Robert (MA)	Path	319
Yousem, Samuel (PA)	Path	323
Yu, George (MD)	U	481
Yu, John S (CA)	NS	238

Name	Specialty	Pg
Yueh, Bevan (WA)	Oto	307
Yuen, James (AR)	PlS	374
Yung, Wai-Kwan (TX)	N	247
Yunus, Furhan (TN)	Onc	174

Z

Name	Specialty	Pg
Zalusky, Ralph (NY)	Hem	133
Zannis, Victor (AZ)	S	450
Zelefsky, Michael (NY)	RadRO	393
Zelenetz, Andrew (NY)	Onc	164
Ziegler, Moritz (CO)	PS	363
Zietman, Anthony (MA)	RadRO	388
Zimmerman, Donald (IL)	PEn	359
Zinner, Michael (MA)	S	426
Zippe, Craig D (OH)	U	488
Zitelli, John (PA)	D	106
Zuckerman, Kenneth (FL)	Hem	136

Acknowledgments

The publishers would like to thank the entire staff for their many hours and days of intense and precise work on this guide in order to further its goal of assisting consumers in making the best healthcare choices.

Castle Connolly Executive Management:

Chairman	John K. Castle
President & CEO	John J. Connolly, Ed.D.
Vice President, Chief Medical & Research Officer	Jean Morgan, M.D.
Vice President, Chief Strategy & Operations Officer	William Liss-Levinson, Ph.D.
Marketing and Public Relations Coordinator	Terese Cecilia

We also would like to extend our gratitude to the American Board of Medical Specialties (ABMS) for allowing us to use excerpts, especially the descriptions of medical specialties and subspecialties, from the text of their publication "Which Medical Specialist for You?"

We wish to thank our research coordinators Maryann Hynd, RN, Sara Belly and Naomi Valensi with additional thanks to our layout/Editorial staff: Stephenie Galvan, Russell Hodgson and Emerson Cooke.

Other Publications from Castle Connolly Medical Ltd.:
America's Top Doctors®; Top Doctors: New York Metro Area;
Top Doctors: Chicago Metro Area; America's Cosmetic Doctors and Dentists;
Cancer Made Easier: New York—Metro Area; Eldercare (Available late 2007)
and others...
Order online at http://www.castleconnolly.com/books

Doctor-Patient Advisor

Doctor-Patient Advisor is a Castle Connolly Medical Ltd., service providing one-on-one consultations with a physician or nurse to individuals who have serious or complex medical problems or to anyone who feels he/she needs assistance finding the right physician for any purpose. Each client will receive personalized assistance in identifying the appropriate specialists for his/her condition utilizing the Castle Connolly Medical Ltd. database of physicians and hospitals, as well as individual searches, to locate the best resources to meet the client's needs.

Fee: $275. For further information call (212) 367-8400 x16.

Strategic Partnerships

Castle Connolly Medical Ltd. has a number of strategic partnerships that may be of interest to consumers and physicians.

Access Medical LLC

Access Medical LLC is a diversified healthcare company that has partnered with Castle Connolly to help expand its top doctors database. Through its various resources and proprietary technologies, Access and Castle Connolly hope to build upon Castle Connolly's core nomination survey, research and selection process, thereby enabling Castle Connolly to identify 2-3 times more top doctors than it currently does.

BML Medical Records Alert

A secure, private and affordable program to electronically store and retrieve your advance directives and personal health care information - 24 hours a day, 7 days a week. MedRecords Alert members carry an ID card, wear an ID bracelet with their personal access code, or even have the option to carry their complete medical records and advance directives at all times on a secure pocket-sized USB memory key that utilizes the latest flash-disc technology. Thus, your physician or other healthcare providers can easily retrieve your information. Through Castle Connolly Medical Ltd., members receive a $5.00 discount from the $36.00 annual fee.

For more information, visit www.medrecordsalert.com.

Castle Connolly Healthcare Navigation Ltd. (CCHN)
This company offers a comprehensive program for individuals and families to assist them with a range of critical healthcare issues and service needs. CCHN identifies top doctors and hospitals through the resources of Castle Connolly Medical Ltd, provides assistance in resolving problems with medical bills and insurance statements, provides a 24/7 electronic medical record, assists in identifying geriatric care managers, provides research on diseases and medical conditions, and assists in the management and care of illness when abroad through health insurance and medical transport.

For further information, visit www.cchealthcarenavigation.com or call (203) 333-2244.

Empowered Doctor

Empowered Doctor develops practice websites for physicians, all of whom must first be screened and vetted by Castle Connolly Medical Ltd.'s physician-led Research Department. Websites are designed for new patients to easily find the physician and request an appointment, as well as to serve as a resource for existing patients. Website features include: practice brochures, appointment and prescription refill request form, patient intake forms, a patient education library and a library of the latest news stories related to the physician's medical specialty.

For further information, call toll-free (866) 375-4007, or visit www.empowereddoctor.net.

Trio Health, LLC

Trio Health is a healthcare services company which is an innovator in the rapidly growing executive health and wellness space. It provides a range of services – including Physician Find and Access and Disease Research provided through Castle Connolly – to its clients at specially designed centers that are created in partnership with some of the nation's most outstanding academic medical centers. The first such center, opened in 2006, is the Center for Partnership Medicine, developed and operated in conjunction with Northwestern Memorial Hospital in Chicago. Trio anticipates creating at least a dozen more centers within the next few years.

For further information visit www.triohealth.com or call (312)-926-9289.

The Castle Connolly National Physician of the Year Awards

Castle Connolly Medical Ltd. hosted its second annual National Physician of the Year Awards on March 13, 2007 at the elegant Pierre Hotel in New York City. This event recognized both the outstanding honorees and the excellence of the many thousands of outstanding physcians throughout the nation.

The Genesis of the Castle Connolly National Physician of the Year Awards

Each year Castle Connolly Medical Ltd. receives thousands of nominations from physicians and the medical leadership of major medical centers, specialty hospitals, teaching hospitals and regional and community medical centers across the U.S. as an integral part of our research, screening and selection process to identify America's Top Doctors®. The selected physicians, while distributed across all fifty states and involved in more than 70 medical specialties and subspecialties, all share one distinguishing professional attribute: an unwavering dedication to their patients and to medicine as a whole. Each and every one of these outstanding medical professionals is a symbol of the clinical excellence that characterizes American medicine. In honor of these exemplary physicians, Castle Connolly Medical Ltd. has created the National Physician of the Year Awards to recognize the thousands of excellent, dedicated physicians across the U.S. Our Medical Advisory Board selected the final honorees from the hundreds nominated in a special nomination process conducted months before the event.

Drs. Cosgrove, McCarthy and Walsh are outstanding examples of excellence in clinical medical practice and were the recipients of the 2007 Clinical Excellence Award. In addition to these recipients Castle Connolly Medical Ltd. honored Dr. Delivoria-Papadopoulos' for her lifetime achievement in the medical community. Her career has spanned almost 50 years and her research, practice and unwavering dedication to neonatal and perinatal medicine have made her the ideal honoree for the Lifetime Achievement Award. The Honorable Nancy G. Brinker, founder of the Susan G. Komen for the Cure, was our 2007 recipient for the National Health Leadership Award. Her dedication and effort in the fight against breast cancer has touched a countless number of lives. Without these individuals contributions to the public and medical community the world would have never reaped the benefits of years of perseverance, research, and medical breakthroughs.

Each honoree received "Imagination," a beautiful and distinctive Lladro statue from the Humanities collection, made of exquisite Spanish porcelain. Portraying an angel with soaring wings, this statue represents the hope and comfort all five honorees have brought to the world through their patients, their profession and their dedication.

2007 National Physician of the Year Awards Honorees For

Delos M. Cosgrove, M.D.
Chairman, Board of Governors, CEO and President
The Cleveland Clinic

Joseph G. McCarthy, M.D.
Lawrence D. Bell Professor of Plastic Surgery and Director,
The Institute of Reconstructive Plastic Surgery
NYU Medical Center

Patrick C. Walsh, M.D.
University Distinguished Service Professor and Director of Urology
The James Buchanan Brady Urological Institute
The Johns Hopkins Hospital

Lifetime Achievement
Maria Delivoria-Papadopoulos, M.D.
Director, The Neonatal Intensive Care Unit
St. Christopher's Hospital for Children
Professor of Pediatrics, Physiology and Obstetrics/Gynecology
Drexel University College of Medicine

For National Health Leadership
The Honorable Nancy G. Brinker
Founder of Susan G. Komen for the Cure;
former U.S. Ambassador to Hungary

Othe[r Books by Castle Con]nolly

Castle Conn[olly]

Titles Include:

- *America's Top Doctors®*
- *Top Doctors: New York Metro Area*
- *Cancer Made Easier*

And Many More

To order other Castle Connolly guides at a 15% discount, please visit:

http://www.CastleConnolly.com/books

When ordering use discount code: **ATDC07VAN**

Castle Connolly's Top Doctors Available Online

- Free Access to 20 -25% of Castle Connolly's Top Doctors
- Purchase Access to the entire database of more than 20,000 doctor profiles

http://www.CastleConnolly.com/membership

Customer Feedback Offer

We would appreciate your help in improving our guide. If you will take a few minutes to complete an online survey, we will give you a free copy of a Healthcare Choice Guide.

Please complete the survey at
http://www.CastleConnolly.com/feedback